LAPAROSCOPIC COLORECTAL SURGERY

Edited by

RAMA M. JAGER, M.D., Ph.D.
Clinical Assistant Professor
Department of Surgery
Indiana School of Medicine
Medical Director
Colon and Rectal Care Inc.
Indianapolis, Indiana

STEVEN D. WEXNER, M.D.
Chairman
Department of Colorectal Surgery
Vice-Chairman
Department of Surgery
Director of Research and Education
Cleveland Clinic, Florida
Fort Lauderdale, Florida

CHURCHILL LIVINGSTONE

New York, Edinburgh, London, Madrid, Melbourne, San Francisco, Tokyo

Library of Congress Cataloging-in-Publication Data

Laparoscopic colorectal surgery / edited by Rama M. Jager, Steven D. Wexner.

p. cm.

Includes bibliographical references and index.

ISBN 0-443-08998-1

1. Colon (Anatomy)—Endoscopic surgery. 2. Rectum—Endoscopic surgery. I. Jager, Rama M. II. Wexner, Steven D.

[DNLM: 1. Colonic Diseases—surgery. 2. Rectal Diseases—surgery. 3. Surgery, Laparoscopic—methods. WI 520 L299 1996]

RD544.L37 1996

617.5′547—dc20

DNLM/DLC

for Library of Congress 95-35115

CIP

Distributed in the United Kingdom by Churchill Livingstone, Robert Stevenson House, 1–3 Baxter's Place, Leith Walk, Edinburgh EH1 3AF, and by associated companies, branches, and representatives throughout the world.

Accurate indications, adverse reactions, and dosage schedules for drugs are provided in this book, but it is possible that they may change. The reader is urged to review the package information data of the manufacturers of the medications mentioned.

The Publishers have made every effort to trace the copyright holders for borrowed material. If they have inadvertently overlooked any, they will be pleased to make the necessary arrangements at the first opportunity.

Acquisitions Editor: *Miranda Bromage*
Production Editor: *Bridgett L. Dickinson*
Production Supervisor: *Laura Mosberg Cohen*
Desktop Coordinator: *Jo-Ann Demas*
Cover Design: *Jeannette Jacobs*

Printed in Hong Kong

First published in 1996 7 6 5 4 3 2 1

This book is dedicated to our wives,
Patricia Ann Jager and Pamela Rosen Wexner,
and our children,
Rama Dev, Lisa Ramani, and Matthew Patrick Jager
and Wesley Myles and Trevor Grant Wexner.

Contributors

H. Randolph Bailey, M.D.

Clinical Professor, Department of Surgery, Chief, Division of Colon and Rectal Surgery, University of Texas Medical School at Houston, Houston, Texas

Garth H. Ballantyne, M.D.

Director, Center for Advanced Laparoscopic Surgery; Chief, Division of Laparoscopic Surgery, St. Luke's-Roosevelt Hospital Center, New York, New York

David E. Beck, M.D.

Clinical Associate Professor, Department of Surgery, Uniformed Services University of the Health Sciences, F. Edward Hébert School of Medicine, Bethesda, Maryland; Chairman, Department of Colon and Rectal Surgery, Ochsner Clinic, New Orleans, Louisiana

Dennis G. Begos, M.D.

Chief Resident, Yale University School of Medicine, New Haven, Connecticut

Irwin R. Berman, M.D.

Clinical Professor, Department of Surgery, Mercer University School of Medicine, Macon, Georgia; Colon and Rectal Clinic, Brunswick, Georgia

Marc Bessler, M.D.

Surgical Research Fellow, Department of Surgery, Columbia University College of Physicians and Surgeons; Surgical Resident, Department of Surgery, Columbia Presbyterian Medical Center, New York, New York

David F. Canal, M.D.

Associate Professor, Department of Surgery, Indianapolis University School of Medicine; Director, Endoscopic Surgical Research Laboratory, Indianapolis Medical Center, Indianapolis, Indiana

Philip F. Caushaj, M.D.

Associate Professor, Department of Surgery, University of Massachusetts Medical School; Chairman, Department of Surgery, Medical Center of Central Massachusetts, Worcester, Massachusetts

P. Jan Chandler, M.D.

Assistant Professor, Department of Surgery, Uniformed Services University of the Health Sciences, F. Edward Hébert School of Medicine; Staff Surgeon, Department of Surgery, National Naval Medical Center, Bethesda, Maryland

Stephen M. Cohen, M.D.

Clinical Fellow, Department of Colorectal Surgery, Cleveland Clinic Florida, Fort Lauderdale, Florida

Stephan J. Cohn, M.D.

Assistant Professor, Department of Anesthesia and Critical Care, University of Chicago Division of the Biological Sciences Pritzker School of Medicine, Chicago, Illinois

John A. Coller, M.D.

Staff Surgeon, Department of Colon and Rectal Surgery, and Director, Ambulatory Surgical Research Center, Lahey Hitchcock Clinic, Burlington, Massachusetts

Ara Darzi, M.D.

Consultant Surgeon, Academic Unit, St. Mary's Hospital Medical School; Consultant Surgeon, Minimal Access Surgical Unit, St. Mary's Hospital London, England

Thomas L. Dent, M.D.

Professor, Department of Surgery, Temple University School of Medicine, Philadelphia, Pennsylvania; Chairman, Department of Surgery, Abington Memorial Hospital, Abington, Pennsylvania

Afonso H. S. e Sousa, Jr., M.D.

Assistant Professor of Surgery, Department of Gastroenterology, São Paulo University School of Medicine; Surgeon, Hospital Oswaldo Cruz, São Paulo, São Paulo, Brazil

Andrea Ferrara, M.D.

Colon and Rectal Surgeon, Colon and Rectal Clinic of Orlando, Orlando, Florida

Abe Fingerhut, M.D.

Associate Professor, Department of Surgery, Louisiana State University School of Medicine in New Orleans, New Orleans, Louisiana; Chief, Department of Surgery, Center Hospitalier Intercommunal, Poissy, France

James W. Fleshman, Jr., M.D.

Associate Professor, Department of Surgery, Washington University School of Medicine; Section of Colorectal Surgery, Washington University Medical Center, St. Louis, Missouri

Kenneth A. Forde, M.D.

Professor, Department of Surgery, Columbia University College of Physicians and Surgeons; Attending Surgeon, Columbia Presbyterian Medical Center, New York, New York

Franz P. Gall, M.D.

Professor, Department of Surgery, University of Erlangen-Nueremberg, Erlangen, Germany

Joaquim Gama-Rodrigues, M.D.

Associate Professor of Surgery, Department of Gastroenterology, São Paulo University School of Medicine; Surgeon, Hospital Oswaldo Cruz, São Paulo, São Paulo, Brazil

Ingo Gastinger, M.D.

Professor, Department of Surgery, University of Erlangen-Nueremberg, Erlangen, Germany

Peter M. Y. Goh, F.R.C.S.Ed.

Associate Professor, Department of Surgery, National University Hospital; Consultant Surgeon, Department of Surgery, National University Hospital, Singapore

Ulf Haglund, M.D.

Professor, Department of Surgery, Uppsala University; Chairman, Department of Surgery, University Hospital, Uppsala, Sweden

James W. C. Holmes, M.D.

Associate Professor, Divisions of Clinical Surgery and Colorectal Surgery, Department of Surgery, Tulane University School of Medicine; Surgeon, Divisions of Clinical Surgery and Colorectal Surgery, Department of Surgery, Tulane University Hospital and Clinic, New Orleans, Louisiana

Rama M. Jager, M.D., Ph.D.

Clinical Associate Professor, Department of Surgery, Indiana University School of Medicine, Indiana University; Medical Director, Colon and Rectal Care Inc., Indianapolis, Indiana

Ferdinand Koeckerling, M.D.

Professor, Department of Surgery, University of Erlangen-Nueremberg; Consultant Surgeon, Department of Surgery, University Hospital Erlangen, Erlangen, Germany

James Kohn, M.D.

Surgical Endoscopy Fellow, Department of Surgery, University of Massachusetts Medical School; Department of Surgery, Medical Center of Central Massachusetts, Worcester, Massachusetts

Cheng-Kiong Kum, F.R.C.S.Ed.

Senior Registrar, Department of Surgery, National University Hospital, Singapore

Sergio W. Larach, M.D.

Assistant Clinical Professor, Division of Colon and Rectal Surgery, Department of Surgery, University of Florida College of Medicine, Gainesville, Florida; Colon and Rectal Surgeon, Colon and Rectal Clinic of Orlando, Orlando, Florida

Richard McCammon, M.D.

Clinical Professor, Department of Anesthesiology, Indiana University School of Medicine; Department of Anesthesiology, Community Hospital North, Indianapolis, Indiana

Robin S. McLeod, M.D.

Professor, Department of Surgery, University of Toronto Faculty of Medicine; Head, Colorectal Surgery Program and Surgical Clinical Epidemiology Program, Mount Sinai Hospital, Toronto, Ontario, Canada

John R. T. Monson, M.D.

Professor and Head, Academic Surgical Unit, University of Hull; Surgeon, Castle Hill Hospital, Cottingham, North Humberside, United Kingdom

David A. Nakata, M.D.

Clinical Assistant Professor, Department of Anesthesia, Indiana University School of Medicine; Department of Anesthesia, Indiana University Hospital, Indianapolis, Indiana

Heidi Nelson, M.D.

Assistant Professor, Department of Surgery, Mayo Medical School; Consultant, Colon and Rectal Surgery, Mayo Clinic and Foundation, Rochester, Minnesota

Ronald Lee Nichols, M.D.

William Henderson Professor of Surgery and Professor of Microbiology and Immunology, Department of Surgery, Tulane University School of Medicine; Department of Surgery, Tulane University Hospital and Clinic, New Orleans, Louisiana

John Northover, M.S., F.R.C.S.

Director, Imperial Cancer Research Fund's Colorectal Cancer Unit, and Consultant Surgeon, St. Mark's Hospital for Intestinal and Colorectal Disorders, London, United Kingdom

Frank G. Opelka, M.D.

Staff Surgeon, Department of Colon and Rectal Surgery, Ochsner Clinic, New Orleans, Louisiana

Lars Påhlman, M.D., Ph.D.

Associate Clinical Professor, Department of Surgery, Uppsala University, Uppsala, Sweden

Petachia Reissman, M.D.

Clinical Fellow, Department of Colorectal Surgery, Cleveland Clinic Florida, Fort Lauderdale, Florida

Michael F. Roizen, M.D.

Professor of Internal Medicine, and Professor and Chairman, Department of Anesthesia and Critical Care, University of Chicago Division of Biological Sciences Pritzker School of Medicine, Chicago, Illinois

Lester Rosen, M.D.

Professor, Department of Clinical Surgery, Pennsylvania State University College of Medicine, Hershey, Pennsylvania; Program Director, Colon and Rectal Residency Program, Lehigh Valley Hospital, Allentown, Pennsylvania

Jonathan M. Sackier, M.D.

Associate Professor, Department of Surgery, George Washington University School of Medicine and Health Sciences, Washington, D.C.

Bernd Schneider, M.D.

Professor, Department of Surgery, University of Erlangen-Nueremberg, Erlangen, Germany

Ignaz Schneider, M.D.

Professor, Department of Surgery, University of Erlangen-Nueremberg, Erlangen, Germany

Susan A. Sgambati, M.D.

Senior Surgical Resident, University of Connecticut Medical Center, Hartford Connecticut

Thomas A. Stellato, M.D.

Professor, Department of Surgery, Case Western Reserve University School of Medicine; Chief, Division of General Surgery, University Hospitals of Cleveland, Cleveland, Ohio

Michael R. Treat, M.D.

Associate Professor of Clincial Surgery, Department of Surgery, Columbia University College of Physicians and Surgeons; Attending Surgeon, Department of Surgery, Columbia Presbyterian Medical Center, New York, New York

Robert D. Tucker, M.D., Ph.D.

Associate Professor, Department of Pathology, Adjunct Associate Professor, Departments of Biomedical Engineering and Pathology, University of Iowa College of Medicine, Iowa City, Iowa

Anthony M. Vernava III, M.D.

Associate Professor of Surgery, Department of Surgery, Saint Louis University School of Medicine; Chief, Section of Colon and Rectal Surgery, St. Louis University Medical Center, St. Louis, Missouri

C. Randle Voyles, M.D.

Associate Clinical Professor, Department of Surgery, University of Mississippi School of Medicine, Jackson, Mississippi

Eric G. Weiss, M.D.

Staff Surgeon, Department of Colorectal Surgery, Cleveland Clinic Florida, Fort Lauderdale, Florida

Steven D. Wexner, M.D.

Chairman, Department of Colorectal Surgery, Vice-Chairman, Department of Surgery, Director of Research and Education, Cleveland Clinic Florida, Fort Lauderdale, Florida

Richard L. Whelan, M.D.

Assistant Professor, Department of Surgery, Columbia University College of Physicians and Surgeons; Attending Surgeon, Department of Surgery, Columbia Presbyterian Medical Center, New York, New York

Norman S. Williams, M.S.

Professor and Director, Academic Surgical Unit, University of London, London Hospital Medical College, London, United Kingdom

Foreword

There are few areas that have generated so much controversy in recent years as the advent of laparoscopic colorectal surgery. The strongly held and expressed views, often in the absence of long-term data on outcome, fall into three camps: the frank enthusiasts, the outright rejecters, and those who regard the new approach as offering substantial benefit when used with careful selection and by the fully trained. In hindsight, this situation is understandable, since the reported literature on the conventional open surgical treatment of colorectal disease has consistently provided evidence that the surgeon is the most important factor in influencing the postoperative morbidity and, in the case of colorectal cancer, the clinical outcome in terms of recurrence rates and long-term survival. Indeed, these reports and surveys have led to the establishment of colorectal surgery as a subspecialty of surgical gastroenterology.

Having read the chapters and the important editorial comments that comprise the three sections, I believe *Laparoscopic Colorectal Surgery* has been edited by Drs. Jager and Wexner with the above considerations in mind. The account is comprehensive, covering the necessary technology and its safe deployment, as well as all the laparoscopic procedures for benign and malignant colorectal disorders currently practiced in various institutions. At the same time, the pitfalls, risks, controversies, and limitations of laparoscopic surgery for colorectal disease are stressed throughout. In this respect, this substantive monograph stands out as different from the many books that have been published on laparoscopic surgery during the past 5 years, since it provides a critical and factual evaluation of the current situation. In stressing the current real or perceived risks and the undoubted limitations, the book points to the progress needed in the speciality of colorectal surgery when the laparoscopic approach is used.

Drs. Jager and Wexner and their internationally recognized contributors are to be congratulated for producing a scholarly account that is timely and sets the scene for future development and evaluation.

Alfred Cuschieri, M.D.
Professor and Chairman
Department of Surgery
Ninewells Hospital and Medical School
University of Dundee
Dundee, Tayside, Scotland

Preface

Over the past five years, the domain of laparoscopic surgery has dramatically expanded. Complex laparoscopic procedures that were initially thought impossible have subsequently become routine. However, the technical feasibility of any surgical operation does not suggest its routine use. One such example may be colorectal surgery. Although laparoscopic colorectal surgical procedures have become ubiquitously adopted, the benefits and advantages are by no means universally accepted. Whether our initial fruitful forays into laparoscopic colorectal surgery are mere ephemeral excitements or epochal eurekas is controversial.

The focus of *Laparoscopic Colorectal Surgery* is therefore to address both sides of the controversy, to sharpen the contrast, and to dissect the conflict between competing beliefs. We believe that controversy is as essential for evolution of surgical knowledge as is concurrence. Thus, we deliberately recruited some surgeons who are very enthusiastic about laparoscopy, others who remain very skeptical, and many who adopt a neutral position. Moreover, we recruited laparoscopic surgeons from around the globe to provide a more universal perspective of the current state of knowledge. Finally, because of the inevitable controversy, most chapters have at least one editorial comment to present a balanced approach.

Laparoscopic Colorectal Surgery is not a deployment of one position and argument, but rather a dialectic presentation of the current state of knowledge and an examination of the cognitive dynamics in the ever fluctuant field of laparoscopic colorectal surgery. Our goal, as editors, is to interpret the current flux in laparoscopic colorectal surgery but not to advocate any particular viewpoint or technique. The ideal of intellectual integrity involves considering all sides of the question and seeking a balanced approach and we have encouraged an overlapping admixture of ideas and concepts to enhance the book's value.

Laparoscopic Colorectal Surgery is divided into 32 chapters in three sections. Each chapter is followed by its respective editorial commentaries. The book begins with a provocative critique of laparoscopic colorectal surgery by Dr. Jager, which is commented on by the coeditor, Dr. Wexner. After this initial introduction, a number of basic topics are addressed, including the history of laparoscopy, preoperative evaluation, positional and anesthetic intraoperative complications, bowel preparation, techniques of pneumoperitoneum, the physiology of pneumoperitoneum, port placement and operative technique, monopolar electrosurgery, and the operating room setup.

The next 12 chapters describe either specific procedures, specific techniques, or results. Dr. Jager discusses the utility of diagnostic laparoscopy and Drs. Caushaj and Wexner comment on the indications and technique. Dr. Beck discusses the function of synchronous laparoscopy and colonoscopy after which Dr. Jager discusses laparoscopic enterostomy. Laparoscopic appendectomy is discussed in great detail by eminent surgeons in Singapore and Brazil. Similarly, the technique and results of stapled laparoscopic rectopexy for prolapse is described by several respected laparoscopic and colorectal surgeons. Other procedures are described in detail and the results of these procedures discussed, including sigmoid colectomy, abdominoperineal resection, total proctocolectomy, and right hemicolectomy. The myriad methods and disparity of indications are highlighted in the accompanying editorial comments to these chapters. The last chapter in this section discusses the recent application of laparoscopic surgery for intestinal obstruction.

The final 10 chapters describe the results of laparoscopic surgery and concentrate on the more controversial areas. Specifically, Professor Fingerhut from France describes the results of a large French trial. Several of the problems of the learning curve are well discussed by Professor Fingerhut and critiqued by Dr. Wexner. Drs. Weiss and Wexner then describe the learning process in laparoscopic colorectal surgery and Dr. Jager offers his comments. Next, Dr. Beck discusses complications of laparoscopic surgery and Drs. Påhlman and Wexner each offer their view on these complications and how they are best avoided. The interesting area of immune function after laparoscopy is detailed by Dr. Whelan and commented on by Drs. Nelson and Jager. Drs. Cohen and Wexner offer a very provocative critique on laparoscopic colorectal surgery, commented on by Professor Williams. Dr. Fleshman then describes the credentialing process for laparoscopic colorectal surgery and Drs. Dent, Rosen, and Jager all add their opinions. Dr. Canal describes the economics of laparoscopic instrumentation and Dr. Larach adds his viewpoint. The role of randomized clinical trials in laparoscopic colorectal surgery is discussed by Dr. Jager. Dr. Larach concludes the section with a discussion on cost analysis, with comments by Dr. Wexner.

Laparoscopic Colorectal Surgery is intended to be a dialogue dealing with the domain of our collective ignorance in the rapidly changing field of laparoscopic colorectal surgery and not a mere documentation of current dogma. Plasticity of belief, when faced with paucity of solid evidence, as is the current status with laparoscopic colorectal surgery, is advantageous and in fact, indispensable for all surgeons because of the need for continuous learning. Intellectual courage in surgical practice not only demands ability to defend one's beliefs, but also maturity to question one's own convictions and a disposition to be tentative when appropriate. The ability to weave the new with the old in order to restructure the whole conceptual web is necessary in proper application of laparoscopic colorectal surgical techniques. As John Locke, the English philosopher comments in his essay concerning human understanding, "He that judges without informing himself to the utmost that he is capable, cannot acquit himself of judging amiss."

We hope that by having amassed this formidable collection of talented surgeons, the reader will be afforded a highly useful, but also controversial, didactic text. We also hope that the reader sees a larger, deeper conceptual unity hidden behind the surface dissimilarity when reading differing opinions from our experienced surgeons, and perceives this textbook as a useful resource in managing colorectal diseases with laparoscopic surgical techniques.

Rama M. Jager, M.D., Ph.D.
Steven D. Wexner, M.D.

Acknowledgments

Obviously, hard work by multiple people was required from the inception of this manuscript to its completion. We thank all the authors of the chapters and editorial commentaries for taking time from their busy surgical practices to assist us in this project. We also thank Ms. Miranda Bromage from Churchill Livingstone International for her invaluable assistance and cooperation with technical aspects of the production. We commend Sherry Cockerham and Elektra McDermott for their expeditious handling of a huge volume of paper from the four corners of the globe. They were able to skillfully type and fax the chapters and commentaries while communicating with each of us and keeping everyone apprised of the progress of the book. Finally, it is appropriate at this juncture to thank Patricia Ann Jager and Pamela Rosen Wexner and our children for having allowed us to take much valuable time away from our families to undertake this formidable project in a timely fashion.

Rama M. Jager, M.D., Ph.D.
Steven D. Wexner, M.D.

Contents

Section II: Procedures

Section III: Current Results and Controversies

1

Laparoscopic Colectomy—Is It Evolutionary or Revolutionary?

Rama M. Jager

The first recorded colonic resection with anastomosis was performed in 1844 by Reybard.[1] The practice of successful transabdominal colorectal resection evolved over the past 150 years to the current state because of medical advances in anesthesia, asepsis, and antisepsis. Transabdominal surgical procedures have been attempted for colonic resection even before the days of anesthesia and asepsis. Because of increased operative risk, they were not conducted universally, and not on a large scale. Advances such as aseptic technique, intravenous fluid therapy, availability of blood transfusions, improved hemostatic modalities, and antibiotics improved the surgeon's ability to conduct transabdominal colorectal resections. Colorectal resections and anastomoses could finally be done with minimal surgical risk.

Satisfactory exposure of every portion of the colon via a long abdominal incision combined with mechanical retractors is feasible in most patients. Thus, the length of the incision never proved to be a limiting factor and enabled extensive and radical resection for colorectal cancer. The incisional pain, tissue trauma, and resultant metabolic stress and postoperative ileus from manual intestinal manipulation were considered necessary evils. Surgeons tolerated them as unavoidable and a small price to pay for the excellent exposure from a long laparotomy incision.

PHENOMENON OF THE 1990s

A new phenomenon caught every surgeon's fancy in the 1990s—laparoscopic cholecystectomy. The unprecedented, universal, and immediate acceptance of laparoscopic cholecystectomy[2] naturally led to extension and extrapolation. The minimally invasive approach spread to the treatment of other intra-abdominal organs, including the colorectum.[3,4]

The major advantage of a laparoscopic approach to any surgical therapy is a reduction in postoperative morbidity. Until recently, current surgical dogma underplayed the morbidity associated with long surgical incisions. Such clichés as "the bigger the incision, the better the surgeon" and "since incisions heal from side to side but not from top to bottom, the length of the incision does not matter" belittle the significant postoperative morbidity from long abdominal incisions. A reduction in incisional injury reduces postoperative pain in the immediate postoperative period. It may also decrease long-term postoperative morbidity. The longer the incision, the greater the incidence of wound infection, incisional herniation, and adhesion formation, thus underscoring the morbidity from long abdominal incisions.[5–7]

Gynecologic surgeons have long appreciated the advantage of minimally invasive surgery.[8] Since the beginning of this century, gynecologic extirpative and reparative surgery via the laparoscope proved that invasive intra-abdominal procedures through a keyhole incision are possible and cause the least morbidity. Procedures such as laparoscopic tubal ligation and oophorectomy have become commonplace. The introduction of videolaparoscopy and well-designed laparoscopic instruments promoted the trend. Although two-dimensional videolaparoscopy still hinders surgeons accustomed to the three-dimensional view of open abdominal operations, most gynecologists currently do many therapeutic pelvic surgical procedures through the laparoscope.

For reasons that may never become fully understood, nongynecologic abdominal surgeons did not immediately extrapolate the minimally invasive techniques to their surgical practice. The laparoscopic approach to cholecystectomy reminded many abdominal surgeons of the marked reduction in postoperative metabolic morbidity from surgical procedures with minimal incisions. The benefits were immediately obvious to our patients who demanded this new operation. Given the private health care system in the United States and associated competitive atmosphere, American health care providers rapidly adopted the new technique.

The surgical instrument industry saw a winner and lent its might to promote the newcomer. Industrial interests led to accelerated training of postgraduate surgeons in laparoscopic techniques. The ease with which a novice endoscopic surgeon can learn laparoscopic cholecystectomy, along with the continuously improving laparoscopic hemostatic and dissecting equipment, made laparoscopic cholecystectomy widespread and the new "gold standard."[2]

A NEW TWIST IN SURGICAL PHYSIOLOGY

Laparoscopic cholecystectomy also introduced a new twist to the understanding of surgical physiology. The dramatic difference in the postoperative course after laparoscopic cholecystectomy as compared with open cholecystectomy requires further analysis.

The intensity of the body's metabolic response to surgical injury—including protein catabolism, carbohydrate intolerance, and acute phase protein synthesis—is directly proportional to the severity of surgical injury.[9] Surgical stress from laparoscopic surgery is noticeably less than that from open operations. The metabolic and neuroendocrine responses are less severe in patients undergoing laparoscopic surgery as compared with open laparotomy.[10–16] Laparoscopic surgery does not suppress the patient's neutrophil function in contrast to a laparotomy.[17]

Which component of the surgical injury contributes most to the surgical stress response has yet to be experimentally determined. Apart from the anesthetic injury, surgical injury consists of both "somatic" incisional injury and the injury from visceral dissection. The visceral dissection in cystic duct transection and the gallbladder dissection in laparoscopic cholecystectomy do not differ significantly from that in open cholecystectomy. The only difference between open cholecystectomy and its laparoscopic counterpart is the length of the incision and the degree of dermomyofascial injury. The reduction in postoperative morbidity after laparoscopic cholecystectomy suggests that the morbidity from visceral dissection may be significantly less than the morbidity from "somatic" dermomyofascial injury. The somatic injury seemingly contributes a great deal more to postoperative neuroendocrine alterations than does the visceral injury.[13,14] The benefit from laparoscopic surgery is most probably from the decreased somatic injury and pain because the laparoscopic visceral injury is similar to that from a laparotomy.[12]

The observed reduction in postoperative morbidity following laparoscopic operations is multifaceted. The skin injury is minimal. Incisional injury to the abdominal wall muscles and fasciae is also diminished with laparoscopic procedures as compared with laparotomy (either vertical or transverse). The peritoneum is disrupted less in laparoscopy than during transabdominal surgical procedures. In addition, the generalized pneumoperitoneum distributes the retraction uniformly for exposure of the operative area as compared with localized mechanical retraction. Thus, the retraction-induced myofascial injury is less concentrated with laparoscopic surgery. The viscera are less manipulated, since the pneumoperitoneum and gravity aid exposure instead of the surgeons' hands or mechanical retractors. Consequently, the postoperative ileus will be less severe.[16] Since patients have less incisional pain, they use less narcotic for analgesia. This, in turn, decreases pharmacogenic gastrointestinal hypomotility.

LAPAROSCOPIC COLECTOMY DIFFERS FROM LAPAROSCOPIC CHOLECYSTECTOMY

Acceptance of laparoscopic colectomy has been slower than acceptance of laparoscopic cholecystectomy. There are many reasons for this phenomenon. Laparoscopic colectomy differs a great deal from laparoscopic cholecystectomy. The area of critical dissection in laparoscopic cholecystectomy involves a 2-cm^2 area of the cystic triangle. Laparoscopic colectomy involves extensive mesocolic and paracolic dissection. Larger vessels such as the right colic artery and the inferior mesenteric artery need ligation. Also, multiple mesenteric and mesocolic vessels need occlusion in laparoscopic colectomy as compared with laparoscopic cholecystectomy. Peritoneal contamination by bile during laparoscopic cholecystectomy leads to minimal long-term complications. By contrast, peritoneal contamination by colonic contents during colonic removal may lead to major postoperative complications. Laparoscopic cholecystectomy is usually necessary for benign gallbladder disease.

Current oncosurgical dogma dictates that the surgeon resect the draining lymph nodes along with the diseased colonic segment. Colon resection for cancer involves more extensive mesocolic dissection. The gallbladder can often be removed through the cannula entrance site without enlarging the incision. Removal of a transected colonic segment often needs an incision larger than that used for cannula insertion. Intestinal staplers obligate the use of larger cannulas, up to 18 mm, than those used with cystic duct clip ligators. Gallbladder removal requires no repair of the cystic duct other than ligation. By contrast, removal of a diseased colonic segment requires re-establishment of gastrointestinal continuity by intraperitoneal anastomosis. With laparoscopic colectomy, a portion of the operation such as the anastomosis may have to be conducted extramurally by delivering the colonic ends through a small incision. In addition, laparoscopic colectomy can be more tedious than laparoscopic cholecystectomy. The patient's obesity does not increase the technical difficulty of a laparoscopic approach to gallbladder surgery. Indeed, a laparoscopic approach is the preferred mode of cholecystectomy in morbidly obese patients.[18] By contrast, laparoscopic colectomy may be unacceptably tedious and frustrating in obese patients.

However, the reduction in incisional morbidity can be as clear-cut with some laparoscopic colorectal surgical operations as with laparoscopic cholecystectomy. The incision for classical open colectomy is significantly longer than the incision for open cholecystectomy. Thus, a proportional reduction in incisional morbidity is noticeable, although more cannulas are needed for laparoscopic colectomy. The postoperative course of a patient who undergoes laparoscopic colostomy or ileostomy as opposed to the classical open operation to achieve the same surgical objective is one demonstration of the advantage of minimally invasive surgery.

SLOW ADOPTION OF LAPAROSCOPIC COLECTOMY

In spite of its potential advantages, multiple factors impeded universal adoption of the laparoscopic approach for the treatment of colorectal disease. Apart from the tedious nature of the surgical procedure, the cost of the operation is another factor. Like any new operation and surgical technique, laparoscopic colectomy costs more to conduct. Postgraduate surgeons need training in the new technique. Hospitals need more equipment—such as monitors, cannulas, and grasping devices—than they need for the classical abdominal surgical procedure.

Conversely, the hospital stay of a laparoscopic surgical patient may be significantly shorter. The patient will lose less time from work, and productivity is restored sooner. Laparoscopic surgery is more precise because of the magnified view, a component of every successful laparoscopic surgery. Small incisions may also decrease the incidence of incisional hernias and postoperative adhesions.

After standard transabdominal colorectal surgical procedures, either epidural analgesia or patient-controlled analgesia is often used. These aggressive analgesic modes become unnecessary after laparoscopic colorectal surgical procedures, since the incision for specimen removal and extramural anastomosis will be significantly smaller.

The other major impediment to adoption of laparoscopic colectomy even for benign colorectal disease is the reluctance of insurance companies to view this operation as a variation in access for standard colectomy. Prima facie, laparoscopic colectomy appears to be a new experimental surgical procedure. On further analysis, however, the only difference between laparoscopic colectomy and its standard abdominal counterpart is the mode of access to the internal organ and mode of dissection.

Use of the yttrium-aluminum-garnet (YAG) laser for tissue dissection and coagulation does not make an operation experimental. When a hepatic surgeon conducts hepatic resection with an ultrasonic dissector, the hepatic resection is not considered experimental solely because of the new equipment used. The laparoscope used for access should not render laparoscopic colectomy experimental. It should be emphasized that the new technique is guided by the same surgical principles—hemostasis, prevention of peritoneal microbial and cancer cell contamination, and satisfactory anastomosis toward the goal of recognition, resection, and reconstruction of the colorectal disease. Laparoscopic colectomy, although it uses laparoscopic visualization and dissection, is similar to classical transabdominal surgical colectomy as long as it follows the standard surgical principles. The claim by various insurance and governmental agencies that laparoscopic colorectal surgery is experimental is debatable.

LAPAROSCOPIC COLECTOMY OR LAPAROSCOPIC-ASSISTED COLECTOMY

Considerable debate exists among laparoscopic surgeons as to whether laparoscopic colectomy is truly laparoscopic colectomy or a laparoscopic-assisted colectomy. This nuance is of little practical significance and is probably meaningless. Surgeons do not hesitate to enlarge the cannula insertion site to remove a large gallbladder with large stones during laparoscopic cholecystectomy. This maneuver does not convert a laparoscopic cholecystectomy to a laparoscopic-assisted cholecystectomy.

Similarly, if a surgeon removes sigmoid colon by enlarging the existing cannula insertion site into a small incision, this operation need not be qualified as a laparoscopic-assisted colectomy. The surgical objective is to reduce the incisional morbidity by limiting the length of the incision while still bringing about an equivalent outcome. Whether the incision made is 1 cm to insert the peritoneal cannula or 5 cm to remove a sigmoid colon, the goal of a reduction in incisional morbidity is achieved. Hence, the discussion and differentiation as to whether an operation is laparoscopic-assisted colectomy or laparoscopic colectomy serve little useful purpose. If a "laparoscopic" colorectal resection requires the same length of incision as the open resection, that operation cannot be classified as laparoscopic or laparoscopic-assisted surgery. It is a "conversion" of a laparoscopic attempt to the standard open technique, which is very appropriate in many patients. The semantics can be discussed at length but are useful only in studies dealing with metabolic morbidity and surgical stress rather than clinical practice. The term *minimally invasive surgery* or *minimal access surgery* may be more appropriate for laparoscopic surgery, although the adjective *laparoscopic* is too well entrenched and convenient to replace.

INDICATIONS AND CONTRAINDICATIONS

Included is a list of the current indications for laparoscopic colorectal surgery. The list is obviously incomplete, since any surgical procedure via an incision should be amenable to laparoscopic conduction.

Indications for Laparoscopic Colorectal Surgery

- Recognition of disease
  - Evaluation of lower quadrant abdominal pain
  - Abdominal mass detected by computed tomography or magnetic resonance imaging
  - Abdominal trauma
  - Metastatic workup to decide operability
  - Second look procedure for colorectal cancer when carcinoembryonic antigen levels are elevated
- Resection of benign colorectal lesions
  - Villous adenoma
  - Colonic lipoma
  - Familial ademomatous polyposis
  - Various premalignant polyposis syndromes
  - Inflammatory bowel disease
  - Colorectal stricture
  - Endometriosis
  - Sigmoid diverticular disease
  - Meckel's diverticulum
  - Idiopathic colonic inertia
- Resection of malignant colorectal lesions
  - Curative resection of superficially invasive cancer after colonoscopic polypectomy
  - Palliative resection of colon cancer with metastases
- Repair
  - Proctopexy
  - Colostomy
  - Ileostomy
  - Iatrogenic colonic injury

The equivalence of a laparoscopic resection to an open resection of invasive colorectal cancer is currently being debated, as reflected in the differing views of authors included in this book. The expanding or limited indications for laparoscopic colorectal surgery may be determined not only by the disease process but also by the availability of surgical instrumentation such as microsensors, ultrasound transducers, radioscintigraphic probes, stereovision, and so forth.[19] Even simpler technological improvements in basic surgical instruments (such as increased steerability and a semirigid shaft axis) enhance the instrumental degree of freedom and, in turn, the technical facility of intraperitoneal dissection.[20] Integration and extrapolation of various technological advances such as stereovision and robotic manipulators make surgeons depend as much on technology as on their manual dexterity to accomplish many of their surgical objectives using minimal access surgery.

Although the contraindications may change in the future, laparoscopic colectomy is currently not universally feasible. Various factors such as obesity and adhesions from previous abdominal surgical procedures preclude laparoscopic colectomy in some patients.

FUTURE COURSE OF LAPAROSCOPIC COLORECTAL SURGERY

Most laparoscopic surgeons notice a reduction in postoperative morbidity and decreased postoperative pain and ileus in patients undergoing laparoscopic colorec tal surgery.[4] In addition, the magnified view with the videolaparoscope enables more satisfactory dissection, especially along the base of the right colic artery in right colectomy, as well as the presacral space in proctopexy. Because of decreased incisional pain and ileus, the patient can be discharged from the hospital sooner and return to a productive life more quickly.

The disadvantages of laparoscopic procedures tend to be mostly secondary to the tedious nature of laparoscopic dissection. Also, since most colorectal surgeons are not familiar with laparoscopic procedures, the

Contraindications to Laparoscopic Surgery

- Obesity
- Extensive intraperitoneal adhesions
- Extension of malignant disease to adjacent organs requiring removal of the adjacent organs
- Inability to tolerate marked intraoperative positional changes
- Surgical inexperience
- Contraindications to laparoscopy such as pregnancy and coagulopathies

learning curve may be longer. The surgical instrumentation of various hospitals may have to change extensively with increased use of laparoscopic colectomy. In essence, laparoscopic surgery is necessitating massive "retooling" of operating rooms. Since the surgeons in the community have to learn this new surgical procedure, the cost of conducting a laparoscopic colorectal surgical procedure is obviously going to be higher than for the standard abdominal surgical procedure, at least in the near future. Unfortunately, at the present time, laparoscopic colectomy cannot replace the transabdominal surgical procedure, since quite a few patients (including patients who are overweight, have intra-abdominal adhesions, are pregnant) still need open standard colorectal surgical resection.

Although comparatively smaller incisions are made, laparoscopy is still abdominal surgery. Any laparoscopic operation may have to be quickly converted into an open surgical procedure for any number of reasons, including complications such as bleeding or visceral injury, difficult peritoneal access, or puzzling anatomy. The laparoscopic surgeon's technical training and skills must be advanced enough that the same surgeon can accomplish the surgical objectives of repair, resection, or reconstruction of the colorectum in the same sitting and with equal facility using the conventional open approach. Although diagnostic laparoscopy has been practiced by various nonsurgeons such as gastroenterologists, complex therapeutic laparoscopic procedures such as colorectal resections should be attempted only by surgeons trained in traditional and conventional abdominal surgery.

As with any new surgical technique, the question of whether the laparoscopic colorectal surgical approach is comparable or superior to conventional techniques needs to be answered. Metamorphosis of a much anticipated and commercially advanced "fashion" into an accepted and affirmed surgical "fact" occurs rapidly in only a few instances such as laparoscopic cholecystectomy. More often, the technical newcomer must go through an arduous process and be proved to achieve the same surgical objective with less morbidity.

Both the natural surgical innovation that goes on in day-to-day clinical practice and the planned, controlled trials in tertiary medical centers will hasten this conversion of the newcomer or dictate its rightful abandonment. It can be argued that the laparoscopic techniques that proved to be so successful in gallbladder surgery should not be extended to colorectal surgery until extensive, multicenter prospective clinical trials prove the advantage. Such caution avoids premature adoption of potentially dangerous surgical procedures. The difference between reckless surgical experimentation and reasonable scientific extrapolation of legitimate surgical concepts traverses a subtle path of which all of us should be aware.

The future role of laparoscopic colectomy depends on multiple factors. Existing surgical instruments need refinement. Active and aggressive involvement by the medical-industrial complex that is evident to every laparoscopic surgeon will help achieve this objective. The problem of specimen retrieval needs to be addressed because an incision is often made for the sole purpose of retrieving the surgical specimen. The role of DNA flow cytometry as a prognostic indicator equivalent to histopathologic staging has been demonstrated in gastric neoplasms.[21] Similar independent prognostic indicators equivalent to pathologic staging of the intact surgical specimen have yet to be identified for colorectal neoplasms. Current application of the laparoscopic approach to colorectal disease is in a process of continuous evolution and improvement.

BASHING OR JUMPING ON THE BANDWAGON

As happens with every new religion, every scientific breakthrough encounters a vigorous but varied response. Some will immediately convert because it is new; some will automatically curse it for exactly the same reason. A similar phenomenon can be observed among surgeons exposed to laparoscopic colorectal surgery. Some may be intent on "bashing" the laparoscopic approach, whereas others enthusiastically jump on the "bandwagon." Most "wait and see." When all the facts are in, the laparoscopic approach may prove to be appropriate for the treatment of most colorectal surgical lesions but inadequate for some abnormalities that will continue to require old-fashioned standard laparotomy.

Various questions still need to be answered regarding laparoscopic colorectal surgery:

1. Is laparoscopic colectomy a satisfactory operation for cancer?
2. Should laparoscopic colectomy be performed by all surgeons or only by specially qualified surgeons who are adept in laparoscopic procedures?
3. Should laparoscopic surgery be done at very few centers rather than in every community hospital?
4. Does laparoscopic surgery actually increase or decrease the expense of colorectal surgery?

With increased diffusion of laparoscopic surgical skills and the accumulation of more extensive data, some of the questions that remain will be answered in the near future or discarded as being anachronistic.

IS LAPAROSCOPIC SURGERY A REVOLUTION OR A PARADIGM SHIFT

Is laparoscopic surgery revolutionary, the dawn of a new era, or is it essentially a logical evolution in application of the fundamental surgical tenet of getting the most healing from a procedure? Laparoscopic surgery can be viewed as a variation of the basic surgical practice of exposing and dissecting intra-abdominal viscera by an incision.[22] The incision is replaced in laparoscopic surgery by thin cannulas. Exposure by retraction is replaced by exposure through pneumoperitoneum and gravity-aided visceral displacement. Intraperitoneal dissection is performed with thin, long instruments. Hemostasis by ligature is replaced by electrocautery, laser photocoagulation, or ultrasonic dissection. Transection of the viscera is done by staplers or long instruments. Intestinal anastomosis is conducted by using staplers or suturing with long instruments. Thus, other than decreasing incisional morbidity and using innovation rather than increasing the length of the incision, laparoscopic techniques achieve the surgical objective of intra-abdominal resection, repair, or reconstruction in the same surgical tradition as classical transincisional surgery. Whether laparoscopic resection for colorectal cancer achieves the same oncologic objectives as open resection is currently being debated.

Laparoscopic surgery, including its application to colorectal diseases, is a major surgical revolution that will be debated for some time to come. Its true role may be in facilitating a "paradigm shift" in traditional surgical thinking. Every significant breakthrough in any science breaks first with the tradition and established ways of thinking or "paradigms."[23] Gynecologic laparoscopy, laparoscopic cholecystectomy, and more recently, laparoscopic colorectal surgery questioned the traditional benignancy of long abdominal incisions and forced surgeons to rethink their conventional techniques and practices toward a reduction in postoperative incisional morbidity. This "paradigm shift" may be the true significance of the era of minimally invasive surgery.

REFERENCES

1. Schwartz SI, Ellis H: Abdominal Operations. Appleton-Century-Crofts, E. Norwalk, CT, 1984
2. Soper NJ, Stockmann PT, Dunnegan DL et al: Laparoscopic cholecystectomy. The new "gold standard?" Arch Surg 127:917, 1992
3. Falk PM, Beart RW, Wexner SD: Laparoscopic colectomy: a critical appraisal. Dis Colon Rectum 36:28, 1992
4. Phillips EH, Franklin M, Carroll BJ et al: Laparoscopic colectomy. Ann Surg 216:703, 1992
5. Santora TA, Roslyn JJ: Incisional hernia. Surg Clin North Am 73:557, 1993
6. Hesselink VJ, Luijendijk RW, deWilt JH et al: An evaluation of risk factors in incisional hernia recurrence. Surg Gynecol Obstet 176:228, 1993
7. Lundorff P, Hahlin M, Kallfelt B et al: Adhesion formation after laparoscopic surgery in tubal pregnancy: a randomized trial versus laparotomy. Fertil Steril 55:911, 1991
8. Semm K: Change in the classic gynecologic surgery. Int J Fertil 24:13, 1979
9. Cruikshank AM, Fraser WD, Burns HJG et al: Response of serum interleukin-6 in patients undergoing surgery of varying severity. Clin Sci 79:161, 1990
10. Joris J, Cigarini I, Legrand M et al: Metabolic and respiratory changes after cholecystectomy performed via laparotomy or laparoscopy. Br J Anaesth 69:341, 1991
11. Mealy K, Gallagher H, Barry M et al: Physiological and metabolic responses to open and laparoscopic cholecystectomy. Br J Surg 79:1061, 1992
12. Jakeways MSR, Mitchell V, Hashim IA et al: Metabolic and inflammatory responses after open or laparoscopic cholecystectomy. Br J Surg 81:127, 1994
13. Lefebvre G, Thirion AV, Vauthier-Brouzes D et al: Laparoscopic surgery versus laparotomy. Comparative analysis of stress markers. J Gynecol Obstet Biol Reprod 21:507, 1992
14. Lind LI: Metabolic gas exchange during gynecological laparotomy and laparoscopy. Can J Anaesth 41:19, 1994
15. Agnifili A, Ibi I, Guadagni S et al: Perioperative pain and stress: a comparison between video laparoscopic cholecystectomy and open cholecystectomy. G Chir 14:344, 1993
16. Schippers E, Ottinger AP, Anurov M et al: Intestinal motility after laparoscopic versus conventional cholecystectomy. An animal experiment study and clinical observation. Langenbecks Arch Chir 377:14, 1992
17. Carey PD, Wakefield CH, Thayeb A et al: Effects of minimally invasive surgery on hypochlorous acid production by neutrophils. Br J Surg 81:557, 1994
18. Miles RH, Carballo RE, Prinz RA et al: Laparoscopy: the preferred method of cholecystectomy in the morbidly obese. Surgery 112:818, 1992
19. Fujimasa I: Micromachining technology and biomedical engineering. Appl Biochem Biotechnol 38:233, 1993

20. Schurr MO, Melzer A, Dautzenberg P et al: Development of steerable instruments for minimal invasive surgery in modular conception. Acta Chir Belg 93:73, 1993
21. Suzuki H, Sugihira N: Prognostic value of DNA ploidy in primary gastric leiomyosarcoma. Br J Surg 80:1549, 1994
22. Editorial: Colons and keyholes. Lancet 340:824, 1992
23. Kuhn T: The structure of scientific revolutions. In: Foundations of the Unity of Science Series. 2nd Ed. Vol. 2. University of Chicago Press, Chicago, 1970

Editorial Comment

Steven D. Wexner

Dr. Jager addressed many interesting and controversial points in this chapter. Although it would certainly be easy to agree with his thoughts, I will instead assume the role of devil's advocate.

Dr. Jager commences by mentioning that incisions for standard laparotomy were exclusively "long" laparotomy incisions. In point of fact, many surgeons routinely use low transverse or Pfannenstiel-type incisions as well as paramedian or oblique incisions when performing right hemicolectomies. I would caution against the latter incision when the indication for ileocolic resection is Crohn's disease. In patients with Crohn's disease, a right iliac fossa ileostomy may at some point in the future become necessary. Creation of a transverse lower quadrant incision may limit optimal placement of that stoma in the future. Accordingly, with the single exception of ileocolonic Crohn's disease, any pathology can be approached through any incision and indeed has been over the years. The midline incision, although the most common, was by no means universally accepted.

Dr. Jager discusses the "phenomenon of the 1990s" and refers to laparoscopic cholecystectomy as having been "immediately accepted." I would beg to differ on this point and note that, although the media disseminated the results of these operations in terms of reduced morbidity as compared with standard cholecystectomy, results were published in the lay press before the scientific press. Furthermore, many academic centers did not adopt the procedure until it had serendipitously been proved superior. This unusual sequence of events included a strong drive by surgical equipment manufacturers and, because of the financial impact, interest by the media was easily obtained. This latter interest made the public acutely aware of this development, which led to the third arm of the push: public demand. Therefore, surgical equipment manufacturers, the media, and the public drove laparoscopic cholecystectomy to be accepted by the entire medical community in the absence of reputable scientific data. Nonetheless, the advantages of laparoscopic cholecystectomy are now historical.

Dr. Jager mentions that the major advantage of laparoscopic surgery is a reduction in postoperative morbidity. Again, although this reduction has been shown relative to cholecystectomy, the generally accepted incidence of postoperative morbidity noted in published series of laparoscopic colectomy hovers in the vicinity of 30 percent. Very few surgeons with whom I am familiar gladly accept that incidence of morbidity after "open" resections. I will be the first to admit that this incidence dramatically decreases with increased experience. My personal morbidity rate after my first 33 laparoscopic colectomies was 42 percent. In cases numbering 66 to 100, the overall morbidity rate was 12 percent, and in my series after the 100th patient, the morbidity decreased to under 10 percent. These data have been well documented by other surgeons. Furthermore, one must be cognizant that my laparoscopic cases account for less than 20 percent of my abdominal procedures. This selective application has also represented part of my learning curve. While my technical abilities have no doubt improved, so too has my ability of predicting who will best benefit from a laparoscopic operation. Finally, one must remember that an "average"-volume practice may not include the performance of 200 to 400 abdominal colorectal procedures per year, which would allow a surgeon to rapidly surmount the steep learning curve. Bear in mind that for the morbidity rate to decrease, the learning curve must be surmounted, presumably within a relatively short period. If the learning curve is not surmounted, the complication rate may never decrease to an acceptable level, thus obviating one of Dr. Jager's stated advantages of laparoscopy.

Dr. Jager quite elegantly discusses points that have been previously alluded to by me.[1–6] Differences among the various laparoscopic procedures are well addressed, and I will not reiterate those areas. Dr. Jager correctly notes that laparoscopic colectomy is, at least initially, more expensive to perform than laparotomy. Numerous authors have proved this point.[7–9] Dr. Jager states that the hospital stay may be significantly shorter and the time lost from work and productivity may be less. One must be very careful to compare apples and apples rather than apples and oranges. Several laparoscopic enthusiasts have cited reductions of 50 percent or more in the length of hospitalization. However, the data that they cite include recently performed laparoscopic procedures and historical control cases. It is inappropriate to make such a comparison as it yields a 5- to 6-day length of stay for the laparoscopic patient and a 10- to 12-day stay after "open" surgery.[10–12] Similarly, other laparoscopic enthusiasts have claimed that patients after laparoscopic colectomy have been discharged home much sooner than patients after standard colectomy. Although never mentioned in publications or during presentations, when queried, one discovers that the patients in the two groups are treated in markedly different fashions. Many of these surgeons who send patients home 4 to 5 days after laparoscopic colectomy send those patients home on a clear fluid or regular diet *before bowel movement.* Their patients who are discharged home after standard "open" surgery are not discharged home until after they are tolerating a regular diet and have had at least one bowel motion. Not surprisingly, when one changes the methods, the results are different.

In point of fact, a recent sampling of 161 consecutive patients who had undergone "open" colorectal procedures in my department revealed that the mean hospital stay was 6.5 days.[10] Thus, many of the proponents who cite these "massive" reductions in hospital stay would be best advised to not keep their standard patients in the hospital as long. I address this issue again later.

The problem with a comparison of pain levels among patients is that pain and return to work are two of the most subjective variables. We are all familiar with self-employed energetic individuals who are back to work almost immediately after major surgery. Conversely, we are all familiar with rather slothful employees who fully utilize all available disability compensation regardless of the magnitude of the procedure performed. Thus, again, some of the "advantages" of laparoscopy may similarly be advantages in either patient selection or patient perception. Furthermore, it is of little interest to the insurance company, which pays only the hospital bill, whether the patient is back to work within 6 weeks or 6 months.

There are several other points with which I must take issue with my co-editor. First, I believe that the semantics among laparoscopic colectomy, laparoscopic-assisted colectomy, and standard colectomy are indeed crucial. Dr. Jager believes that these terms are only useful "in studies dealing with metabolic morbidity and surgical stress." With current reforms in the health care system, the availability of data on cost and length of stay, and the mandating of diagnosis-related groups (DRGs), it behooves us to distinguish these three groups so that we can gather accurate statistics that will assist in assigning lengths of stay and in remuneration. Dr. Jager believes that enlargement of an existing cannula incision into a "small" incision is a laparoscopic rather than a laparoscopic-assisted procedure. The problem is that the word *small* has different connotations in different surgeons' minds. For instance, Senagore et al[13] have stated that a "small" incision ranges from 4 to 10 cm. Alternatively, Caushaj[14] has stated that any incision greater than 5 cm entails a conversion. My personal definition is based on the phases of the operation and the incision size. I define a laparoscopic procedure as one in which all the phases of the operation are performed through cannulas. Specifically, for me to qualify an operation as laparoscopic, all vessel division, bowel transection, anastomosis creation, and specimen extraction must occur through ports. The ports may range in size from 10 to 33 mm. Generally speaking, sigmoid colectomy, anterior resection, Hartmann's reversal, creation of an ileostomy or colostomy, rectopexy, and enterolysis are all well suited to be performed as laparoscopic procedures. In none of these operations is any incision made other than those necessary for the ports. In general, these procedures are performed through two to four 10-mm ports and one 18- or 33-mm port.

In my vernacular, a laparoscopic-assisted procedure is one in which vascular division, bowel transection, anastomosis creation, or some combination of these phases is performed through an incision. The incision may be one made through an already existing port site but nonetheless represents enlargement of a port site or delivery of bowel for extracorporeal performance of one or more of the above-cited phases of the procedure. Thus, an ileocolic resection, right hemicolectomy, small bowel resection, abdominoperineal resection, sigmoid colectomy with rectopexy, or total proctocolectomy are all well suited to be performed as laparoscopic-assisted procedures. These procedures are generally performed using between three and six 10-mm ports and an abdominal or perineal incision. A right hemicolectomy is usually performed through a 2- to 4-mm transumbilical incision, a sigmoid colectomy with rectopexy through a 4- to 6-cm true Pfannenstiel incision, and an abdominoperineal resection or total proctocolectomy through only the perineal incision.

The third category in the definition sequence is the laparoscopic converted case. Again, as stated in numerous places in this textbook, conversion should not be followed by shame or embarrassment. Conversion should instead be followed by the sound knowledge that one has saved the patient from potential morbidity. My definition of conversion is a situation in which I have had to perform any phase of the operation through either an unplanned incision, an enlarged incision, or an incision made earlier in the procedure than I had initially intended. For instance, if I have performed laparoscopic mobilization for an ileocolic resection for Crohn's disease but discover that because of a thick mesentery I am unable to deliver the specimen through the 2-cm incision I have made, I might enlarge the incision to 4 cm. While many surgeons might consider such a maneuver a triumph, I would consider it a conversion. Alternatively, if I planned to perform a sigmoid colectomy to include intracorporeal vascular ligation, bowel division, and anastomosis but I am unable to complete one of these phases laparoscopically and instead perform extracorporeal vascular ligation, that procedure would be considered a conversion. If the specimen cannot be delivered through the 33-mm port and requires enlargement of the 33-mm incision to 40 cm, the procedure is deemed to have been converted.

Unlike Dr. Jager, I believe it is crucial that we all speak the same language so that we may communicate our results to each other and those results can be understood by our peers, our patients, our hospital administrators, and perhaps most importantly, third party payers.

Both the readers and Dr. Jager will no doubt be pleased to know that I do agree with him on at least one issue. Laparoscopic colectomy is by no means experimental. It merely represents another method of performing the operation. The specific indications and contraindications are still debatable, but use of the technique is not. I also agree with him that the laparoscopic surgeon must be fully adept at "standard" surgery in case conversion is necessary. Furthermore, when the only tool one possesses is a hammer, the whole world resembles a nail. If a surgeon is a "laparoscopic" surgeon, the patient who might be best suited to a "standard" operation might be denied that approach. Laparoscopic surgery should be considered yet another tool in the surgeon's armamentarium. Certain colorectal pathology might be addressed through a trans-sphincteric incision, others through a trans-sacral incision, others transanally, others colonoscopically, others through a laparotomy, and still others laparoscopically. It would be foolish to think that every pathology or every patient is uniformly best dealt with through any single intervention.

Regardless of specific indications or contraindications, many lessons learned from laparoscopic colorectal surgery can be applied to "standard" practice. First, Dr. Jager alludes to laparoscopic colectomy being more hemostatic. It is not the technique itself that is more hemostatic, but that most surgeons prefer electrocautery dissection rather than sharp dissection. The reason for this preference is that even minute amounts of blood can absorb light and severely impede visualization. Although such impairment is not crucial during a relatively brief laparoscopic cholecystectomy, appendectomy, or herniorrhaphy, the same amount of blood loss per hour during laparoscopic colectomy can mean the difference between safely completing the procedure and causing complications or needing to convert. Thus, many surgeons who previously preferred sharp dissection during "open" surgery have now adopted electrocautery dissection. I personally have always used electrocautery during all phases of open surgery and find the technique particularly well suited to rectal mobilization. After high ligation of the inferior mesenteric vessels and marginal vessels of Drummond, the remainder of the entire procedure, whether an anterior resection or an abdominoperineal resection, is performed with electrocautery without any ligatures or clips in the vast majority of cases.

Another laparoscopic principle well suited to open surgery is the use of video. Again, I have always used an operating room headlight. I have now purchased a video headlight that one of my assistants wears during surgery. During certain phases, such as splenic flexure mobilization or low pelvic dissection in a male patient, I find myself looking not directly at the field but instead at the monitor while I am performing the surgery. Alternatively, instead of purchasing a video headlight, one might use the laparoscopic camera to facilitate certain phases of an "open" operation.

The most universally applicable lesson we have learned from laparoscopic surgery is that it is unnecessary to starve patients after surgery. We performed two prospective randomized trials[15,16] that accumulatively included approximately 250 consecutive patients who underwent standard "open" colorectal surgery. In both trials, patients were randomly assigned to either an early oral feeding group or a standard feeding group. In the former trial, the former group was given clear fluids the day of surgery. In both studies, the latter group of patients had diet withheld until flatus was passed, at which time clear fluids were commenced. After a bowel movement, patients in the latter group in both of these studies were then advanced to a regular diet. In both studies, the group of patients fed early did not have a significantly higher incidence of nasogastric tube insertion than did patients fed in the standard manner. Moreover, the patients in the early fed group in both trials were discharged home 0.6 to 1.2 days sooner than their counterparts in the standard feeding group. Since these trials have been completed, we have adopted a practice of routinely feeding all of our "open" colectomy patients a clear fluid diet the day of surgery. As soon as they request a regular diet, they are advanced to one. Most patients are now discharged between 4 and 6 days after a standard "open" colectomy, including patients who have undergone restorative proctocolectomy.

Various questions still need to be answered, as Dr. Jager mentions. He raises four specific points:

1. *Is laparoscopic colectomy a satisfactory operation for cancer?* To date, no prospective randomized trials exist to prove the acceptability of the laparoscopic approach for cure of cancer. There should certainly be no argument that laparoscopy is an acceptable alternative for palliation of malignancy. However, the data "supporting" laparoscopy for cancer are tenuous at best. First, the mean number of lymph nodes harvested in most series ranges from 4 to 14 nodes.[1] Although the mean number of nodes may be acceptable, the lower end of the range in these same series ranges from 0 to 8 nodes, clearly unacceptable nodal harvest. Obviously, numerous factors have an impact on the number of nodes reported. While surgical prowess and radicalness of surgery are factors to be recognized, so too are the diligence and enthusiasm of the pathologist. Even in the standard open setting, there is tremendous variability in the number of nodes identified through standard step-sectioning techniques.[17]

   Only one study has addressed distal margins when resecting rectosigmoid cancers. Tate and co-workers[18] clearly showed that the margins obtained during laparoscopic "anterior resection" were inadequate. Although the mean margin was 2.0 cm, the minimum margin was 5 mm, a clearly unacceptable level. Finally, not a single reference exists to suggest that the incidence of isolated wound implantation of malignant cells soon after curative laparotomy is within the 3.2- to 4.5-percent incidence range noted after laparoscopy.[8,19] Thus, Dr. Jager mentions the word "satisfactory" in his question. While satisfactory may connote a technically satisfactory operation to the surgeon, I believe that it should connote a long-term satisfactory outcome for the patient. Since the answer to this question is not yet known, I believe that laparoscopic colectomy for cure of malignancy should be confined to prospective randomized trials at the present time. The American Society of Colon and Rectal Surgeons endorses this view.[20]
2. *Should laparoscopic colectomy be done by all surgeons or only specially qualified surgeons who are adept in laparoscopic procedures?* Although the issue is addressed elsewhere in this book, there are two groups of surgeons who are qualified to perform laparoscopic procedures. One group includes surgeons who exclusively or almost exclusively perform surgery of the colon, rectum, and anus and who choose to incorporate the laparoscope as one of many possible modes of addressing the pathology in their patients. The second group of surgeons includes those who frequently use the laparoscope to address a wide array of pathology and may, with varying frequency, address pathophysiology and pathology of the colon, rectum, and anus. Regardless of which of these groups a surgeon belongs to, the learning curve is sufficiently arduous for both the surgeon and the patient. Unless surgeons are facile with the laparoscope and have a high-volume colorectal practice, it is probably better for them to not perform it at all.
3. *Should laparoscopic surgery be done at very few centers rather than in every community hospital?* This issue will most likely be decided by third-party payers rather than by physicians. However, again the situation is analogous to that of restorative proctocolectomy. Because of very high complication rates, these operations were, at least initially, developed only at tertiary referral centers. Only after techniques were refined was the operation disseminated to the community at large. Undoubtedly, such a parallel course of development is occurring with laparoscopic colorectal surgery.
4. *Does laparoscopic surgery actually increase or decrease the expense of colorectal surgery?* This last issue is contingent on which facet of the expense is in question and who is paying for that facet. Specifically, the "in-hospital" expenses may eventually decrease to levels below those noted for "open" surgery. While this savings may interest the insurance company, the company paying the disability insurance may be less interested. Conversely, if the patient remains in the hospital for as long as a counterpart patient undergoing a similar open procedure but returns to work 2 weeks sooner, the company paying the disability insurance would find the procedure to be of cost benefit. In order to answer this last question, costs must be further dissected. Currently, these data are not available. The few publications that have addressed the issue have failed to show a significant cost benefit to laparoscopic colectomy.[7,9,13,21]

Clearly, I have tried to introduce as much controversy as possible into my editorial for this particular chapter. While no answers are available to support either Dr. Jager or myself, trials are evolving that will, I hope, solve the mystery as to whether the technique is evolutionary or revolutionary.

REFERENCES

1. Teoh TA, Wexner SD: Laparoscopic surgery in colorectal cancer. In Williams N (ed): Colorectal Cancer. Churchill Livingstone, London (in press)
2. Verzaro R, Wexner SD: Laparoscopic colorectal surgery. In Brune I (ed): Laparoendoscopic Surgery. Blackwell Scientific Publications, Boston (in press)
3. Weiss EG, Wexner SD: A recommended training schema for laparoscopic surgery. Surg Oncol Clin North Am 3:759, 1994
4. Weiss EG, Wexner SD: Training and preparing for laparoscopic colon surgery. Semin Colon Rectal Surg 5:224, 1994

5. Wexner WD, Cohen SM, Johansen OB et al: Laparoscopic colorectal surgery: a prospective assessment and current perspective. Br J Surg 80:1602, 1993
6. Wexner SD, Cohen SM: Laparoscopic procedure in the appendix and colon. In Condon RE, Zudema GD (eds): Shackleford's Surgery of the Alimentary Tract. 4th Ed. WB Saunders, Philadelphia (in press)
7. Hoffman GC, Baker JW, Fitchett CW: Laparoscopic-assisted colectomy: initial experience. Ann Surg 219:732, 1994
8. Ngoi SS: Laparoscopic colorectal surgery. Presented at the International Society of University Colon and Rectal Surgeons 15th Biennial Congress, Singapore, July 1994
9. Reiver D, Kmiot WA, Cohen SM et al: A prospective comparison of laparoscopic procedures in colorectal surgery, abstracted. Dis Colon Rectum 37:22, 1994
10. Falk PM, Beart RW, Wexner DS et al: Laparosopic colectomy: a critical appraisal. Dis Colon Rectum 36:28, 1993
11. Ortega A, Beart R, Anthone G et al: Laparoscopic bowel resection: a consecutive series, abstracted. Dis Colon Rectum 37:22, 1994
12. Ortega A, Beart R, Winchester D et al: Laparoscopic bowel surgery registry: preliminary results, abstracted. Dis Colon Rectum 37:21, 1994
13. Senagore AJ, Luchtefeld MA, Mackeigan JM et al: Open colectomy versus laparoscopic colectomy: are there differences? Am J Surg 59:549, 1993
14. Caushaj P: Laparoscopic colon and rectal surgery: pitfalls and complications. Presented at the 5th Annual International Colorectal Disease symposium, Ft. Lauderdale, FL, February 1994
15. Binderow S, Cohen SM, Wexner SD et al: Must early oral intake be limited to laparoscopy. Dis Colon Rectum 37:584, 1994
16. Reissman P, Teoh TA, Weiss EG et al: Is early oral feeding safe after elective colorectal surgery?, abstracted. Dis Colon Rectum 37:22, 1994
17. Cohen SM, Wexner SD, Schmitt SL et al: Does xylene fat clearance improve lymph node harvest after colon resection? Eur J Surg 60:693, 1994
18. Tate JJ, Kwok S, Dawson JW et al: Prospective comparison of laparoscopic and conventional anterior resection. Br J Surg 80:1396, 1993
19. Wexner SD, Cohen SM: Port site metastases after laparoscopic colorectal surgery for cure of malignancy. Br J Surg 82:295, 1995
20. American Society of Colon and Rectal Surgeons: Policy statement on laparoscopic colectomy. Dis Colon Rectum 37:13A, 1994
21. Vayer AJ, Larach SW, Williamson PR et al: Cost effectiveness of laparoscopic-assisted colectomy. Coloproctology 16:190, 1994

2

History of Minimally Invasive Colorectal Surgery

Susan A. Sgambati and Garth H. Ballantyne

Surgical procedures that treat diseases of the colon and rectum have been plagued by high rates of morbidity and mortality throughout history. Undoubtedly, this resulted from the high bacterial counts within the colon. In fact, during the classical period, surgeons rarely operated on the abdominal cavity, but confined their intervention to indirect methods such as diet changes, cathartics, and purgatives. When confronted with diseases requiring more invasive therapy, surgeons attempted to develop minimally invasive techniques that not only treated the disease process but also minimized patient morbidity. Minimally invasive surgery thus has a rich history spanning thousands of years.

In the modern era, surgeons continued to develop minimally invasive techniques, particularly to treat colorectal diseases. Perineal approaches to rectal prolapse allowed the treatment of elderly patients before the advent of modern anesthesia. Use of the rigid sigmoidoscope for nonoperative decompression of sigmoid volvulus dramatically decreased the mortality from this form of colonic obstruction. The flexible endoscope provided intraluminal access to the colon and allowed the development of polypectomy techniques. Through minimally invasive techniques, surgeons could safely and effectively treat a larger population of patients.

The introduction of laparoscopic cholecystectomy in 1987 clearly illustrates the potential benefits of minimally invasive approaches to gastrointestinal disease. Patients suffer less postoperative pain, have fewer infections, resume oral intake earlier, and are discharged sooner than after cholecystectomy performed through a standard Kocher incision. Laparoscopic cholecystectomy's tremendous success, along with the flood of new technology into general surgery, stimulated surgeons to apply laparoscopic techniques to treat other gastrointestinal diseases.

Within 2 years of the first successful videolaparoscopic cholecystectomy, the first laparoscopic-assisted colectomy was accomplished. Preliminary reports suggested that many of the same benefits accrued by patients following laparoscopic cholecystectomy were reaped by patients with colorectal diseases. As such, the current efforts in the development of videolaparoscopic techniques represent the continuation of an ancient tradition of surgeons' attempts to treat colorectal diseases with minimally invasive techniques to decrease the morbidity associated with colorectal procedures. Nonetheless, innovative efforts to develop minimally invasive techniques for colorectal operations have been met with a groundswell of controversy. Many surgeons have questioned whether the expense of this new technology and the required retraining of practicing surgeons can be justified by the improved results reported in early series.

Surgeons have traditionally attempted to find new methods to treat their patients' afflictions, methods that would concomitantly reduce injury caused by the treatment. The application of minimally invasive techniques to operations for colorectal diseases follows in this tradition. Consequently, the purpose of this chapter is to trace the evolution of minimally invasive techniques for gastrointestinal diseases over the past 3,000 years and to highlight recent successes in the application of these techniques to diseases of the colon and rectum and will demonstrate that videolaparoscopic colorectal surgery represents the arrowhead of an ancient tradition pointing surgery toward the third millennium.

MINIMALLY INVASIVE THERAPEUTICS

Classical physicians were limited in their invasive therapeutic options. Religious prohibition against cadaveric dissections resulted in limited knowledge of human anatomy. Surgical procedures on anything but superficial structures carried high rates of infection and death. Consequently, classical physicians directed their efforts toward the stimulation of the patient's own ability to fight off the disease. Classical physicians believed that the symptoms of disease were produced by the response of the patient's natural faculties to the disease. They believed that disease resulted from putrefaction of humors within the body. Therefore, the principal role of the physician was to moderate symptoms and assist in the neutralization and disposal of malevolent humors.

Classical physicians attentively studied the progression of symptoms in both acute and chronic illnesses. In particular, they focused on the divergence of symptoms between patients who recovered and those who succumbed to the disease. It was the role of the physician to promote such symptoms as vomiting and diarrhea when the response of the patient was judged inadequate or when the symptoms became too extreme. The role of the physician, then, was to assist nature in the fight against disease.[1–3]

The importance of nature in the battle against disease remained explicitly the central postulate of therapeutics until the 19th century. This doctrine was deemed the *vis medicatrix naturae.* William Cullen, Professor of Medicine at the University of Edinburgh in the late 18th and early 19th centuries, defined this important concept. Cullen[4] wrote the following while addressing the phenomena of fevers:

> How the state of debility produces some of the symptoms of the cold stage, we cannot particularly explain, but refer it to a general law of the animal economy, whereby it happens, that powers, which have a tendency to hurt and destroy the system, often excite such motions as are suited to obviate the effects of the noxious power. This is the *vis medicatrix naturae,* so famous in the school of physic; and it is probable, that many of the motions excited in fever are the effects of this power.

Thus, classical physicians did not believe that they could directly treat a disease. Instead, they believed that their role was to support and assist the natural response of their patients to the illness. Physicians guided the powers of nature in the struggle against disease. In other words, they strived to use minimally invasive therapies to avoid compromising the patient's response to disease.

USE OF THE GASTROINTESTINAL TRACT IN CLASSICAL THERAPEUTICS

The gastrointestinal tract played a central role in classical medical therapeutics. Classical physicians recognized that alterations in gastrointestinal activity produced important effects on the natural history of acute and chronic illnesses. Hippocrates[5] (460 to 375 BC) wrote in *Aphorism* LXVIII of Section VII that in acute diseases,

> and with respect to the alvine [alimentary] evacuations . . . it is then necessary to purge; but if instead of this nutritive, liquids be administered, the disease will be proportionally increased.

Thus, stimulation of the colon ameliorated the disease, whereas stimulation of the proximal portion of the gastrointestinal tract worsened it. The classical Greeks did not identify the mechanisms by which the colon might produce these beneficial actions, but they did attempt to treat patients by affecting gastrointestinal function. This minimally invasive approach avoided the very real dangers of more invasive approaches.

The interest of Galen (AD 133 to 199), physician and surgeon to Emperor Marcus Aurelius, was directed toward the lower portion of the gut, because he believed it played an important role in health. The production and elimination of excrement was a fundamental requirement for the preservation of health. Galen[6] emphasized the following in *De Sanitate Tuenda:*

> Now our discussion has shown these two objectives of wholesome living, one the replacement of wastes, the other the elimination of excrements. And the third, that the animal should not age prematurely, follows of necessity those aforesaid. For if there were no failure, either in replacing the wastes or in the excrements remaining within, the animal would be healthy and would flourish for a long time.

In Book I of this treatise, Galen[6] devoted Chapter XIII to "Causes and Prevention of Excrementary Retardation" and Chapter XIV to "Evacuation of Retained Excrements." Difficulties with retention or evacuation of excrement could be avoided by careful management of diet and exercise. By careful regulation of the evacuation process, patients could help to preserve their own health.

Function of the lower portion of the gut played an important role not only in the preservation of health but also in the diagnosis and treatment of disease. In illness, for example, the normal process of concoction becomes unbalanced. The normal sources of nutrition are not fully separated from the excrement, and this condition can lead to retention of yellow bile and suppression of the excretion of black bile and excrement.[6]

Physicians could obtain insight into the cause of the patient's disease by another noninvasive technique: examination of stool. Stool color and thickness were indicative of the specific imbalance in the process of concoction.

Galen taught that "nature itself at the first onset [of sickness] often expels bile or pituita through vomit and through the bowel; therefore, it might be harmful not to imitate the actions of nature."[7] Thus, it was the physician's responsibility to restore normal concoction, thereby re-establishing health. The physician accomplished this through the administration of syrups. Galen's noninvasive therapeutics used syrups (1) to concoct, (2) to alter the disease by a contrary quality, (3) to extenuate and to comminute, (4) as a diuretic, (5) to control the bowels, (6) to bind the bowels, and (7) to strengthen the patient.[7] The physician carefully timed the administration of syrups to accomplish these different goals at different times in the natural history of the disease.

MINIMALLY INVASIVE SURGERY

Some diseases, however, failed to respond to noninvasive modalities. When patients were afflicted with intestinal obstruction, more direct means of treatment were required. The Greeks used the term *ileus* for intestinal obstruction. Hippocrates detailed one fatal case of ileus in a woman in whom no remedy would work.[8] Hippocrates did not specifically discuss the anatomic basis of ileus, but his writings suggest several etiologies. In his *Affections,* Hippocrates wrote that this malady supervened when a great quantity of fecal material accumulated within the intestines. In the *Third Book of Diseases* he explained that ileus might occur when the upper part of the abdomen was heated and the lower portion cooled.

Some treatments that Hippocrates practiced also lend insight into the possible etiologies of ileus. In *Affectations,* he advised injecting a large quantity of air into the intestines through the anus.[8] In *Diseases,* Hippocrates advocated the insertion of a suppository 10 digits long (approximately 2 cm). Modern experience has proved the efficacy of reducing an intussusception with insufflation and reducing a volvulus with a proctoscope that is 25 cm long. These descriptions suggest that Hippocrates equated ileus with intestinal obstruction and thought that there were several possible etiologies, including fecal impaction, intussusception, and sigmoid volvulus. Moreover, Hippocrates treated these life-threatening conditions with minimally invasive approaches.

Hippocrates' treatment of another colorectal disease further illustrates his minimally invasive surgical technique. The Hippocratic corpus suggested several remedies for the treatment of rectal prolapse. The most dramatic calls for suspending the patient in the air[8]:

> If procidentia ani takes place, having fomented the part with a soft sponge, and anointed it with a snail, bind the man's hands together, and suspend him for a short time, and the gut will return.*

Hippocrates also describes a technique for maintaining permanent reduction of the prolapse. A caustic potash is applied to the rectal mucosa, and after reduction of the prolapse, the thighs are bound together for 3 days. The inflammation and scarring serve to fix the rectum in place.[6] A similar remedy is also suggested for children. Other methods are advocated if the major symptom is bleeding, and yet another if the patient complains mostly of pain. The Greek physicians developed several different minimally invasive therapeutic modalities to treat the specific clinical manifestations of rectal prolapse.

EARLY ATTEMPTS AT MINIMALLY INVASIVE ACCESS: DEVELOPMENT OF ENDOSCOPY

Physicians have always attempted to gain additional information about the afflictions of their patients through careful physical examination. Direct visualization of accessible internal organs such as the mouth or rectum often provided important supplemental insight into the etiology of various symptoms.

Descriptions of minimally invasive techniques date to ancient times and include endoscopic examination of internal structures such as the anus and rectum. Innovative physicians, frustrated with the intrinsic limitations of endoscopy, introduced the endoscope directly into the peritoneal cavity, and named the procedure "organoscopy." This procedure gained access to additional organs and the serosal surface of the gut, providing important diagnostic information.

The earliest recorded references to endoscopy date to ancient times with Hippocrates' description of examination of the rectum with a speculum. Hippocrates[8] wrote in Section 5 of *On Hemorrhoids:*

> But if the condyloma be higher up, you must examine it with the speculum, and you should take care not to be deceived by the speculum; for when expanded, it renders the condyloma level with the surrounding parts, but when contracted, it shows the tumor right again.

*Until the 18th century, rectal prolapse was universally termed *prolapsus ani* or *procidentia ani.*

Classical physicians used speculums for examination but did not describe their use in operations.

The transfer of Greek teachings of medicine to the Arabs included the use of speculums. The Arabian Abulkasim (AD 936 to 1013) improved on Hippocrates' method by using reflected light to examine the cervix[9] (Fig. 2-1). In 1585, Tulio Caesare Aranzi fostered the next evolutionary step. Aranzi was the first to use a light source for an endoscopic procedure. He focused sunlight through a flask of water and projected the light into the nasal cavity.[10–13] Throughout the historical era, surgeons have used endoscopes to gain access to cavities of the human body. The industrial revolution provided the means to improve these instruments.

The modern era of endoscopy began in the early 18th century. In 1806, Bozzini used an aluminum tube to visualize the genitourinary tract. The tube, illuminated by a wax candle, had fitted mirrors to reflect images. Unfortunately, Bazzini's invention was poorly received, and the idea of "a magic lantern in the human body" was ridiculed.[14]

In 1867, Desormeaux, "the father of cystoscopy," used an open tube to examine the genitourinary tract. He combined alcohol and turpentine with a flame to generate a brighter, more condensable beam of light. In Dublin, Francis Cruise improved on Desmoreaux's model by enhancing illumination through a paraffin lamp, essentially making cystoscopy a practical technique. Cruise's instrument had attachments for examination of the rectum, uterus, auditory meatus, pharynx, and larynx. Also, Cruise envisioned that it might be adapted for investigation of the esophagus and stomach[14,15] (Fig. 2-2).

In 1869, Commander Pantaleoni used a modified cystoscope to cauterize a hemorrhagic uterine growth. Pantaleoni thus performed the first diagnostic and therapeutic hysteroscopy. Nitze, in 1877, developed a cystoscope with a distal light source and designed the first modern-type endoscope.[11,14,15]

In 1868, Kussmaul performed the first esophagogastroscopy on a professional sword swallower, which was the initiation of efforts at instrumentation of the gastrointestinal tract. Mikulicz and Schindler, however, are credited with the advancement of gastroscopy, having designed gastroscopes equipped with both an optical system and a means to insufflate air[16] (Fig. 2-3).

The use of rigid endoscopic instruments severely limited access to the gastrointestinal tract. A flexible instrument was required to gain entrance into the duodenum or the colon proximal to the rectosigmoid junction. The necessary technology took more than 100 years to be developed. In 1870, the British physicist John Tyndall demonstrated that light would follow a curved path. J.L. Baird of England and C.W. Hansell of the United States proposed using flexible glass fibers to propagate light in 1927 and 1930, respectively. It was not until 1954, however, that Lawrence Curtiss, an undergraduate physics student at the University of

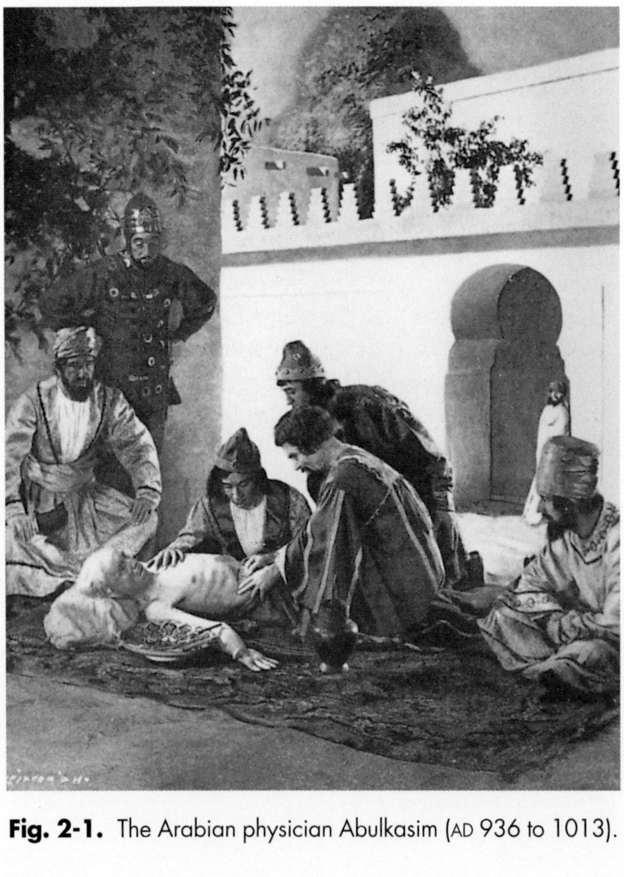

Fig. 2-1. The Arabian physician Abulkasim (AD 936 to 1013).

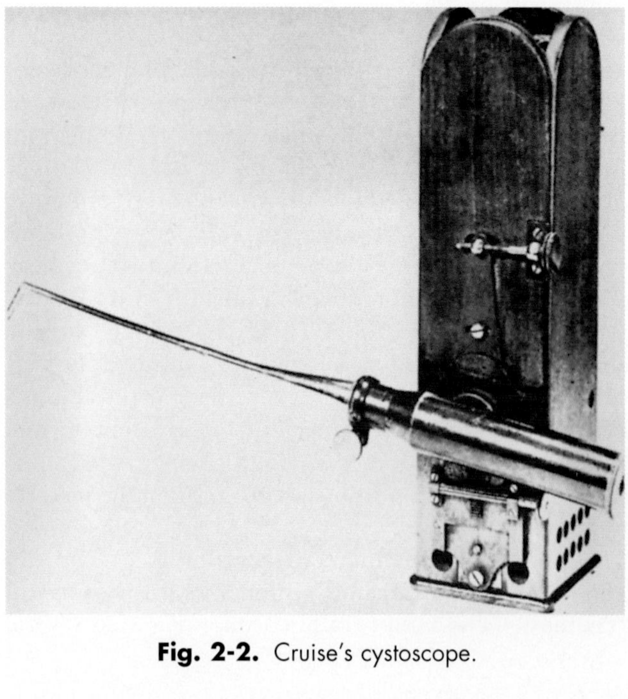

Fig. 2-2. Cruise's cystoscope.

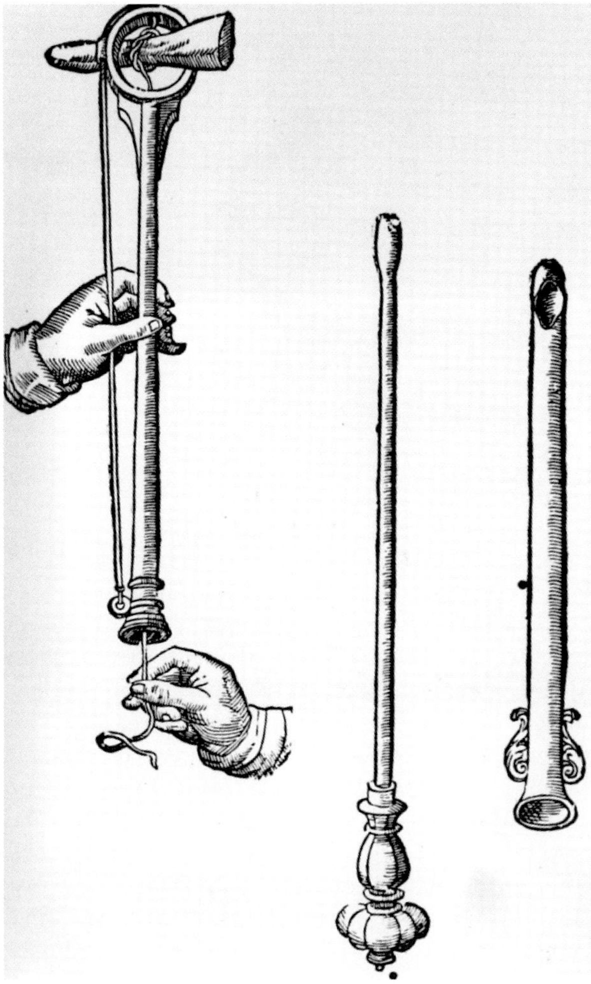

Fig. 2-3. Early gastroscope.

Michigan, invented the process by which fine glass fibers could be coherently bundled to convey an entire image. The prototype fiberscope, initially adapted as a gastroscope, was introduced at the University of Michigan by Basil Hirshowitz in 1957.[16]

The tortuosity of the rectosigmoid colon limited application of the fiberscope to the distal portion of the gastrointestinal tract. Advances in fiberoptics along with the persistence of Bergein F. Overholdt led to the introduction of the first fiberoptic sigmoidoscope in 1963[16] (Fig. 2-4). It was not until 1967, however, when Overholdt presented his experience to a skeptical American Society of Gastrointestinal Endoscopists, that colonoscopy was officially embraced. Technical refinements eventually led to advanced endoscopic surgical techniques consistent with the goal of minimally invasive surgery.

DEVELOPMENT OF LAPAROSCOPY

The earliest reference to laparoscopy dates to Biblical history, where Ezekiel (Ezekiel 21:21) wrote,

> For the king of Babylon stood at the parting of the way, at the head of the two ways, to use divination: He made his arrows bright, he consulted with images, he looked into the liver.

During ancient times, the peritoneal cavity was a central focus, with the umbilicus symbolizing the connection to life and the liver representing the "cradle of the soul."[12]

As previously discussed, classical Galenic medical tradition was based on the concept of maintaining balanced production and excretion of bodily waste, as imbalances led to disease states. Classical medical therapy attempted to restore normal balance through purgatives and cathartics. Alternatively, balance could be restored through surgery by inserting a trocar into the abdominal cavity and draining the bad humors. Celsus[17] (25 BC to AD 50) detailed the procedure:

> Some perform it below the navel at the distance of about four digits to the left; some perforate the navel itself; some cauterize the integument and make their opening into the abdomen by incision. . .
>
> A leaden or copper cannula with its lips curved outwards, or one that has a circular rim at its middle to prevent its slipping into the cavity is then introduced through the aperture. When the latter is used, that part of the instrument which is introduced should be no longer than that which remains external to the aperture, in order that it may proceed beyond the peritoneum.

Instruments closely resembling laparoscopic trocars have been recovered from Roman ruins (Fig. 2-5). Similarly, Albukasim described an "exploring needle with a groove" mounted on a handle. The term *trocar,* however, was not coined until 1706 and is thought to be derived from *trochartor trois-quarts,* a three-faced instrument consisting of a perforator enclosed in a metal cannula[18] (Fig. 2-6).

The first endoscopic examinations of the peritoneal cavity were accomplished early in the 20th century. In 1901, Dimitri Ott, a German gynecologist, described "ventroscopy," a technique in which a speculum was introduced through an incision in the posterior vaginal fornix. Ott wore head mirrors to reflect light and augment visualization. Also in 1901, George Kelling, a German surgeon, reported using a cystoscope to examine the intra-abdominal viscera of a dog after insufflating the peritoneal cavity with air, and coined the term *celioscopy.* Jacobeus performed the first human celioscopy in Sweden in 1910 and advocated the technique for the evaluation of patients with ascites. In 1911

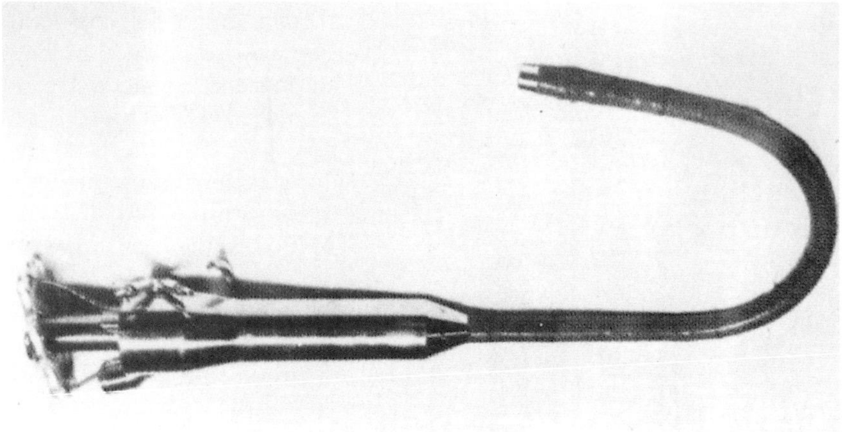

Fig. 2-4. The first fiberoptic sigmoidoscope.

in the United States, Bernheim published his laparoscopic experiences in an article titled "Organoscopy" in the journal *Annals of Surgery*[10–14,16,19] (Fig. 2-7).

World War I interrupted technological advances, and it was not until the mid-1920s that enthusiasm for "organoscopy" was renewed and photographic documentation attempted. In 1923, Kelling reported his 22 years of experience with laparoscopy to the German Surgical Society. Kelling became one of the earliest advocates of minimally invasive surgery. He encouraged surgeons to use diagnostic laparoscopy to spare patients the prolonged and costly stay of a laparotomy.[11,19,20]

TECHNICAL ADVANCES

The pioneers of laparoscopy believed that the technique was an important adjunct to surgical practice. Nonetheless, inadequate technology limited their vision, both literally and figuratively. Light sources in the first laparoscopes consisted of a distal light bulb with a rheostat to control the intensity. The danger of thermal burns to intra-abdominal contents from these primitive devices significantly limited their use. The laparoscope was introduced directly into the peritoneal cavity and pneumoperitoneum established by instilling air through the scope. Understandably, bowel perforations and vascular injuries posed very real risks in these early procedures.[13,16,20] In 1929, Kalk introduced the Foroblique (135-degree) lens system and advocated the use of a separate pneumoperitoneum needle and a second puncture site. These refinements in technique, along with Kalk's descriptions of therapeutic laparoscopic interventions, earned him the designation as the "father of modern laparoscopy."[11] In 1938, Veress developed a needle with a spring-loaded obturator that allowed safe insertion and insufflation of the peritoneal cavity. Thereafter, pneumoperitoneum was established before instrumentation of the abdomen.[13]

Despite such advances in laparoscopic imaging and technique, several troublesome problems persisted. Bowel and vascular injuries during trocar insertion continued to occur. No scientific knowledge existed regarding the dangers of increased intra-abdominal pressure. Finally, and most distressingly, unipolar cautery was associated with a high rate of thermal injury to the bowel. These dangers severely restricted the use of laparoscopy. Few surgeons judged that the advantages of laparoscopy outweighed the inherent risks of the technique.

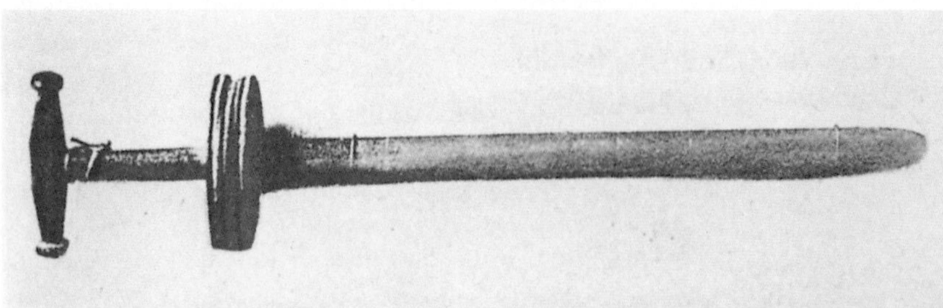

Fig. 2-5. Ancient trocar recovered from the Pompeian ruins.

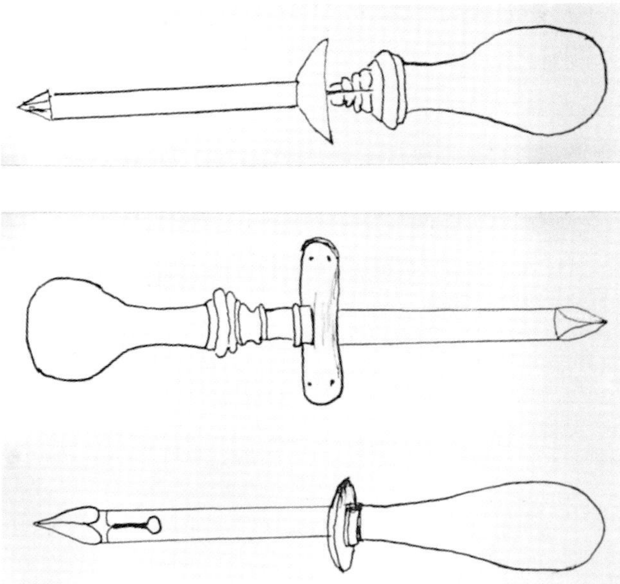

Fig. 2-6. Early trocars were described as three-faced instruments consisting of a perforator enclosed in a metal cannula.

MODERN LAPAROSCOPY

In 1952, Fourestier, Gladu, and Valmiere developed a new imaging system that revolutionized endoscopy. The system used a quartz rod to transmit an intense light beam distally along a telescope. This development solved many of the aforementioned problems and allowed the light intensity to be concentrated enough to photograph images. Closed-circuit television was added in 1959.[11,13,14]

Another decade was required, however, before the dangers of insufflation of the abdomen were overcome. In 1966, Kurt Semm introduced an automatic insufflation device capable of monitoring intra-abdominal pressure. This allowed for safer laparoscopy, and bowel perforations and retroperitoneal vascular injuries subsequently declined. Semm developed thermocoagulation, which revolutionized laparoscopic surgery by virtually eliminating thermal injuries. Semm also designed a high-volume irrigation/aspiration system and perfected the EndoLoop applicator as well as intra- and extracorporeal knot-tying techniques and instruments.[11,13,21] These technical advances elevated laparoscopy to a safe procedure that could be used in common clinical settings.

A

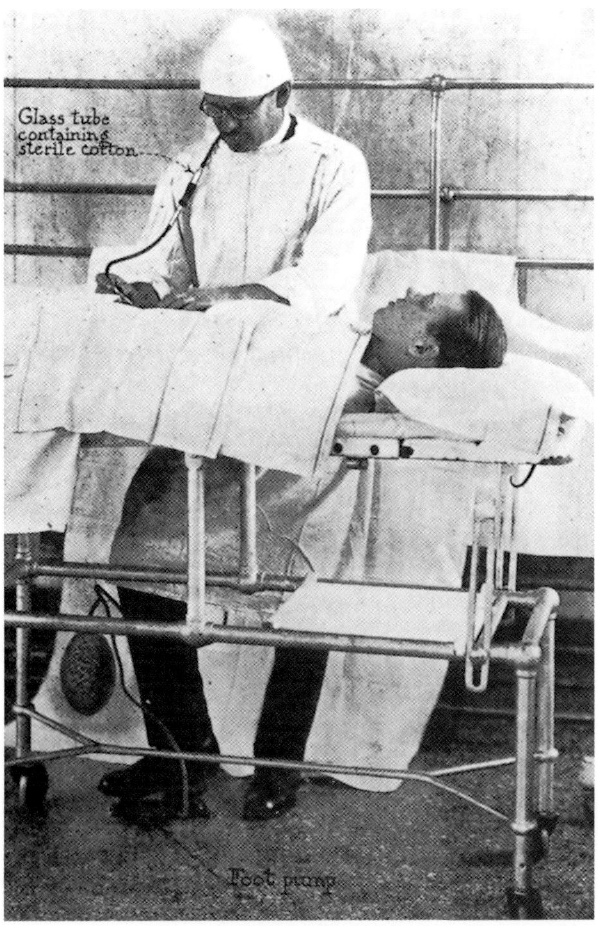

B

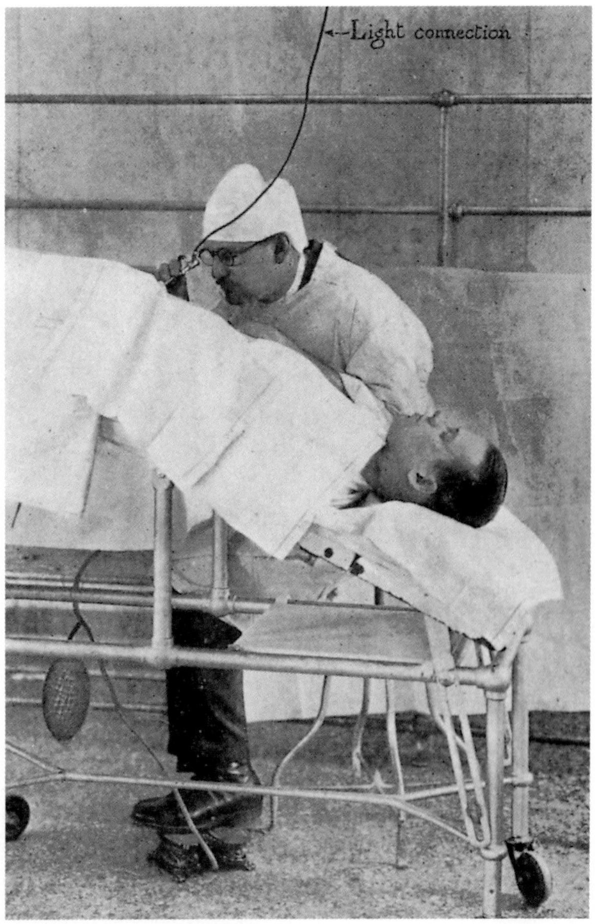

Fig. 2-7. (A & B) Early laparoscopy. (From Bernheim,[19] with permission.)

Therapeutic uses of laparoscopy were rapidly developed. Along with the technical advances, Semm adapted numerous surgical procedures to laparoscopic techniques, including tubal sterilization, salpingostomy, oophorectomy, salpingolysis, and tumor reduction therapy. Beyond the realm of gynecologic surgery, Semm popularized such laparoscopic procedures as omental adhesiolysis, bowel suturing, tumor biopsy and staging, and notably, incidental appendectomy.[13,21] Although interest was piqued, general surgeons still considered laparoscopy a "blind" procedure fraught with risks of intra-abdominal injuries and thus did not incorporate the technique into the practice of general surgery.

LAPAROSCOPY IN GENERAL SURGERY

By the late 1970s, gynecologic surgeons had embraced laparoscopy and thoroughly incorporated the technique into their practice. General surgeons, despite exposure to laparoscopy in consultation with gynecologic colleagues, remained skeptical and staunchly supported traditional open surgery. In 1978, Hasson[22] introduced an alternative method of trocar placement that permitted direct visualization of trocar entrance into the peritoneal cavity. Subsequent to the development of the Hasson technique, general surgeons became more receptive to laparoscopic surgery, as the open technique allayed fears of bowel and vascular injury.[22]

Liver biopsies were the first laparoscopic procedures attempted by general surgeons in 1982.[23] Laparoscopy was applied to the staging of pancreatic cancer by Warshaw and associates[24] in 1986, who reported a 93-percent accuracy rate. In 1987, Mouret performed the first human laparoscopic cholecystectomy in France.[25] McKernam and Saye performed the first laparoscopic cholecystectomy in the United States in 1988, but the technique was refined and popularized by Reddick and Olsen,[26] who also developed the technique of laparoscopic cholangiography.[27]

MINIMALLY INVASIVE COLON SURGERY

Despite the advances in other areas of the gastrointestinal tract, many surgeons have remained reluctant to apply videolaparoscopy to colorectal surgery. It must be kept in mind, however, that efforts to develop minimally invasive techniques in colorectal surgery are merely a continuation of an ancient tradition. A striking example of the continuous effort toward minimally invasive colon surgery is seen in the history of the treatment of rectal procidentia. The vast majority of patients affected with rectal prolapse are elderly, with associated medical problems that make them poor surgical candidates. In addition to the method offered by Hippocrates (see above), modern surgeons have struggled to find better means of treating these patients. Since the 1890s, more than 100 procedures have been proposed to treat rectal prolapse, all aimed at definitive treatment through the least invasive means possible.

Several perineal procedures were designed to avoid laparotomy, namely, the Thiersch procedure in 1891, the Delorme procedure (mucosal sleeve resection) in 1900, and perineal rectosigmoidectomy. The latter procedure, originally advocated by Miles in 1933 and Gabriel in 1948, was popularized by Altemeier in 1952. Altemeier's success with the technique resulted in the association of his name with perineal rectosigmoidectomy (i.e., the Altemeier procedure).[28–30]

Colonoscopy further illustrates recent efforts to develop minimally invasive modalities for the treatment of colorectal diseases. Colonoscopy became a vital component of colon and rectal surgery in the late 1970s, and improvements in technique and instrumentation permitted aggressive endoscopic treatment of colonic neoplasms. In many cases, formal laparotomy could be avoided, as polyps could be resected both safely and effectively through the colonoscope. Christopher Williams, Hiromi Shinya, and Jerome Way led the world in the development and promotion of colonoscopy as a minimally invasive surgical technique.[16] The application of laparoscopy to colorectal diseases follows naturally in this same tradition.

LAPAROSCOPIC APPENDECTOMY

The first laparoscopic appendectomy was performed by DeKok[31] in 1977. This was a laparoscopic-assisted procedure, with a minilaparotomy performed to remove the noninflamed appendix. Semm[32] performed the first complete laparoscopic appendectomy in 1983. His technique, recommended only for nonacute cases, consisted of extracorporeal ligation of the mesoappendix and endoscopic ligation of the appendix with a pretied loop. The appendix was transected across its base with electrocautery.[32] Laparoscopy subsequently became a practical and popular technique used by general and gynecologic surgeons alike for the evaluation and treatment of right lower quadrant pain in women.[33,34]

LAPAROSCOPIC COLON SURGERY

Patients who require colorectal surgery are often elderly and debilitated by chronic diseases. The abdominal wound has always been a source of major morbidity for these patients. The high concentration of bacteria within stool contributes to the high rate of wound infection, dehiscence, and evisceration associated with colorectal surgery. In addition, the pain from the abdominal wound often compromises pulmonary function and may limit the mobility of these patients in the immediate postoperative period, as well as after hospital discharge. As a result, minimally invasive techniques, which limit the size of the abdominal wound, theoretically offer distinct advantages to patients requiring colorectal operations.

Application of videolaparoscopic techniques to colorectal operations was initially limited by the lack of appropriate instruments. Consequently, the first laparoscopic colon resections were "laparoscopic-assisted" colectomies (i.e., minilaparotomies were used for ligation of mesenteric vasculature, extracorporeal anastomoses, and specimen removal). The first laparoscopic colonic resection using this technique was a right hemicolectomy, which was accomplished by Moises Jacobs in Miami, Florida, in June of 1990. Similarly, closure of a colostomy required few specialized laparoscopic instruments. Joseph Uddo performed a laparoscopic colostomy closure on November 14, 1990. The anastomosis was constructed with a circular stapling device.

The introduction of laparoscopic intestinal staplers, allowed intraperitoneal transection of the bowel. Using this instrument for ligation of the mesentery and transection of the colon, Dennis Fowler performed the first laparoscopic sigmoid resection in October of 1990. The anastomosis was constructed with a stapling device. The following month, using a similar technique, Patrick Leahy was able to resect a proximal rectal cancer and to construct a low anterior anastomosis. Several months later on July 26, 1991, Joseph Uddo performed an entirely laparoscopic right hemicolectomy; the ileocolic anastomosis was constructed intracorporally. In rapid succession, virtually all types of colorectal procedures were accomplished using minimally invasive techniques (Table 2-1).

The natural extension of minimally invasive techniques beyond colonoscopic polypectomy was the development of laparoscopic-assisted polypectomy. In 1991, Saclarides et al[35] reported the laparoscopic removal of a colonic lipoma. The accomplishment of Saclarides and associates added a technique to the growing armamentarium of minimally invasive surgery, as lesions not heretofore resectable colonoscopically required laparotomy for removal. A lesion deemed nonresectable through the colonoscope could now be resected laparoscopically, thereby extending the benefits of minimally invasive surgery to a larger patient population.

LAPAROSCOPIC COLECTOMY: ADVANTAGES AND DISADVANTAGES

Initial reports indicate that laparoscopic colectomy can be performed safely with significant patient benefits. Advantages of laparoscopic colectomy include decreased postoperative ileus, pain, and disability; fewer pulmonary complications; improved cosmesis; shorter hospitalization; and reduced costs of care.[36–38]

Several controversial issues surround the application of laparoscopic techniques to colonic surgery. The biggest and potentially most severe issue concerns the propriety of laparoscopic colectomy for malignancy. The present standard of care dictates that generous mesenteric lymphadenectomy be performed when resecting for carcinoma. Resection through the laparoscope is thought to provide a less extensive lymphadenectomy, and thus concerns arise regarding the adequacy of laparoscopic colon resection for carcinoma.[39,40]

Institutional differences in reporting the lymph node content of pathology specimens further complicate this issue. The small sample groups and large standard deviations of existing studies add to the problem. Clearly, long-term clinical studies, including stage-specific survival data, are required. The American Society of Colon and Rectal Surgeons established a laparoscopic colectomy registry to gather and analyze data from surgeons performing laparoscopic colorectal procedures. This body of data should provide the information needed to evaluate the therapeutic value and cost-effectiveness of laparoscopic colorectal procedures.[40] A second issue concerns the granting of privileges for surgeons to perform these operations in individual hospitals. Laparoscopic colectomy is significantly more complicated than laparoscopic cholecystectomy and has a very steep learning curve. Adequate

Table 2-1. Milestones in Laparoscopic Colorectal Surgery

Procedure	Surgeon	Date
Right hemicolectomy	Moises Jacobs	June 1990
Sigmoid resection	Dennis L. Fowler	October 1990
Low anterior resection	Patrick Leahy	November 1990
Abdominoperineal resection	Robert W. Beart	April 1991
Total abdominal colectomy	Steven Wexner David G. Jagelman	August 1991
Transverse colectomy	Garth H. Ballantyne	February 1992

instruction, animal model experience, and proctoring by individuals skilled in advanced laparoscopic techniques are required to minimize complications and optimize patient outcome. This complex issue also encompasses economic concerns such as restraint of trade. Several peer groups, most notably the Society of American Gastrointestinal Endoscopic Surgeons, have issued policy statements regarding privileging. Presently, however, privileging decisions remain with institutional credentialing boards.[41–43]

SUMMARY

This historical overview has traced the evolution of minimally invasive surgery from ancient times through the present. Minimally invasive approaches to diseases of the colon and rectum were developed because of the high rates of septic complications associated with invasive bowel procedures. Similarly, endoscopes were developed to gain minimally invasive access to the gastrointestinal tract. Throughout the 20th century, surgeons have struggled to design surgical procedure that minimally injured their patients, yet adequately treated the gastrointestinal afflictions. Perineal approaches to rectal prolapse and endoscopic reduction of sigmoid volvulus exemplify this strategy. More recently, laparoscopy evolved out of endoscopic principles, gaining minimally invasive access to the abdominal cavity, and technological refinements led to the birth of laparoscopic intestinal surgery. These technological advances allowed the accomplishment of traditional gastrointestinal operations through small incisions. This approach produced a significant reduction in the injury inflicted on patients—decreasing pain, decreasing rates of wound infection, and shortening the length of hospitalization. As these advantages became evident, surgeons naturally directed videolaparoscopic techniques toward the performance of colorectal operations. These attempts at the development of minimally invasive colorectal procedures represent only the most recent endeavors in a truly ancient tradition. Nonetheless, laparoscopic colectomy is currently in its infancy and will inevitably undergo many evolutionary stages. Each of these stages, however, will serve to improve the results of treatment and strive to decrease patient morbidity. The chapters that follow illustrate just how far minimally invasive colorectal surgery has progressed.

REFERENCES

1. Guthrie D: A History of Medicine. JB Lippincott, Philadelphia, 1946
2. Kutumbiah P: The Evolution of Scientific Medicine. Orient Longman, Madras, India, 1971
3. Stubbs SGB, Bligh EW: Sixty Centuries of Health and Physick. Sampson, Low, Marston, London, 1931
4. Cullen W: First Lines of the Practice of Physic. William Creech, Edinburgh, 1777
5. Hippocrates (Coar T, trans): The Aphorisms of Hippocrates: With a Translation into Latin and English. A Valpy, London, 1822
6. Galen (Green RM, trans): A Translation of Galen's Hygiene (De Sanitate Tuenda). p. III:9, Book 1, Charles C Thomas, Springfield, IL, 1951
7. Michael Servetus (O'Malley CD, trans): Christianismi Restitutio and Other Writings. The Classics of Medicine Library, Birmingham, 1989
8. Hippocrates (Adams F, trans): The Genuine Works of Hippocrates. The Sydenham Society, London, 1849
9. Benton P, Hewlett JH: Surgery Through the Ages: a Pictorial Chronicle. Hastings House, New York, 1944
10. Organ CH: Historical contributions to gasless laparoscopy. In Smith RS, Organ CH (eds): Gasless Laparoscopy With Conventional Instruments: The Next Phase in Minimally Invasive Surgery. Norman Publications, San Francisco, 1933
11. Gunning JE, Rosenzweig BA: Evolution of endoscopic surgery. In White RA, Klein SR (eds): Endoscopic Surgery. Mosby–Year Book, St. Louis, 1991
12. Saleh JW: Laparoscopy. WB Saunders, Philadelphia, 1988
13. Philipi CJ, Fitzgibbons RJ, Salerno GM: Historical review: diagnostic laparoscopy to laparoscopic cholecystectomy and beyond. In Zucker KA (ed): Surgical Laparoscopy. Quality Medical Publishing, St. Louis, 1991
14. Berci G: History of endoscopy. In Berci G (ed): Endoscopy. Appleton-Century-Crofts, E. Norwalk, CT, 1976
15. Coakley D: The Irish School of Medicine: Outstanding Practitioners of the 19th Century. Townhouse Publications, Dublin, Ireland, 1988
16. Haubrich WS: History of endoscopy. In Sivak MV (ed): Gastroenterologic Endoscopy. WB Saunders, Philadelphia, 1987
17. Celsus (Spencer WG, trans): De Medicina. Book VII, Ch. 15. Harvard University Press, London, 1979
18. Thompson CJ: The History and Evolution of Surgical Instruments. Schuman, New York, 1942
19. Bernheim BM: Organoscopy. Ann Surg 53:764, 1911
20. Nadeau OE, Kampmeier OF: Endoscopy of the abdomen: abdominoscopy. A preliminary study, including a summary of the literature and description of the technique. Surg Gynecol Obstet 41:259, 1925
21. Semm K (Friederich ER, trans): Operative Manual for Endoscopic Abdominal Surgery. Year Book Medical Publishers, Chicago, 1987
22. Hasson HM: Open laparoscopy vs. closed laparoscopy: a comparison of complication rates. Adv Planned Parenthood 13:41, 1978
23. Lightdale CJ: Laparoscopy and biopsy in malignant liver disease. Cancer, suppl. 11:2672, 1982
24. Warshaw AC, Tepper JE, Shipley WU: Laparoscopy in staging and planning therapy for pancreatic cancer. Am J Surg 151:76, 1986
25. Dubois F, Icard P, Berthelot G et al: Celioscopic cholecystectomy: preliminary report of 36 cases. Ann Surg 211:60, 1990

26. Reddick EJ, Olsen DO: Laparoscopic laser cholecystectomy: a comparison with nonlaparoscopic cholecystectomy. Surg Endosc 3:131, 1989
27. Soper NJ: Laparoscopic cholecystectomy. Curr Probl Surg 28:583, 1991
28. Miles WE: Rectosigmoidectomy as method of treatment for procidentia recti. Proc R Soc Med 26:1445, 1933
29. Altemeier WA, Giuseffi J, Hoxworth PI: Treatment of extensive prolapse of rectum in aged and debilitated patients. Arch Surg 65:72, 1952
30. Altemeier WA, Cuthbertson WR, Schowengerdt C et al: Nineteen years experience with the one-stage perineal repair of rectal prolapse. Ann Surg 173:993, 1971
31. DeKok H: A new technique for resecting the noninflamed not-adhesive appendix through a mini-lapa-rotomy with the aid of a laparoscope. Arch Chir Neerl 29:195, 1977
32. Semm K: Endoscopic appendectomy. Endoscopy 15:59, 1983
33. Schreiber J: Early experience with laparoscopic appendectomy in women. Surg Endosc 1:211, 1987
34. Whitworth CM, Whitworth PW, Sanfillipo J et al: Value of diagnostic laparoscopy in young women with possible appendicitis. Surg Gynecol Obstet 107:187, 1988
35. Saclarides TT, Ko ST, Airen M et al: Laparoscopic removal of a large colonic lipoma. Report of a case. Dis Colon Rectum 34:1027, 1991
36. Fowler DC, White SA: Brief clinical report: laparoscopic-assisted sigmoid resection. Surg Laparosc Endosc 1:183, 1991
37. Corbitt JD: Preliminary experience with laparoscopic-guided colectomy. Surg Laparosc Endosc 2:79, 1992
38. Phillips EH, Franklin M, Carroll BJ et al: Laparoscopic colectomy. Ann Surg 216:703, 1992
39. Senagore A, Luchtfeld MA, Mackeigan JM et al: Open colectomy vs. laparoscopic colectomy: are there differences? Am Surg 59:549, 1993
40. Falk PM, Beart RW, Wexner SD et al: Laparoscopic colectomy: a critical appraisal. Dis Colon Rectum 36:28, 1993
41. Society of Gastrointestinal Endoscopic Surgeons: Guidelines for granting privileges for laparoscopic (peritoneoscopic) general surgery: SAGES guidelines. Surg Endosc 7:67, 1993
42. Dent TL, Forde KA, Greene FL: Training and credentialing: who should monitor the quality of endoscopic surgery? In Schrock TR (ed): Insights Today: Endosurgery for the 90's. Health Learning Systems, Little Falls, NJ, 1992
43. Forde KA: Hospital credentialing. In Ballantyne GH, Leahy PF, Modlin LM (eds): Laparoscopic Surgery. WB Saunders, Philadelphia, 1994

Editorial Comment I

Thomas A. Stellato

Drs. Sgambati and Ballantyne have presented a fascinating portrait of the literature and personalities relevant to colorectal disease and gastrointestinal endoscopy from classical Greece to current attempts at laparoscopic colorectal surgery. Other examples of "minimally invasive" surgery abound; two familiar examples include rubber band ligation of internal hemorrhoids and percutaneous endoscopic gastrostomy (PEG), the latter serving as an alternative to open gastrostomy. The spectrum of management of colorectal and gastrointestinal disorders certainly includes a myriad of nonoperative options and "minimally invasive" procedures, as well as major surgical interventions. Drs. Sgambati and Ballantyne have imaginatively woven a historical fabric implying that a thread of collective surgical consciousness actively worked from classical times to the present to identify and develop "minimally invasive" surgery. Their interpretation of this history makes for enjoyable and interesting reading; however, I would offer three criticisms: (1) not all of their examples represent a "minimally invasive" approach, (2) expediency rather than tradition may be more reasonable as an explanation for many of these less invasive procedures, and (3) the appellation "minimally invasive surgery" is inappropriate and premature at this time for diseases of the colon and rectum.

Drs. Sgambati and Ballantyne suggest that the classical Greek physicians stimulated the colon to produce "beneficial actions . . . by affecting gastrointestinal function. This minimally invasive approach avoided the very real dangers of more invasive approaches." These measures can be traced to ancient Egypt, where the rectum was considered a dangerous center of decay and prophylactic purging enemas were routinely practiced.[1] Thus, although the historical validity of these remedies is unquestioned, the actual benefits are uncertain. The suggestion that these treatments represented a "minimally invasive approach" implies that other more invasive approaches were available. There is little evidence to suggest that alternatives were available. Guido Majno,[2] in *The Healing Hand,* constructs the ancient Egyptian body as follows:

> All vessels came from the heart, but they had a second assembly center around the anus. . . . . Air entered the nose, poured through the heart, and went to the anus. . . . . It [the anus] could become flooded with excrement and carry [the excrement] elsewhere.

Thus, the purges may be seen as a very aggressive (rather than minimally invasive) approach to maintain total body health. These are two differing interpretations—one suggests that the classical physician had a somewhat purposeful effort to employ less invasive maneuvers in treating disease; the other interpretation suggests that based on the understanding of health and disease at that time, the treatments employed were simply those available.

Evidence that Hippocrates treated anorectal diseases is unquestioned. That his treatment illustrates "minimally invasive surgical technique" is debatable. Drs. Sgambati and Ballantyne describe the Hippocratic method as reducing prolapse by suspending the patient in the air and maintaining reduction of the prolapse by applying a caustic potash to the rectal mucosa and binding the patient's thighs together for 3 days. Does this represent the beginning of a "historical tradition of minimally invasive surgery" as the authors suggest?

Finally, Drs. Sgambati and Ballantyne address the history of laparoscopy and the development of laparoscopic approaches to colorectal disease. George Kelling is credited with performing the first celioscopy in a canine in 1901. He also performed the first laparoscopy in humans,[3] although Drs. Sgambati and Ballantyne have credited Jacobeus with this distinction. Nonetheless, surgeons ignored laparoscopy for nearly 90 years. There is absolutely no evidence that surgeons in any way accepted or developed laparoscopy despite its "minimally invasive" appeal. There was an occasional surgeon who tried to promote laparoscopy, but it was not until the late 1980s, when laparoscopic cholecystectomy emerged, that surgeons developed any interest in this important modality. Applications other than gallbladder removal then developed at a rapid pace. Literally every abdominal operation performed as an open procedure has been attempted laparoscopically. However, the appellation *minimally invasive* is not synonymous with *laparoscopic.*

For example, few would agree that a laparoscopic pancreaticoduodenectomy (Whipple resection) is less invasive than an open Whipple procedure. Although some procedures, when performed laparoscopically, are less painful and more cosmetic and allow quicker recovery (i.e., less or minimally invasive), not all procedures performed laparoscopically are necessarily minimally invasive. The phrase "minimally invasive" has a special connotation for the patient and the nonsurgical physician. Controlled prospective trials are not available that compare open and laparoscopic colon resection. Although these may not have been necessary for laparoscopic cholecystectomy, they will be essential for laparoscopic colon resection. Until evidence is available that laparoscopic colon surgery is comparable in effectiveness and less morbid than open colon surgery, the phrase "minimally invasive" should be avoided. Despite these criticisms, Drs. Sgambati and Ballantyne provide us with a thoughtful and provocative essay. As with any worthwhile reading, it compels us to question and reflect.

REFERENCES

1. Magner L: A History of Medicine. p. 30. Marcel Dekker, New York, 1992
2. Majno G: The Healing Hand. Man and Wound in the Ancient World. Plate 3.8. Harvard University Press, Cambridge, MA, 1975
3. Stellato T: History of laparoscopic surgery. Surg Clin North Am 72:997, 1992

Editorial Comment II

Rama M. Jager

The craft of surgery is a paradox. Surgery achieves healing by hurting. All surgeons aim to heal the most by hurting the least. Laparoscopic surgery and its application to the treatment of colorectal diseases are logical extensions of this basic surgical tenet of achieving the most healing from the least hurting. As Drs. Sgambati and Ballantyne relate, surgeons have been trying for the past many centuries to reduce the tissue trauma of surgery. Some examples are gastrointestinal endoscopy and minimal incisional surgery to achieve the traditional surgical goal of resecting or repairing the diseased organ. The success of minimally invasive surgical techniques—such as laparoscopic cholecystectomy, laparoscopic oophorectomy, and arthroscopic surgery—validates the appropriateness of the idea of the smallest incision. Whether laparoscopic colorectal surgery using small incisions will replace traditional open abdominal techniques is unknown. This question may not even be proper. The true significance of the laparoscopic approach to the management of colorectal disease is the surgeon's appreciation or re-appreciation of morbidity from the peritoneal access and stimulation of attempts to improve surgical treatment by alleviating the access injury.

A PASSING PHENOMENON OR A PARADIGM SHIFT

Laparoscopic colorectal surgery, like other forms of surgery, may be a passing phenomenon. All surgical attempts are at best the physician's crude maneuvers to repair an organ at a macroscopic level, whereas the disease starts at a cellular or molecular level. Once a simpler means of healing becomes available, even the most sophisticated operation is only of historical interest. Two examples include (1) surgical treatment of peptic ulcer disease has been displaced to a secondary role by H_2 blockers and proton inhibitors; and (2) thyroidectomy for hyperthyroidism is rarely necessary with current medical treatment using radioactive iodine and antithyroid agents. A similar fate awaits laparoscopic cholecystectomy when a "magic pill" will permanently dissolve the gallstones and promote emulsification of bile. Restorative proctocolectomy may become archaic if genetic therapy for familial adenomatous polyposis and curative therapy for inflammatory bowel disease ever become available. Possible future medical advances in no way belittle the significance of currently available surgical treatment. In fact, they point to the supreme conceptual importance of laparoscopy as a "paradigm shift" in the surgical thought-world rather than the latest fad bewitching every surgeon who wants to stay current with progress.

CATASTROPHE THEORY

Change and progress in human history are not always linear and chronologically predictable. They go through sporadic bursts of dramatic change. The invention of the printing press, the industrial revolution, and the development of nuclear weapons and microcomputers are not examples of continuous and linear progress. Echoing the French mathematician Rene Thom, who proposed the catastrophe theory, such events represent a sharply discontinuous process superimposed on the more prevalent linear and continuous progress. To cite a few examples in the field of medicine, the discovery of microbial causes of disease, surgical asepsis, antibiotics, and H_2 blockers do not represent gradual progress. They are dramatic, abrupt changes and extraordinary events that strikingly influenced the extant medical practice. Laparoscopic surgery is a similar dramatic step in the gradual progression of the idea of minimal invasion and a "catastrophic" ripple in the stream of surgical innovation to reduce access-induced morbidity.

As Dr. Stellato comments, abdominal surgeons have ignored laparoscopy for almost a century. The current explosive interest in laparoscopic surgery is secondary to the demonstrated success of laparoscopic gynecologic extirpative surgery and cholecystectomy. Whether extrapolation of laparoscopic techniques from cholecystectomy to colectomy is appropriate or beneficial will be answered over the next few years by the rapidly accumulating clinical experience, some of which is reported in the next few chapters.

3
Preoperative Evaluation

Stephan J. Cohn and Michael F. Roizen

In the current cost-conscious medical environment, many of the patients scheduled for laparoscopic procedures will come to the hospital on the morning of surgery. Concern for cost efficiency has created a preoperative assessment environment that severely limits a physician's time to achieve the goals of preoperative evaluation: reduce the morbidity of surgery, discuss with the patient the risks and benefits of the procedure, and allay patient anxiety. When patients who are not hospitalized before the day of surgery undergo laparoscopic surgery, a "system change" is needed for the preoperative anesthetic assessment to be effective and efficient. The evaluation system can be implemented in the surgeon's office or a preanesthetic clinic. With a good system for assessment in place, the patient is more confident, and the surgeon's operating schedule is not disrupted with unexpected delays or cancellations.

The first goal of the preoperative evaluation is to reduce the morbidity of surgery. Ostensibly, this goal seems to encourage the use of tests to uncover hidden conditions that may contribute to perioperative morbidity. From the 1940s to the 1960s, physicians accomplished this goal by relying primarily on an accurate patient history and physical examination. Then, in the early 1960s, Kaiser and Technicon introduced batteries of tests for multiphasic screening with the idea that, if a disease could be identified by screening before it became clinically evident, morbidity could be prevented. The ease and low cost of ordering and obtaining many tests made the process seem logical and desirable. As a result, many anesthesia departments made rather arbitrary rules—recommendations that became requirements—regarding the tests that should be performed before elective surgery. When, with good intentions, anesthesiologists and surgeons tried to follow the rules, problems arose. Physicians believed that with inexpensive batteries of tests they could efficiently screen for disease. Instead, they were still trying to determine which tests to order before surgery, what to do about an unexpectedly abnormal result on the morning of surgery, and how abnormal a test result had to be before seeking the advice of a consultant. The system of preoperative multiphasic screening with multiple nonselective tests proved impractical.

Soon, the hypothesis that nonselective testing benefits patients by uncovering hidden conditions was challenged (by Kaiser itself and others). Inadequate or inappropriate care sometimes resulted from the time-consuming follow-up of abnormal test results. In addition to the increased patient risk caused by random batteries of tests, the medicolegal risk for physicians could also increase. The practice of ordering batteries of tests preoperatively was not cost-effective and diminished health care resources for others.

Because perioperative mortality and morbidity increase with the severity of pre-existing disease,[1–7] careful evaluation and treatment should reduce their occurrence.[3,8,9] We first review the scientific evidence demonstrating that, with an accurate history and physical examination, one can select the preoperative tests for patients that can reduce perioperative morbidity.

ROUTINE LABORATORY TESTING

Leonard and co-workers[10] reported that biochemical screening tests had no significant value in the preoperative screening of pediatric patients expected to be hospitalized for less than 1 week. In another study, Korvin and associates[11] reviewed biochemical tests given routinely to 1,000 patients on hospital admission. None of the tests produced a new diagnosis that was unequivocally beneficial to the patient. In an ambitious, controlled trial of multiphasic screening in 1,500 patients, Olsen and co-workers[12] found no difference in morbidity between control groups and groups having screening tests. Durbridge and colleagues[13] compared 1,500 patients who were randomly assigned to undergo or not undergo screening tests on admission. No benefit resulted from the 8,363 tests that were performed with respect to duration of hospitalization or patient outcome. Narr et al[14] found that more than 3,000 patients of ASA (American Society of Anesthesiologists) physical status I or II who underwent elective surgical procedures at the Mayo Clinic did not benefit from laboratory testing. Apfelbaum et al[15] reviewed data from a multicenter study showing that asymptomatic individuals were more likely to be harmed by, than to benefit from, unwarranted tests and physicians' actions in response to the abnormal results of those tests.

Some testing is indicated to uncover disease in high-risk groups (i.e., electrocardiography [ECG] in men older than 40 years or women older than 50 years of age, chest radiography for smokers with a productive cough) or to optimize therapy (glucose levels in a diabetic patient, prothrombin time for a patient receiving sodium warfarin).[16,17] However, even for the elderly, for whom testing is likely to be of most benefit, nonselective screening has not been of great value. Domoto et al[18] examined the yield and effectiveness of a battery of 19 screening laboratory tests performed routinely in 70 functionally intact elderly patients (average age, 82.6 years) who resided at a chronic care facility. The 70 patients underwent 3,903 screening tests. "New abnormal" results primarily occurred in 5 of the 19 screening tests; most of these "new abnormalities" were only minimally outside the normal range. Only 4 (0.1 percent of all tests ordered) led to changes in patient management, none of which, Domoto and colleagues concluded, benefited any patient in an important way.

Wolf-Klein and colleagues[19] retrospectively studied the results of annual laboratory screening on a population of 500 institutionalized and ambulatory elderly patients (average age, 80 years). From the 15,000 tests performed, 756 new abnormalities were discovered, 690 of which were ignored. Sixty-six of the new abnormalities were evaluated; 20 new diagnoses resulted, 12 of which were treated. Of the 500 patients, 2 may ultimately have benefited from eradication of asymptomatic bacteriuria (although eradication of asymptomatic bacteriuria has not been shown to improve the quality of life or extend the life span).[20–23]

Studies show that the history and physical examination are the best measures for screening for disease. Delahunt and Turnbull[24] evaluated patients who were assessed preoperatively for varicose vein stripping or inguinal herniorrhaphy. For 803 patients who underwent 1,972 tests, only 63 abnormalities were uncovered in those patients whose history or physical findings had not indicated the need for tests, but in no instance did the discovery of these abnormalities influence patient management. Rosselló and associates[25] retrospectively evaluated 690 admissions for elective pediatric surgical procedures. The history and physical examination indicated the probability of abnormalities in all 12 patients in whom an abnormality was found through laboratory testing. Clinical diagnosis, not laboratory testing, was the apparent basis for any change in operative plans.

Several studies have compared the outcomes of groups of hospitalized patients who had routine laboratory screening tests performed to supplement the history and physical examination with the outcomes of patients who did not have routine screening tests. Wood and Hoekelman[26] found that 28 of 1,924 children examined had changes in their preoperative clinical course (all had surgery postponed) because of abnormal history, physical examination, or laboratory examination results. Of the 28 patients whose surgery was postponed, 3 had abnormal laboratory tests that were not indicated by the history or physical examination. Thus, the history or physical examination dictated appropriate laboratory testing for all but 3 of 1,924 patients. The abnormalities discovered for these 3 patients pertained to their chest radiographs. (These children were part of a study comparing perioperative outcome at two hospitals, one of which required chest radiographs as a screening test for elective surgery in children and one of which did not.) There were no differences noted in anesthetic or perioperative complications between the two groups. Therefore, Wood and Hoekelman recommended that chest radiographs not be obtained routinely for apparently healthy children.

Even in a referral population, the history and physical examination determine the clinical course in more than 90 percent of cases after consultation about cardiovascular, neurologic, or respiratory diseases.[27] Other studies have also demonstrated that the history and physical examination accurately indicate all areas in which subsequent laboratory testing proves beneficial to patients. For example, Rabkin and Horne[28,29] examined the records of 165 patients with "new" (i.e., a change from a previous tracing) abnormalities on the ECG that were potentially "surgically significant" (i.e., that might affect perioperative management or outcome). In only two instances were the anesthetic or surgical plans altered by the discovery of new abnormalities on an ECG that were not indicated by the history. Thus, for these 165 patients, for whom the benefits of a laboratory test should have been maximal (because a new abnormality was detected during the preoperative assessment), the history or physical examination determined case management most of the time. Even in one of the two instances of altered case management—a patient having atrial fibrillation—the physical examination should have indicated that an ECG needed to be performed. A history or physical examination was not available for the other patient.

Repeating laboratory tests when the results were normal within the previous 2 months does not appear to benefit patients. MacPherson et al[30] found that only 13 tests of more than 3,000 repeated within 1 year of surgery yielded new information, and the 13 new results could have been predicted from a new event in each patient's history.

In summary, the aforementioned studies point to the inadequacy of routine laboratory tests as an independent means of assessing patients preoperatively. Most of these laboratory tests are superfluous to patient care management. The evidence supports the primacy of history and physical examination to screen for disease; laboratory tests can be used to screen for disease when such tests have proved to be effective but are better used to confirm clinical diagnoses or to optimize a patient's condition before surgery.

RANDOM TESTING

Additional Patient Risk

Unnecessary testing may lead physicians to pursue and treat abnormalities based on borderline positive and false-positive results. Few studies have examined whether increased tests and the follow-up of false-positive test results adversely affect patients. Roizen et al[31] retrospectively examined the adverse effects of chest radiography on patients. In this study population of 606 patients, 386 extra chest radiographs were ordered without indication. In those 386 patients, one elevated hemidiaphragm and probable phrenic nerve palsy was found that may have resulted in improved care for that patient. In addition, three lung shadows were found that resulted in three sets of invasive tests, including one thoracotomy without discovery of any disease. These procedures caused considerable morbidity for those patients, including one pneumothorax and 4 months of disability. Tape and Mushlin[32] found that chest radiographs performed without indication or symptoms of disease, even in an elderly population, resulted in less benefit than harm.

In another study, Turnbull and Buck[33] examined the charts of 2,570 patients undergoing cholecystectomy to determine the value of preoperative tests. The history and physical examinations successfully indicated all tests that ultimately benefited the patients with four possible exceptions. But again, in those four patients it is doubtful whether any benefit actually occurred. Among them was one patient whose emphysema was detected only by chest radiography; he underwent preoperative physiotherapy without subsequent postoperative complications. Two patients had unsuspected hypokalemia (3.2 and 3.4 mEq/L, respectively) and received potassium treatment before surgery. Data in the literature now indicate that no harm occurs to patients undergoing an operation with this degree of hypokalemia and that severe potential harm may be caused by treating such patients with oral or intravenous potassium.[34–38] The fourth patient in whom possible benefit occurred received a blood transfusion before cholecystectomy for an asymptomatic hemoglobin concentration of 9.9 g/dl. Since cholecystectomy is not normally associated with major blood loss, this patient also received no benefit but only the risks associated with the transfusion.

In another study, only two patients at most (who had eradication of asymptomatic bacteriuria) benefited from the 9,270 screening tests that were performed.[39] At least one patient was seriously harmed from the pursuit of abnormalities on screening tests and their treatment; atrial fibrillation and congestive heart failure developed after thyroid therapy was instituted for borderline low thyroxine and free thyroxine index tests. It is unclear whether these investigators examined other patients for potential harm arising similarly from the pursuit and treatment of abnormalities.

Increased Medicolegal Risks for Physicians

When batteries of laboratory tests yield abnormal results that are neither pursued nor noted, the medicolegal risk for physicians increases. Extra testing—testing that is not warranted by findings on the medical history—does not serve as medicolegal protection against liability. A series of studies reviewed by Roizen[40] shows that 20 to 95 percent of all unexpected abnormalities found on preoperative laboratory tests are not noted on the chart preoperatively. Many reports of preoperative radiographs, for example, are not on the chart before anesthesia is administered. This lack of notation occurs not only at university medical centers but in community hospitals as well. Data show that failure to pursue an abnormality that has been detected poses a greater risk of medicolegal liability than does failure to detect an abnormality.[41] In this way, extra testing results in extra medicolegal risk for physicians.

Three true anecdotes illustrate the pitfalls:

1. An asymptomatic woman scheduled for a tubal ligation with no indication for a chest radiograph received one on the morning of surgery. The radiograph showed a solitary nodule to the left of the hilum. Three months

(Continues)

later, after removal of the upper left lobe of her lung, she returned to work. She did not receive a tubal ligation nor any benefit from the removal of this benign cyst. The anesthesiologist and surgeon were successfully sued.

2. A litigator underwent a series of preoperative laboratory tests. No history of bleeding diathesis existed, but test results showed an abnormal prothrombin time. The anesthesiologist discussed the abnormal result with the surgeon's first assistant and with the patient. It was decided that the abnormality posed no significant risk. Before the procedure, but after anesthesia had been administered, the surgeon, fearing potential bleeding around a facial nerve in a litigator, requested a hematology consultation. Surgery was postponed for 2 weeks, and the litigator underwent $1,900 worth of factor assays. His prothrombin time remains a laboratory test abnormality without explanation.
3. A patient received a preoperative chest radiograph that showed a cancer. The radiograph result was not sought by the anesthesiologist or the surgeon. The surgeon was successfully sued because he failed to pursue that abnormality.

Inefficient Operating Room Schedules

According to informal surveys, surgeons say that they order preoperative tests to satisfy the anesthesiologist: they find it easier to order all the tests and let the anesthesiologist sort them out. Surgeons also believe that it is much more efficient to order batteries of tests than to have the anesthesiologist, who sees the patient the night before or the morning of surgery, try to get the tests performed on an emergency basis. These surgeons, who want predictable surgical schedules, apparently do not realize that abnormalities detected by tests done in this battery fashion are not discovered until the night before or the morning of surgery, if at all. Thus, any abnormal results on these tests delay or postpone schedules because extra effort and time are wasted in obtaining consultant reviews of false-positive or slightly abnormal results.

LAPAROSCOPIC SURGERY CONSIDERATIONS

Approximately 500,000 cholecystectomies are performed each year in the United States.[42] Laparoscopic cholecystectomy is preferred to traditional laparotomy[43] because of the benefits of a shorter hospital stay, a more rapid return to normal activities, less pain from smaller incisions, and less postoperative ileus.[44–47] General anesthesia is often administered for laparoscopic cholecystectomy to eliminate the patient discomfort associated with pneumoperitoneum or body positioning changes from the Trendelenburg to the reverse Trendelenburg position.[44,48] Although most patients undergoing laparoscopic surgery tend to be relatively healthy, in the present age of cost containment, old (age greater than 64), very old (age greater than 74), and sicker patients may be scheduled to arrive at the hospital on the day of surgery. Same-day admission severely limits the time for test selection or discussion with patients about the risks or alternatives of perioperative care. If a system to see patients before the day of surgery is not in place, a time-limited environment may tempt surgeons and anesthesiologists to return to ordering batteries of tests preoperatively. Because carbon dioxide is used for insufflation of the abdomen during laparoscopic cholecystectomy, physicians may be tempted to order chest radiographs, pulmonary function tests, and ECGs routinely in anticipation of a patient's altered hemodynamic and pulmonary function during the perioperative period. As discussed above, such random testing in asymptomatic patients may increase the risk to both the patient and physician. To avoid these risks and to ensure a predictable surgical schedule, we believe that a clinic should be established to perform preoperative assessments in a cost-effective manner. The remainder of this chapter is devoted to a discussion of the use of guidelines and patient questionnaires in a preoperative clinic to determine what laboratory tests are needed to reduce patient morbidity, as well as a discussion of some specific tests.

GUIDELINES AND PATIENT QUESTIONNAIRES

At the University of California, San Francisco, Kaplan et al[49] found that even a partial history, combined with the expert rules provided in Tables 3-1 and 3-2, conveyed enough information to indicate correctly all but 22 abnormalities (none of which affected patient outcome) in more than 2,785 preoperative blood tests obtained (counting the complete blood count and the simultaneous multichannel analysis of six variables [SMA 6] as one test). Knowing only the admission diagnosis, previous discharge diagnoses, and scheduled operation, and using previously determined indications for laboratory testing enabled the detection of virtually

Table 3-1. Laboratory Test Recommendations for Asymptomatic Healthy Patients Scheduled to Undergo Peripheral Surgery Involving No Major Blood Loss

	Tests Indicated	
Age (yr)	For Men	For Women
≤40	None	Pregnancy test[a]
40–49	ECG	Hematocrit Pregnancy test[a]
50–64	ECG	ECG Hemoglobin or hematocrit
65–74	ECG Hemoglobin or hematocrit BUN and glucose level Chest radiograph[b]	ECG Hemoglobin or hematocrit BUN and glucose level Chest radiograph[b]
≥75	ECG Hemoglobin or hematocrit BUN and glucose level Chest radiograph[b]	ECG Hemoglobin or hematocrit BUN and glucose level Chest radiograph[b]

Abbreviations: ECG, electrocardiogram; BUN, blood urea nitrogen.
[a]If the patient cannot rule out pregnancy with certainty.
[b]Although the benefit/risk ratio of chest radiographs for asymptomatic individuals >60 years of age is not clear, the risk appears to exceed the benefit until age >74 years.

Table 3-2. Simplified Strategy for Preoperative Testing[a]

	Hemoglobin												
Preoperative Condition	Male	Female	WBC	PT/ PTT	PLT/ BT	Elect	Creat/ BUN	Blood Glucose	SGOT/ Alk PO_4	Radio-graph	ECG	Pregnancy Test	T/S
Procedural blood loss													
Yes	X	X											X
No													
Neonates	X	X											
Adult age													
<40 yr		X											
40–49		X									M		
50–64		X									X		
≥65–74	X	X					X	X		P	X		
≥75	X	X					X	X		P	X		
Cardiovascular disease							X			X	X		
Pulmonary disease										X	X		
Malignancy	X	X	L	L						X			
Radiotherapy			X							X	X		
Hepatic disease				X					X				
Hepatitis exposure									X				
Renal disease	X	X				X	X						
Bleeding disorder				X	X								
Diabetes						X	X	X			X		
Smoking ≥20 pack-yr	X	X								X			
Possible pregnancy												X	
Drug use													
Diuretics						X	X						
Digoxin						X	X				X		
Steroids						X		X					
Anticoagulants	X	X		X									
CNS disease			X			X	X	X			X		

Abbreviations: WBC, white blood [cell] count; PT, prothrombin time; PTT, partial thromboplastin time; PLT, platelet count; BT, bleeding time; Elect, electrolytes (i.e., sodium, potassium, chloride, carbon dioxide, and proteins); Creat/BUN, creatinine or blood urea nitrogen; SGOT/Alk PO_4, serum glutamic-oxaloacetic transaminase/alkaline phosphatase; ECG, electrocardiogram; T/S, blood typing/screening for unexpected antibodies; P, perhaps obtain; L, obtain for leukemias only; X, obtain; M, obtain for men only; CNS, central nervous system.
[a]Not all diseases are included here; the physician's own judgment is needed regarding patients with diseases not listed.
(Data from Roizen,[40] Kaplan et al,[49] and Blery et al.[73])

all abnormalities that would have been detected by routine screening or would have affected patient care.

Several groups have tested the effect and sensitivity of orally administered or written questionnaires as a means of linking the selection of laboratory tests with a patient's medical history.[40,50] In 1987, McKee and Scott[51] used an orally administered set of 17 questions and patient demographics to select preoperative tests for 400 patients. They found that age was the best predictor of abnormalities on preoperative tests. Complications occurred most commonly in patients who reported positive symptoms on the questionnaire and who were older.

One study determined that the responses of patients to written questions can be used to predict which laboratory tests will yield abnormal results for those patients. After the patient answers the questionnaire, a plastic overlay reveals what tests are indicated. If the patient cannot answer the questions, a standard group of tests is ordered. Even in a tertiary care hospital that admits very sick patients, more than 60 percent of those laboratory tests now routinely performed could be eliminated. The elimination of such tests could result in more than an 80-percent reduction in patient charges and hospital costs[52] (Cohen SN, personal communication).

The protocols outlined in Tables 3-1 and 3-2 offer guidelines for using clinical judgment in ordering laboratory tests. A careful history and physical examination of the patient are required, with special attention to testing whenever indicators of the disease entities listed in Tables 3-1 and 3-2 are discovered. The protocol clearly places the burden on an accurate history. We do not recommend that all standard screening tests be discontinued. Some are beneficial: the ECG for diabetic patients, men older than 40 years, and women older than 50 years of age; the fecal occult blood test for individuals older than 40 years of age (every 2 years, every year in high-risk groups); the Papanicolaou smear (every 3 years for sexually active women, every year for women at high risk); and the mammogram (every year for women 50 years of age and older and for women older than 40 years in high-risk groups).[16,17,53,54] This is the point of the screening history, to identify individuals likely to benefit from testing. The rationale for the choice of some specific tests deserves further comment.

Specific Tests

White Blood Cell Count, Hemoglobin, and Hematocrit

How many asymptomatic patients have a degree of abnormality on the hematocrit or the white blood cell (WBC) count that alters perioperative management? We define the following values as not meriting intervention perioperatively: a hematocrit of 27 to 54 for patients undergoing operations during which major blood loss is unlikely and a WBC count of 2,400 to 16,000/mm^3 for individuals not undergoing insertion of a prosthesis. When values fall outside these ranges, we recommend seeking alternative diagnoses before the institution of anesthesia or surgery. The data available in the literature indicate that either preoperative hematocrit or hemoglobin levels should be determined for all surgical patients older than 60 years of age.[40] Hematocrit and red blood cell antigen screening is warranted for all patients undergoing procedures involving possible blood loss of more than 2 U/70 kg of body weight. WBC counts appear to be rarely indicated in asymptomatic individuals but might be considered when a prosthesis is to be inserted.

Blood Chemistries and Urinalysis

What blood chemistries would have to be abnormal and how abnormal would they have to be to justify changing perioperative management? Abnormal hepatic or renal function might change the choice and dose of anesthetic or adjuvant drugs. About 1 in 700 supposedly healthy patients is actually harboring hepatitis, and 1 in 3 of those will become jaundiced. However, our group, using data from 3,500 patients in a prospective study, did not find any asymptomatic patient who denied exposure to hepatitis and who then became jaundiced after uneventful surgery.[15] These data imply that either the screening history suffices or the incidence of asymptomatic hepatitis is decreasing. Unexpected abnormalities are reported for 2 to 10 percent of patients with multiphasic screening, and these abnormalities lead to many additional tests that in approximately 80 percent of cases have no significance for the patient. Unexpected abnormalities that are significant arise in 2 to 5 percent of patients studied. Of these abnormalities, approximately 70 percent are related to blood glucose and blood urea nitrogen (BUN) levels. The 2 to 20 additional tests on the screening SMA 6–21 panels lead to very few discoveries important enough to affect anesthesia. In fact, the false-positive rate is so high (96.5 percent for the test for calcium) that the value representing cost/benefit for most of these tests (even when the initial tests are free) is negative, as is the value representing benefit/risk.

If a screening test for hepatitis is desired because the incidence of hepatitis is 0.14 percent or because one wishes to avoid the potential legal problems of postanesthetic jaundice, only three tests appear to be justified: serum glutamic-oxaloacetic transaminase (SGOT), blood glucose, and BUN. Even then, the last two are indicated only for patients older than 64 years of age. In fact, if the data from our group on asymptomatic liver disease can be generalized, no blood chemistry tests are warranted for patients younger than 64 years of age. Furthermore, if the antibody test that detects hepatitis C (formerly non-A, non-B hepatitis) proves as useful after infection has occurred, the medicolegal risk posed by postanesthetic jaundice will be even less.

Abnormalities are commonly found on urinalysis.[40] The quality of urinalysis results obtained by the dipstick technique has been variable at best. In addition, these abnormal results usually do not lead to beneficial changes in management unless an implant operation is planned. Most of the results that do lead to beneficial changes could have been obtained from the history or by a determination of BUN and glucose levels, tests that are already recommended for all patients older than 64 years of age. Thus, urinalysis, although initially inexpensive, becomes an expensive test to justify on a cost/benefit or benefit/risk basis.

Chest Radiography

What abnormalities on chest radiographs would influence the management of anesthesia? Before proceeding to anesthesia and surgery it may certainly be important to know about the existence of tracheal deviation; mediastinal masses; pulmonary nodules; a solitary lung mass; aortic aneurysm; pulmonary edema; pneumonia; atelectasis; new fractures of the vertebrae, ribs, or clavicles; dextrocardia; or cardiomegaly. However, a chest radiograph would probably not detect the degree of chronic lung disease requiring a change in anesthetic technique any better than would the history and physical examination. Data reviewed by Roizen[40] show that abnormalities are rare in asymptomatic individuals. In fact, if the patient is asymptomatic and younger than 74 years of age, the risks of a chest radiography examination probably exceed the potential benefits. This analysis is, of course, predicated on maximizing benefit to society in general, since one cannot predict in advance which patients will benefit or which will be harmed.

Screening for Cardiac Disease

Although individual episodes of myocardial ischemia may not produce symptoms, almost all patients (excluding diabetic patients and patients with autonomic insufficiency) have symptoms that lead one to screen for myocardial disease. Identifying patients with coronary artery disease, aortic valvular disease, or a low left ventricular ejection fraction to alter their perioperative care may improve their outcome. Identification of these cardiac conditions by low-risk tests is often followed by percutaneous transluminal coronary angioplasty (PTCA), coronary artery bypass grafting (CABG), or a recommendation for increased perioperative monitoring and more aggressive pain management to improve their outcome and the chance of survival. While such reasoning is logical, it has not been tested by rigorous prospective trials. Rao et al[55] found that scrupulously maintaining the hemodynamics of patients in an intensive care unit for 3 days after surgery reduced the reinfarction and mortality rates by more than 60 percent. Hertzer et al[56,57] followed 1,000 vascular surgery patients who either did or did not undergo coronary revascularization preoperatively. Initially, mortality rates increased for the former, but that group had a lower 5-year cardiac death rate. Similar results have emerged from the multicenter Coronary Artery Surgical Study[58] (CASS) and from a study of patients who underwent PTCA before noncardiac surgery.[59] Thus, attempts have been made to identify factors in the history that lead to increased risk. The 12 factors in the history that correlate with ECG abnormalities and the 5 factors, including ECG abnormalities, that have been correlated with outcome after vascular surgery are depicted in Figure 3-1.[58] The following generalizations can be made from the data: an ECG is not needed preoperatively for women younger than 50 years nor for men younger than 40 years of age who are without chest pain, congestive heart failure, hypertension, diabetes, dysrhythmia, or shortness of breath and they do not need vascular surgery, do not smoke, and are able to exercise. For procedures more likely to be associated with cardiovascular events, men and women with a history of three of the following should undergo cardiac catheterization: myocardial infarction, congestive heart failure, hypertension, diabetes, or angina. Individuals with one or two of these conditions would probably benefit from Holter monitoring to determine their risk group.

A simple approach to preoperative cardiac evaluation is the use of Holter monitoring for the detection of ischemia during daily life. After ambulatory Holter monitoring of patients for 24 hours, Raby et al[60] documented complications in one-third of those with 1 hour or more of preoperative ischemia and in only 1 percent of nonischemic patients. There is some evidence that Holter monitoring may be an inexpensive way of evaluating patients before proceeding to the tests described below.[61]

A determination of systolic left ventricular function may provide prognostic information for major surgery, given the association of congestive heart failure with morbid postoperative events. Radionuclide angiography can define systolic and diastolic function. Most investigators attempting to predict operative risk have evaluated only systolic function; however, we are becoming increasingly aware that diastolic failure is also a problem, particularly for hypertensive patients.

Kazmers et al[62] studied 60 patients undergoing abdominal aortic aneurysm repair. Although patients with a low ejection fraction survived the operation and had no higher incidence of perioperative myocardial infarction (a tribute to modern perioperative management), their long-term survival rate was poor (50 percent versus 86 percent at 20 months).

Pasternack et al[63] showed that patients with an ejection fraction above 55 percent had no myocardial infarctions, whereas four of five patients with an ejection fraction below 35 percent sustained a myocardial infarction postoperatively within 48 hours. Their

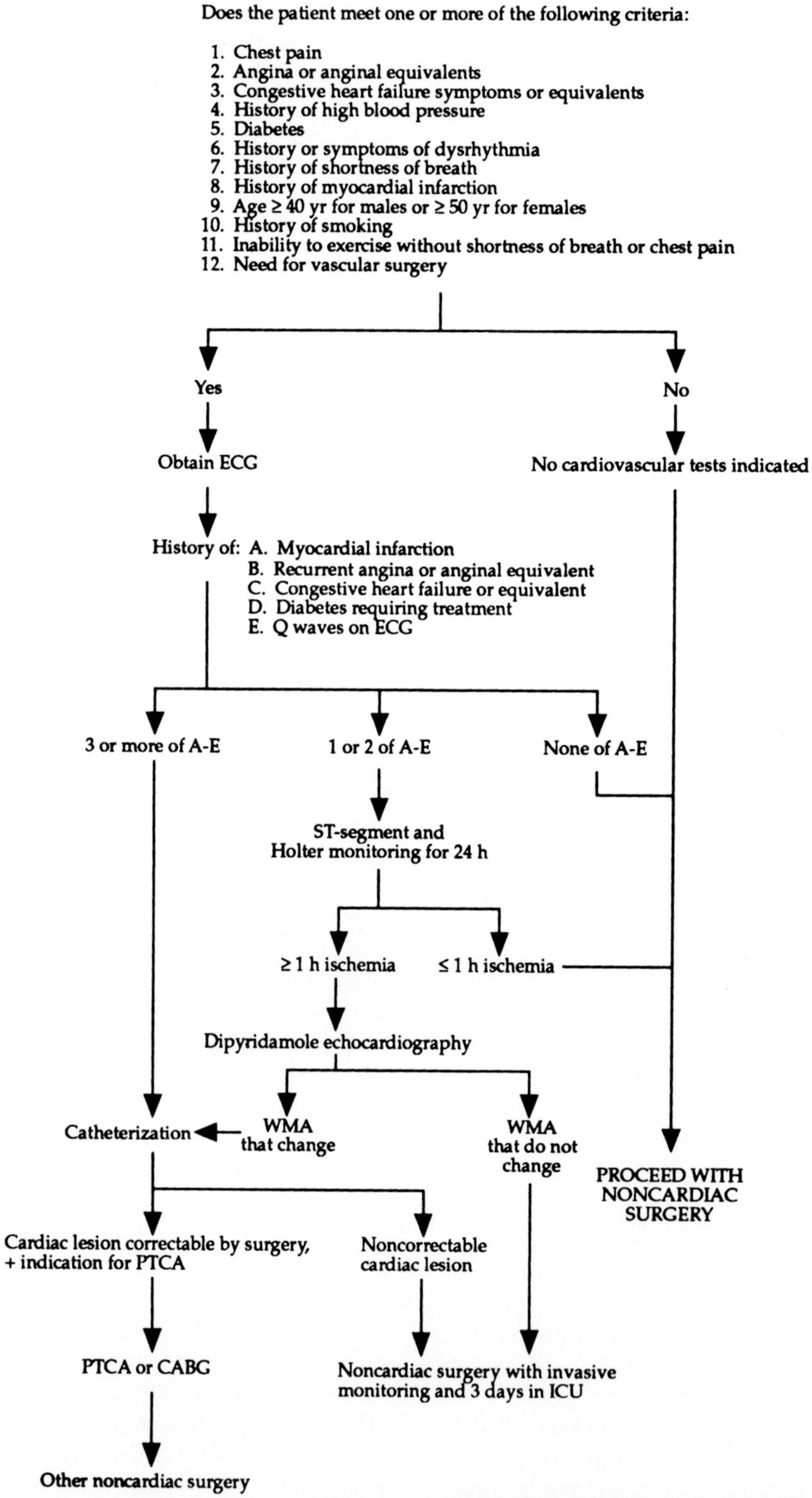

Fig. 3-1. Procedure for determining which cardiovascular laboratory tests are necessary. The history is used to segregate patients into groups for testing or invasive monitoring, or both. WMA, wall motion abnormalities; PTCA, percutaneous transluminal coronary angioplasty; CABG, coronary artery bypass grafting; ICU, intensive care unit.

patients did not fare as well in the perioperative period as did those of Kazmers' group; still, a previous myocardial infarction predicted a 26-percent probability of reinfarction, and 50 percent of the patients older than 80 years sustained an infarction perioperatively.

Del Guercio and Cohn[64] studied 148 elderly patients who had been cleared for major surgery by their internists. Preoperatively, the patients were admitted to the intensive care unit for insertion of a pulmonary artery catheter. Cardiac output, pulmonary capillary wedge pressure, and oxygen delivery were measured. The patients were classified into one of four stages, from normal to having severe, uncorrectable deficits. In 34 patients, severe hemodynamic abnormalities were detected, and for most of these, surgery was canceled. Of 8 high-risk patients who underwent the planned surgical procedure, all died, whereas the mortality was 0 percent for stage 1 and 8.5 percent for stage 2 and stage 3 patients.

Another method advocated for preoperative risk assessment is dipyridamole-thallium scanning (DTS). Dipyridamole is a potent coronary vasodilator that produces coronary steal by increasing blood flow to normal areas and diminishing collateral flow to poststenotic areas. Areas that are prone to ischemia are hypoperfused after dipyridamole administration; several hours later, when the "steal" has subsided, the areas are perfused normally. Such areas are said to have a redistribution defect. Fixed defects represent old myocardial infarctions.

The Massachusetts General Hospital experience[65] with DTS has yielded two important observations: an old myocardial infarction is not a risk factor in itself, and an area of redistribution (i.e., myocardium at risk) is associated with an adverse outcome. Recent results of a meta-analysis suggest that stress echocardiography is even more helpful than DTS in risk stratification of patients at intermediate risk.[66] If a patient has a negative DTS, a negative stress echocardiogram, or a low clinical risk based on patient factors and the type of operation, given the low rate of adverse cardiac events, we might choose to forego extensive invasive monitoring and extended intensive care unit stay with the potential for reducing costs and iatrogenic complications.

Patients who are at high risk because of individual and surgical risk factors should probably not have a stress echocardiogram or DTS. They should have coronary angiography and revascularization or give informed consent that addresses the high risk of their surgery. Preoperative CABG or coronary angioplasty may be useful, although some dismiss them as survival tests and debate their capacity to decrease perioperative mortality.

Patients with a markedly positive DTS or stress echocardiogram should probably undergo myocardial revascularization. Lette et al[67] demonstrated in a study of 66 patients that those with markedly positive scans (16 patients) tended to die (7 of 10 patients who underwent surgery) if surgery was not canceled. Recently, Mangano et al[68] challenged the effectiveness of DTS for preoperative screening of vascular surgery patients, but the limitations of their study (noted in an accompanying editorial[69]) make their challenge less compelling. Furthermore, diabetic patients undergoing vascular surgery commonly (80 percent) have positive DTS results; only by quantifying the degree of redistribution is it possible to stratify the risk of diabetic patients by means of DTS. Lane et al,[70] who studied 101 diabetic patients, found that neither the type of anesthesia (regional versus general), the use of pulmonary artery catheters, the site of surgery (aortic versus femoral), nor the use of nitroglycerin infusions predicted outcome. The presence of angina and a high Goldman classification[71] predicted cardiac complications, as did the presence of more than two reversible effects and defects in distribution in the left anterior descending artery. In Figure 3-1, we present an algorithm for pursuing laboratory testing for cardiovascular disease.[40] The data do not support the use of the algorithm as a guideline or a standard but only as one option. Until these procedures gain widespread acceptance and until extensive trials show that they reduce overall mortality, the goal of optimizing care and minimizing myocardial morbidity seems logical.

Pulmonary Function Testing

These expensive tests are rarely needed but are useful for determining which patients may benefit from bronchodilator therapy and for predicting the risk of thoracic operations before obtaining informed consent. The indications for pulmonary function tests seem justified by the data.[40]

Indications for Pulmonary Function Tests

- History of at least one of the following
  - Chronic obstructive pulmonary disease
  - Shortness of breath
  - Orthopnea
- Or at least one of the following needs to be determined
  - Reversibility of bronchospasm
  - Baseline condition if intubation is expected postoperatively[a]
  - Risk of lung resection (maximal mid-expiratory flow rate, maximum breathing capacity, diffusing capacity for carbon monoxide)[a]

[a]Not likely for most patients undergoing laparoscopic colon resection.

Clotting Function Studies

Virtually no asymptomatic patient in the literature has had unequivocal benefit from clotting function studies preoperatively. Most patients who benefit show symptoms or have a medication history suggesting that clotting function tests may be necessary. Aspirin at 60 mg/day/70 kg of body weight does not seem to pose a risk of bleeding, but the data are not available for 300 mg of aspirin or more within 12 hours of surgery. Since the pharmacology of aspirin changes when more than 2 g/day/70 kg body weight is consumed, patients should be evaluated if they cannot stop taking aspirin early enough to have no appreciable acetylsalicylic acid level for 24 hours before surgery (the period without acetylsalicylic acid necessary to generate the approximately 50,000/mm^3 of new platelets needed for normal platelet aggregation), if surgical hemostasis cannot be ensured, or a regional procedure into a closed space is planned. Figure 3-2 presents an algorithm for determining whether coagulation tests are indicated.

Other Tests

Tests for acquired immunodeficiency syndrome (AIDS) and pregnancy and screening for hemoglobinopathy and malignant hyperthermia raise ethical issues that may require close attention to institutional policy and the immediate availability of counseling services. Moreover, all these tests have associated risks. The physician may therefore decide to limit testing to only at-risk populations (e.g., for pregnancy testing, only women who believe they may be pregnant).

Testing of the asymptomatic population for AIDS is not likely to be the most effective way of uncovering the disease. One program that screened for human immunodeficiency virus (HIV) in asymptomatic individuals was able to produce an "acceptably low false-positive rate" by diagnosing HIV infection only after one sample of blood produced positive results on four different tests and after a second sample of blood had been used for verification. Thus, for pregnancy, hemoglobinopathies, malignant hyperthermia, and AIDS, the history is still best at identifying those at risk of the condition.

We believe that because we biased the analysis to favor laboratory testing, the guidelines in Table 3-1 provide the upper limits of tests to be performed in asymptomatic individuals. Just as good an argument could be made for no testing of asymptomatic individuals in low-risk groups.

TEST SELECTION BASED ON MEDICAL HISTORY

We firmly believe that a clinic can be set up to perform preoperative assessment reliably and cost-effectively. In the clinic, history taking can be accomplished in one of several ways. Patients may complete a questionnaire or a check-off list on paper, enter their responses by computer, or respond orally to questions asked by a health professional.* Alternatively, a computerized history can be taken from each patient in the surgeon's office. The history summary, which may include preoperative test suggestions, can be transferred electronically (directly or by facsimile) to the anesthesiologist. Figure 3-3 is a sample of a patient summary report. This information can be reviewed far enough in advance of surgery for tests or other surgery-related appointments to be scheduled if they are needed. The involvement of the anesthesiologist can actually ensure fewer delays in operating room schedules. In our Sports Medicine Clinic, for example, approximately 1 in 20 patients requires further medical evaluation before surgery as determined by preoperative evaluation. Our system has thus reduced delays and turnover time.

Whatever the method, the goal is a thorough history, which the anesthesiologist or surgeon can then use to determine the necessary tests and perioperative care. The charge for the physician's assessment time will be offset by elimination of the cost of unwarranted tests and operating room expense when surgery is delayed.[72] For cost savings alone, hospitals, surgical centers, payers, and managed care providers should favor a clinic for preoperative assessment.

Knowing which abnormal results are likely to affect patient management is of great importance.[73] Tables 3-1 and 3-2, the box titled *Indications for Pulmonary Function Tests,* and Figures 3-1 and 3-2 present the most appropriate choices for testing based on published evidence. These recommendations were made after an examination of the potential for abnormalities in each risk group and after assumptions about the benefits and harm proceeding from the abnormalities.[53,54] Randomized trials proving the benefits and harm, however, are rare. To institute selective testing while avoiding the four hazards of batteries of tests requires either a preoperative clinic or provision for an assessment system in the offices of the surgeon or primary care physician. The rewards for such a system are fewer tests, reduced medicolegal risk, and improved patient out-

*Dr. Roizen developed a preoperative automated health questionnaire at the University of Chicago to help solve the problem of inefficient preoperative assessment and test selection methods. The University owns the rights to commercialize the product and has transferred the U.S. rights to the Anesthesia and Critical Care Research Foundation and the non-U.S. rights to Dr. Roizen. If the product is successful, the Foundation and Dr. Roizen will benefit financially. Royalties to the Foundation will be used to support research in preoperative evaluation. Both the University of Chicago and Johns Hopkins University may also benefit from commercialization of this technology.

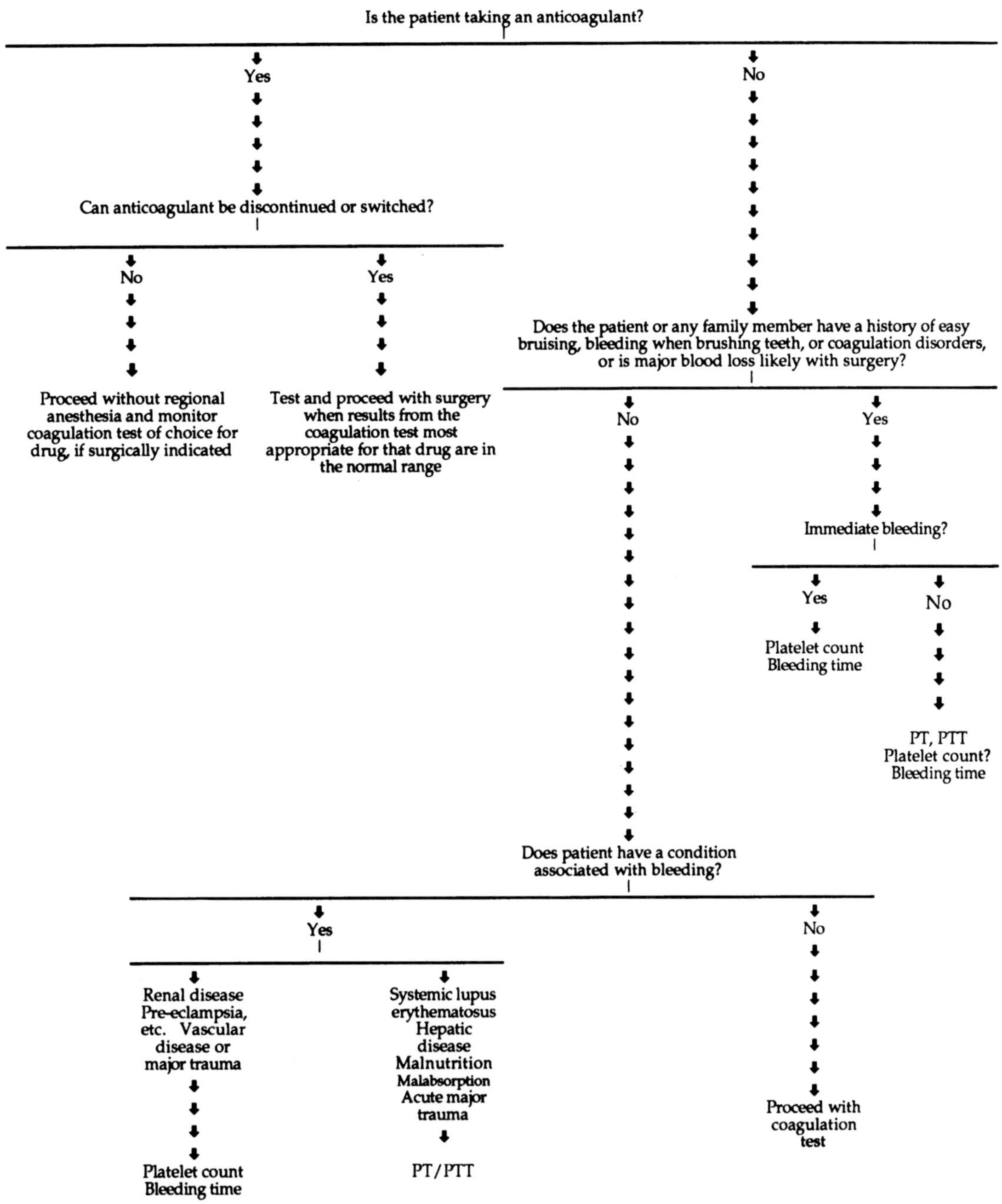

Fig. 3-2. Procedure for determining whether coagulopathy or coagulation tests are needed.

Prescreen Version 2.1 Patient Summary Report (© 1993, 1994 Nellcor)

Patient:
41-year-old white male

ID #

Dr:

Systems Review:

CNS	Hx nerve injury, tremor, or headache
CNS	Hx migraine headaches
CNS	Hx numbness over 2 hr
GI	Hx of hepatitis/liver disease
GI	Reflux esophagus

DOB:	03/08/52
Date:	01/31/94
HT:	182.88 cm
WT:	93.0 kg
BMI:	27.80
BP:	NA /NA
HR:	NA min
HQASA:	1.50
Validity:	Good

Allergies:

None

Suggested Laboratory Tests:

SGOT/SGPT ECG

May Consider:

WBC count Ca^{2+}

Medications:

NSAID
Pain medications
Other medications

Pertinent Anesthesia Care Items:

Caps or bridge	No loose/chipped teeth
Denies past anesthesia	Hx snoring
Drink <72 hr	

Tobacco / ETOH / IVDA:

Current smoker

Fig. 3-3. A sample of a summary report after preoperative assessment of a 41-year-old male patient. CNS, central nervous system; GI, gastrointestinal, Hx, history of; DOB, date of birth; HT, height; WT, weight; BMI, body mass index; BP, blood pressure; HR, heart rate; HQASA, Health Quiz rating of physical status according to guidelines by the American Society of Anethesiologists; SGOT/SGPT, serum glutamic-oxaloacetic transaminase/serum glutamic-pyruvate transaminase; WBC, white blood [cell] count; Ca^{2+}, calcium ion; NSAID, nonsteroidal anti-inflammatory drug; ETOH, ethyl alcohol; IVDA, intravenous drug abuse.

come. The reward will also be evident in the physician's pride in delivering quality care and, ultimately, in the patient's satisfaction.

REFERENCES

1. Vacanti CJ, VanHouten RJ, Hill RC: A statistical analysis of the relationship of physical status to postoperative mortality in 68,388 cases. Anesth Analg 49:564, 1970
2. Lewin I, Lerner AG, Green SH et al: Physical class and physiologic status in the prediction of operative mortality in the aged sick. Ann Surg 174:217, 1971
3. Goldman L, Caldera DL, Nussbaum SR et al: Multifactorial index of cardiac risk in noncardiac surgical procedures. N Engl J Med 297:845, 1977
4. Keats AS: The ASA classification of physical status—a recapitulation. Anesthesiology 49:233, 1978
5. Rehder K: Clinical evaluation of isoflurane: complications during and after anesthesia. Can Anaesth Soc J, suppl. 29:S44, 1982
6. Cohen MM, Duncan PG: Physical status score and trends in anesthetic complications. J Clin Epidemiol 41:83, 1988
7. Ziffren SE, Hartford CE: Comparative mortality for various surgical operations in older versus younger age groups. J Am Geriatr Soc 20:485, 1972
8. Okelberry CR: Preadmission testing shortens preoperative length of stay. Hospitals 49:71, 1975
9. Duckett JB: Preoperative assessment of the patient for outpatient anesthesia. p. 21. In Brown BB Jr (ed): Outpatient Anesthesia. FA Davis, Philadelphia, 1978
10. Leonard JV, Clayton BE, Colley JRT: Use of biochemical profile in children's hospital: results of two controlled trials. BMJ 2:662, 1975
11. Korvin CC, Pearce RH, Stanley J: Admission screening: clinical benefits. Ann Intern Med 83:197, 1975
12. Olsen DM, Kane RL, Proctor PH: A controlled trial of multiphasic screening. N Engl J Med 294:925, 1976
13. Durbridge TC, Edwards F, Edwards RG et al: Evaluation of benefits of screening tests done immediately on admission to hospital. Clin Chem 22:968, 1976
14. Narr BJ, Hansen TR, Warner MA: Preoperative laboratory screening in healthy Mayo patients: cost-effective elimination of tests and unchanged outcomes. Mayo Clin Proc 66:155, 1991
15. Apfelbaum J, Roizen MF, Robinson D et al: How frequently do asymptomatic patients benefit from the pursuit of abnormalities in their preoperative test results? Anesthesiology 73:A1254, 1990
16. Sox HC Jr (ed): Common Diagnostic Tests: Use and Interpretation. American College of Physicians, Philadelphia, 1987
17. Hayward RSA, Steinberg EP, Ford DE et al: Guideline for periodic preventive care. In Eddy DM (ed): Common Screening Tests. American College of Physicians, Philadelphia, 1991
18. Domoto K, Ben R, Wei JY et al: Yield of routine annual laboratory screening in the institutionalized elderly. Am J Public Health 75:243, 1985
19. Wolf-Klein GP, Holt T, Silverstone FA et al: Efficacy of routine annual studies in the care of elderly patients. J Am Geriatr Soc 33:325, 1985
20. Dontas AS, Kasviki-Charvarti P, Chem L et al: Bacteriuria and survival in old age. N Engl J Med 304:939, 1981
21. Boscia JA, Kobasa WD, Knight RA et al: Epidemiology of bacteriuria in an elderly ambulatory population. Am J Med 80:208, 1986
22. Boscia JA, Kobasa WD, Knight RA et al: Therapy versus no therapy for bacteriuria in elderly ambulatory nonhospitalized women. JAMA 257:1067, 1987
23. Nordenstam GR, Brandberg CA, Odén AS et al: Bacteriuria and mortality in an elderly population. N Engl J Med 314:1152, 1986
24. Delahunt B, Turnbull PRG: How cost effective are routine preoperative investigations? N Z Med J 92:431, 1980
25. Rosselló PJ, Cruz AR, Mayol PM: Routine laboratory tests for elective surgery in pediatric patients. Bol Asoc Med P R 72:614, 1980
26. Wood RA, Hoekelman RA: Value of the chest x-ray as a screening test for elective surgery in children. Pediatrics 67:447, 1981
27. Sandler G: Costs of unnecessary tests. BMJ 2:21, 1979
28. Rabkin SW, Horne JM: Preoperative electrocardiography: its cost-effectiveness in detecting abnormalities when a previous tracing exists. Can Med Assoc J 121:301, 1979
29. Rabkin SW, Horne JM: Preoperative electrocardiography: effect of new abnormalities on clinical decisions. Can Med Assoc J 128:146, 1983
30. MacPherson DS, Snow R, Lofgren RP: Preoperative screening: value of previous tests. Ann Intern Med 113: 959, 1990
31. Roizen MF, Kaplan EB, Schreider BD et al: The relative roles of the history and physical examination, and laboratory testing in preoperative evaluation for outpatient surgery: the "Starling" curve of preoperative laboratory testing. Anesth Clin North Am 5:15, 1987
32. Tape TG, Mushlin M: The utility of routine chest radiographs. Ann Intern Med 104:663, 1986
33. Turnbull JM, Buck C: The value of preoperative screening investigations in otherwise healthy individuals. Arch Intern Med 147:1101, 1987
34. Hirsch IA, Tomlinson DL, Slogoff S: The overstated risk of preoperative hypokalemia. Anesth Analg 67:131, 1988
35. Vitez TS, Soper LE, Wong KC: Chronic hypokalemia and intraoperative dysrhythmias. Anesthesiology 63:130, 1985
36. Harrington JT, Isner JM, Kassirer JP: Our national obsession with potassium. Am J Med 73:155, 1982
37. Lawson DH: Adverse reactions to potassium chloride. Q J Med 43:433, 1974
38. Lawson DH, Hutcheon AW, Jick H: Life threatening drug reactions amongst medical inpatients. Scott Med J 24:127, 1979
39. Levinstein MR, Ouslander JG, Rubenstein LZ: Yield of routine annual laboratory tests in a skilled nursing home population. JAMA 258:1909, 1987
40. Roizen MF: Preoperative evaluation. p. 743. In Miller RD (ed): Anesthesia. 3rd Ed. Vol. 1. Churchill Livingstone, New York, 1990
41. Robertson WM: Medical Malpractice: A Preventive Approach. University of Washington Press, Seattle, 1985
42. McSherry CK: Cholecystectomy: the gold standard. Am J Surg 158:174, 1989

43. Way LW: Changing therapy for gallstone disease. N Engl J Med 323:1273, 1990
44. Cunningham AJ, Brull SJ: Laparoscopic cholecystectomy: anesthetic implications. Anesth Analg 76:1120, 1993
45. Dubois F, Icard P, Berthelot G et al: Celioscopic cholecystectomy. Preliminary report of 36 cases. Ann Surg 211:60, 1990
46. Grace PA, Quereshi A, Coleman J et al: Reduced postoperative hospitalization after laparoscopic cholecystectomy. Br J Surg 78:160, 1991
47. Jones RM, Fletcher DR, MacLellan DG et al: Laparoscopic cholecystectomy: initial experience. Aust N Z J Surg 61:261, 1991
48. Brown DR, Fishburne JI, Roberson VO et al: Ventilatory and blood gas changes during laparoscopy with local anesthesia. Am J Obstet Gynecol 124:741, 1976
49. Kaplan EB, Sheiner LB, Boeckmann M et al: The usefulness of preoperative laboratory screening. JAMA 253:3576, 1985
50. Roizen MF, Kaplan EB, Sheiner LB et al: Elimination of unnecessary laboratory tests by preoperative questionnaire. Anesthesiology 61:A455, 1984
51. McKee RF, Scott EM: The value of routine preoperative investigations. Ann R Coll Surg Engl 69:160, 1987
52. Finkler SA: The distinction between cost and charges. Ann Intern Med 96:102, 1982
53. U.S. Preventive Services Task Force: Guide to Clinical Preventive Services. An Assessment of the Effectiveness of 169 Interventions. Williams & Wilkins, Baltimore, 1990
54. Hayward RSA, Steinberg EP, Ford DE et al: Preventive care guidelines. Ann Intern Med 114:758, 1991
55. Rao TLK, Jacobs KH, El-Etr AA: Reinfarction following anesthesia in patients with myocardial infarction. Anesthesiology 59:499, 1983
56. Hertzer NR, Beven EG, Young JR et al: Coronary artery disease in peripheral vascular patients: a classification of 1000 coronary angiograms and results of surgical management. Ann Surg 199:223, 1984
57. Hertzer NR, Young JR, Beven EG et al: Late results of coronary bypass in patients with peripheral vascular disease. Cleve Clin Q 53:133, 1986
58. Roizen MF, Ellis JE: Anesthesia for vascular surgery. p. 1059. In Barash PG, Cullen BF, Stoelting RK (eds): Clinical Anesthesia. 2nd Ed. JB Lippincott, Philadelphia, 1992
59. Huber KC, Evans MA, Bresnahan JF et al: Outcome of noncardiac operations in patients with severe coronary artery disease successfully treated preoperatively with coronary angioplasty. Mayo Clin Proc 67:15, 1992
60. Raby KE, Goldman L, Creager MA et al: Correlation between preoperative ischemia and major cardiac events after peripheral vascular surgery. N Engl J Med 321:1296, 1989
61. Fleisher LA, Rosenbaum SH, Nelson AH et al: The predictive value of preoperative silent ischemia for postoperative ischemic cardiac events in vascular and nonvascular surgery patients. Am Heart J 122:980, 1991
62. Kazmers A, Cerqueira MD, Zierler RE: The role of preoperative radionuclide ejection fraction in direct abdominal aortic aneurysm repair. J Vasc Surg 8:128, 1988
63. Pasternack PF, Imparato AM, Bear G et al: The value of radionuclide angiography as a predictor of perioperative myocardial infarction in patients undergoing abdominal aortic aneurysm resection. J Vasc Surg 1:320, 1984
64. Del Guercio LRM, Cohn JD: Monitoring operative risk in the elderly. JAMA 243:1350, 1980
65. Eagle KA, Singer DE, Brewster DC et al: Dipyridamole-thallium scanning in patients undergoing vascular surgery: optimizing preoperative evaluation of cardiac risks. JAMA 257:2185, 1987
66. Mantha S, Roizen MF, Barnard J et al: Relative effectiveness of four preoperative tests in predicting adverse cardiac outcome after vascular surgery: a meta-analysis. Anesth Analg 79:422, 1994
67. Lette J, Waters D, Lassonde J et al: Postoperative myocardial infarction and cardiac death: predictive value of dipyridamole-thallium imaging and five clinical scoring systems based on multifactorial analysis. Ann Surg 211:84, 1990
68. Mangano DT, London MJ, Tubau JF et al: Dipyridamole thallium-201 scintigraphy as a preoperative screening test: a re-examination of its predictive potential. Circulation 84:493, 1991
69. Pohost GM: Dipyridamole-thallium test. Is it useful for predicting coronary events after vascular surgery? Circulation 84:931, 1991
70. Lane SE, Lewis SM, Pippin JJ et al: Predictive value of quantitative dipyridamole-thallium scintigraphy in assessing cardiovascular risk after vascular surgery in diabetes mellitus. Am J Cardiol 64:1275, 1989
71. Goldman L, Caldera DL, Southwick FS et al: Cardiac risk factors and complications in noncardiac surgery. Medicine (Baltimore) 57:357, 1978
72. Rupani G, Roizen MF, Glosten B et al: Can a system change improve operating room efficiency? Anesthesiology 71:A930, 1989
73. Blery C, Szatan M, Fourgeaux B et al: Evaluation of a protocol for selective ordering of preoperative tests. Lancet 1:139, 1986

Editorial Comment I

David A. Nakata

Preoperative evaluation of patients undergoing laparoscopic surgery is addressed in this chapter. Additional aspects of anesthesia in laparoscopic colorectal surgery are discussed further in this commentary. These issues include laboratory assessment, myocardial evaluation, pulmonary status, and nutritional concerns.

LABORATORY ASSESSMENT

Drs. Cohn and Roizen reaffirm the importance of conducting a thorough history and physical examination as the primary means of determining which laboratory tests to obtain. They also point out the hazards—to both the patient and physician—of using a "shotgun" approach for obtaining preoperative laboratory tests. These hazards might be better understood in the light of how most "normal" laboratory values are defined. Normal laboratory values are defined as being two standard deviations (SD) from the mean, which constitutes 95 percent of a gaussian distribution. In other words, 5 percent of the "normal" population is by definition abnormal. In a panel containing 20 different tests, one of those test values would likely be "abnormal" even in an absolutely healthy patient. What do we do with these unexpected abnormal values? Do we perform further laboratory tests or invasive tests, or do we do nothing and hope that the abnormal value represents a normal variant?

MYOCARDIAL EVALUATION

The evaluation and management of patients with known myocardial disease are also discussed. Rao and Jacobs[1] reported in a prospective study that the incidence of postoperative myocardial reinfarction was decreased by aggressive hemodynamic monitoring. In addition, they reported that the incidence of myocardial reinfarction was decreased by prolonging the time between the myocardial infarction and surgery. Anesthesiologists still embrace these results—perhaps for good reason because of good results overall. Yet at the same time there have been marked advances in various modalities of assessing myocardial function and dysfunction. Newer, less invasive, less costly, more sensitive, and more specific tests have been introduced that may improve our ability to risk-stratify these patients.

Recently an article by Fleisher and Barash[2] described an approach that uses some of these newer diagnostic modalities. Even though this means of assessing the risk of perioperative ischemia has yet to be evaluated in a prospective, randomized, double-blind, placebo-controlled fashion, it is based on solid principles.

The review of Fleisher and Barash suggests that we consider risk-stratifying patients according to the "impact of surgical procedure on cardiovascular morbidity." This approach entails dividing patients into groups depending on whether a surgical procedure is likely to increase the risk of perioperative ischemia. Examples of high-risk surgical procedures include intrathoracic and major abdominal procedures such as aortic aneurysm repairs. The exact risk of perioperative cardiac ischemia in patients undergoing laparoscopic surgical procedures has yet to be defined. However, one would certainly expect the risk of perioperative myocardial ischemia to be lower in this group of individuals than in the previously mentioned high-risk group.

An algorithm using this strategy has been proposed that does not necessarily mandate that a patient who had a recent myocardial infarction (within the last 6 months) be excluded from low- to moderate-risk surgical procedures. This algorithm, as previously mentioned, has yet to undergo formal clinical trials, but further progress in this area is expected in the future.

PULMONARY CONSIDERATIONS

Preoperative assessment of a patient's pulmonary status with regard to the effect of pneumoperitoneum must be considered. Pneumoperitoneum can lead to decreased functional residual capacity, increased work of breathing, and pulmonary atelectasis—conditions that can worsen shunt and ventilation/perfusion abnormalities. In addition, carbon dioxide is directly absorbed from the peritoneal cavity and can cause hypercarbia and respiratory acidosis. These changes are usually not clinically significant. However, adverse effects can be seen in patients with pre-existing pulmonary and cardiac pathology. To decrease these complications, general anesthesia is often instituted to minimize many of the effects of pneumoperitoneum.

The aforementioned cardiovascular and pulmonary concerns assume that laparoscopic interventions will be successful, an assumption that will not always be correct. Considerations for this possibility should be made before surgery and might include aborting the planned procedure in lieu of further cardiopulmonary evaluation if more invasive intervention is necessary.

NUTRITIONAL CONSIDERATIONS

Patients undergoing colorectal surgery—depending on their underlying pathology—may present with poor gastric motility, malfunctioning gastroesophageal and gastrojejunal sphincter mechanisms, and partial or frank obstruction. These conditions can lead to an increased risk of gastroesophageal reflux and aspiration and appropriate preventive measures should be taken. These may include the use of nasal or oral gastric suction, nonparticulate antacids, H_2 blockers, and gastrointestinal prokinetic drugs such as metoclopramide. In any case, these patients should, in most instances, be considered to have a full stomach regardless of their fasting (NPO) status. Awake or rapid sequence induction of anesthesia should be considered in some patients.

Vomiting, diarrhea, and generally poor oral intake may also lead to marked hypovolemia. Hypovolemia can be of particular concern during induction, where many of the currently used anesthetic induction drugs can cause marked hypotension. If hypovolemia is present during the preoperative evaluation, fluid administration to correct deficiencies in intravascular volume should be instituted before induction of anesthesia.

In addition to hypovolemia, malnutrition can be a serious concern in this group of individuals. Malnutrition can have a wide range of adverse physiologic effects. Some of these effects include decreases in cardiac reserve, leading to potentially increased myocardial depression from the inhalational and intravenous anesthetic drugs. Pulmonary manifestations can include a decline in the concentration of surfactant, a decrease in diaphragmatic muscle mass, and a decreased ability to compensate for increased demand during the postoperative period. Renal manifestations include a loss of renal concentrating ability, leading to abnormal excretion of free water and metabolic waste products. Hepatic decreases in glycogen stores and protein synthesis can affect both glucose hemostasis and drug binding. Immunologic effects can be manifested by a decrease in T-cell counts, resulting in an increased susceptibility to infection.

Concerns for patients undergoing colorectal surgery should not be limited to events that affect only the immediate perioperative time course, but rather must take into account each patient's co-existing disease states. The particular concerns for each patient will obviously differ, but a wide variety of clinical concerns may be manifested—from coronary artery disease to malnutrition and all of its associated problems.

REFERENCES

1. Rao TLK, Jacobs KH: Reinfarction following anesthesia in patients with myocardial infarction. Anesthesiology 59:499, 1983
2. Fleisher LA, Barash PG: Preoperative cardiac evaluation for noncardiac surgery: a functional approach. Anesth Analg 74:586, 1992

Editorial Comment II

Rama M. Jager

PREGNANCY TESTING

The authors propose that preoperative pregnancy testing be limited to patients who believe that they may be pregnant. This practice may vary depending on institutional policy. Reliance on the clinical history without laboratory confirmation of nonpregnancy exposes the surgeon and the medical institution to avoidable medicolegal risk. The hospitals and freestanding surgical centers where I practice require that pregnancy be excluded by human chorionic gonadotropin (hCG) testing before any operation requiring general anesthesia or intravenous sedation. While the cost-inefficiency of similar practice is apparent, the argument of cost avoidance carries the least protection to the anesthesiologist, the surgeon, or the institution if the patient were to be pregnant when she had the operation.

INEFFICIENT OPERATING ROOM SCHEDULES

This chapter discusses the problem of routine preoperative testing and its effect on a predictable operating room schedule from an anesthesiologist's perspective. Here is my perspective as a surgeon. Last minute cancellations of scheduled elective operations such as laparoscopic colectomy affect the patient's time and work plans. Such scheduling inefficiency is also unwanted and unpleasant to the anesthesiologist and the surgeon. Surgeons may have problems filling gaps in their schedules more than anesthesiologists. The anesthesiologist is usually based at a hospital and controls the entire work schedule of the hospital operating room. The surgeon may not have that convenience. I concede that some anesthesiologists take issue with this argument of convenience.

Multiple factors come into play in ensuring a predictable operating room schedule and preventing last minute cancellations of scheduled operations. The ultimate goal of avoiding postoperative surgical complications from existing preoperative medical abnormalities dictates careful preoperative medical and laboratory evaluation. Attention to efficient and timely preoperative evaluation by the surgeon, the anesthesiologist, and the hospital improves the quality of care at an acceptable cost. The concept of a preoperative outpatient clinic to evaluate the surgical patient efficiently before the patient comes to the hospital for the operation has great merit. Logistic questions such as whether the clinic should be staffed by primary care physicians, anesthesiologists, or surgeons, as well as how the providers' time is compensated, are important issues to be resolved in this era of cost controls. However, they are beyond the scope of this book. The possible strategy and solutions are too dependent on institutional policies to make generalizations.

4

Anesthetic and Positional Complications

Richard McCammon

This chapter reviews and calls to the attention of practicing anesthesiologists and surgeons the various perioperative anesthetic and surgical complications associated with laparoscopic colorectal surgical procedures. Some of these complications are reasonably common and can be prevented or at least their impact lessened. Others, although rare, can lead to significant morbidity and even mortality. Both surgeons and anesthesiologists must anticipate and recognize such rare events and have a clear plan of action ready to lessen the likelihood of a significant adverse outcome. This chapter does not intend to review common anesthetic considerations and problems associated with regional and general anesthesia. Many excellent texts are available and fulfill that purpose.[1]

Insufflating Needle or Trocar Placement Complications

- Vasovagal response
- Subcutaneous, preperitoneal, and retroperitoneal insufflation of gas
- Insufflation of gas into mesentery and bowel
- Gas embolization with hypotension or paradoxical embolization
- Sudden and severe hemorrhage
- Insidious blood loss
- Viscus perforation

INSUFFLATING NEEDLES AND TROCARS

Various complications have been associated with the placement of either insufflating needles or the trocars needed to initiate a pneumoperitoneum. A vasovagal response can indeed be manifested as profound sinus bradycardia or even asystole. This may occur at the time of placement of the insufflating needle or trocars, as a result of abdominal distension with the insufflating gas. A vasovagal response can develop during the operation itself secondary to traction on the various viscera. The patient's bradycardia will reverse if the surgeon stops the visceral traction. Nevertheless, profound bradycardia that does not quickly reverse after cessation of visceral traction may require immediate treatment with an anticholinergic medication such as atropine. In its extreme manifestation, the operating room team must be prepared to initiate cardiopulmonary resuscitation should the dysrhythmia not be reversed with the anticholinergic agent.

Incorrect placement of the insufflating needle with extraperitoneal insufflation of gas can result in a number of sequelae. Subcutaneous and preperitoneal insufflation of gas results in the appearance of crepitance, which may occur over the abdomen and chest. Unrecognized extraperitoneal insufflation of larger volumes of gas can even result in crepitance over the neck, face, perineum, and extremities, depending on the volume and duration of insufflation and the patient's position on the operating table. Although this complication does not result in any long-term disability, it is annoying to the patient postoperatively and may cause mild discomfort. Extraperitoneal carbon dioxide insufflation may also create difficulty for the surgeon in subsequent correct placement of the insufflating needle or the trocars because of the increased width of the preperitoneal space. Posterolateral extension of the extraperitoneally insufflated carbon dioxide may displace the ureters medially, increasing the risk of ureteral injury during trocar placement or laparoscopic dissection.

The problem of extraperitoneal insufflation can be avoided or at least ameliorated by careful surgical technique and awareness of the insufflating pressures and the quantity of carbon dioxide used throughout the surgical procedure. Once extraperitoneal insufflation is recognized, the surgeon may try to evacuate the extraperitoneal carbon dioxide. The anesthesiologist should discontinue the use of nitrous oxide because it will expand the size of this unwanted gas space in direct proportion to the concentration and duration of nitrous oxide administration. The duration of subcutaneous emphysema will depend on the gas used for insufflation as well as the amount insufflated. Because of its high blood solubility, carbon dioxide will be the most quickly resorbed of the commonly used insufflating gases.

Incorrect placement of the insufflating needle can also result in gas accumulation in the retroperitoneal space, mesentery, and bowel. Retroperitoneal insufflation of gas may also result in the appearance of crepitance of the abdominal and thoracic walls. Similarly, insufflation of gas into the mesentery or bowel wall or bowel lumen will result in anatomic distortion that may make subsequent surgical dissection difficult or impracticable.

A potentially devastating complication of incorrect placement of the insufflating needle is that of gas embolism. Intravenous insufflation of gas via the inferior vena cava, mesenteric veins, or a highly vascular organ such as the uterine wall results in gas embolism. Although gas embolism rarely occurs with laparoscopic surgical procedures,[2] it remains an ever-present and potentially fatal danger. Gas embolism can lead to cardiovascular collapse secondary to an air lock within the central vascular tree or to paradoxical gas embolization across the foramen ovale with subsequent embolization of the central nervous system, coronary vasculature, and other vital organ systems.

Clearly, prevention and early recognition are the keys to avoiding significant injury. The surgeon should aspirate the insufflating needle before connecting the inflow gas line. The insufflating pressure and flow rate, as well as the clinical signs of successful abdominal distension, should be monitored and a high index of suspicion with corrective responses initiated if all is not proceeding as expected. The sequelae of gas embolism are dependent on the rate and amount of gas entering the vascular tree. A sudden decrease in end-tidal carbon dioxide as detected via mass spectrometers or freestanding end-tidal carbon dioxide monitors should lead the anesthesiologist to suspect this problem. Pulmonary edema and reflex bronchoconstriction may be noted, as well as progressive hypoxemia. If the embolism is of sufficient magnitude, it will result in hypotension or even complete cardiovascular collapse. The incidence of gas embolization is so low, however, as to not justify the institution of measures such as Doppler probe placement, central venous catheterization, or transesophageal echocardiography—the diagnostic and potentially therapeutic modalities used in surgical procedures associated with a much higher incidence of gas or air embolization.

If gas embolism is clinically suspected, insufflation of gas should be immediately stopped. Clearly, nitrous oxide should be discontinued, as it will rapidly enlarge any existing intravascular gas. The need and urgency of subsequent responses following gas embolization will depend on the degree of cardiovascular compromise. The operating room team must be prepared to initiate cardiopulmonary resuscitation. Similarly, an emergent effort to aspirate air from the right-sided circulation can be initiated by placing a central venous catheter in the superior vena cava or right atrium. One may or may not be successful in aspirating trapped air. Classically, a patient severely compromised as a result of venous gas embolization should be placed in the Trendelenburg position and turned to the left side down position. This position theoretically traps the insufflated gas in the apex of the right ventricle and subsequently unblocks the right ventricular outflow tract, thus re-establishing flow to the lungs. Such a maneuver should be undertaken only if other efforts at cardiovascular support via drugs and cardioresuscitation have been unsuccessful.

Sudden and severe hemorrhage may result from perforation of a large intra-abdominal vessel. Again, from a preventive standpoint the anesthesiologist should ensure that the patient will not move at the time of needle or trocar placement. The surgeon should be comfortable with the degree of abdominal distension and site of placement of the insufflating needle and the trocars. Nevertheless, the operating room team should always be prepared to perform an emergent exploratory laparotomy when doing laparoscopic abdominal surgical procedures. In addition to these preventive and preplanned emergency procedures, a call for more help is invaluable to assist in obtaining more vascular access and for handling fluid resuscitation. In addition, the team should be familiar with the resuscitative protocol that will be instituted in terms of fluid resuscitation and potential use of O-negative or type-specific blood.

Insidious hemorrhage either from the site of surgery, from adhesions that have been lysed, or from the abdominal wall presents another clinical dilemma. A high index of suspicion must be maintained to minimize or avert disaster. Many times these patients are in significant head-down positions during the operation, and thus relative hypovolemia secondary to ongoing hemorrhage may go unrecognized. Only when the patient's legs are taken out of the stirrups or leg holders and the patient is returned to a relatively level position may hypotension be evident. Similarly, recurring hypotension in the recovery room—despite what appears to be adequate fluid administration perioperatively—should raise warning flags. Pain out of proportion to the usual degree of surgical pain may be a clinical clue in patients in whom an abdominal wall hematoma is developing. Serial hematocrit values or the placement of intravascular catheters to measure filling pressures adds evidence to clinical suspicion and may necessitate a return to the operating room.

Finally, incorrect placement of an insufflating needle or trocars or problems associated with the use of other laparoscopic instruments may result in viscus perforation. Perforations of the stomach, bowel, bladder, and uterus have all been described in the literature. Once again, prevention is the treatment of choice. Not only should the patient not move in response to the needle or trocar placement, but also many advocate decompression of the stomach by an orogastric tube and the bladder by a urethral catheter before needle or trocar placement. If viscus perforation is recognized at the time of laparoscopy, it may be successfully repaired via the laparoscope or a laparotomy. Problems arise if the visceral injury is not recognized at the time of the operation. Again, a high index of suspicion postoperatively is very helpful. Patients may have abdominal pain, tenderness, fever, or other signs of peritonitis or sepsis. Residual air from the initial laparoscopic surgery may persist for several days, especially if the distending gas is other than carbon dioxide. The residual air may confound the diagnosis of viscus perforation because such gas may reflect either the retained gas or free air on abdominal radiograms.

PNEUMOPERITONEUM

Several complications associated with the creation of a pneumoperitoneum have been reported. Originally it was feared that the use of carbon dioxide for an insufflating gas might result in hypercarbia. In practicality, this result has not proved to be a clinical problem, particularly if the patient is undergoing general anesthesia with controlled ventilation. Again, end-tidal carbon dioxide monitoring should allow an adequate assessment of ventilation. If end-tidal carbon dioxide levels increase, a rather standard assessment by the anesthesiologist should lead to appropriate diagnostic and corrective actions.

More troublesome, intraoperative problems arising from the creation of a pneumoperitoneum are those of respiratory embarrassment and decreased venous return. Overdistension of the abdominal cavity, especially if combined with a steep Trendelenburg's position, can result in marked cephalad displacement of the diaphragm. In a spontaneously ventilating patient, these changes may be very dramatic and cause clinically significant compromise of ventilation. In a patient undergoing general anesthesia in whom ventilation is being controlled, however, such changes are usually overcome rather easily. Nevertheless, the anesthesiologist should be aware of the ventilating pressures required to adequately ventilate the patient as well as the intra-abdominal pressure noted on the insufflating machine. In general, intra-abdominal pressures should not have to exceed 20 mm Hg and should always be reduced to a level as low as is appropriate for the patient. In addition, high intra-abdominal pressures can compromise venous return and thus result in hypotension. Thus, the anesthesiologist should suspect high intra-abdominal pressure as a possible cause of intraoperative hypotension and recommend appropriate corrective action.

Rare, but potentially life-threatening, complications reportedly associated with pneumoperitoneum include the occurrence of pneumomediastinum and pneumothorax.[3] The purported mechanism of these rare occurrences is secondary to the passage of insufflated gas from the intra-abdominal cavity through congenital diaphragmatic defects into the pleural or mediastinal space. A pneumothorax must be suspected if significant hypotension ensues during a laparoscopic procedure. The ongoing pressure gradient from the intra-abdominal cavity, combined with the common usage of nitrous oxide as a part of most general anesthesia, makes the conversion of a small pneumothorax into a cardiovascularly compromising tension pneumothorax a real threat. Should a pneumothorax be suspected, the usual clinical signs should be sought quickly. Suggestive signs include a marked increase in peak ventilatory pressure, a decrease in oxygen saturation, absent breath sounds and hyperresonance to percussion on the affected side, possible wheezing, and hypotension. Treatment includes the immediate discontinuance of nitrous oxide, institution of 100 percent oxygen, and relief of the pneumothorax. The latter may be accomplished by piercing the involved side with a large-bore angiocatheter or by the more formal placement of a chest tube surgically.

PATIENT POSITIONING

Laparoscopic-assisted bowel surgical procedures often necessitate placement of the patient in a significant head down or otherwise modified Trendelenburg's position. The Trendelenburg position, particularly in combination with the creation of a pneumoperitoneum, can result in significant cardiopulmonary changes. The usual or expected cardiovascular changes

Positioning Complications

Adverse cardiovascular changes, including hypotension and left ventricular failure
Increased intracranial or intraocular pressure
Respiratory compromise
Passive regurgitation and aspiration
Dislocation of the tip of the endotracheal tube
Deep vein thrombosis
Neurovascular and soft tissue injuries

associated with Trendelenburg's position are well described in the literature. In healthy patients, there is usually an initial increase in venous return with a concomitant increase in cardiac output. Increased central blood volume and cardiac output activate stretch receptors on the aortic arch and carotid sinus, often reflexly lowering the blood pressure and cardiac output slightly. In most patients, the hemodynamic changes associated with the combination of head-down or lithotomy positioning and the creation of a pneumoperitoneum are clinically unremarkable.

It is, however, clinically important to recognize and treat unexpected cardiovascular compromise in fit patients or to anticipate those patients in whom cardiovascular compromise might be expected from positioning or the creation of a pneumoperitoneum. For example, hypotension can occur secondary to decreased venous return in some patients. After the initial autotransfusion of blood from the lower extremities associated with lithotomy positioning, venous return may be compromised by the combination of pooling of blood in suspended lower extremities, high intra-abdominal pressure occluding the vena cava secondary to the pneumoperitoneum, and patient manipulation during the surgical procedure. Likewise, the surgeon may place the patient in a reverse Trendelenburg's position to facilitate dissection. This position, in combination with blunted cardiovascular reflexes associated with general anesthesia, can further decrease venous return. Finally, as previously noted, insidious blood loss can go unrecognized. Hypotension can therefore result in a diagnostic dilemma. Patients with normal preoperative cardiovascular status do not need central venous pressure or pulmonary artery catheter monitoring perioperatively when undergoing laparoscopic-assisted bowel surgical procedures. However, when the differential diagnosis or evolving picture of intraoperative hypotension is unclear, more aggressive monitoring should be instituted. In addition, left ventricular failure secondary to increased venous return resulting in increased ventricular filling pressure may occur in patients with compromised cardiovascular reserve. Thus, because of the unpredictable nature of hemodynamic changes that can occur during laparoscopic-assisted bowel surgical procedures with the patient in a marked Trendelenburg's position, patients with preoperative compromise in their cardiovascular status should ideally be monitored with central venous or preferably pulmonary arterial catheters. Patients at particular risk include those with mitral stenosis or significant left ventricular dysfunction.

Other cardiovascular changes that should be anticipated and appreciated include those in cerebrovascular and ocular dynamics. Prolonged head-down positioning can result in increases in intracranial pressure and cerebral edema. These conditions are usually of little clinical concern. In the rare patient with cerebrovascular disease or concomitant intracranial abnormalities, these hydrodynamic changes can result in a very real problem. Case reports cite patients in whom both retinal detachment as well as attacks of acute glaucoma have been attributed to changes in hemodynamics associated with a head-down position for lengthy periods.[4] Anticipation of the problems in at-risk patients and minimal time in the head-down position are the most effective means of reducing these problems. In the case of intracranial pathology, mild to moderate hyperventilation may be of some value. Similarly, patients with glaucoma should receive their glaucoma medications perioperatively.

Respiratory changes associated with the Trendelenburg or lithotomy position are also well described in the literature. In general, these include a decrease in vital capacity and other lung volumes. This decrease is the result of restriction of diaphragmatic movement by the abdominal contents, as well as decreased pulmonary compliance due to increased pulmonary blood volume. Clearly, such changes result in an increase in the work of breathing. Again, such changes are compounded with the creation of a pneumoperitoneum. Thus, spontaneous ventilation in awake or anesthetized patients is clinically unacceptable in all but the fittest of patients. In fact, in laparoscopic bowel surgical procedures, the level of block necessary for adequate anesthesia (usually a solid T4 sensory level), in combination with the respiratory stress from the pneumoperitoneum, makes regional anesthesia alone a poor choice.

Other changes or considerations associated with steep Trendelenburg's positioning and laparoscopic surgical procedures include the occurrence of regurgitation, changes in location of the endotracheal tube, and the occurrence of deep vein thrombophlebitis.

Passive regurgitation of gastric contents can obviously occur in patients with pre-existing anatomic problems such as a hiatal hernia. Compounding the problems are the increases in intra-abdominal pressure associated with the creation of a pneumoperitoneum. The real danger is aspiration of gastric contents with resultant pulmonary infection. This problem can be obviated or at least minimized by using endotracheal intubation with a cuffed tube when general anesthesia is employed.

Not always commonly appreciated is that a steep Trendelenburg's position can result in caudad displacement of the tip of the endotracheal tube. This displacement can result in intubation of the right main stem bronchus and can cause significant hypoxemia. Intraoperative hypoxemia as picked up via the intraoperative use of pulse oximetry should alert the anesthesiologist to the problem of endotracheal tube displacement and result in appropriate confirmatory and corrective action.

Deep vein thrombophlebitis is an ever-present risk perioperatively that has received much interest in the past several years. Patients undergoing sometimes lengthy laparoscopic-assisted bowel surgeries in odd positions are certainly at risk and ideally deserve utilization of prophylactic measures such as support hose or some of the newer lower extremity sequential compression devices.

A rare intraoperative complication associated with the use of electrocautery in laparoscopic bowel surgical procedures is the risk of an intraperitoneal explosion. Indeed, intestinal gas contains high concentrations of both hydrogen and methane gases. Inadvertent and unrecognized puncture of the bowel may cause these gases to diffuse into the abdominal cavity. If nitrous oxide is used as the insufflating gas, it can sustain combustion and yield a highly explosive mixture in combination with intestinal gas.[5] Thus, nitrous oxide is not a good choice of insufflating gas if electrocautery is to be used.

Finally, a variety of neurovascular and soft tissue injuries may be associated with laparoscopic-assisted bowel surgery. Although not unique to laparoscopy, because of the duration and positioning requirements of some procedures, these injuries must be anticipated and prevented. Peripheral nerve injuries likely occur much more commonly than appreciated by many practicing surgeons and anesthesiologists.[6] They are certainly one of the most frequent causes of malpractice judgments. In most instances, they are the result of either stretch or direct compression of the neurovascular bundle. A number of excellent reviews discuss peripheral nerve injuries.

The peripheral nerves most likely to be injured are the ulnar nerve or the brachial plexus itself. The preferred position for prevention of either ulnar nerve or brachial plexus injury is to tuck the arms at the side of the patient. Likewise, many try to pad the ulnar groove or ensure (usually through pronation of the arm) that the patient is not lying on the ulnar nerve itself as it passes through the ulnar groove at the elbow. Nevertheless, injuries to the ulnar nerve still occur. A recent excellent editorial addressed the issue of whether such injuries are indeed preventable.[7]

Positioning for laparoscopic-assisted bowel surgical procedures may, however, necessitate that the arms be extended from the body in certain patients. If abducted, care should be taken to not extend the arms beyond 90 degrees. Abduction beyond 90 degrees, rotation of the head away from the extended arm, improper placement of shoulder rests, or braces too far medially over the clavicle can stretch the brachial plexus and cause injury. It should be noted that shoulder pain following laparoscopy is a common complaint. It is usually benign and self-limited, lasting no more than 12 to 24 hours. It is most commonly attributed to diaphragmatic irritation from residual insufflated gas. Pain persisting beyond 24 hours is worrisome and may indicate a brachial plexus or shoulder injury. Any motor or sensory deficits involving the brachial plexus should receive immediate and full attention as outlined below.

A number of lower extremity peripheral nerve injuries have been associated with lithotomy and head-down positioning. Among these are injuries to the femoral and obturator nerves, as well as the sciatic nerve, in particular, the common peroneal branch. Injury to the common peroneal nerve has been the one most commonly associated with surgeries requiring patients to be placed in stirrups or leg supports. The common peroneal nerve can be injured if its nutrient vessels are directly compressed as it wraps around the head of the fibula on the lateral aspect of the knee (Fig. 4-1). Motor loss of this nerve results in footdrop, whereas sensory loss results in numbness to the sole of the foot.

Stretching of the sciatic nerve can occur as a result of extension of the knees when the thighs are flexed. Additional tension is placed on the sciatic nerve by external rotation of the hip with the thighs and knees flexed. Hyperflexion of the hip joint aggravates this problem of sciatic stretch. Prevention by careful patient positioning is the only effective means of reducing the likelihood of injury to the sciatic nerve and its branches. Preventive measures include flexing the knees before flexing the hips, avoiding hyperflexion of the hips, allowing only limited external rotation of the hip, raising and lowering both legs at the same time when changing the patient's position, and ensuring that no external pressure is applied to the lateral aspect of the fibula near the course of the common peroneal nerve.

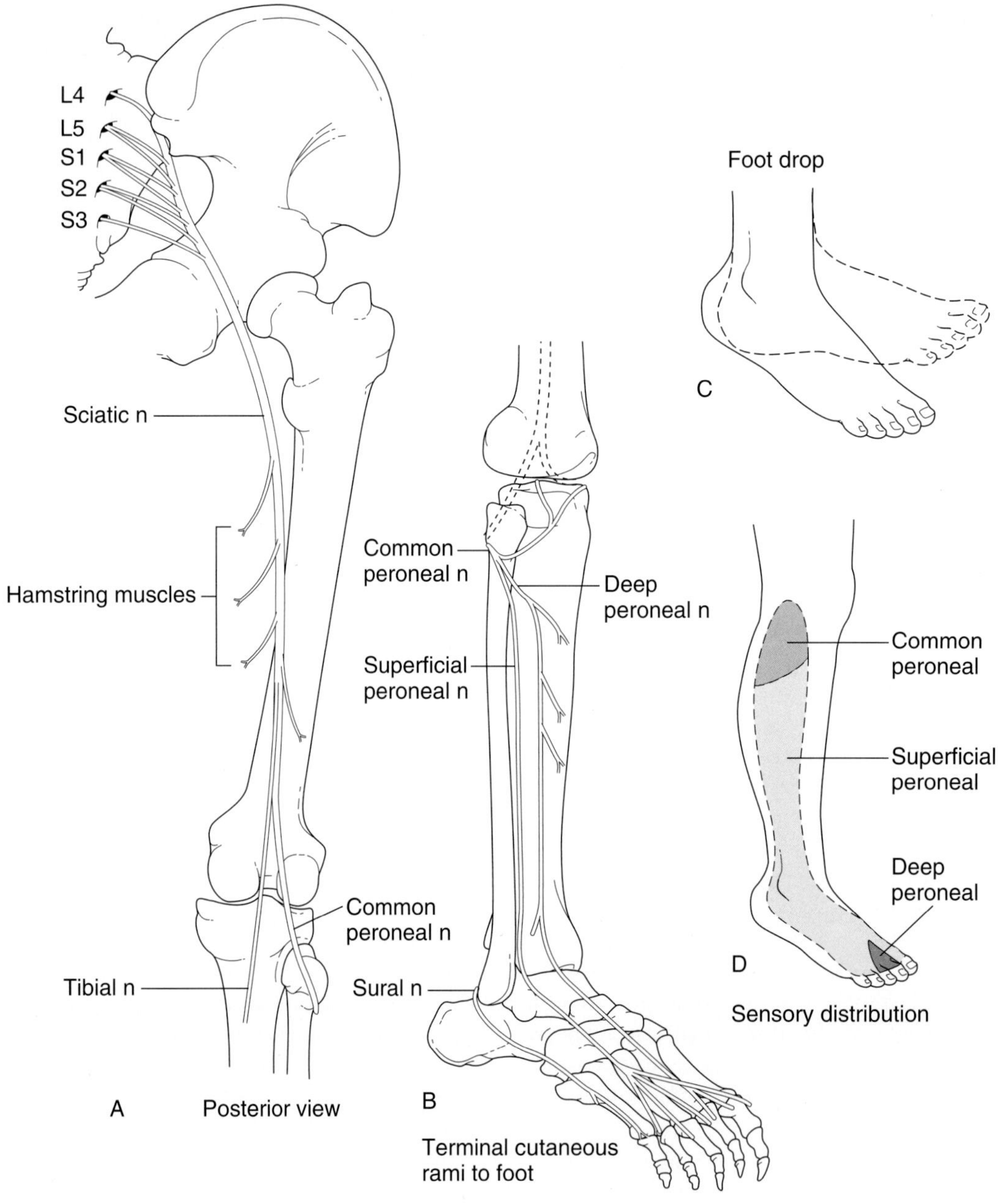

Fig. 4-1. Sciatic nerve (insertion, L4-L5 and S1–S3): **(A)** posterior view, **(B)** common peroneal nerve and its major branches, **(C)** footdrop from peroneal nerve injury, and **(D)** sensory deficit associated with peroneal nerve injury. (From Nicholson and McAlpine,[11] with permission.)

Injuries to peripheral nerves are often manifested as a mixed picture with both partial and complete motor and sensory deficits. Early and thorough evaluation in conjunction with a consulting neurologist or neurosurgeon is important to rule out other etiologic factors before positioning trauma is assumed to be the sole cause. Patients often have pre-existing diseases of peripheral nerves that either predispose them to injury or have not previously been appreciated by the patient. Similarly, other perioperative trauma—such as misplaced intramuscular injections, direct surgical trauma, or spontaneous or traumatic hematomas—may cause these nerve injuries. Fortunately, many of these injuries resolve over the course of days or months with appropriate interim care and therapy.

Another injury not widely appreciated that can result from improper positioning is compartment syndrome, recently the subject of increased interest in the literature.[8,9] Compartment syndrome is a condition in which the circulation and function of tissues within a closed space are compromised by increased pressure within that space. Instances of compartment syndrome have been reported to follow the use of several versions of the lithotomy position, particularly if the patient has remained in that position for a lengthy time. Almost all variations of the different leg holders or supports available have been associated with this injury; thus, no single type of leg holder that is clearly superior exists. Again, besides careful positioning and padding, minimizing the duration of lithotomy positioning may be the most important preventive step. Maintenance of blood pressure intraoperatively is important. Detecting the onset of compartment syndrome intraoperatively is not clinically feasible. Detection of distal pulses in an extremity, as well as capillary refill in the ipsilateral nail beds, has not proved to be a reliable prognosticator.

Manifestations of a compartment syndrome may be noted on awakening of the patient or may not appear for several hours. Physical signs of a compartment syndrome include sensory loss, muscle weakness, painful passive movement, and local tissue distension. Early decompression decreases postischemic swelling, tissue devitalization, and the likelihood of infection. Unfortunately, functional impairment and permanent structural damage to compartmental contents are more common with these injuries than with most peripheral nerve injuries.

Finally, other miscellaneous injuries that frequently occur include back strain or injury and alopecia. Back strain is fairly common and responds to analgesics, anti-inflammatory agents, rest, and physical therapy. It is probably an unavoidable side effect of prolonged surgery in the steep Trendelenburg position. Both ligamentous relaxation during anesthesia and muscle relaxation allow the loss of natural lumbar lordosis. Likewise, uncoordinated elevation or lowering of the legs has been implicated in producing spinal torsion with an increased risk of disc extrusion.

Occipital alopecia may occur if the head is allowed to rest in one dependent position for a long duration.[10] Prevention is the treatment of choice and is accomplished by padding the head carefully at its pressure point and intermittently turning the head slightly to change the actual site of pressure. The onset of hair loss may occur any time during the first postoperative month. Hair regrowth is often slow to occur, and in fact, hair loss may be permanent.

REFERENCES

1. Stoelting RK, Dierdorf SF (eds): Anesthesia and Co-Existing Disease. 3rd Ed. Churchill Livingstone, New York, 1993
2. Borten M (ed): Laparoscopic Complications. BC Decker, Toronto, 1986
3. Doctor NH, Hussain Z: Bilateral pneumothorax associated with laparoscopy. Anesthesia 28:75, 1973
4. Martin JT (ed): Positioning in Anesthesia and Surgery. 2nd Ed. WB Saunders, Philadelphia, 1987
5. Drummond GB, Scott DB: Laparoscopy explosion hazards with nitrous oxide. BMJ 1:586, 1976
6. Dawson DM, Krarup C: Perioperative nerve lesions. Arch Neurol 46:1355, 1989
7. Stoelting RK: Postoperative ulnar nerve palsy. Is it a preventable complication? Anesth Analg 76:7, 1993
8. Martin JT: Compartment syndromes: concepts and perspectives for the anesthesiologist. Anesth Analg 75:275, 1992
9. Adler LM, Loughlin JS, Norin CJ et al: Bilateral compartment syndrome after a long gynecologic operation in the lithotomy position. Am J Obstet Gynecol 162:1271, 1990
10. Patel KD, Henschel EO: Postoperative alopecia. Anesth Analg 59:311, 1980
11. Nicholson MJ, McAlpine FS: Neural injuries associated with surgical positions and operations. p. 193. In Martin JT (ed): Positioning in Anesthesia and Surgery. WB Saunders, Philadelphia, 1978

Editorial Comment I

David A. Nakata

The completeness of this chapter's contents highlights the perioperative complications associated with laparoscopic bowel surgery. Dr. McCammon points out that multiple adverse events can be directly associated with laparoscopic surgery. Some can be life-threatening. It is imperative that we not only be aware of these various complications but also plan to deal with these eventualities. This commentary discusses the etiology, prevention, detection, and treatment of venous gas embolism and associated complications of patient positioning.

VENOUS GAS EMBOLISM

One of the more devastating complications of laparoscopic surgery is venous gas embolism. Venous gas embolism is a rare occurrence that can be immediately life-threatening. Detection may be obscured by its ability to mimic other more common hemodynamic events such as obstruction of venous return from pneumoperitoneum and a steep reverse Trendelenburg's position. In addition, its rare and unexpected nature can catch even the most astute by surprise.

Venous gas embolism differs from air embolism. Venous air embolization most commonly occurs during sitting craniotomies when the patient's head is elevated above the level of the right atrium. Multiple open venous sinuses can facilitate the entry of air into the central circulation. The driving force for entry of air is the difference between the atmospheric and central venous pressures. By contrast, venous gas embolism occurs when pressurized gas is actively pumped into the central venous compartment. This condition can lead to immediate hemodynamic compromise. Therefore, extreme care must be exercised during the insufflation of gas into the peritoneal cavity for the production of a pneumoperitoneum.

Because gas embolism is rare during laparoscopic procedures, transesophageal echocardiography and precordial Doppler ultrasound—the two most sensitive means of detecting gas embolism—are not routinely used. Other less sensitive means of detecting air embolism include monitoring end-tidal nitrogen and carbon dioxide. The concentration of these two gases is routinely measured using standard gas monitoring techniques. Measurement of end-tidal nitrogen has been found to be more sensitive than measurement of end-tidal carbon dioxide in detecting venous air embolization. Since carbon dioxide is used for insufflation of the peritoneal cavity during laparoscopic surgery, nitrogen would not be detected during gas embolism, possibly making the diagnosis and treatment more difficult.

Successful treatment of venous gas embolism begins with the recognition that embolization has occurred. Because of the previously mentioned events that can mimic embolism, a heightened level of suspicion must always be maintained. If gas embolism does occur, the insufflation of gas, as well as nitrous oxide, should be immediately discontinued. Full cardiac life-support measures may need to be instituted, including external cardiac massage. The left lateral position has been proposed as the position that facilitates the best forward cardiac flow, but if cardiac massage is necessary, it may not be feasible to maintain this position. In addition, the placement of a large-bore central lumen catheter to aspirate gas should be considered, although placement of this catheter can be fraught with complications, especially during the performance of cardiac massage. If these maneuvers fail, open chest cardiac massage and direct aspiration of gas from the central circulation should be considered.

PATIENT POSITIONING

Complications from positioning of patients during laparoscopic surgical procedures are addressed in this chapter. Other complications not directly associated with patient positioning but with the movement of patients with respect to laparoscopic equipment should also be considered. The operating suites of many older hospitals were not designed to accommodate the new and space-consuming plethora of equipment being introduced. This limitation can be a hazard to both the patient and the operating room personnel.

Standard equipment in today's operating rooms consists of an operating table, electrocautery unit, sterile supply table, Mayo stand, anesthesia machine, and related equipment. During laparoscopic procedures, this list grows to include laparoscopic video and gas insufflating equipment and an extra sterile supply table to accommodate the specialized laparoscopic equipment. Further congestion is added by the electrical, vacuum, irrigation, and compressed gas lines attached to this conglomeration of equipment. These can make movement about the operating suite cumbersome at best and, in some instances, nearly impossible.

Furthermore, the operating table is often repositioned after anesthetic induction to optimize surgical access and visualization. This repositioning can lead to accidental extubation of the trachea, disconnection of monitors, extraction of intravenous catheters, and blunt physical trauma from impact with the operating room equipment. Even if the patient's location is not altered after induction of anesthesia, table height and tilt are often changed one or more times during the operation, with the potential of causing crush injuries to susceptible areas.

This wide array of equipment can also block the anesthesiologist's view of suction canisters and the operating room floor, thus increasing the chance of not appreciating both blood loss and disconnection of vascular access lines. In addition, operating room lights are often extinguished to further optimize video contrast, further limiting the anesthesiologist's ability to assess patient color and evaluate the surgical and nonsurgical fields for blood loss.

As the complexity of laparoscopic surgical procedures increases, the potential for major blood loss and fluid shifts increases. With the increased likelihood of blood loss comes the increased possibility that an emergent open laparotomy will need to be performed. This event, when considered in the face of the previously mentioned array of equipment, tubes, and cramped quarters, can lead to disastrous consequences. Maintaining vigilance is therefore of extreme importance, even in the seemingly simplest of cases.

Editorial Comment II

Rama M. Jager

Dr. McCammon details various perioperative complications that can occur in patients undergoing laparoscopic colorectal surgery. Some additional comments follow.

MANAGING EXTRAPERITONEAL INSUFFLATION

Preperitoneal placement of a Veress needle during the initiation of pneumoperitoneum is more likely in obese patients. The site of insertion may have to be the center of the umbilicus or superior rim rather than the inferior rim as is commonly used. The angle of insertion is less acute and more perpendicular to the skin in obese patients to avoid preperitoneal placement. If a significant amount of carbon dioxide enters the preperitoneal space, insertion of the needle should be abandoned, and an open Hasson technique used to get into the peritoneal cavity. The technique of using the laparoscope to aid insertion after the preperitoneal space is described elsewhere.[1]

NITROUS OXIDE USE

The surgeon should preoperatively discuss with the anesthesiologist the choice of anesthetic agents and request that nitrous oxide not be used. There are many advantages to using nitrous oxide for balanced anesthesia. The disadvantages such as prolonged enlargement of the preperitoneal space from nitrous oxide diffusion, dilation of small intestinal loops, and promotion of intraperitoneal combustion during the use of electrocautery far outweigh any advantages.[2] There are multiple means of inducing balanced anesthesia without using nitrous oxide. I request my anesthesiologist to avoid nitrous oxide during laparoscopic surgical procedures.

RISK OF MAJOR VESSEL INJURY

The most catastrophic complication during the initiation of pneumoperitoneum is penetration of the aorta or iliac vessels by the Veress needle or the laparoscopic trocar. In agreement with Semm,[3] a surgeon who tries to palpate the aorta before plunging the needle or cannula rarely injures the aorta. Laparoscopic surgeons should be aware of the proximity of the aorta to the anterior abdominal wall and the relationship of the umbilicus to the aortic bifurcation. Although the aorta may be proximal to the umbilicus in some patients, the left iliac vein crosses the midline in all patients and is at risk of injury. Pointing the needle and the sharp trocar away from the aortic bifurcation is one approach. Some surgeons propose the use of an open laparoscopic insertion technique and avoid blind puncture with the Veress needle completely.

END-TIDAL CARBON DIOXIDE AND INVASIVE ARTERIAL BLOOD GAS ANALYSIS

As Dr. McCammon suggests, hypercarbia from carbon dioxide pneumoperitoneum is rarely a clinical problem unless the patient has preoperative risk factors such as a decreased forced expiratory volume in 1 second (FEV_1) of below 70 percent of the predicted value and a diffusion capacity of less than 80 percent of predicted. Preoperative evaluation may alert the anesthesiologist to the degree of intensity needed in monitoring carbon dioxide metabolism intraoperatively. End-tidal carbon dioxide monitoring is quite satisfactory in many patients. In patients with poor cardiopulmonary reserve, arterial blood gas monitoring may be needed because the end-tidal carbon dioxide may not accurately reflect the arterial carbon dioxide partial pressure.

Twenty to 40 percent of the carbon dioxide may remain intraperitoneally after the completion of laparoscopic procedures. The residual intraperitoneal carbon dioxide and the extraperitoneally insufflated carbon dioxide may affect postoperative ventilation, more so if the patient is given opioids for postoperative analgesia. It is a good practice for the surgeon to take extra effort to desufflate carbon dioxide at the end of the laparoscopic procedure if a mini-incision is not part of the operation. Young and healthy patients with good pulmonary reserve will have no problems with retained carbon dioxide, but an elderly patient with chronic obstructive pulmonary disease may exhibit hypercarbia.[4]

DISPLACEMENT OF CARINA WITH TRENDELENBURG'S POSITION AND PNEUMOPERITONEUM

The tip of the endotracheal tube is displaced into the right main stem bronchus not only by a steep Trendelenburg's position but also from the superior mediastinal shift induced by the pneumoperitoneum.[5] Most laparoscopic left colonic and abdominoperineal resections involve both of these causal factors. The anesthesiologist should be vigilant to detect such displacement and correct the problem either by withdrawing the tube, by removing the patient from the Trendelenburg position, or by partially deflating the pneumoperitoneum.

LUMBAR LORDOSIS LOSS

The lumbosacral torsion and stretching produced by the lithotomy position can be reduced by placing the patient in the lithotomy position before induction of anesthesia. The patient can voice any back pain or discomfort resulting from the positioning, and the surgeon can take appropriate steps to reduce the strain. Prolonged laparoscopic procedures, even in the supine position, can produce postoperative back pain from the loss of lumbar lordosis. Placing foam rubber pads or intravenous fluid bags inflated with air to provide a sublumbar air cushion may reduce the severity of this problem.

COMPARTMENT SYNDROME

Crural compartment syndrome from prolonged dorsolithotomy Trendelenburg's positioning is difficult to detect,[6,7] although various measures of ischemia such as pedal pulse palpation, capillary refill, and intraoperative lower extremity oximetry have been used. Sensors to monitor compartmental pressures have been devised (Innerspace Medical Company, Irvine, CA). Whether the intraoperative use of sensing devices avoids postoperative compartment syndrome is unknown. Other positional problems such as femoral neuropathy occur after prolonged dorsolithotomy positioning.[8] However, most of the laparoscopic colorectal procedures require that the thighs be flexed as little as possible to avoid femoral interference with instrumental freedom. This measure may reduce the problem of position-related femoral neuropathy.

REFERENCES

1. Kabukoba JJ, Skillern LH: Coping with extraperitoneal insufflation during laparoscopy: a new technique. Obstet Gynecol 80:144, 1992
2. West ST, Haring L: Laparoscopy explosion hazards with nitrous oxide. Anesthesiology 78:875, 1993
3. Semm K: Operative Manual for Endoscopic Abdominal Surgery. Year Book Medical Publishers, Chicago, 1987
4. Tolksdorf W, Strang CM, Schippers E: The effects of the carbon dioxide pneumoperitoneum in laparoscopic cholecystectomy on postoperative spontaneous respiration. Anesthetist 41:199, 1992
5. Hamm P, Lang C, Fornecker ML: Recurrent selective bronchial intubation in laparoscopic cholecystectomy. Ann Fr Anesth Reanim 12:67, 1993
6. Schwartz LB, Stahl RS, DeCherney AH: Unilateral compartment syndrome after prolonged gynecologic surgery in the dorsolithotomy position. A case report. J Reprod Med 38:469, 1993
7. Mulhall JP, Drezner AD: Postoperative compartment syndrome and the lithotomy position: a report of three cases and analysis of potential risk factors. Conn Med 57:129, 1993
8. Hakim M, Katirji B: Femoral mononeuropathy induced by the lithotomy position: a report of five cases with a review of literature. Muscle Nerve 16:891, 1993

5
Bowel Preparation

James W. C. Holmes and Ronald Lee Nichols

Preoperative preparation of the gastrointestinal tract is the hallmark of modern elective colorectal surgery.[1] Traditionally, preparation has been done within the hospital environment, thus adding to the total cost of the procedure by lengthening the hospital stay. It also increases the risk factors for postoperative surgical infection, primarily by exposing the patient to hospital-acquired microbial pathogens before surgery.[2] The two major components of elective preoperative bowel preparation can most frequently be done on an outpatient basis, which permits admission of patients for elective colorectal surgery through a same-day surgery system. The mechanical cleansing of the large bowel done preoperatively is identical to that routinely done on an outpatient basis before colonoscopy. Adequate preoperative patient education, including instruction sheets written in simple, clear, and concise terms, allows for administration of the preoperative oral antibiotic bowel preparation on an outpatient basis. Perioperative parenteral antibiotic prophylaxis is then given in the operating room following admission of the patient to the hospital. Such an approach enhances patient comfort by allowing the preoperative mechanical and oral antibiotic bowel preparation to be done in the privacy of the home, decreases risk factors for postoperative infection by reducing the time spent in the hospital before surgery to a few hours, and further lessens the cost of this hospitalization by decreasing the total length of stay as an inpatient.[3]

BOWEL PREPARATION BEFORE ELECTIVE SURGERY

Preoperative Mechanical Cleansing

Preoperative bowel preparation, including mechanical cleansing and antibiotics, should be the same before laparoscopic colorectal operations as before traditional surgical procedures. The protocols followed while mechanically cleansing the gastrointestinal tract before elective colorectal surgery differ considerably but include certain basic practices:

1. A clear liquid diet, which should be translated as a "no residue" diet
2. Removal of formed fecal elements in the intestinal tract
3. Evaluation of the patient for fluid and electrolyte abnormalities and their prevention and treatment

Traditionally, a 3- to 5-day fast was imposed on patients during their bowel preparation before elective colorectal surgery. Such prolonged fasting with purgation and enemas frequently caused moderate to severe metabolic disturbances secondary to iatrogenically produced losses of body fluids and salts. This approach also ignored the daily nutritional requirements of the patient, thus potentiating the morbidity of preoperative bowel preparation. A more modern approach can reduce the duration of preoperative bowel preparation to a 24- to 36-hour period and allows for the addition of no-residue caloric supplements to the traditional clear liquid, low caloric diet of juices, tea, water, and broths.

Having decided on the need for elective colorectal surgery, we routinely discuss two methods of preoperative mechanical bowel preparation with the patient. We select one of them on the basis of patient preferences and convenience, as well as on the presence of associated health factors such as renal insufficiency and cardiovascular disease (Table 5-1). Since we recommend outpatient preparation, every effort must be made to achieve the degree of patient education, information, and compliance needed to accomplish this task. One of the cleansing approaches recommended is an oral antegrade lavage using a polyethylene glycol solution.[4] The rate of consumption of this solution is critical for the success of the preparation. Four liters of this preparation must be drunk over a 3- to

Table 5-1. Preoperative Preparation for Elective Laparoscopic Colorectal Surgery

Method	Facility	Diet	Mechanical Cleansing	Oral Antibiotics
One	Usually as outpatient	Clear liquids with "no-residue" caloric supplements beginning at noon or midnight on preoperative day 2	Isotonic polyethylene glycol-based solution, 4 L PO over 3- to 4-h period beginning at 6 PM on preoperative day 2 or at 6 AM on preoperative day 1[a]	1 g erythromycin base PO and 1 g neomycin PO at 1, 2, and 11 PM on preoperative day 1
Two	As above	Begin as above at noon on preoperative day 2	45 ml of sodium phosphate solution (Fleet phosphosoda) mixed with an equal volume of clear liquid at 6 PM on preoperative day 2 and at 6 AM on preoperative day 1	As above

[a]Preoperative mechanical bowel preparation is done on preoperative day 1 if no testing is scheduled that day that would conflict with purgation. Otherwise, it is begun on preoperative day 2 after initiating the clear liquid diet at noon on that day.

4-hour period to achieve the best results. Accelerated consumption of the 4-L solution can result in violent emesis and, rarely, the development of Boerhaave syndrome. Decelerated consumption over more than a 4-hour period can result in increased absorption of fluids and salts. This also results in clinically significant fluid and electrolyte disturbances, and the mechanical bolus effect needed to effectively purge the bowels is decreased. Both the clear liquid diet and antegrade gastrointestinal lavage are initiated 24 to 36 hours before surgery. If no additional testing (such as colonoscopy) is required the morning before surgery, it is possible to shorten this form of preoperative bowel preparation to a 24-hour period. The other protocol for mechanical cleansing that we recommend to the patient uses a Fleets phosphosoda solution given orally at 6 PM on preoperative day 2 and at 6 AM on preoperative day 1. The clear liquid diet is started at noon on preoperative day 2. Each dose of purgative consists of 45 ml of Fleets phosphosoda mixed with an equal volume of water. Patient acceptance is enhanced by following each dose with a 300-ml drink of a favorite clear liquid (nonalcoholic). It is very important that patients who use this method of purgation consume 1 to 2 L of a balanced salt solution (such as Gatorade, 10-K, or other brand) on each of the 2 days before surgery to avoid intravascular volume depletion. A recent prospectively randomized trial of 450 patients compared the phosphosoda preparation with polyethylene glycol and with sulfate-free polyethylene glycol.[5] Patient acceptance to the sodium phosphate solution was vastly superior ($P < 0.001$). This technique should be used carefully, if at all, in patients with cardiac disease. It is contraindicated in those with significant renal dysfunction because it can produce hyperphosphatemia.

Various personal, physical, and environmental factors should be considered in selecting the form of bowel preparation. These factors range from a patient's wish to enjoy solid foods until the morning before surgery to the presence of a stoma, which creates problems in managing the rapidly evacuated intestinal contents produced by mechanical preoperative cleansing of the bowel. Patients with stomas are provided with an irrigation sleeve that is placed over the stoma so that the patient can sit next to a commode with the distal conduit end of the sleeve placed in the toilet bowl. This allows early controlled passage of the liquified stool from the patient's stoma to the commode. In normal patients, protective perineal care during the preoperative period is important because excoriation of the perianal skin can result from the frequent evacuation of stool caused by mechanical purgation. Perineal cleansing after defecation should be done with the softest of toilet paper or cleansing pads to avoid further irritation of the skin secondary to the abrasion of frequent wiping. The patient must also have prompt and easy access to toilet facilities. Patients undergoing preparation at home preoperatively must be warned to stay at home or at least in close proximity to bathroom facilities. Last-minute shopping sprees are contraindicated once consumption of the mechanical bowel preparation has begun. For the hospitalized patient with a semiprivate room, bathroom access can be difficult, but bedside commodes are a good solution to this problem.

Preoperative Oral Antibiotic Prophylaxis

The goal of preoperative oral antibiotic prophylaxis is to produce a high level of bactericidal activity against the endogenous aerobic and anaerobic colonic microflora while at the same time producing minimal local and systemic toxicity by using drugs with limited absorption from the bowel lumen.[6] Most preoperative oral antibiotic prophylaxis consists of neomycin in combination with one of three agents, each having excellent coverage of the anaerobic microflora: erythromycin base, tetracycline, or metronidazole. Our preference is erythromycin base and neomycin sulfate. The timing of administration is very important and must be initiated only after the mechanical bowel preparation is finished so that the antibiotics do not undergo purgation with the fecal contents. We recommend beginning preoperative oral antibiotic prophylaxis 19 hours before the anticipated time of surgery. For an 8:00 AM start, 1 g of erythromycin base and 1 g of neomycin sulfate in combination should be taken orally by the patient at 1, 2, and 11 PM the day before surgery. If surgery is to begin later than 8 AM, the timing of administration for the oral antibiotics should be altered appropriately to preserve the time intervals between dosing with prophylactic oral antibiotics and the start of surgery.

PERIOPERATIVE PARENTERAL ANTIBIOTIC PROPHYLAXIS

A recent survey of board-certified colorectal surgeons has shown that the vast majority favor using perioperative parenteral antibiotic prophylaxis during elective colorectal surgery following the successful completion of preoperative mechanical and oral antibiotic bowel preparation.[7] The preoperative oral antibiotic preparation (see previous section for our preference) should be enhanced by preoperative parenteral administration of a single dose of antibiotic with the required aerobic and anaerobic antimicrobial coverage appropriate to suppress the large bowel microflora. This parenteral agent should be given within 30 minutes of the incision time and should be repeated in procedures lasting more than 2 hours.[8]

Selected Antibiotics With Dual Activity Against Aerobic and Anaerobic Colonic Microflora

- Ampicillin and sulbactam (combined form)
- Cefotetan
- Cefoxitin
- Ceftizoxime
- Piperacillin and tazobactam (combined form)
- Ticarcillin and clavulanic acid (combined form)

PREOPERATIVE BOWEL PREPARATION BEFORE URGENT SURGERY

Patients being prepared for urgent (nonelective) surgery usually require observation and treatment in a hospital setting. Such patients often present with signs and symptoms of partial bowel obstruction. These patients do not tolerate well the rapid mechanical bowel preparation outlined in Table 5-1 because such preparation can impact formed stool proximal to the stenotic area, thereby converting a partial obstruction to a complete one. Such a patient, who is otherwise in good and stable clinical condition, usually requires admission to the hospital for observation and resuscitation, as well as for correction of any fluid and electrolyte imbalances during the preoperative preparatory period. Support with parenteral administration of fluids and electrolytes is usually necessary, although some patients can hydrate themselves with clear liquids alone. Biochemical and hematologic studies should be obtained as needed, as should serial flat and erect abdominal radiographs. Often these patients will tolerate a decelerated mechanical bowel preparation using fractionated oral doses of a sodium phosphate solution such as Fleets phosphosoda given on preoperative days 2 and 3. Ten-milliliter aliquots of Fleets phosphosoda are given at hourly intervals for six doses on preoperative day 3 and then repeated on preoperative day 2 starting at 6 AM.

Should the patient develop increased abdominal pain or distension or signs of complete bowel obstruction, the decelerated oral mechanical bowel preparation should be terminated and the patient taken to urgent or emergency surgery. Appropriate parenteral perioperative antibiotic therapy should be administered and may require continuation into the postoperative period.

Those patients who tolerate the decelerated bowel preparation well, should continue to receive fluid and electrolyte support and should be given preoperative oral antibiotic prophylaxis with erythromycin base and neomycin sulfate with the usual timing on preoperative day 1. Surgery should follow the next day with appropriate parenteral antibiotic prophylaxis administered as suggested in the previous section.

PREOPERATIVE BOWEL PREPARATION BEFORE EMERGENCY SURGERY

Emergency situations requiring immediate surgical intervention seldom permit preoperative mechanical bowel preparation or oral antibiotic prophylaxis. An exception is the rare patient who undergoes surgery for complications following colonoscopy who has undergone mechanical bowel cleansing before endoscopy. Optimally, most patients should receive preoperative volume resuscitation with correction of biochemical or hematologic abnormalities before proceeding to surgery. Parenteral antibiotic therapy should be initiated at the time of admission if the underlying disease is of an infectious origin (e.g., diverticulitis, peritonitis) or is likely to result in infectious complications (e.g., bowel obstruction, perforation). The antimicrobial selected must have coverage for both the aerobic and anaerobic microflora of the gastrointestinal tract and often should be re-administered intraoperatively or continued into the postoperative period. This decision will depend on the intraoperative findings and the patient's subsequent postoperative course.[9]

Parenteral Antibiotic Therapy

The vast majority of colorectal surgeons currently advocate the use of parenteral perioperative antibiotic therapy whether the patient has undergone preoperative mechanical bowel preparation and oral antibiotic prophylaxis or not. It is essential that the agent or agents administered parenterally have adequate coverage of both the aerobic and anaerobic microflora of the gastrointestinal tract. Current consensus recommends that the parenteral agent be administered within 30 minutes of the incision. The custom of ordering its administration "on call to the operating room" should be avoided because unpredicted events may delay initiation of the surgical procedure.[10] Other factors such as the length of the operation, location of the portion of large bowel resected (intraperitoneal colon versus rectum), excessive blood loss intraoperatively, and the presence of a colonic perforation have been identified as prime risk factors for the development of postoperative infections.[2,8] The presence of any of these warrants consideration of the administration of a second dose of antibiotic 2 hours into the operation or its continuation into the postoperative period, or both.

Antibiotics That in Combination Provide Coverage of Colonic Microflora

- Aerobic coverage—to be used with a drug having anaerobic activity
  - Amikacin
  - Aztreonam
  - Cefotaxime
  - Ceftriaxone
  - Ciprofloxacin
  - Gentamicin
  - Tobramycin
- Anaerobic coverage—to be used with a drug having aerobic activity
  - Chloramphenicol
  - Clindamycin
  - Metronidazole

No single antibiotic agent or combination thereof should be relied on for prophylaxis in all operations. The patient's history of drug allergies may contraindicate the use of cephalosporins, which are the most widely used antibiotics for surgical prophylaxis worldwide.[9] It is also important to maintain an up-to-date hospital analysis of the antimicrobial sensitivities of isolates from surgical wound infections or intraoperative cultures. For colorectal surgery and appendectomy, the *Medical Letter on Drugs and Therapeutics* prefers cefoxitin or cefotetan because both are more active against bowel anaerobes than is cefazolin.[11] The use of third-generation cephalosporins for antibiotic prophylaxis of surgical wound infections is not generally recommended. Rather, they should be reserved for the treatment of infections caused by sensitive microorganisms. When an aminoglycoside is used for aerobic coverage, serum peak and trough levels should be monitored so as to achieve therapeutic but nontoxic drug levels. If antibiotic polypharmacy is chosen, the combination of antimicrobial agents selected should be limited to the fewest number possible and must provide appropriate aerobic and anaerobic coverage of the intestinal microflora.

CONCLUSION

That colorectal surgery is to be done laparoscopically rather than as a traditional "open" procedure should have little influence on the type of bowel preparation used perioperatively. Modern developments in preoperative mechanical bowel cleansing techniques and in preoperative oral antibiotic prophylaxis have resulted in a decreased rate of postoperative infectious complications.[2,12] Most colorectal surgeons complement these preoperative regimens with perioperative parenteral antibiotic prophylaxis, usually with a second-generation cephalosporin, although the use of other agents is appropriate if the necessary aerobic and anaerobic antimicrobial activities are present. The presence of associated risk factors encountered intraoperatively influences the duration of administration of perioperative and postoperative antimicrobial agents.

Most patients tolerate outpatient preoperative preparation for an elective colorectal surgical procedure well and in the process accrue savings to themselves and to the health care delivery system. In this situation, special attention must be paid to patient instruction to guarantee patient understanding of the techniques used and the medicines involved in preoperative mechanical bowel preparation and preoperative oral antibiotic bowel prophylaxis. Careful instruction will enable the patient to be fully compliant with the preoperative bowel preparation protocol selected and thereby decrease the risk of postoperative infections.

REFERENCES

1. Nichols RL, Condon RE: Preoperative preparation of the colon: collective review. Surg Gynecol Obstet 132:323, 1971
2. Nichols RL: Surgical wound infection. Am J Med, suppl. 3:S54, 1991
3. Frazee RC, Roberts J, Symmonds R et al: Prospective randomized trial of inpatient versus outpatient bowel preparation for elective colorectal surgery. Dis Colon Rectum 35:223, 1992
4. Fleites RA, Marshall JB, Eckhauser ML et al: The efficacy of polyethylene glycol electrolyte lavage solution versus traditional mechanical bowel preparation for elective colonic surgery: a randomized, prospective, blinded clinical trial. Surgery 98:708, 1985
5. Cohen SM, Wexner SD, Binderow SR et al: A prospective randomized endoscopic-blinded trial comparing precolonoscopy bowel cleansing methods. Dis Colon Rectum 37:689, 1994
6. Nichols RL: Bowel preparations. In Wilmore DW, Brennan MF, Harken AH et al (eds): Care of the Surgical Patient. VI. Preoperative Care. 2nd Ed. Scientific American, New York, 1990
7. Solla JA, Rothenberger DA: Preoperative bowel preparation—a survey of colon and rectal surgeons. Dis Colon Rectum 33:154, 1990
8. Coppa GF, Eng K: Factors involved in antibiotic selection in elective colon and rectal surgery. Surgery 104:853, 1988
9. Gorbach SL, Condon RE, Conte JE Jr et al: General guidelines for the evaluation of new anti-infective drugs for prophylaxis of surgical infections: evaluation of new anti-infective drugs for surgical prophylaxis. Clin Infect Dis, suppl. 15:S313, 1992
10. Classen DC, Evans RS, Pestonik SL et al: The timing of prophylactic administration of antibiotics and the risk of surgical wound infection. N Engl J Med 326:281, 1992
11. Antimicrobial prophylaxis in surgery. Med Lett Drug Ther 35:91, 1993
12. Nichols RL, Condon RE, Gorbach SL et al: Efficacy of preoperative antimicrobial preparation of the bowel. Ann Surg 176:227, 1972

Editorial Comment I

David E. Beck

Mechanical bowel cleansing and preoperative antibiotic preparation are essential to safe colorectal surgical resection. The developmental nature and the current limitations of laparoscopic bowel surgery result in increased bowel manipulation and a greater potential for intra-abdominal bacterial contamination. Thus, an intestine that is clean and decompressed is extremely important. Drs. Holmes and Nichols have produced a comprehensive review of current practices. With appropriate patient instruction and an efficient support staff, these preparations can be accomplished in an outpatient setting. This status is especially important in laparoscopic surgery, as one of its goals is to shorten the hospital stay. Several areas merit additional comment and are listed below:

1. Readers should be reminded that neither of the mechanical preparations described by Drs. Holmes and Nichols has received approval from the U.S. Food and Drug Administration for use as a preoperative bowel preparation.[1]
2. To ensure a clean colon for patients scheduled for surgery on the left colon,[1] many surgeons use rectal irrigation after induction of anesthesia. This technique identifies and eliminates any residual stool in the left colon. If the catheter used for irrigation is left in place, any additional gas or liquid stool can be expressed out through the catheter. Others have routinely employed preoperative colonoscopy to confirm a clean, dry, and decompressed colon[2] (see also Ch. 12).
3. Many surgeons use metronidazole (Flagyl) instead of Drs. Holmes and Nichols preference of erythromycin. Metronidazole eliminates the gastric distress associated with erythromycin.
4. Two surveys of board-certified colorectal surgeons have shown that the vast majority of surgeons favor the use of perioperative parenteral antibiotic prophylaxis during elective colorectal surgery after the successful completion of preoperative mechanical and oral antibiotic bowel preparation.[3,4] Several studies have also demonstrated that antibiotics with extended half-lives such as cefotetan (Cefotan) require only a single preoperative dose to obtain perioperative wound prophylaxis.[5,6] The second dose recommended by Drs. Holmes and Nichols may not be necessary if cefotetan or a similar long-acting antibiotic is used.

REFERENCES

1. Beck DE: Mechanical bowel cleansing for surgery. Prospect Colon Rectal Surg 7:97, 1994
2. Franklin M Jr, Ramos R, Rosenthal D et al: Laparoscopic colonic procedures. World Surg 17:51, 1993
3. Beck DE, Fazio VF: Current preoperative bowel cleansing methods. Results of a survey. Dis Colon Rectum 33:12, 1990
4. Solla JA, Rothenberger DA: Preoperative bowel preparation: a survey of colon and rectal surgeons. Dis Colon Rectum 33:154, 1990
5. Jagelman DG, Fabian TC, Nichols RL et al: Single dose cefotetan versus multiple dose cefoxitin as prophylaxis on colorectal surgery. Am J Surg, suppl. 155:71, 1988
6. Perti P, Mazzei T, Toneli F et al: Single dose cefotetan versus multiple dose cefoxitin—antimicrobial prophylaxis in colorectal surgery. Dis Colon Rectum 32:121, 1989

Editorial Comment II

Rama M. Jager

There are many physiologic advantages of gut lavage with a polyethylene glycol solution for preoperative bowel preparation. Disadvantages of this technique of bowel preparation include low patient acceptance and dilation of small bowel loops with retained gut lavage solution. The use of agents such as cisapride or metoclopramide just before the patient starts drinking the polyethylene glycol solution may facilitate rapid transit of the solution. These gastrokinetic agents also reduce the gastric fullness and nausea from rapid ingestion of the gut lavage solution. Having the patient take 15 mg of bisacodyl orally just before ingestion of the polyethylene glycol solution also promotes faster passage of the gut lavage solution.

Many patients also have difficulty in tolerating the oral antibiotics and experience nausea and epigastric distress. The problem of nausea, vomiting, and epigastric distress is more common with erythromycin than the related clindamycin. Since the antibacterial spectrum of both agents is similar, patients may tolerate clindamycin if they cannot take erythromycin. Oral metronidazole has also been used for oral antibiotic bowel preparation before colorectal surgical procedures.

Accidental injury to the colon during laparoscopic mobilization can lead to uncontrollable spillage of colonic contents into the peritoneal cavity. Thus, effective bowel preparation is an absolute requirement for laparoscopic colorectal surgery. If the colon is not properly prepared in patients undergoing open abdominal colectomy, intraoperative colonic lavage can be done. The laparoscopic surgeon does not have that option. Suboptimal bowel preparation may force the abandonment of the laparoscopic approach. Some laparoscopic surgeons go to the extent of verifying adequate bowel preparation by intraoperative colonoscopy before proceeding with laparoscopic mobilization. If there is any question as to the adequacy of mechanical bowel preparation, intraoperative colonoscopy before starting the laparoscopic mobilization is necessary. A colonoscopy should be performed after the establishment of pneumoperitoneum to avoid distension of the colon and small bowel from the insufflated air. Occluding the terminal ileum with an atraumatic endoscopic clamp prevents small intestinal insufflation in patients with an incompetent ileocecal valve. Problems with the intestinal insufflation interfering with the establishment of the pneumoperitoneum and the laparoscopic dissection become less important if the colonoscope is equipped to use carbon dioxide as an insufflating agent (see Ch. 12 for discussion of intraoperative colonoscopy).

6

Technique of Pneumoperitoneum

Jonathan M. Sackier

The peritoneal cavity is merely a potential space. The introduction of gas into this space produces the room in which the surgeon may manipulate instruments and perform surgical procedures. Therefore, the creation of this pneumoperitoneum is of vital importance to the completion of a laparoscopic operation. Several aspects of the pneumoperitoneum technique are considered in this chapter, including creation of the pneumoperitoneum (by either the closed or open technique), choice of gas and speed of insufflation, introduction of the trocars, maintenance of the pneumoperitoneum and its physiologic effects, and release of the abdominal gas.

HISTORY

Laparoscopy has its earliest recorded beginnings at the turn of the century with Ott in Petrograd[1] and Kelling in Dresden[2] reporting their experimental findings. In Stockholm, Jacobaeus[3] amassed a large clinical experience and laparoscopy was firmly on the clinician's map. The pneumoperitoneum was obtained with a foot pump and room air, until Fervers,[4] in 1933 proposed the use of carbon dioxide. The introduction of the pneumoneedle by Janos Veress[5] also proved to be a valued advance. Recent developments have been high-flow insufflators,[6] disposable trocar/cannula assemblies, alternate gases such as helium, and the suggested abandonment of pneumoperitoneum with abdominal lift devices for so-called gasless laparoscopy.[7–9]

PNEUMOPERITONEUM CREATION

Before surgery, completion of a full history and physical examination will alert the surgeon to potential problems such as adhesions, inguinal hernia, or liver disease.[10,11] Preoperative mapping of adhesions may be performed with ultrasound as described by Siegel et al.[12] The choice of position for needle insertion will depend on the findings found at the history and physical examination. Usually the umbilicus is ideal, but other sites include the iliac fossa or the hypochondrium in the midclavicular line. The abdominal wall should be palpated to assess the distance from the skin to the aorta. It is often surprising how negligible this distance is in very slim patients. There are a number of tests of needle position. None are foolproof, but together they do render the operation safer.

The first is the "hiss" test; the surgeon opens the top of the Veress needle and lifts the abdominal wall so that the negative pressure sucks air through the needle. The surgeon should then attach a syringe to aspirate and then inject sterile saline. If a little blood is retrieved, the needle position should be changed and the examination continued. If blood gushes out, the surgeon should assume that a major vessel has been injured and perform laparotomy to correct the problem as a matter of urgency. The retrieval of intestinal contents should lead to replacement of the needle, continuation of the laparoscopy, and evaluation of the injury. Often the puncture is so small that it will suffice to treat the patient conservatively with nasogastric suction and intravenous antibiotics and keep the patient nil per os (NPO). Certainly, a large hole will merit surgical repair either by laparoscopy or open surgery, depending on the surgeon's proficiency. If on aspiration, saline is returned, the tip of the needle is almost certainly in the preperitoneal space and must be reinserted.

The next test is to place a "hanging drop" of saline in the hub of the needle, open the top, and see whether it disappears. The disappearance of saline into the peritoneal cavity reflects the negative intraperitoneal pressure and confirms intraperitoneal placement of the needle tip.

The Palmer test[13] (sequentially sucking and aspirating saline) can be used to ascertain whether there are any adhesions near the needle. This is best done once the pneumoperitoneum has been completed.

INSUFFLATION

Once the needle is correctly inserted, the insufflation tubing should be joined to the needle. If the needle is free within the peritoneal cavity, low pressures and high flow rates will be seen. If the pressures are high but previous tests suggest that the needle is within the peritoneum, the surgeon may rotate the needle circumferentially or alter its position to disentangle the attached omentum. However, the surgeon should not change the depth to which the needle has been introduced because at this stage a blood vessel may inadvertently be punctured. The use of a filter between the insufflator and the patient has been suggested to stop the transfer of microorganisms to the patient and to prevent contamination by transfer of body fluids from one patient to another (Hunter JG, personal communication, 1991).

Some surgeons believe that a pneumoperitoneum is unnecessary and choose to insert sharp trocars immediately. This technique is dangerous and should be decried because the pneumoperitoneum provides a safety cushion into which the trocar may more safely be inserted. An alternative technique used routinely by some but selectively by myself is open laparoscopy. Originally described by Hasson,[14] this technique involves making a circumferential incision under the umbilicus and dissecting parallel to the upper tissue plane. By elevating the subumbilical skin, a vertical raphe may be palpated, grasped between two Kocher clamps, and incised, leading into the peritoneal cavity.[15] The open laparoscopy cannula has a sliding olive seal to which sutures are attached to ensure that no gas leaks during the procedure. This technique is valuable when adhesions or an umbilical hernia are suspected or when Veress needle insertion fails (Fig. 6-1).

A good indication that the needle is in the preperitoneal space is if the insufflation pressure is initially about 8 mm Hg, which then drops after 1 L of carbon dioxide is insufflated and then steadily climbs. A consistently high pressure should lead the surgeon to change the position of the needle. If the insufflation pressure remains low despite good flow rates and after a large volume of gas is infused, there is a leak in the system, the needle is within the lumen of the bowel or in the bladder, or the patient has an inguinal or hiatal hernia. If a hiatal hernia is suspected from the patient's medical history, the anesthesiologist should be informed to very carefully monitor the patient because filling a large hiatal hernia with carbon dioxide can lead to cardiorespiratory complications.

The maximum flow rate one can achieve through a Veress needle is not much over 2.5 L, but as an added safeguard, the surgeon should insufflate at about 1.5 L/min. At this flow rate it is extremely unlikely that there will be any cardiorespiratory problems; if they do occur, the anesthesiologist has an opportunity to cor-

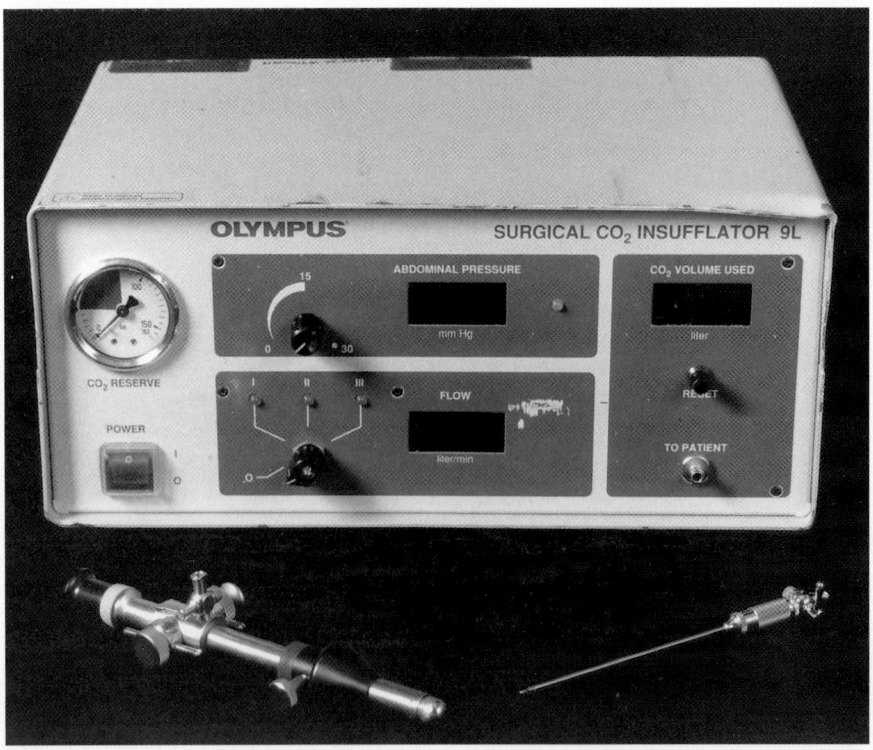

Fig. 6-1. Equipment needed to create the pneumoperitoneum: Veress needle, Hasson cannula, and high-flow insufflator.

rect them. In addition, if the needle is inadvertently inside the lumen of a blood vessel, the lower the infusion rate, the greater the patient's chance of absorbing the gas. It is my practice to convert to the higher flow rates (6 to 10 L/min) only after a steady pressure state has been reached and the cannula is within the abdomen. This may seem like an extremely conservative approach, but by taking the extra 1 or 2 minutes to create the pneumoperitoneum, potentially fatal complications are avoided.[16,17]

GAS

The choice of gas for insufflation now rests between carbon dioxide and nitrous oxide. Historically, air and oxygen were used, but the former was aborted because of the time taken for the gas to be absorbed, the pain it caused, and the support of combustion. There are some who maintain that nitrous oxide causes less postoperative pain, but that may be related to the time taken for the procedure, which causes diaphragmatic stretching and phrenic nerve irritation. Carbon dioxide is cheaper, more available, and more rapidly absorbed from the circulation but does have some inherent problems: it causes vasodilation, which can be misinterpreted by the neophyte laparoscopist as peritonitis. This dilation may very rarely cause vascular collapse in an elderly patient. The absorption will cause a decrease in the pH and an increase in the partial pressure of oxygen (PCO_2). Therefore, the anesthesiologist should monitor the patient carefully.

Recently, it has been suggested that inert gases, such as helium, may obviate some of these concerns, but there are insufficient data at the moment. A number of authors have proposed the use of mechanical retractors to hold the abdominal wall up and away from the viscera.[7–9] This technique may have some value for certain procedures, especially operations expected to take a long time or ones in which the patient has problems with cardiorespiratory compromise or morbid obesity.

MAINTENANCE

After the pneumoperitoneum has been created, it is time to insert the trocar/cannula assembly. A number of safety features should be considered. First, the barrel of the cannula should always be held with one hand to prevent accidentally introducing the trocar too far and risking the chance of injuring the viscera or major vessels. In addition, since the surgeon is most concerned about hitting the aorta, the simple safety step of not aiming at it should be taken. It is extremely important to have sharp trocars, as less force is required to insert them, diminishing the chance of iatrogenic injury. Some trocars have retractable safety shields, which may prove advantageous, but the shields should not lower the surgeon's level of caution during this vital stage of the operation.

PHYSIOLOGIC CONSIDERATIONS

The pneumoperitoneum limits the return of blood from the legs. During extended procedures like laparoscopic cholecystectomy, there may be an increased risk of deep venous thrombosis. Therefore, I routinely use sequential compression stockings. In addition, the increased abdominal pressure interferes with ventilation pressures; the anesthesiologist should be made aware of this.[18] These effects could also have an impact on cardiac function by causing hypo- or hypertension or dysrhythmias, the most common of which is bradycardia. As noted above, the absorption of carbon dioxide will cause acidosis and hypercapnia. For this reason, the ventilatory rate may need to be increased, and those patients likely to be more sensitive (such as those with chronic obstructive pulmonary disease) should have a thorough preoperative workup.

For the above reasons, the anesthesiologist should very carefully monitor the patient by heart rate, cardiogram, pulse oximetry, and possibly end-tidal carbon dioxide. If any problems are noted, the surgeon should *immediately* cease insufflation and desufflate the abdomen by opening one of the valves and aspirating the gas.

A major concern is gas embolism. Care with insertion of the Veress needle and trocar avoids this problem. The anesthesiologist should be aware of the clinical signs and management of this potentially fatal complication (see also Ch. 4).

RELEASE

At the end of the operation, the pneumoperitoneum should be released by opening one of the cannula valves and placing the suction tubing near the cannula to aspirate the gas. The surgeon should not breathe in this gas, as it may contain particulate matter such as viruses. The aim should be to completely desufflate the abdomen, as this limits the patient's shoulder discomfort due to phrenic nerve irritation postoperatively. Occasionally, some subcutaneous emphysema occurs. This is more likely if one of the cannulas accidentally slips out during the operation or if the gas seal between the cannula and skin is poor. Although this condition may produce anxiety in some patients, they should be reassured. The subcutaneous emphysema will be rapidly absorbed and cause no problems. All patients should be thoroughly examined before the operation to exclude the presence of an inguinal hernia. If one is discovered, it should be covered with a truss perioperatively. However, if a small hernia is missed, a pneumoscrotum may develop. This is a distressing condition for the patient, but one that does not usually cause any sequelae.

REFERENCES

1. Ott D: Die direkte Beleuchtung der Bauchhole, der Harnblase, des Dickdarms und des Uterus zu diagnostichen Zwecken. Rev Ned Tcheque (Prague) 2:27, 1909
2. Kelling G: Zur Coelioskopie. Arch Klin Chir 126:226, 1923
3. Jacobaeus HC: Kurze Ubersicht uber meine Erfahrungen mit der Laparoskopie. Munch Med Wochenschr 58:2017, 1923
4. Fervers C: Die Laparoskopie mit dem Cystoskope. Med Klin 29:1042, 1933
5. Veress J: Neues Instrument zue Aufuhrung von Brust oder Bauchpunktionen. Dtsch Med Wochenschr 41:1480, 1938
6. Berci G, Cuschieri A: Practical Laparoscopy. Baillierre Tindall, London, 1986
7. Nagai H, Kondo Y, Yasuda T et al: A new method of laparoscopic cholecystectomy and other abdominal surgery: an abdominal wall-life technique not utilizing peritoneal insufflation. Surg Endosc 6:87, 1992
8. Kitano S, Moriyama M, Sugimachi K: A newly designed U-shaped retractor for laparoscopic cholecystectomy. Surg Endosc 6:10l, 1992
9. Banting S, Shimi S, Van der Velpen G et al: Abdominal wall lift: low-pressure pneumoperitoneum laparoscopic surgery. Surg Endosc 7:57, 1993
10. Sackier JM, Berci G: Diagnostic and interventional laparoscopy for the general surgeon. Contemp Surg 37:15, 1990
11. Sackier JM, Berci G, Paz-Partlow M: Elective diagnostic laparoscopy. Am J Surg 161:326, 1991
12. Siegel B, Golub RM, Loiacano L et al: Technique of ultrasonic detection and mapping of abdominal wall adhesions. Surg Endosc 5:161, 1991
13. Palmer R: Security in laparoscopy. p. 17. In Phillips JM, Keith L (eds): Gynecological Laparoscopy: Principles and Techniques. Symposia Specialists Medical Books, New York, 1974
14. Hasson HM: Open laparoscopy vs. closed laparoscopy. A comparison of complication rates. Adv Planned Parenthood 13:41, 1978
15. Sackier JM: Laparoscopic cholecystectomy. In Hunter JG, Sackier JM (eds): Minimally Invasive Surgery. McGraw-Hill, New York, 1993
16. Lindemann HJ: Atlas der Hysteroskopie. Fischer, Stuttgart, 1980
17. Doctor HN, Hussain Z: Bilateral pneumothorax associated with laparoscopy: a case report of a rare hazard and review of the literature. Anesthesiology 28:75, 1973
18. Wittgen CM, Andrus CH, Fitzgerald SD et al: Analysis of the hemodynamic and ventilatory effects of laparoscopic cholecystectomy. Arch Surg 126:997, 1991

Editorial Comment

Rama M. Jager

Although surgeons generally use pneumoperitoneum for laparoscopic surgery, pneumoperitoneum is not indispensable for laparoscopic technique. The objective is to displace the abdominal wall away from the viscera by one means or another. Intraperitoneal or extraperitoneal carbon dioxide, nitrous oxide, and more recently, helium are the gases most commonly used to displace the abdominal wall from the viscera and create a working space for the surgeon to maneuver the surgical instruments. Unless "gasless" laparoscopy with the aid of various abdominal wall lifting devices completely replaces the need for pneumoperitoneum, laparoscopic surgeons need to understand the various techniques of pneumoperitoneum, its establishment and maintenance, and the potential complications associated with insufflation of the peritoneum with carbon dioxide or other gases.

ABDOMINAL WALL HEMATOMAS

Abdominal wall hematoma secondary to insertion of a Veress needle or peritoneal cannula is not an uncommon occurrence. Bleeding from the puncture site often stops spontaneously. By contrast, continued bleeding may require intraoperative measures such as suture ligation of the bleeding vessel under laparoscopic guidance and Foley balloon tamponade (Fig. 6-2) or postoperative abdominal wall exploration to drain the hematoma and stop continued bleeding.

Abdominal wall hematomas develop from injury to the inferior epigastric, superficial epigastric, and superficial circumflex iliac arteries by the peritoneal puncturing instrument. Insertion of the Veress needle or the trocars lateral to the lateral margins of the rectus muscle reduces the chance of hematomas; however, this may not be feasible in all patients. The anatomic location of the abdominal wall vessels at risk of injury during the establishment of pneumoperitoneum have been studied by abdominal computed tomography (CT).[1] Superior to the symphysis pubis, the inferior epigastric vessels are 5.6 ± 1.0 cm, and the superficial epigastric vessels are 5.5 ± 2.0 cm from the midline. At the umbilical level, the superficial epigastric arteries are 4.6 ± 1.4 cm, the circumflex iliac vessels 10.7 ± 1.7 cm, and the lateral rectus muscle margins 7.6 ± 1.5 cm from the midline. When the abdominal wall puncture must be through the rectus muscle and the laparoscopic landmarks are not visible to guide placement, lateral trocars should be at least 8 cm away from the midline and 5 cm above the symphysis to reduce the risk of abdominal wall hematomas.[1]

PORT SITE HERNIAS

Port site hernias are another common problem following laparoscopic surgery. Incisional hernias often develop at the sites of port insertion either immediately postoperatively or during the first year after the operation. Incomplete emptying of carbon dioxide pneumoperitoneum and leaving a large amount of irrigation fluid in the peritoneal cavity may promote the formation of incisional hernias.[2] Closure of fascial defects, especially those from trocars larger than 10 mm, and careful deflation of pneumoperitoneum at the end of the laparoscopic operation may reduce the risk of these port site hernias. (This topic is also addressed in the editorial comments following Chs. 8 and 21.)

OPEN VERSUS CLOSED TECHNIQUE

Blind insertion of the Veress needle or a trocar can lead to various complications such as bowel or blood vessel injury, at times with catastrophic consequences.[3] Some gynecologists use the technique of blind insertion of a trocar without initial pneumoperitoneum induced with a Veress needle.[4,5] I agree with Dr. Sackier that blind trocar insertion can be dangerous and has little to recommend for less experienced laparoscopic surgeons.

Some of the problems associated with blind insertion of a Veress needle or trocar make some opt for the open insertion technique. There are various advantages to open insertion of a blunt-tipped cannula through a small incision to introduce pneumoperitoneum. This open technique avoids the problem of visceral and vascular trauma by the puncturing instrument. However, there are also certain disadvantages to the open tech-

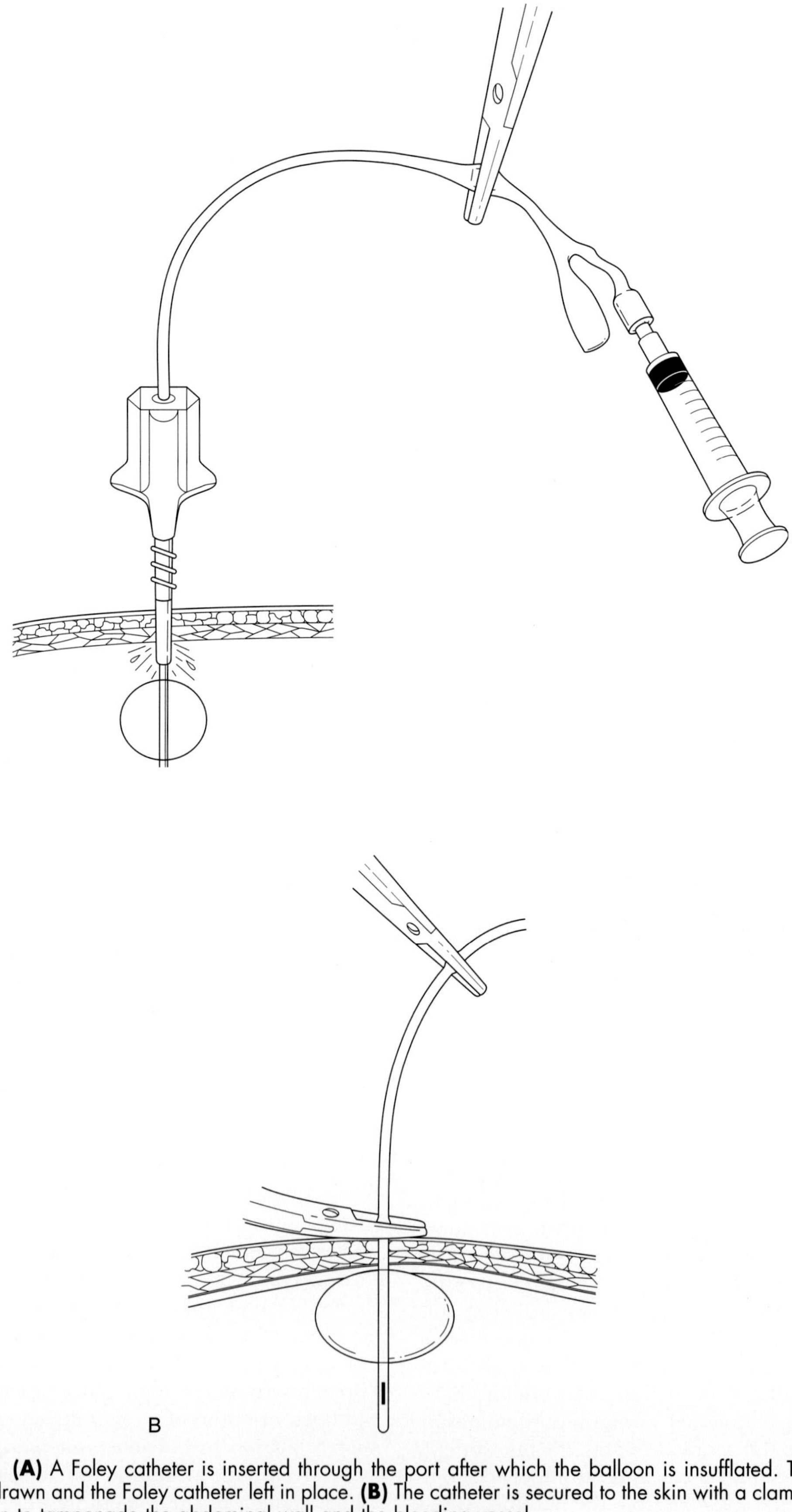

A

B

Fig. 6-2. (A) A Foley catheter is inserted through the port after which the balloon is insufflated. The port is then withdrawn and the Foley catheter left in place. **(B)** The catheter is secured to the skin with a clamp to allow the balloon to tamponade the abdominal wall and the bleeding vessel.

nique. The open technique can be difficult in extremely obese patients. In addition, it requires the placement of fascial sutures to prevent gas leakage around the cannula. Visceral injury from fascial sutures has been described.[6] I prefer to use the open technique of cannula placement for initiation of pneumoperitoneum only in patients who have had previous abdominal surgery. Surgeons who are not trained in the use of Veress needle initiation of pneumoperitoneum may find it safe to use the open placement of a blunt cannula in all patients. Some surgeons report blunt cannula placement in less than 5 minutes,[7] even in obese patients, although I often require quite a bit more time to achieve the same objective.

OPTICAL TROCARS

Various ingenious devices have been described, such as an insufflation needle with a transparent conical tip and an attached endoscope to permit puncture of the abdominal wall under direct vision.[8,9] Similar instruments to achieve direct optical visualization during the abdominal wall puncture are currently available at most North American hospitals, although I fail to see the need for such instruments for most patients. By contrast, patients with previous abdominal operations and consequent intra-abdominal adhesions may benefit from the use of such instruments. However, caution must be exercised because major complications such as visceral and vascular injury can occur from the use of the visible port devices. Open placement of a blunt-tipped cannula achieves the same objective of avoiding visceral or vascular injury as these optical devices. The former technique also avoids the expense of the optical cannulas.

CARBON DIOXIDE WARMING

Warming the carbon dioxide to 37°C before instillation into the peritoneal cavity can reduce intraoperative hypothermia. Some authors have reported a reduction in tachycardia from 40 to 11 percent by use of the warming technique.[10] (The issue of hypothermia and the advantages of warming the carbon dioxide are also addressed in the editorial comments in Ch. 7.)

GASLESS LAPAROSCOPY

Multiple problems associated with the technique pneumoperitoneum initiation and maintenance raise the option of avoiding pneumoperitoneum use by using various abdominal wall lifting devices to achieve "gasless" laparoscopy. One such device includes an electric-powered abdominal wall lifter.[11] Mechanical lifting of the abdominal wall away from the viscera establishes a working space for the surgeon to see and manipulate the viscera as needed. Some authors propose that the planar ceiling achieved by abdominal wall lifting, in contrast to the domed ceiling of a carbon dioxide sealed pneumoperitoneum, brings the abdominal organs closer to the surgeon. They suggest that this shortens the needed instrument length.[12] Since no gas is used to lift the abdominal wall away from the viscera, gas leakage at the port sites poses no difficulty. Also, right-angle clamps can be used through the original mini-incision or through separate stab wounds. In patients with a pneumoperitoneum, advancing the right-angle clamps through the rigid peritoneal cannulas is difficult. Other proposed advantages include the avoidance of the physiologic side effects of pneumoperitoneum, as well as the ability to digitally palpate the intra-abdominal organs through the mini-incision after lifting the abdominal wall away from the viscera. I have little experience with gasless laparoscopy.

CONCLUSION

The pneumoperitoneum needed for laparoscopic surgery is not benign. Most of the complications from laparoscopic surgery occur during the initiation and maintenance of the pneumoperitoneum. Whichever technique is used for the pneumoperitoneum, care and attention to detail is essential to reduce the risk of complications.

REFERENCES

1. Hurd WW, Bude RO, DeLancey JO, Newman JS: The location of abdominal wall blood vessels in relationship to abdominal landmarks apparent at laparoscopy. Am J Obstet Gynecol 171:642, 1994
2. Howard FM, Sweeney TR: Omental herniation after operative laparoscopy. A case report. J Reprod Med 39:415, 1994
3. Kaali SO, Barad DH: Incidence of bowel injury due to dense adhesions at the sight of direct trocar insertion. J Reprod Med 37:617, 1992
4. Byron JW, Markenson G, Miyazawa K: A randomized comparison of Veress needle and direct trocar insertion for laparoscopy. Surg Gynecol Obstet 177:25, 1993
5. Nezhat FR, Silfen SL, Evans D et al: Comparison of direct insertion of disposable and standard reusable laparoscopic trocars and previous pneumoperitoneum with Veress needle. Obstet Gynecol 78:148, 1991
6. Sadeghi-Nejad H, Kavoussi LR, Peters CA: Bowel injury in open technique laparoscopic cannula placement. Urology 43:559, 1994
7. Hurd WW, Ohl DA: Blunt trocar laparoscopy. Fertil Steril 61:1177, 1994
8. Riek S, Bachmann KH, Gaiselmann T, Hoernstein F et al: A new insufflation needle with a special optical system for use in laparoscopic procedures. Obstet Gynecol 84:476, 1994
9. Melzer A, Weiss U, Roth K, Loeffler M et al: Visually controlled trocar insertion by means of the optical scalpel. Endosc Surg Allied Technol 1:239, 1993

10. Trappe M, Kube D: Pain reduction after pelvi-laparoscopic interventions by insufflation of CO_2 gas at body temperature (Flow-Therme). Geburtshilfe Frauenheilkd 54:300, 1994
11. Tsoi EK, Smith RS, Fry WR, Henderson VJ et al: Laparoscopic surgery without pneumoperitoneum. A preliminary report. Surg Endosc 8:382, 1994
12. Eaton J, Tsoi EK, Smith RS, Fry WR et al: Gasless laparoscopy using a planar lifting technique. J Am Coll Surg 178:401, 1994

7

Physiology of Pneumoperitoneum

P. Jan Chandler and H. Randolph Bailey

For many years laparoscopy has been used primarily for gynecologic procedures, which are, in general, operations of brief duration performed on young, healthy women with few systemic consequences.[1,2] Even in this patient population, however, occasional reports of intraoperative hypotension and cardiac arrest have appeared.[3] Cognat et al[4] estimated the incidence of acute cardiovascular collapse during gynecologic laparoscopy to be 1 in 2,000, and fatal in 1.2 in 10,000.

With the advent of improved technology, including high-resolution video camera systems, better light sources, and high-flow insufflators, the scope of laparoscopic surgery has rapidly expanded.[5] The ability to perform more complex operations has resulted in procedures of longer duration and the inclusion of older patients and those with pre-existing cardiopulmonary diseases. Evidence that patients with diagnosed cardiac or pulmonary disease (or both) have a higher operative morbidity and mortality from laparoscopic surgery than do otherwise healthy patients is not surprising.[6] Although patients with significant pre-existing diseases may benefit the most from the reduced invasiveness and faster postoperative recovery, the physiologic stresses associated with laparoscopic surgery may cause more severe physiologic disturbances than open surgery in this group.[7,8]

Many factors contribute to the circulatory instability during laparoscopy. The most important seems to be increased intra-abdominal pressure associated with maintaining adequate pneumoperitoneum.[1,9] It is important therefore to understand the physiology of pneumoperitoneum in order to minimize its adverse effects and reduce the morbidity and mortality associated with laparoscopic surgery.

PULMONARY EFFECTS

Increased intra-abdominal pressure elevates the diaphragm, which results in increased ventilation pressure,[1,3,5] decreased pulmonary compliance that is progressive throughout the period of insufflation,[9,10] and a reduction in functional residual capacity (FRC).[11] The chest wall component of total compliance in the Trendelenburg position is particularly affected, decreasing to about 50 percent of preoperative values.[12] The reverse Trendelenburg position, however, may reduce these effects in that the FRC is increased,[13] as is compliance,[12] when compared with measurements in the supine or Trendelenburg positions.

Decreased compliance and altered ventilation result in increased pulmonary shunting, which may result in hypoxia.[14] Adequate oxygenation can be maintained by minimizing peritoneal insufflation pressure, increasing the inspired oxygen fraction (FIO_2), and ventilating with large tidal volumes to prevent progressive alveolar atelectasis.[7] The use of positive end expiratory pressure (PEEP) has also been recommended but should be used cautiously, since the associated increase in intrathoracic pressure may significantly reduce cardiac output.[7,15]

Both ventilation-perfusion mismatch and a decrease in cardiac output may cause a significant increase in dead space ventilation.[2] The resulting impaired elimination of carbon dioxide is evidenced by a large increase in the arterial partial pressure of carbon dioxide ($PaCO_2$) without an associated increase in the end-tidal carbon dioxide ($ETCO_2$) level.[2] These changes may be seen with any of the gases used for insufflation but are particularly pronounced with carbon dioxide because of its peritoneal absorption.

With carbon dioxide insufflation for laparoscopic surgery, hypercarbia and accompanying respiratory acidosis are common occurrences.[14] Hypercarbia may result from carbon dioxide embolism or from subcutaneous emphysema from slippage of a trocar into a subcutaneous position.[5,16] It is usually, however, the result of peritoneal absorption of the insufflated gas. Increased minute ventilation is necessary to enhance the elimination of absorbed carbon dioxide and to counteract the mechanical and ventilatory effects of increased intra-abdominal pressure.[12]

Although the need for increased minute ventilation is well established,[12,14] the degree of increase needed to maintain normal $PaCO_2$ levels is influenced by the position of the patient,[12] the presence of underlying cardiopulmonary disease,[2,14] and the duration of the operation. In a study of healthy patients undergoing pelvic laparoscopy in the Trendelenburg position, a 20 to 30 percent increase in minute ventilation was necessary to maintain normal $PaCO_2$ levels,[17] whereas in a study of healthy patients undergoing laparoscopic cholecystectomy in the reverse Trendelenburg position, increasing minute ventilation by only 12 to 16 percent maintained the $PaCO_2$ at acceptable levels.[12] Hypercarbia, however, occurred in spite of increases in minute ventilation of up to 30 percent in patients with pulmonary disease who underwent laparoscopic surgery.[2,14]

The increased carbon dioxide elimination associated with carbon dioxide insufflation[9] is associated with an increase in $ETCO_2$.[2] Alveolar PCO_2 ($PACO_2$) and therefore $ETCO_2$ is determined by multiple factors, including carbon dioxide production and absorption, delivery of carbon dioxide to the lungs (cardiac output), effective ventilation (minute ventilation minus dead space ventilation), and diffusion capacity.[14]

Although an increase in minute ventilation does not necessarily cause a proportionate increase in alveolar ventilation, it is the most common method of dealing with the extra carbon dioxide absorbed through the peritoneum and the effects of reduced compliance.[8] One danger in this approach is that the increased ventilation may decrease cardiac output, paradoxically increasing dead space ventilation and resulting in an increasing $PaCO_2$ that is not reflected in the $ETCO_2$.[12] It is well established that $ETCO_2$ does not always reflect $PaCO_2$ changes.[12,14] It has been demonstrated that $ETCO_2$ values greater than 41 mm Hg are not satisfactory indicators of $PaCO_2$. Values less than 41 mm Hg can, however, be used as an index of $PaCO_2$ (with the awareness that an increase in $PaCO_2$ due to decreased cardiac output may exist in some patients).[12,16] Attempts have been made to identify those patients at risk of developing intraoperative hypercarbia and acidosis during carbon dioxide pneumoperitoneum.[14,18] In one study, a forced expiratory volume in 1 second (FEV_1) of less than 1 L and a maximal voluntary ventilation of less than 50 percent of predicted values were high-risk indicators for pulmonary complications associated with anesthesia regardless of the operative site.[18] In another study, a diffusion capacity of less than 80 percent of predicted values was associated with a 50 percent chance of acidosis developing as compared with 12 percent in the absence of a diffusion defect.[14] Unfortunately, arterial blood gas analysis and simple bedside spirometry did not accurately identify patients at risk of developing these complications.[14]

CARDIOVASCULAR EFFECTS

The hemodynamic effects of increased intra-abdominal pressure and pneumoperitoneum have been extensively examined, often with widely divergent findings. This variability is readily explained by the many factors that have an effect on these cardiovascular changes. Among these factors are the following: type and depth of anesthesia, presence or absence of cardiopulmonary disease, intravascular volume status, gas selected for insufflation (carbon dioxide, nitrous oxide, helium), insufflation pressures, duration of insufflation, position (Trendelenburg's vs. reverse Trendelenburg's), and degree of surgical trauma.[19]

Cardiac Arrhythmias

Cardiac arrhythmias may occur as a complication of the initial creation of pneumoperitoneum.[20] Cardiac events may be sympathetically or parasympathetically mediated.[1,5] The sympathetic reflex response generally results in tachycardia with or without associated hypertension, whereas the vasovagal response is associated with bradycardia and hypotension.[3,5] Pretreatment with atropine is recommended to prevent vasovagal complications.[5] Treatment consists of exsufflation of the pneumoperitoneum and stabilization of the patient. If the baseline status is quickly restored, then pneumoperitoneum may be re-established in a slow fashion.[5]

Cardiac Function

Evaluation of the effect of increased intra-abdominal pressure on cardiac output has resulted in variable outcomes. Two studies in the early 1970s reported an increase in cardiac output in young, healthy women undergoing laparoscopy for gynecologic conditions.[10,21] Three other studies reported no significant change in cardiac output in healthy adults.[3,22,23] Most clinical and experimental studies, however, show evidence of decreased cardiac output.[1,9,24–28] One recent representative clinical study[28] found that cardiac output decreased in most (53 to 80 percent) patients by 20 to 26 percent, but the magnitude of the reduction decreased with the duration of the pneumoperitoneum. The two factors responsible for decreased cardiac output are increased systemic vascular resistance (SVR)[26,27] and decreased venous return.[25] There is little controversy surrounding the changes in other parameters, with most studies reporting an increased heart rate, increased mean arterial pressure, increased central venous pressure, increased pulmonary artery wedge pressure, and decreased stroke index.[2,9,21,25–27]

PERIPHERAL VASCULAR EFFECTS

Increased SVR is a consistent finding associated with elevated intra-abdominal pressure.[1,3,9,25–27] Proposed mechanisms of development include direct compression of the abdominal aorta, increased sympathetic activity with arteriolar contraction, and increased splanchnic venous resistance.[1,9,24,27] It is likely that all three factors contribute to some degree. The end result is a significant increase in SVR, measured in one study at 30 percent.[25]

Increased intra-abdominal pressure results in a notable increase in lower extremity venous pressure[29] and impedance to venous flow in the common femoral vein.[30] The decreased venous flow contributes to decreased cardiac output on the basis of decreased venous return.[25,27] Because of the associated risk of deep venous thrombosis (DVT), prophylaxis is important.[5] Although the effectiveness of different methods of DVT prophylaxis for laparoscopic surgery have not been studied, one report demonstrates a return to normal venous flow at an intra-abdominal pressure of 13 to 15 mm Hg in a 30-degree reverse Trendelenburg's position using intermittent pneumatic compression devices.[30]

It was demonstrated in 1987 that an intra-abdominal pressure of 20 mm Hg caused a decrease in tissue blood flow in all intra-abdominal organs except the adrenal gland.[26] The reduction was greater than could be explained by the measured decrease in cardiac output. Two recent studies in dogs have confirmed these results, documenting impairment of blood flow in the superior mesenteric artery and portal vein at intra-abdominal pressures of 14 to 16 mm Hg for 1 to 3 hours.[1,24] There was a rapid decrease in jejunal mucosal blood flow to 50 percent of baseline associated with decreased tissue pH (consistent with tissue ischemia).[1]

Several mechanisms have been proposed to explain the decreased splanchnic blood flow.[24] Mechanical compression of the splanchnic veins results in increased resistance and decreased flow. Humorally induced vasoconstriction may be due to the release of vasopressin stimulated by increased intra-abdominal pressure and peritoneal distension. Splanchnic arteriolar vasoconstriction is caused by elevated venous outflow pressures due to compression. Hypercapnia may also produce increased portal pressure and mesenteric vasoconstriction.[24] Although the clinical significance of the observed decrease in splanchnic blood flow remains to be defined, the results suggest the possibility of intestinal ischemia, gastric mucosal ulceration, and organ dysfunction as potential complications of laparoscopic surgery, especially in cases of long duration.[1,26]

RENAL FUNCTION AND NEUROHUMORAL CHANGES

For most of this century it has been known that increased intra-abdominal pressure has an adverse effect on renal function.[31] More recent clinical and experimental data have confirmed this early work. An intra-abdominal pressure of 15 to 20 mm Hg produces oliguria, and anuria ensues at pressures greater than 20 mm Hg, even in the absence of hypotension or hypovolemia.[32] Several mechanisms have been proposed to explain this phenomenon, with the most likely possibilities being direct renal compression, inferior vena cava and renal vein obstruction, and compression of the intra-abdominal aorta resulting in increased arterial vascular resistance and lower renal blood flow.[32] Caldwell and Ricotta[26] subsequently showed that decreased renal blood flow does occur with increased intra-abdominal pressure, but urine output was not measured in their study.

Three recent clinical investigations have looked at the renal effects of increased intra-abdominal pressure associated with laparoscopic surgery. The first study compared healthy patients undergoing laparoscopic and open cholecystectomy.[23] There was a significant decrease in urine output, effective renal plasma flow, and glomerular filtration rate in the laparoscopy group 60 minutes after carbon dioxide insufflation at 12 mm Hg. These effects reversed immediately after exsufflation. These results were attributed to increased intra-abdominal pressure alone, since there was no concomitant decrease in blood pressure, cardiac output, or circulatory volume. Another study compared a group of patients with known heart disease with a group of healthy patients undergoing laparoscopic cholecystectomy.[33] Urine output 30 to 60 minutes after the initiation of pneumoperitoneum in the group with heart disease was significantly lower than that in the healthy control group, although urine output was decreased in both groups. A third study looked at the effect on creatinine clearance when carbon dioxide pneumoperitoneum was maintained at 10 mm Hg for laparoscopic cholecystectomy.[34] Even at this low pressure, creatinine clearance decreased in 29 of 48 patients, falling to less than 50 percent of preoperative values in 8 of these patients. Postoperative renal function was normal in all cases. Although neurohumoral factors are thought to play a role in regulating many of the physiologic changes encountered during periods of increased intra-abdominal pressure, these effects have not yet been adequately studied.

At this time it appears that the renal effects in patients with normal renal function are immediately reversible on return to normal intra-abdominal pressure. For patients with pre-existing renal dysfunction or decreased cardiac output, consideration should be given to intermittent exsufflation during operations requiring prolonged pneumoperitoneum.[24]

GAS EMBOLISM

Gas embolism is a rare but potentially fatal complication of laparoscopic surgery.[7,35–37] In gynecologic laparoscopy, the incidence ranges from 1 in 63,845 cases to 8 in 50,247 cases.[36] Occurring most frequently in the initial phase of laparoscopic procedures,[38] gas embolism is usually due to the direct intravenous injection of gas through a misplaced Veress needle.[37] Although insufflation-induced puncture wounds in blood vessels, the liver, and the uterus are frequently identified after these occurrences,[38] evidence of these direct or indirect vascular injuries is sometimes absent.[7,38]

In addition to direct blood vessel puncture, it has been proposed that increased intra-abdominal pressure may force gas into an injured vessel if the opening is kept patent by surrounding tissue.[7] This mechanism seems more likely to apply to neurosurgical procedures on the cranium than in the abdominal cavity, where pressure would be more likely to result in the collapse of soft tissue and blood vessels. Another proposed mechanism suggests that blood flow across an opening in an injured vessel entrains gas by the venturi effect.[7]

The clinical consequences of venous gas embolism depend on the rate of passage into the vascular system, the volume of gas introduced, and the nature of the gas introduced.[7,38] Gas injection of significant volume commonly produces cardiovascular collapse on the basis of pulmonary outflow tract obstruction, causing decreased venous return and decreased cardiac output.[35,36,38] If smaller gas bubbles pass through the right heart and enter the pulmonary circulation, however, the result is pulmonary hypertension, right ventricular failure, and noncardiogenic pulmonary edema, as is seen during neurosurgical procedures with slow air entrainment.[38] Although the effects of embolization are usually immediately apparent, passage through the portal system has delayed the onset of symptoms by up to 1 hour.[37]

Carbon dioxide is highly soluble and therefore rapidly absorbed. With a carbon dioxide embolus, symptoms are rapidly reversed unless complete cardiovascular collapse has occurred.[35] Experimental studies have demonstrated that the body should be able to absorb carbon dioxide at the rate of 1 L/min from the systemic venous circulation without forming emboli.[5] Initiating carbon dioxide insufflation through the Veress needle at a rate of less than 1 L/min should therefore theoretically eliminate the most common cause of embolization.[5]

The most sensitive method of identifying air embolism is Doppler ultrasonography, which can detect as little as 0.1 ml of air in the right ventricle.[37] Because gas embolism is so rarely encountered in laparoscopic surgery, it is unlikely, however, that this device will be used routinely for intraoperative monitoring. Clinical signs associated with gas embolism are relatively nonspecific and include tachycardia, acute hypotension, and decreased oxygen saturation.[39] A rapid but transient increase in $ETCO_2$ may be an early sign of carbon dioxide embolus[16,39] that goes unnoticed. This brief increase is followed by a significant decrease in $ETCO_2$, which occurs as a result of the ventilation-perfusion mismatch and increase in physiologic dead space.[36,37] However, this finding is nonspecific and may be associated with any cause of decreased cardiac output.[36] The one distinctive clinical sign of gas embolism is the "millwheel" murmur caused by gas in the right ventricle.[5,35,36,39] At least in two cases, this abnormal heart sound was detected before changes in any other parameters measured intraoperatively.[36,38]

If gas embolism is suspected, one should immediately exsufflate the pneumoperitoneum to restore normal intra-abdominal pressure.[38,39] The patient should be hyperventilated with 100 percent oxygen and placed in the left lateral decubitus and Trendelenburg position (head and left side down).[5,35,36,38,39] Nitrous oxide anesthesia should be discontinued to promote absorption of the carbon dioxide embolus and avoid diffusion hypoxia.[35] Central venous line insertion should be performed for right atrial aspiration.[35–37,39] Supportive care includes treatment of cardiac arrhythmias[36] and resuscitation[35] as indicated on the basis of the clinical course. If external cardiac massage is needed for circulatory support, beneficial dispersion of the gas embolus may result.[36] In at least one case, resuscitation with cardiopulmonary bypass has been successfully employed.[35]

GASES USED FOR INSUFFLATION

As laparoscopy has evolved, a number of gases have been used for insufflation. Air was one of the earliest gases employed because of its ready availability. However, the ability of air to support combustion has eliminated its current use. Nitrous oxide produces less peritoneal irritation than carbon dioxide and minimizes hypercarbia,[7] but it also supports combustion, which may cause an explosion if used with electrocautery or lasers.[7,40] Therefore, its use is limited to diagnostic laparoscopy.

Carbon dioxide is currently the most commonly used gas for insufflation. Even though it has the disadvantage of producing significant hypercarbia and respiratory acidosis,[1,7,35,39] it has several advantages. It is readily available.[41] It is rapidly absorbed from the bloodstream, which may reduce the risk associated with gas embolism.[39] It does not support combustion,[5,7,39] thus allowing the use of electrocautery or lasers for therapeutic procedures. Although well tolerated by young healthy patients, the difficulty of using this agent in patients with cardiopulmonary disease has resulted in an active search for other methods of providing laparoscopic visualization.

Helium is an inert gas that may be a safer alternative to carbon dioxide in patients with pre-existing cardiopulmonary disease.[1,42] Hypercapnia and respiratory acidosis would be reduced or eliminated.[1,14] One group used helium initially in animal studies and then successfully progressed through a clinical trial in healthy patients undergoing laparoscopic cholecystectomy with good results.[41–43] Additional studies, however, are needed before widespread use of this agent is recommended. The direct influences of helium on the myocardium and on hemodynamic parameters have not yet been clearly defined.[1]

Because of the significant adverse effects associated with establishing and maintaining a pneumoperitoneum, others are vigorously exploring the use of mechanical retractors to eliminate the need for pneumoperitoneum in laparoscopic surgery. Reports of several successful clinical trials have been published.[44–47] If these mechanical concepts and devices can be generally adapted, they may significantly reduce or eliminate many of the adverse physiologic stresses associated with laparoscopic surgery.

CONCLUSION

Because of the physiologic effects of pneumoperitoneum on the patient, it is incumbent on both the surgeon and the anesthesiologist to understand the changes so that their effects can be prevented or minimized. A great deal of investigational work continues to be done in the area of the physiology of pneumoperitoneum. The use of alternative gases, as well as techniques that avoid pneumoperitoneum altogether, is being studied and used in some clinical practices. The recent reports of port site recurrences in patients undergoing laparoscopic resection of intra-abdominal malignancy are quite disturbing. It has been widely speculated that this problem is somehow related to pneumoperitoneum use. The true incidence and mechanism of these recurrences must be better understood before laparoscopic resection of malignant disease can become accepted and widely practiced.

REFERENCES

1. Kotzampassi K, Kapanidis N, Kazamias P et al: Hemodynamic events in the peritoneal environment during pneumoperitoneum in dogs. Surg Endosc 7:494, 1993
2. Wittgen CM, Andrus CH, Fitzgerald SD et al: Analysis of the hemodynamic and ventilatory effects of laparoscopic cholecystectomy. Arch Surg 126:997, 1991
3. Motew M, Ivankovich AD, Bieniarz J et al: Cardiovascular effects and acid-base and blood gas changes during laparoscopy. Am J Obstet Gynecol 115:1002, 1973
4. Cognat M, Gerald D, Vigneaud A: Le resque d'arret cardiaque au cours de la caelioscopie. J Gynecol Obstet Biol Reprod (Paris) 7:925, 1976
5. Dent TL, Duppler D, Soper N et al: 1991 Scientific session and postgraduate course: advances in laparoscopic general surgery. Surg Endosc 6:47, 1991
6. Wittgen CM, Andrus JP, Andrus CH et al: Cholecystectomy. Which procedure is best for the high-risk patient? Surg Endosc 7:395, 1993
7. Chiu PT, Gin T, Oh TE: Anesthesia for laparoscopic general surgery. Anesth Intensive Care 21:163, 1993
8. Safran DB, Orlando R 3rd: Physiologic effects of pneumoperitoneum. Am J Surg 167:281, 1994
9. Johannsen G, Andersen M, Juhl B: The effect of general anesthesia on the hemodynamic events during laparoscopy with CO_2 insufflation. Acta Anaesthesiol Scand 33:132, 1989
10. Kelman GR, Swapp GH, Smith I et al: Cardiac output and arterial blood-gas tension during laparoscopy. Br J Anaesth 44:1155, 1972
11. Drummond GB, Martin LV: Pressure-volume relationships in the lung during laparoscopy. Br J Anaesth 50:261, 1978
12. Wahba RW, Mamazza J: Ventilatory requirements during laparoscopic cholecystectomy. Can J Anaesth 40:206, 1993
13. Heneghan CPH, Bergman NA, Jones JG: Changes in lung volume and (pAO-paO_2) during anesthesia. Br J Anaesth 56:437, 1978
14. Wittgen CM, Naunheim KS, Andrus CH et al: Preoperative pulmonary function evaluation for laparoscopic cholecystectomy. Arch Surg 128:880, 1993
15. Luz CM, Polarz H, Bohrer H et al: Hemodynamic and respiratory effects of pneumoperitoneum and PEEP during laparoscopic pelvic lymphadenectomy in dogs. Surg Endosc 8:25, 1994
16. Bhavani-Shankar K, Moseley H, Kumar AY et al: Capnometry and anesthesia. Can J Anaesth 39:617, 1992
17. Tan PL, Lee TL, Tweed WA: Carbon dioxide absorption and gas exchange during pelvic laparoscopy. Can J Anaesth 39:677, 1992
18. Barnett RB, Clement GS, Drizin GS et al: Pulmonary changes after laparoscopic cholecystectomy. Surg Laparosc Endosc 2:125, 1992
19. Lenz RJ, Thomas TA, Wilkens DG: Cardiovascular changes during laparoscopy. Anesthesiol 31:4, 1976
20. Ponsky JL: Complications of laparoscopic cholecystectomy. Am J Surg 161:393, 1991
21. Smith I, Benzie RJ, Gordon NL et al: Cardiovascular effects of peritoneal insufflation of carbon dioxide for laparoscopy. BMJ 3:410, 1971
22. Liu SY, Leighton T, Davis I, et al: Prospective analysis of cardiopulmonary responses to laparoscopic cholecystectomy. J Laparoendosc Surg 1:241, 1991
23. Iwase K, Takenaka H, Ishizaka T et al: Serial changes in renal function during laparoscopic cholecystectomy. Eur Surg Res 25:203, 1993
24. Ishizaki Y, Bandai Y, Shimomura K et al: Changes in splanchnic blood flow and cardiovascular effects following peritoneal insufflation of carbon dioxide. Surg Endosc 7:420, 1993
25. Torrielli R, Cesarini M, Winnock S et al: Hemodynamic changes during celioscopy: a study carried out using thoracic electric bioimpedance. Can J Anaesth 37:46, 1990
26. Caldwell CB, Ricotta JJ: Changes in visceral blood flow with elevated intra-abdominal pressure. J Surg Res 43:14, 1987
27. Kashtan J, Green JF, Parsons EQ et al: Hemodynamic effect of increased abdominal pressure. J Surg Res 30:249, 1981
28. Breton G, Poulin E, Fortin C et al: Clinical and hemodynamic evaluation of cholecystectomies performed under laparoscopy. Ann Chir 45:783, 1991
29. Shimomura K, Ohtomo Y, Ishizaki Y: Peripheral venous pressure analysis in the lower limb during pneumoperitoneum in clinical laparoscopic cholecystectomy, abstracted. Surg Endosc 6:87, 1992

30. Millard JA, Hill BB, Cook PS et al: Intermittent sequential pneumatic compression in prevention of venous stasis associated with pneumoperitoneum during laparoscopic cholecystectomy. Arch Surg 128:914, 1993
31. Thorington JM, Schmidt CF: A study of urinary output and blood pressure changes resulting in experimental ascites. Am J Med Sci 165:880, 1923
32. Richards WO, Scovill W, Shin B et al: Acute renal failure associated with increased intra-abdominal pressure. Ann Surg 197:183, 1983
33. Iwase K, Takenaka H, Yagura A et al: Hemodynamic changes during laparoscopic cholecystectomy in patients with heart disease. Endoscopy 24:771, 1992
34. Kubota K, Kajiura N, Teruya M et al: Alterations in respiratory function and hemodynamics during laparoscopic cholecystectomy under pneumoperitoneum. Surg Endosc 7:500, 1993
35. Moscop RJ, Lubarsky DA: Carbon dioxide embolism during laparoscopic cholecystectomy. JAMA 87:414, 1994
36. DePlater RMH, Jones ISC: Nonfatal carbon dioxide embolism during laparoscopy. Anaesth Intensive Care 17:359, 1989
37. McMahon AJ, Baxter JN, O'Dwyer PJ: Preventing complications of laparoscopy. Br J Surg 80:1593, 1993
38. Beck DH, McQuillan PJ: Fatal carbon dioxide embolism and severe hemorrhage during laparoscopic salpingectomy. Br J Anaesth 72:243, 1994
39. Christ DW, Gadacz TR: Complications of laparoscopic surgery. Surg Clin North Am 73:265, 1993
40. Cunningham AF, Brull SJ: Laparoscopic cholecystectomy: anesthetic implications. Anesth Analg 76:1120, 1993
41. Bongard FS, Pianim NA, Leighton TA et al: Helium insufflation for laparoscopic operation. Surg Gynecol Obstet 177:140, 1993
42. Bongard FS, Pianim N, Liu S-Y et al: Using helium for insufflation during laparoscopy. JAMA 299:3131, 1991
43. Leighton TA, Liu S-Y, Bongard FS: Comparative cardiopulmonary effects of carbon dioxide versus helium pneumoperitoneum. Surgery 113:527, 1993
44. Chin AK, Eaton J, Tsoi EK et al: Gasless laparoscopy using planar lifting technique. J Am Coll Surg 178:401, 1994
45. Kitano S, Tomikawa M, Moriyama M et al: A prospective randomized trial comparing pneumoperitoneum and U-shaped retractor elevation for laparoscopic cholecystectomy. Surg Endosc 7:311, 1993
46. Hashimoto D, Nayeem SA, Kajiwara S et al: Laparoscopic cholecystectomy: an approach without pneumoperitoneum. Surg Endosc 7:54, 1993
47. Banting S, Shimi S, Vander Velpen G et al: Abdominal wall lift (low pressure pneumoperitoneum laparoscopic surgery). Surg Endosc 7:57, 1993

Editorial Comment I

Ulf Haglund

The cardiovascular and pulmonary physiology of carbon dioxide pneumoperitoneum is complex and incompletely understood. Many variables, including the level of intra-abdominal pressure, the volume status of the patient, the pharmacologic effect of anesthetic drugs, changes in patient position, and the presence of underlying cardiac and pulmonary disease, interact to produce the final physiologic result. The respiratory effects of pneumoperitoneum are caused primarily by increased intra-abdominal pressure elevating the diaphragm. The cardiovascular effects of carbon dioxide pneumoperitoneum include increased $PaCO_2$ and respiratory acidosis due to carbon dioxide absorption during laparoscopic procedures. Increased $PaCO_2$ is more pronounced in patients with pre-existing cardiopulmonary disease.

As detailed by Drs. Chandler and Bailey, arterial blood pressure and total peripheral resistance are usually increased during intra-abdominal pressure elevation. Decreased venous return giving a reduced cardiac output is seen during laparoscopy, especially if an excessively high intra-abdominal pressure (greater than 20 mm Hg) is employed. The decrease in cardiac output might be exaggerated by the reverse Trendelenburg position. It has been demonstrated in animal experiments that portal venous blood pressure is increased and portal venous blood flow reduced on establishment of the pneumoperitoneum. The change is proportional to the magnitude of the intra-abdominal pressure and does normalize on desufflation of the abdomen.

Although regional anesthesia is possible, laparoscopic surgical procedures are most often performed with general anesthesia and endotracheal intubation. Especially in prolonged laparoscopic procedures, patient discomfort, limited visualization, and poor tolerance of prolonged Trendelenburg's positioning in an awake patient limit the use of regional anesthesia. The anesthesiologist must be aware of the physiologic responses to pneumoperitoneum. Proper oxygenation/ventilation is mandatory to compensate for the cardiopulmonary changes caused by carbon dioxide pneumoperitoneum. Routine monitoring includes electrocardiography, arterial blood pressure and pulse oximetry, continuous $ETCO_2$ monitoring, and preferably, esophageal stethoscopy for the detection of new cardiac murmurs. In patients with underlying heart or lung disease, it is often necessary to perform repeated intraoperative arterial blood gas analyses in addition to the $ETCO_2$ monitoring. During prolonged and complex procedures, pulmonary arterial pressure and blood gas monitoring may be necessary.

Cardiac arrhythmia is common during laparoscopic procedures, but the underlying mechanism is uncertain. Gas embolism is a serious and potentially life-threatening complication. The estimated incidence, however, is quite low. Nevertheless, it has been suggested that an esophageal stethoscope should be used to ensure the rapid diagnoses and resuscitation necessary to prevent cardiac arrest.

Patients undergoing prolonged laparoscopic surgical procedures should be considered to be high risk from an anesthetic standpoint. Appropriate preoperative evaluation and intraoperative monitoring are essential for successful anesthetic management. For anesthetic reasons, open procedures might be an attractive alternative in patients with severe cardiopulmonary disease. Lifting techniques, which provide visibility without establishing increased intra-abdominal pressure, might be an attractive alternative to conventional pneumoperitoneum. However, lifting techniques are at present still developmental, and more experience is necessary to provide proper evaluation.

Editorial Comment II

Rama M. Jager

Every laparoscopic surgeon should understand the physiology and pathophysiology of artificial pneumoperitoneum, the most commonly used method of peritoneal access in laparoscopic surgery. Laparoscopic surgery is less traumatic than conventional open laparotomy but carries its own special brand of morbidity. Surgeons who understand the physiologic implications of pneumoperitoneum can correctly decide whether the laparoscopic technique is truly minimally invasive in a given patient.

PULMONARY RISK

Whether open surgery is preferable to laparoscopic surgery in a patient with colorectal disease complicated by cardiopulmonary abnormalities is a question the surgeon will face often. The decision is based on the patient's cardiopulmonary reserve status, especially if the preoperative pulmonary function tests show a FEV_1 of less than 70 percent of predicted values and diffusion defects of more than 80 percent of the predicted value. Other pertinent factors that enter the decision process are the duration of laparoscopic surgery, the intraoperative positioning, and the type of planned colorectal surgery.

The following are a few specific examples. Laparoscopic sigmoidectomy in a patient with an FEV_1 of less than 1 L may increase the incidence of postoperative pulmonary complications more so than open sigmoidectomy through a Pfannenstiel incision. The increased pulmonary stress in laparoscopic surgery from carbon dioxide pneumoperitoneum with the patient in the Trendelenburg position and the considerably longer surgical time for laparoscopic dissection and anastomosis make open sigmoidectomy more acceptable. By contrast, a second look laparoscopy may be the preferred approach to open laparotomy in a patient with elevated carcinoembryonic antigen (CEA) values who has also had a previous colonic resection. Laparoscopic enterostomy is similarly less risky than the open approach in a patient with severe underlying cardiopulmonary disease. The former technique avoids the need for a separate incision and the surgical time is not any longer than in the open approach.

The pulmonary stress from carbon dioxide pneumoperitoneum, as pointed out by Drs. Chandler and Bailey, is not small. It influences the choice of peritoneal access in the management of colorectal disease. It is worth noting, however, that the hemodynamic parameters return toward preoperative baseline values after exsufflation of pneumoperitoneum with no significant perioperative cardiac sequelae, even in patients with chronic cardiopulmonary disease.[1] Aggressive and invasive intraoperative cardiopulmonary monitoring of the significant hemodynamic stress from pneumoperitoneum may enable a high-risk patient to benefit from the advantages of laparoscopic surgery.

Monitoring $ETCO_2$ with a mass spectrometer does not replace the use of an arterial catheter for intraoperative arterial blood gas measurement of absorbed carbon dioxide, especially in patients with poor cardiopulmonary reserves.[2] Preoperative consultation with the anesthesiologist or a pulmonologist (or both) may be the optimal method of reducing the risk of acute pulmonary decompensation from the pneumoperitoneum.

SIGNIFICANCE OF REMAINING CARBON DIOXIDE

Laparoscopic surgeons should remember that up to 20 to 40 percent of the carbon dioxide may remain in the peritoneal cavity after the completion of colorectal surgery that is totally laparoscopic.[3] The residual peritoneal carbon dioxide after laparoscopic surgery may deleteriously affect postoperative spontaneous respiration. The respiratory rate and expiratory carbon dioxide may increase for up to a period of 3 hours following laparoscopy. The effect of retained carbon dioxide on postoperative ventilation is more prolonged and pronounced if the patient is given opioids for postoperative analgesia. Every attempt should be made to exsufflate carbon dioxide at the end of the laparoscopic procedure to reduce the effects of the remaining carbon dioxide on postoperative spontaneous respiration if an abdominal mini-incision is not a part of the surgical operation.

HYPOTHERMIC STRESS

Hypothermic stress from insufflation of cold carbon dioxide has been discussed but may not lead to significant postoperative complications. A decrease of 0.3°C in the core temperature was noticed for every 50 L of carbon dioxide infused.[4] Warming insufflated carbon dioxide to 30.0 to 30.5°C has been proposed as a means of decreasing the risk of hypothermia,[5] and various manufacturers of insufflators are introducing warming devices to accomplish this objective. Whether laparoscopic hypothermia plays a role in cardiopulmonary complications from pneumoperitoneum is unknown. Infusion of warmed carbon dioxide does, however, offer a novel and alternate means of preventing intraoperative hypothermia, a perennial problem with prolonged abdominal surgical procedures.

CARDIOVASCULAR EFFECTS

The reduction in cardiac output induced by pneumoperitoneum is more significant in patients with hypovolemia. A decrease in stroke volume to 75 percent of baseline can occur in hypovolemic patients after pneumoperitoneum.[6] It is difficult to monitor blood loss away from the visual field in prolonged laparoscopic procedures. The deleterious hypovolemic influence on the pneumoperitoneum-induced decrease in cardiac output is especially significant in prolonged laparoscopic procedures that require extensive dissection.

MEDIASTINAL SHIFT

Diaphragmatic elevation and mediastinal shift during pneumoperitoneum may push the carina upward. An endotracheal tube too close to the carina may be displaced by the mediastinal shift into the right bronchus and lead to left lung collapse. A steep Trendelenburg's position—as is commonly needed in laparoscopic left colonic and abdominoperineal resections—also promotes a superior mediastinal shift and selective bronchial intubation. Chapter 4 of this book discusses some related complications. The anesthesiologist can correct this problem of endotracheal tube displacement by pulling the tube out a few centimeters or by periodic exsufflation of the pneumoperitoneum.[7]

REFERENCES

1. Safran D, Sgambati S, Orlando R III: Laparoscopy in high-risk cardiac patients. Surg Gynecol Obstet 176:548, 1993
2. Wittgen CM, Andrus CH, Fitzgerald SD et al: Analysis of the hemodynamic and ventilatory effects of laparoscopic cholecystectomy. Arch Surg 126:997, 1991
3. Tolksdorf W, Strang CM, Schippers E at al: The effects of the carbon dioxide pneumoperitoneum in laparoscopic cholecystectomy on postoperative spontaneous respiration. Anesthetist 41:199, 1992
4. Ott DE: Laparoscopic hypothermia. J Laparoendosc Surg 1:127, 1991
5. Ott DE: Correction of laparoscopic insufflation hypothermia. J Laparoendosc Surg 1:183, 1991
6. Ho HS, Sanders C, Corso FA et al: The effects of CO_2 pneumoperitoneum on hemodynamics in hemorrhaged animals. Surgery 114:381, 1993
7. Hamm P, Lang C, Fornecker ML et al: Recurrent selective bronchial intubation in laparoscopic cholecystectomy. Ann Fr Anesth Reanim 12:67, 1993

Editorial Comment III

James Kohn and Philip F. Caushaj

Drs. Chandler and Bailey have presented a clear and concise review of the physiologic alterations associated with carbon dioxide pneumoperitoneum in laparoscopic surgical patients. They have evaluated the physiology of pneumoperitoneum by addressing the cardiovascular and pulmonary sequelae. All surgeons who perform laparoscopic surgery should understand the physiologic consequences of pneumoperitoneum in order to manage potential alterations in homeostasis that may occur after carbon dioxide pneumoperitoneum.

This chapter begins appropriately with an introductory warning of the potential for cardiovascular complications in laparoscopy and stresses that these complications may occur even in young healthy patients. Historically, the gynecologic patient who has a laparoscopic procedure has been a relatively healthy individual undergoing a relatively basic procedure. Complication analyses of these patients, which have generally been performed by gynecologic surveys, have demonstrated minimal morbidity. However, the risk associated with laparoscopy in a general patient population has not been epidemiologically studied. One of the most important principles in this chapter explains the hemodynamic difference that may occur in different patient populations due to pneumoperitoneum. Young healthy patients may become hyperdynamic as a consequence of pneumoperitoneum, in contrast to patients with a marginal cardiac reserve or significant coronary artery disease, who may have a reduction in cardiac output as a result of the pneumoperitoneum. Importantly, cardiac output is a gross estimation of the end point of the stress response imposed and alone offers little insight into the potential for alleviating the stress placed on the cardiovascular system. Nevertheless, this basic information is fundamentally important in enabling the anesthesiologist to monitor the patient effectively. As laparoscopic indications expand to advanced laparoscopic procedures, which will occur with increasing frequency in aged populations, we need to understand the physiologic consequences of pneumoperitoneum to enable appropriate hemodynamic intraoperative and perioperative monitoring for our patients.

Advances in monitoring techniques are likely to have an impact on morbidity, as well as enable surgeons to minimize the physiologic alterations associated with pneumoperitoneum in several ways. First, it will extend patient selection criteria and enable surgeons to predict appropriate candidates for laparoscopic procedures. Second, it will enable appropriate physiologic monitoring of patients. Chandler and Bailey stress that the duration of a laparoscopic procedure, the insufflation pressure, the insufflation agent, and patient positioning are all of primary importance in establishing the physiologic response to the pneumoperitoneum as well as the patient response to a laparoscopic procedure. Consequently, the patient's physiologic response may possibly be modulated by appropriate monitoring and understanding of the physiology of the pneumoperitoneum. For example, a lower insufflation pressure or gasless laparoscopy may allow adequate exposure and yet lessen the stress response of the patient and allow a longer operation. Similarly, reverse Trendelenburg positioning may aid the pulmonary dynamics enough that respiratory acidosis is not problematic during long operations. Understandably, the physiology of pneumoperitoneum is an initial step in understanding the basics of a procedure that we perform, as well as ultimately enabling safer laparoscopic procedures.

8

Port Placement and Operative Technique

Ara Darzi and John R. T. Monson

The arrival of videoendoscopy has facilitated a wide range of endoscopic operative procedures across a variety of surgical disciplines, including gynecology, otorhinolaryngology, orthopedics, and general surgery. More recently, laparoscopic colectomy has been described.[1,2] Laparoscopic colonic resection requires extensive mobilization of the colon from its retroperitoneal attachments and meticulous separation of its mesentery from adjacent vital structures before resection. In this chapter we describe the technique of laparoscopic-assisted procedures in colonic surgery as developed in our unit for right and left hemicolectomy.

PATIENT PREPARATION

Preoperative preparation should include documentation of the site of the lesion with contrast radiology. This should be done because of the inaccuracy of colonoscopy in providing accurate information concerning the site of the pathology.[3] All patients should give consent for possible conversion to an open procedure. In addition, routine antithrombotic precautions using heparin and thromboembolotic disease support (TED) stockings is taken because of the increased operative time. Routine bowel preparation is employed, and all patients receive standard antibiotic prophylaxis. In all left-sided procedures, the ideal site for any potential colostomy is marked preoperatively and subsequently serves as the site of the left iliac fossa port.

INSTRUMENTATION

Full videoendoscopy facilities are required. For routine laparoscopic colonic surgery, the following specialized instruments are required in addition to routine equipment: two Babcock-type bowel grasping instruments, EndoShears and EndoSciz (United States Surgical Corporation, Norwalk, CT), and disposable endoscopic scissors. An EndoGauge (United States Surgical Corporation) is used to measure bowel wall thickness and a linear stapling device, EndoGIA (either 30 mm or 60 mm) (United States Surgical Corporation), is used to divide the mesenteric vessels and the bowel.

OPERATIVE TECHNIQUE

A nasogastric tube and urinary catheter are inserted when the patient is anesthetized. All procedures are performed with the patient in the Lloyd-Davies position with the legs flat to avoid interfering with the insertion of instruments into ports. A pneumoperitoneum is created, using a standard technique for insufflation with a Veress needle, and is maintained at 12 to 16 mm Hg by an automatic high-flow carbon dioxide insufflator. A 10-mm, 0-degree telescope is inserted through a subumbilical port, and the initial laparoscopy is performed.

We use 10- or 12-mm endoscopic ports throughout, one subumbilically and potentially one in each of the four quadrants, depending on individual requirements. In all ports, Surgigrips (United States Surgical Corporation) are essential to prevent air leaks and to maintain an efficient pneumoperitoneum throughout the operation. An optional 12-mm port may be inserted supraumbilically to facilitate the use of an EndoGIA for intracorporeal mesenteric and bowel division. At the initial laparoscopy, the lesion to be resected is identified, and both surfaces of the liver and the remainder of the abdominal cavity are examined. If the lesion cannot be identified laparoscopically, intraoperative colonoscopy may be useful in determining the location. The sequence of events in performing laparoscopic colonic surgery is retraction of the bowel, before mobilization and division of, first, the mesenteric vessels and, subsequently, of the bowel. Delivery of the resected specimen is usually performed through a small abdominal incision before anastomosis of the bowel ends. Alternatively, transanal delivery is performed during a total laparoscopic procedure. During an abdominoperineal resection, the specimen is delivered through the perineal wound as in the conventional procedure.

RIGHT HEMICOLECTOMY

The operating room layout and port sites are shown in Figures 8-1 and 8-2.

Retraction

Retraction of the right side of the colon is achieved by grasping the bowel with Babcock instruments. One is

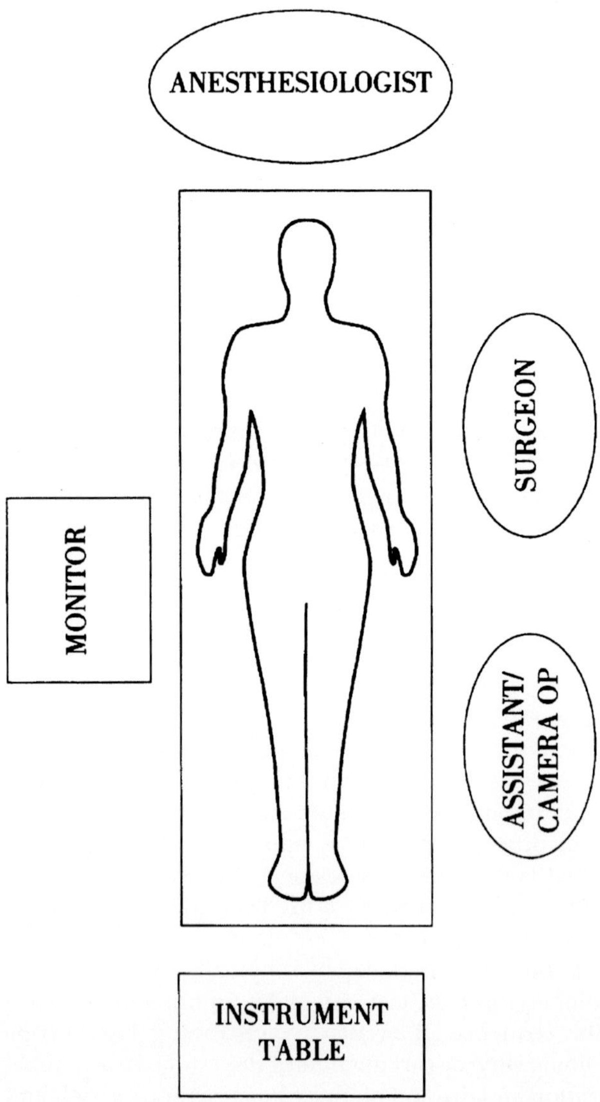

Fig. 8-1. Operating room setup for a right hemicolectomy.

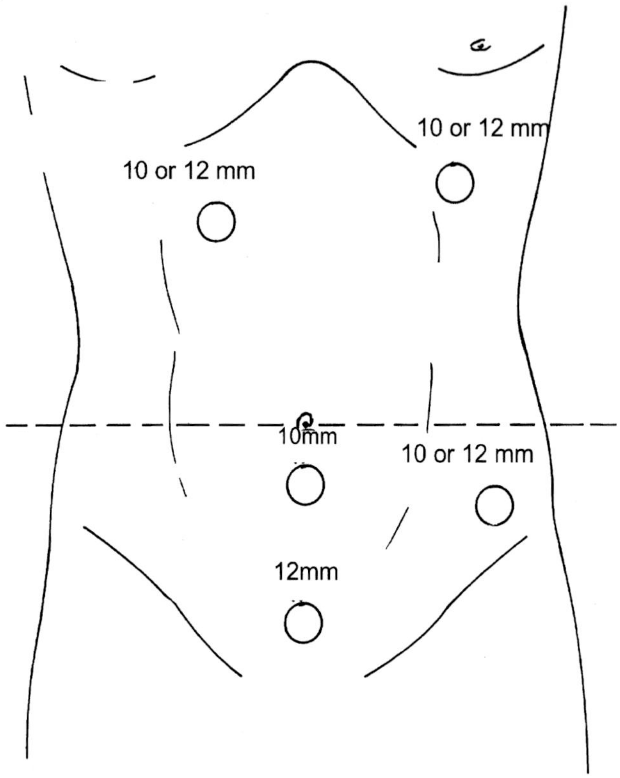

Fig. 8-2. Port positioning for a right hemicolectomy.

passed via the port in the left hypochondrium to hold the ascending colon upward and toward the midline. The second Babcock instrument is passed via the left iliac fossa port and holds the cecum downward and toward the midline (Fig. 8-3). Tilting the table to position the patient with the right side upward facilitates retraction of the colon and exposure of the right paracolic gutter.

Mobilization

Cecal mobilization is commenced with the laparoscope in the subumbilical port. The dissecting scissors are passed via the right upper quadrant. Mobilization is performed along the right paracolic gutter by moving toward the cecum. Meticulous hemostasis is important to avoid blood contaminating the field and reducing light intensity. This blood-free operative field also aids identification of vital structures such as the ureter and duodenum.

The hepatic flexure is then mobilized by placing a Babcock instrument through the right iliac fossa port on the ascending colon proximal to the hepatic flexure and pulling downward and toward the midline. A second Babcock instrument is passed through the left iliac fossa to hold the transverse colon distal to the hepatic flexure downward and to the left. The camera is positioned subumbilically, and the dissecting scissors are inserted via the

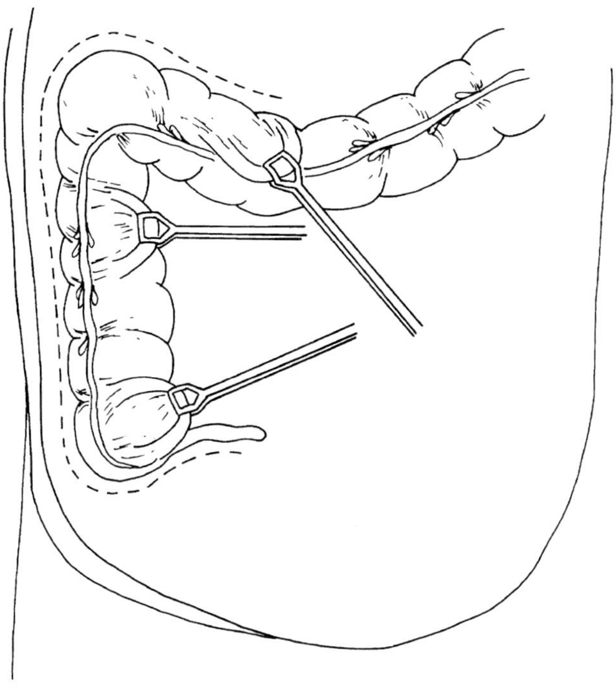

Fig. 8-3. Instrument positioning for a right hemicolectomy.

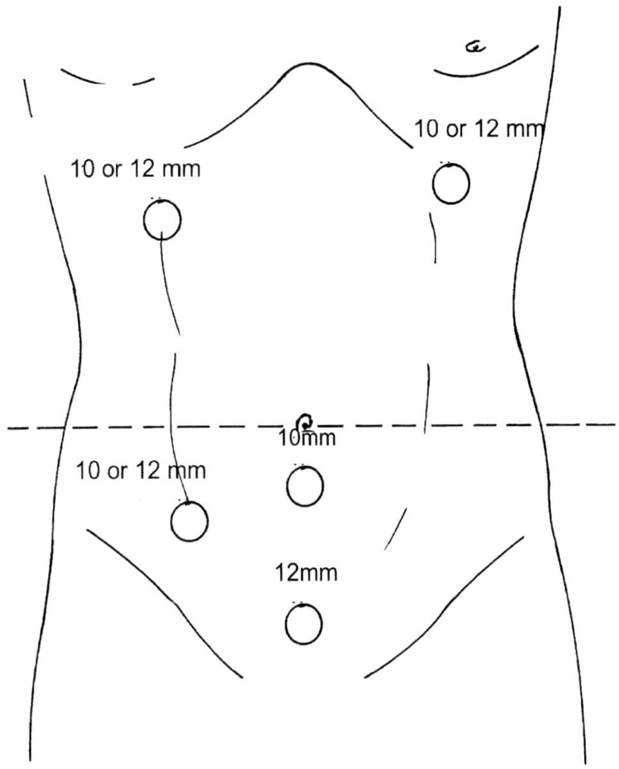

Fig. 8-4. Port positioning for a left hemicolectomy and anterior resection.

left or right upper quadrant port. Mobilization is commenced close to the bowel wall from the midtransverse colon to the hepatic flexure. Hook dissectors are useful at this stage to elevate the omentum off the transverse colon and the hepatic flexure before diathermy and cutting. Visualization of the hepatic flexure is sometimes facilitated by using a 30-degree telescope; however, the 30-degree telescope has the disadvantage of decreasing the light intensity and picture quality.

Bowel Division and Anastomosis

After mobilization of the bowel, the remainder of the operation may be completed extracorporeally if desired. The mobilized colon is delivered through a small transverse upper abdominal incision, followed by division of the vessels and bowel. The anastomosis is completed in the traditional fashion and the bowel returned to the abdomen. Alternatively, an intracorporeal approach may be used in which the terminal ileum is divided proximal to the ileocecal valve with a 30-mm EndoGIA introduced through a 12-mm laparoscopic port. The mesentery is then divided up to the level of the distal resection margin by using the EndoGIA or simple diathermy. The distal transverse colon is then divided again with the EndoGIA. At this stage the specimen is free in the peritoneal cavity.

An incision is made over the predicted position of the bowel anastomosis. Two fingers are placed into the peritoneal cavity to assess tumor size and determine whether the incision should be extended. In our experience, the average size of the incision for a right hemicolectomy has been 7 cm. We always attempt to place the incision above and to the right of the umbilicus. It is important to grasp the bowel ends in Babcock forceps before making the incision so that they can be easily located and positioned for anastomosis.

Bowel Anastomosis

After withdrawing the bowel through the incision, it is reanastomosed with sutures or staples in the standard manner. After returning the anastomosed bowel to the peritoneal cavity, the wound edges are washed with hydrogen peroxide, the trocars are removed, and the abdomen is closed without a drain.

LEFT HEMICOLECTOMY

The port sites for a left hemicolectomy and anterior resection are demonstrated in Figure 8-4. The operating room layout is as seen in Figure 8-5.

Retraction

In resection of the left side of the colon, the same principles of laparoscopic colonic surgery as for right hemicolectomy are applied—beginning with retraction of the

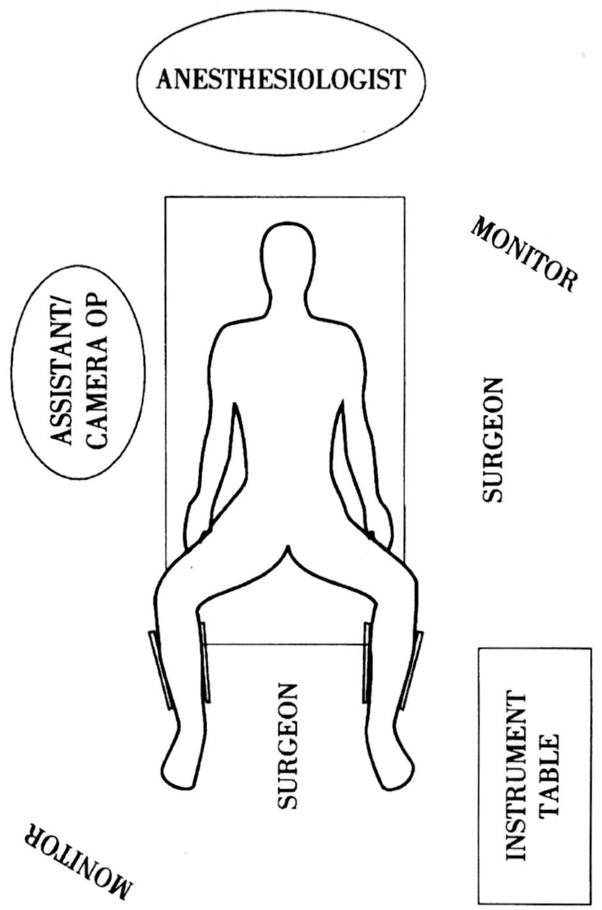

Fig. 8-5. Operating room setup for a left hemicolectomy and anterior resection.

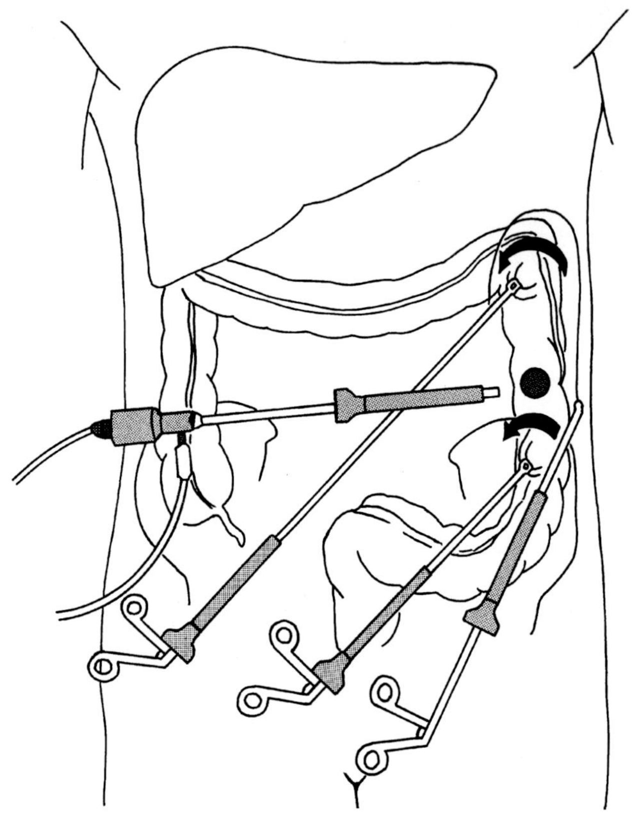

Fig. 8-6. Instrument positioning for a left hemicolectomy.

bowel, mobilization, mesenteric vessel division, and finally division and anastomosis of the bowel. Retraction of the left side of the colon is achieved by grasping the bowel with a Babcock instrument passed via the trocar in the right hypochondrium to hold the descending colon upward and toward the midline (Fig. 8-6). The second Babcock instrument is passed via the right iliac fossa port and holds the sigmoid colon downward and toward the midline. Judicious tilting of the operating table can facilitate retraction of the colon and exposure of the paracolic gutter. The dissecting scissors are inserted via the port in the left iliac fossa.

MOBILIZATION AND MESENTERIC HEMOSTASIS

The dissection is started by dividing the congenital adhesions commonly seen between the sigmoid colon and the abdominal wall. Care must be taken at this stage to identify both ureters and not injure the gonadal vessels. Mobilization of the bowel is continued proximally toward the splenic flexure. For mobilization of the splenic flexure, the bowel should be grasped on the mid-transverse colon, and tension should be applied downward and to the right via the right upper quadrant port. A second grasping instrument should be applied to the descending colon via the right iliac fossa port, with tension applied downward and toward the midline. Dissection is via the left iliac fossa port with the surgeon standing between the patient's legs. If desired, the inferior mesenteric vessels may be isolated and divided using a linear stapler as an initial step before mobilization of the bowel. This technique facilitates subsequent retraction and mobilization of the bowel and reduces blood loss. The mesenteric vessels are divided using the EndoGIA in the same manner as for a right hemicolectomy—via a 12-mm trocar inserted suprapubically to divide the vessels and bowel intracorporeally.

Bowel Division and Anastomosis

Transection of the rectum is easily performed at the rectosigmoid junction using a linear stapler. Through a small suprapubic incision, the mobilized bowel is then delivered to allow proximal transection. End-to-end anastomosis is then performed (usually under direct vision) using a circular stapler passed through the stapled rectum in the traditional fashion.

CONCLUSION

Laparoscopic surgery has had an enormous impact on the practice of general surgery. Laparoscopic colonic surgery has the same potential benefits as laparoscopic cholecystectomy with a potentially shorter postoperative stay and less postoperative pain.[4] However, laparoscopic colonic surgery as described here is essentially laparoscopic-assisted colonic surgery. In our unit, techniques vary with regard to the amount of the procedure performed laparoscopically. In the vast majority of cases, the mobilization of the colon and mesenteric vascular ligation is done laparoscopically. In some, however, the colon is mobilized laparoscopically, but vascular ligation is performed extracorporeally. The length and orientation (midline or transverse) of the incision used to make the anastomosis also vary, depending on the position of the cut ends of the bowel.

Whether laparoscopic colectomy provides adequate clearance of malignant tumors remains to be seen. It is our philosophy that tumors should be delivered intact for the purpose of staging the disease. The oncologic safety of laparoscopic colonic surgery cannot be properly addressed in the short term, and the appropriateness of laparoscopic technology for the treatment of colorectal carcinoma is a legitimate concern. In the short term it is reasonable to make some assessment of the effectiveness of laparoscopy by evaluating for completeness of resection. Since a generous excision of lymph node-bearing tissue is the current standard of care for colorectal cancer, one reasonable assessment may be to compare lymph node yield between laparoscopic and nonlaparoscopic cancer operations. In our experience, the yield following laparoscopic colectomy is no different from that obtained following conventional resection. Unfortunately, the quantity of lymph nodes identified in each specimen is highly variable from institution to institution. Therefore, this assessment may be considered at best a very crude criterion to judge the adequacy of resection. Long-term local and recurrence rates and overall survival rates over the long term will help determine the oncologic adequacy of laparoscopic colectomy for cancer.

One disadvantage of laparoscopic colonic surgery is that small lesions may be difficult to identify without the ability to palpate the colon as in open surgery. In a Dukes' A carcinoma, for example, which may be difficult to identify laparoscopically, this problem might be solved with preoperative colonoscopy and the injection of methylene blue at the site of the lesion, which can be seen laparoscopically through the serosa. Alternatively, simultaneous intraoperative colonoscopy may be used to locate laparoscopically occult lesions.

REFERENCES

1. Sclinkert RT: Laparoscopic-assisted right hemicolectomy. Dis Colon Rectum 34:1030, 1991
2. Monson JRT, Darzi A, Carey PD et al: Feasibility and preliminary results of laparoscopic assisted colectomy in a prospective unselected group of patients. Lancet 340:831, 1992
3. Cotton PB, Williams CB (eds): Colonoscopy. In: Practical Gastrointestinal Endoscopy. Blackwell Scientific Publications, Cambridge, 1990
4. Neugerbaur B, Troidl H, Spangenberger W et al: Conventional versus laparoscopic cholecystectomy and the randomized trial. Br J Surg 78:150, 1991

Editorial Comment I

Rama M. Jager

Optimal and safe port placement is essential for safe and swift laparoscopic colectomy. Various factors affect the optimal location of the ports. The location of the lesion, position of the patient on the operating table, dominant hand of the surgeon, and the vascular anatomy of the anterior abdominal wall all influence the choice of sites for port placement. After introduction of the umbilical port for the videolaparoscope, some laparoscopic surgeons use specific predetermined port locations and rarely change the pattern. Others determine the location of the accessory ports on the basis of the visceral anatomy. They introduce one accessory port at a time depending on need and choose the site "on the fly."

No one pattern of port placement is ideal. The surgeon usually stands on the contralateral side of the lesion (the patient's right side during left hemicolectomy and the left side during right hemicolectomy). If a right-handed surgeon is controlling the camera (laparoscope) port (because a good assistant comfortable with the camera use is not available), the dissecting port should be superior to the umbilical port in the midline when dissecting the right hemicolon. The dissecting port should be inferior to the umbilical port when dissecting the left hemicolon and rectum for a right-handed surgeon. The reverse holds true for a left-handed surgeon, unless the side on which the surgeon stands is reversed.

The surgeon should use both hands, one to dissect and the other to retract the colon or hold the videolaparoscope. The ports for such instruments as endoscopic Babcock forceps to retract the colon are usually placed lateral to the rectus sheath in the upper or lower quadrants of the abdomen. The lateral ports should not be placed too far inferior or too far superior so as not to affect the degree of their freedom from the unyielding iliac crest and costal margin. Placing the ports too far lateral limits their freedom. Port placement too close to the midline and through the rectus sheath may injure the epigastric vessels.[1]

When the patient is placed in the lateral decubitus position, ports cannot be placed in the dependent quadrants of the abdominal wall. Multiple ports may have to be placed in the midline. Proper spacing of ports diminishes intraperitoneal port "fencing," which can become annoying. By contrast, dissecting ports can be close to the camera port, since the dissecting instrument usually travels parallel to the laparoscope.

The most common complication from lateral port placement under direct vision is injury to the epigastric vessels. The anatomy and distribution of the inferior epigastric artery has been studied at great length and in voluminous detail because of its significance in coronary artery revascularization and abdominal wall transverse rectus abdominis musculocutaneous (TRAM) flap procedures in plastic surgery.[2] The actual location of the inferior epigastric vessels can often be identified by laparoscopic visualization and transillumination in most patients. Ultrasonographic localization of these abdominal wall vessels is feasible, although rarely is it necessary to use transoperative ultrasound.[3]

Understanding the anatomy of these vessels reduces the occurrence of annoying and, at times, severe rectus sheath hematoma from the trocar injury. The exact location of the vessels in the rectus sheath varies. Forty-nine percent of the inferior epigastric arteries are located laterally within the rectus sheath, with 34 percent in a mid-sheath site and 17 percent in a medial location. The deep inferior epigastric artery bifurcates into lateral and medial branches. The lateral branch is usually larger and has many skin perforators slightly lateral to the midline of the rectus abdominis.[4] One should remember that the inferior epigastric artery enters the rectus sheath from the lateral side of the rectus abdominis. Bleeding can also develop from trocar injury of perforator vessels near the periumbilical region, which contains 81 percent of the perforators.[5] Hemostasis of epigastric vessels injured by the trocar may require tamponade by passing an inflated Foley catheter balloon or by using a hernia stapler to occlude the vessels from inside the peritoneal cavity. Instances of uncontrolled bleeding from injured epigastric vessels leading to a large rectus sheath hematoma may require laparotomy.

Port site fascial defects should be closed if at all possible. The rate of incisional hernias increases with the size of the trocar used. All the fascial defects at sites where 10-mm or larger trocars are used require careful fascial closure. The surgeon should be aware and avoid

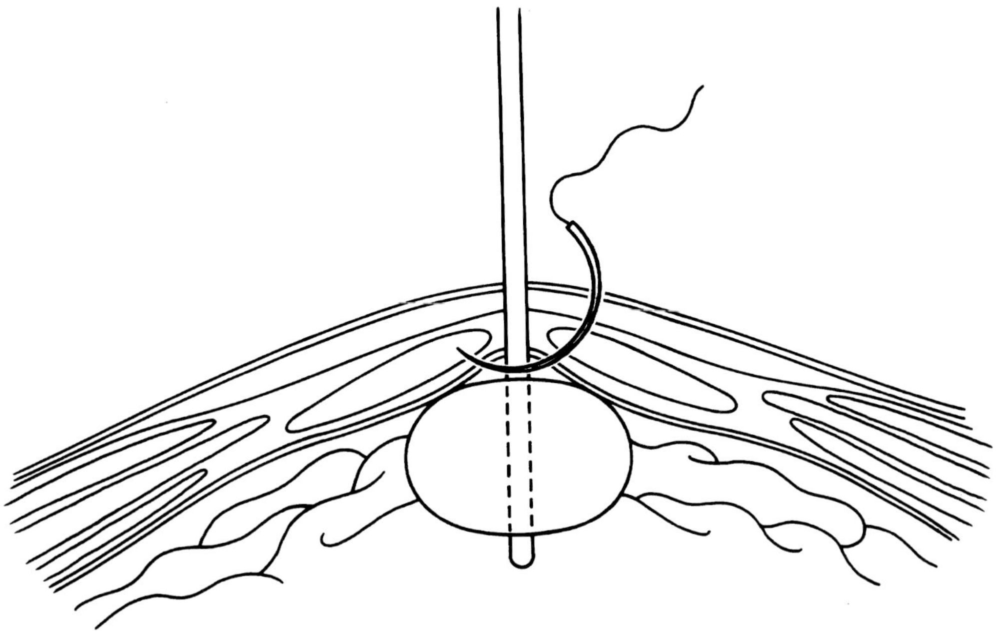

Fig. 8-7. Inflated Foley balloon used to displace subjacent bowel loops during closure of fascial defects at trocar sites.

injury to any subfascial bowel loops when placing fascial sutures. The technique of placing a Foley catheter through the fascial defect and using the inflated Foley balloon to displace the subjacent bowel loops (Fig. 8-7) is a simple and effective maneuver.[6] Other techniques such as using TruCut or other disposable long needles to place fascial sutures may also be appropriate.[6]

REFERENCES

1. Hurd WW, Pearl ML, DeLancey JO et al: Laparoscopic injury of abdominal wall blood vessels: a report of three cases. Obstet Gynecol, suppl. 82:673, 1993
2. Cremer J, Mugge A, Schulze M et al: The inferior epigastric artery for coronary bypass grafting. Functional assessment and clinical results. Eur J Cardiothorac Surg 7:423, 1993
3. Petrossian E, Menegus MA, Issenberg HJ et al: Ultrasound evaluation of the inferior epigastric artery. Ann Thorac Surg 57:895, 1994
4. Itoh Y, Arai K: The deep inferior epigastric artery free skin flap: anatomic study and clinical application. Plast Reconstr Surg 91:853, 1993
5. Rand RP, Cramer MM, Strandness DE Jr: Color-flow duplex scanning in the preoperative assessment of TRAM flap perforators: a report of 32 consecutive patients. Plast Reconstr Surg 93:453, 1994
6. Jager RM: Rectus sheath hematoma from laparoscopic trocar injury to inferior epigastric vessels. J Laparoendosc Surg 1995 (in press)

Editorial Comment II

Petachia Reissman and Steven D. Wexner

As laparoscopic colorectal procedures are more commonly performed, several unique complications that were uncommon after open surgery have been reported. One of those complications is bowel herniation through the fascial defect at the port sites.

Initially, the issue of port site closure after laparoscopic procedures was only vaguely addressed. When mentioned, fascial closure was recommended only at the umbilical port site because the abdominal wall muscles were believed to prevent incisional hernias at the lateral port sites.[1,2] However, an increasing number of midline, as well as lateral port site hernias, have recently been reported.[3–8] The clinical presentation has varied from an asymptomatic lump at the port site to an acute incarcerated hernia with intestinal obstruction requiring emergency laparoscopic or open surgery.[9] The time of onset has also varied between hours,[7] days,[5,6] and months[8] after surgery. In most cases, the involved ports were 10 mm in size or larger. However, as detailed by Drs. Darzi and Monson, in laparoscopic colorectal procedures only 10/12 mm or larger (18 and 33 mm) ports are used to provide maximal flexibility in scope and instrument positioning, insertion of the laparoscopic stapler devices, and removal of a large specimen. Therefore, in such procedures, special attention for closure of the fascial defect is required.[10]

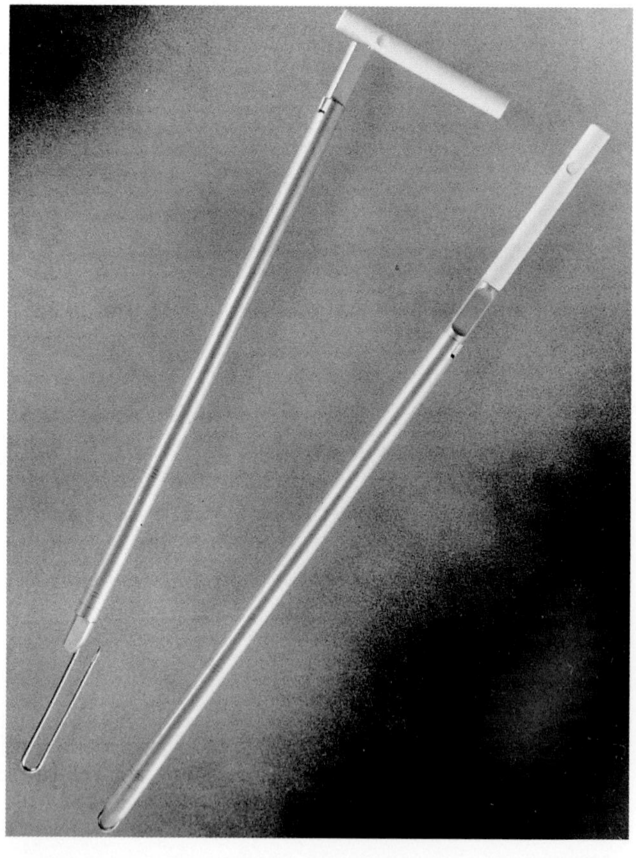

Fig. 8-8. Port site closure instrument (Disposable Puncture Closure Device BCD10, Advanced Surgical, Inc., Princeton, NJ). The device fits a 10/12-mm port. The J-shaped needle is long enough to be withdrawn parallel to the port while the port is still in place (for details see text).

For larger ports such as 18 or 33 mm, the fascia may be exposed by retracting the skin and direct suturing carried out in an ordinary fashion after completion of the procedure. For smaller ports, however, this option may not be feasible and therefore a large variety of port site fascia closure instruments have been introduced. The basic principle of these instruments is to place a fascial suture under laparoscopic video guidance at each port. After all the sutures are placed and the procedure is completed, they are tied in consecutive order after removal of the port under laparoscopic vision except for the last one. One of the disposable simple instruments that is currently available is shown in Figure 8-8. The instrument consists of a plastic rod that fits through a 10/12 mm trocar and a long J-shaped needle that can be turned 360 degrees. The device is introduced with the needle in the "secured" position, which is then turned 180 degrees and withdrawn through the fascia while the trocar is still in place. The device is tilted to drive the tip of the needle through the fascia and out of the abdominal wall between the skin and the trocar body. As the tip is seen, a suture is introduced through the eyehole at the tip of the needle, which is now introduced back into the abdominal cavity, turned 180 degrees, and pulled out through the opposite edge of the fascia. The other end of the suture is now pulled; the needle, which is now free of the suture, is introduced back into the abdomen and turned back to the safe position, and the device is withdrawn. This maneuver is repeated in all ports, and the sutures are tied after the ports are removed. The camera can be repositioned to visualize each port site, including the umbilical camera port during suturing. Before tying, it is important to lift each suture before the trocar is completely removed to prevent inadvertent trapping of the bowel. The suture is tied as soon as the trocar is completely removed. All sutures but the one at the site of the laparoscope may be directly inspected by the laparoscope while tying. In our experience, although it may be time-consuming, it is easier to place the fascial sutures at the beginning of the procedure, since the fascial opening has a tendency to distort and grow during the procedure.

The necessity of fascia closure at port sites 10 mm in size or larger has recently been recognized, as even a 10-mm port site may carry the risk of early or late bowel herniation and incarceration. We strongly believe that the fascia at all 10-mm or larger port sites should be closed after performing a laparoscopic colorectal procedure.

REFERENCES

1. Schirmer BD, Edge SB, Dix J et al: Laparoscopic cholecystectomy: treatment of choice for symptomatic cholelithiasis. Ann Surg 213:665, 1991
2. Dubois F, Icard P, Berthelot G, Levard H: Coeliscopic cholecystectomy: preliminary report of 36 cases. Ann Surg 211:60, 1990
3. Thomas AG, McLymont F, Moshipur J: Incarcerated hernia after laparoscopic sterilization: a case report. J Reprod Med 35:639, 1990
4. Mealy K, Hylant J: Small bowel obstruction following laparoscopic cholecystectomy. Eur J Surg 157:675, 1991
5. Hass BE, Schrager RE: Small bowel obstruction due to Richter's hernia after laparoscopic procedures. J Laparosc Surg 3:421, 1993
6. Patterson M, Walters D, Browder W: Postoperative bowel obstruction following laparoscopic surgery. Am Surg 59:656, 1993
7. Reissman P, Shiloni E, Gofrit O et al: Incarcerated hernia in a lateral trocar site: an unusual early postoperative complication of laparoscopic surgery. Eur J Surg 160:191, 1994
8. Storms P, Stuyven G, Vanhemelen G, Sebrechts R: Incarcerated trocar-wound hernia after laparoscopic hysterectomy. Surg Endosc 8:901, 1994
9. Kopelman D, Schein M, Assalia A, Hashmonai M: Small bowel obstruction following laparoscopic cholecystectomy. Surg Laparosc Endosc 4:325, 1994
10. Reissman P, Bernstein M, Verzaro R, Wexner SD: Port site fascia closure in laparoscopic-assisted colectomy. J Laparoendosc Surg (in press)

9

Monopolar Electrosurgery for Laparoscopic Colectomy

C. Randle Voyles and Robert D. Tucker

The challenge of laparoscopic colon resection is to perform complex tasks within the peritoneal cavity from extraperitoneal sites. Tissue transection and hemostasis can be accomplished by either mechanical or thermal means, but radio frequency (RF) electrical energy appears to have been settled on as the gold standard for energy sources.[1–3] When electrosurgery is combined with laparoscopy (particularly with colon resection), a better understanding of biophysics is essential to improve efficacy and safety.

Minimal access mandates maximum utility of the energy source. The fully developed "art of electrosurgery" combines the appropriate use of electrode design, waveform, and tissue manipulation for effective tissue dissection, cutting, and hemostasis.

The entire peritoneal cavity is incompletely viewed during laparoscopy. The potential for unintended visceral injury from stray or induced electrical currents out of the view of the laparoscope is real. Although the incidence of unrecognized electrosurgical or traumatic injury during laparoscopic electrosurgery is quite low, the occasional complication leaves the surgeon groping for an explanation.[4–6] It is impossible to understand and prevent the occasional unexpected burn—out of the view of the laparoscope—without a better appreciation of the science associated with RF energy.

Most general surgeons have learned laparoscopy with cholecystectomy; fortunately, the bowel is generally well out of the operating field during cholecystectomy. During more aggressive laparoscopic procedures, such as colon resection, surgical instruments are in close proximity to the bowel, thus increasing the potential for injury, which mandates a better understanding of the gold standard energy source: monopolar electrosurgery. Our purpose is to provide an overview of the biophysics of electrosurgery necessary (1) to improve efficacy, with the recognition that the best application is an art form, and (2) to outline the potential mechanisms of "stray current" outside the view of the laparoscope.

BASIC SCIENCE OF ELECTROSURGERY

A complete review of the biophysics of electrosurgery is beyond the scope of this chapter; additional references are available.[7–9] In general terms, the effect of RF electrical energy occurs because an electrical charge is driven through tissue, the tissue resists the current flow, and heat is generated. All the tissue effects of electrosurgery (and laser energy) occur as a result of the conversion of electrical energy (or laser energy) to heat. Electrons or electrical charges are transmitted most readily by tissue with a high electrolyte content, such as blood and muscle; such tissues have a low resistance to the transmission of electrical charges. Good tension and countertension increase local tissue resistance as well as concentrate the electrical current in dissection.

The force pushing electrons through tissue (measured in volts) is analogous to the head of pressure forcing water through a pipe. The current reflects a quantity of electrical charge that is pushed through a tissue and is measured as the charge per unit of time, or amperes. Current can be increased by increasing the voltage (height of the water tower) or by decreasing resistance (enlarging the diameter of the water pipe).

In an electrosurgical generator unit (ESU), the voltage "pushing" the electrical charge is not constant; rather, it alternates between positive and negative. In Figure 9-1, the voltage shift varies between a positive 2,000 V and a negative 2,000 V (a "peak-to-peak" voltage of 4,000 or a "peak" voltage of 2,000 V).

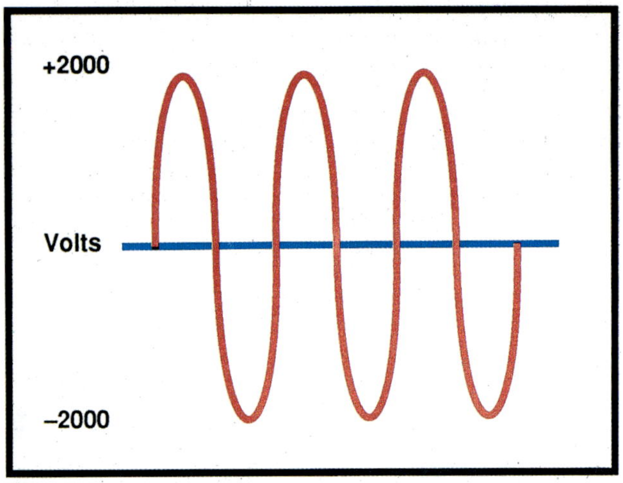

Fig. 9-1. Alternating current with voltage changes.

The electrical power in homes is provided by an alternating current at 60 cycles per second (cps), but typical ESUs in operating rooms provide an alternating current with a frequency of 300,000 to 2,000,000 cps. The high frequency (RF) from the generator is essential to prevent neuromuscular contraction. Lower frequencies, such as the 60 cps in homes, can cause tetany and electrocution, even though the voltage is considerably lower than what is used daily in the operating room. Lower-frequency currents may develop in laparoscopy with the sporadic arcing between the electrode and other metal devices (clips, instruments, cannulas) in the abdomen; such lower-frequency currents are routinely associated with video interference and often cause stimulation of the abdominal wall or diaphragm.

Current from the surgical electrode traverses tissue en route to the dispersive or return pad (inappropriately referred to as a "ground pad"). Because of the alternating current, there is really no "flow," rather just a rapid alternation of electrical charge at all points in the circuit. The intended tissue effect occurs at the surgical electrode/tissue interface—the point in the patient with the highest concentration of current (or power density). Burns at the return pad site (the most common electrosurgical injury 10 years ago) have been virtually eliminated by dynamic electronic monitoring of the adequacy of the skin/pad interface.

A watt is a unit of power delivered by the ESU that reflects the power dissipated by resistance at the electrode/tissue interface, as well as at all other points within the circuit. The wattage is a product of continuously changing voltage and current:

$$P = IV \quad (1)$$

where P is power (watts), I is current (amperes), and V is voltage. Although the generator may be set at 40 W "coag," the voltage and current change continuously as a function of varying tissue/circuit resistance. As tissue is desiccated, resistance increases and current decreases. To maintain a given power, voltage increases. The wattage that is indicated by the digital readout of the ESU represents an "average" (root mean square [RMS]) value. This average value allows for waveform differences when making direct comparisons between "cut" and "coag" powers. The maximum voltage varies according to the manufacturer and product line (Table 9-1).

The rate of change in tissue temperature correlates with the concentration of current or power per unit of tissue. As the RF current spreads from the electrode through the tissue, the concentration of current (and temperature change) decreases dramatically. Theoretically, tissue heating at the tissue/electrode interface is proportional to the following[7]:

$$\Delta T \sim (I^2/r^4)\ R\ t \quad (2)$$

where T is temperature, I is current, r is the radius of tissue/electrode contact, R is resistance, and t is time. Thus, the most important determinant of tissue heating is the radius of electrode contact; the absolute current is second in importance; tissue resistance and time are linear functions. (Doubling the current increases heating by a factor of 4; doubling the radius leads to a change of 16.) Accordingly, a skilled surgeon can achieve the desired tissue effect much more effectively by altering the radius of contact than by increasing the wattage of the generator (which increases the potential for complications). Appropriate tension and countertension of tissue increase the power density by decreasing the amount of tissue receiving the electrical or mechanical energy; tension makes the knife or electrode appear "sharper." The depth of necrosis (and, indeed, the safety of using monopolar electrosurgery) is reflected by the rapid decrease in tissue heating at points remote from the tissue/electrode interface (as a result of the radius to the fourth power). Points in the circuit with a very low power density (i.e., the dispersive "ground pad" or, perhaps, the

Table 9-1. Maximum Peak-to-Peak Voltage and Frequency of Commonly Used Generators

Generator	Peak-to-Peak Voltage	Frequency (kHz)
Valleylab SSE2L	4,070	450
Valleylab Force 2	7,000	500
Valleylab Force 4B	8,000	750
Valleylab Force 40	9,000	500
Aspen Excalibur	10,500	417

all-metal cannula with inadvertent electrode contact) have minimal temperature change in tissue during electrode activation.

A prediction of the extent of tissue change is at best difficult. However, we do know that if cellular temperatures of 70°C or greater are reached, collagen is denatured. Above 100°C, liquids are converted to vapor. Above 200°C, tissues are carbonized. In addition, the inadvertent arcing of current to surgical clips or staples can lead to even higher temperatures of the metal clip. It may be surprising how little power can cause unintended serious burns. Overt tissue necrosis and full-thickness bowel burns have been created experimentally by only 12 W of capacitively coupled power coming off the cannula after 5 seconds.[10]

ELECTROSURGICAL WAVEFORMS

Examples of the varying waveforms created by the ESU are depicted in Figure 9-2. The operating modes of ESUs vary in voltage, current, frequency, and waveform. The labels of "cut" and "coag" incompletely describe the full application of RF energy. The "cut" mode will "coag" quite well when a broad-based electrode/tissue contact is maintained in a static position. The "coag" mode will also cut, given an adequate concentration of power.

The "cut" waveform has a continuous cycle with a peak voltage of only 500 V at 50 W power. Although the precise mechanism of cutting is not fully understood, the cutting effect is best achieved when a fine edge or tip of an electrode is in close proximity to, but not touching, the tissue. It is believed that the uninterrupted movement of ions within cells generates intense intracellular heat within the superficial layer of cells, which causes the cellular contents to boil and vaporize. In the noncontact "cut" mode, deeper tissues are not heated, and poor hemostasis results. However, when the "cut" mode is used and the electrode is in firm contact with the tissue, desiccation rather than cutting occurs because the energy is directly transferred into the tissue, causing drying and hemostasis rather than cutting. Thus, the most effective cutting occurs with a light stroking action and a fine-edged electrode; the feedback for the surgeon is visual and not tactile. Alternatively, when "cut" is used in a contact mode, desiccation occurs with a low-voltage waveform.

Why does the "coag" mode lead to tissue desiccation? Figure 9-2 shows the high-voltage, low-current waveform of the "coag" mode. Note that there is an initial burst of electrical activity with a voltage that is greater than the peak-to-peak voltage change with cutting current. However, the current is "on" for only 6 percent of

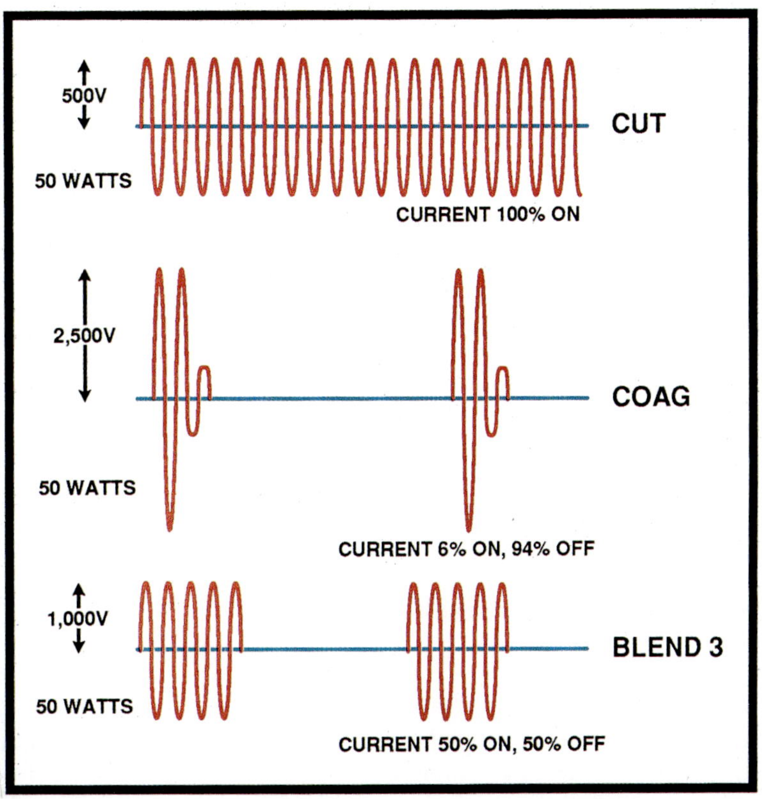

Fig. 9-2. Diagram of "cut," "coag," and "blend" waveforms.

the time; the balance of time, the generator is not generating a current. (This "coag" waveform is often called a "dampened waveform.") The base frequency of both "cut" and "coag" is typically 500 kHz, varying with different generators and models. The initial short burst of high-voltage energy leads to cellular insult (but not vaporization, as occurs with the continuous waveform of cutting). During the "off" interval, a drying effect or cellular desiccation occurs. In the subsequent electrical burst, the "dry cells" have an increased resistance to electron flow, which leads to more local heat dissipation and further cellular desiccation. The progressive insult to deeper layers of tissue from the higher voltage leads to tissue coagulation and hemostasis. As the desiccation increases, tissue resistance continues to increase until the current may actually cease. We see this demonstration when charred tissue coats the electrode, rendering "coag" ineffective. (With a "charred" electrode, why does "coag" work better than "cut"? If you do not know the answer, re-read this section.)

Coaptive coagulation is a useful electrosurgical technique. A vessel is grasped by a hemostat (or atraumatic dissector) and compressed. At open surgery, the hemostat is touched by the activated electrode; at laparoscopy, the atraumatic dissector electrode is activated. As a result of compression of the tissue, the tissue is rendered less vascular and tissue resistance is increased. Electrical energy applied to the tissue locally will promote a collagen weld of the vessel. Larger arteries can be controlled more effectively with coaptive coagulation than by the simple application of electrical energy to a bleeding vessel. When coaptive coagulation is used, the "cut" mode is preferred to "coag" because there is a lower voltage with less lateral tissue damage and a more local tissue effect.

Fulguration (Webster's definition: to give off flashes like lightning) is accomplished by setting the generator in the "coag" mode and holding the electrode off the tissue. Sparks ("minilightning") are given off from the electrode and strike through the path of least resistance. As with lightning, the burst of energy burns, dries, or desiccates the target tissue. The key point for the surgeon is that the tissue desiccation is very superficial because the current actually delivered to the tissue is low and the energy is rapidly dissipated (by the tissue as well as by the heat and light seen in the flashes). Tissue contact will cause deeper desiccation. Use of the argon beam may facilitate the distribution of the energy, in large part by blowing fluid from the target tissue.

With proper fulguration, the surgeon can desiccate and avoid mechanical disruption of friable tissue. Fulguration is enhanced by a higher-wattage and a high-voltage ESU. However, because fulguration occurs with an open circuit and with the high voltage of the "coag" mode, the stray current of capacitive coupling and insulation failure will also be increased (see the section, *Capacitive Coupling*).

The blend modes offer varying combinations of the "cut" and "coag" waveforms (Fig. 9-2). As the relative amount of the "coag" current is increased in different "blend settings," the tissue desiccation is enhanced and tissue cutting is lessened.

POTENTIAL PROBLEMS

The incidence of unintended electrosurgical injury has been relatively low. However, significant injuries have occurred[4–6] within the past 2 years and are likely to increase as general surgeons pursue more aggressive laparoscopic procedures, such as colon resection.

> Features common to these injuries include the following:
>
> 1. Mechanism of injury frequently unknown
> 2. Site of injury not seen during the procedure
> 3. Recognition of injury delayed
> 4. Poor outcome likely; with unrecognized bowel injury, the mortality rate may exceed 25 percent
> 5. Litigation common
> 6. Biophysics of the energy source not fully appreciated
> 7. Surgeons reluctant to discuss the poorly understood complications

Because of the difficulties in retrospectively studying the characteristics and mechanisms of bowel injury during laparoscopy, it is important to categorize potential mechanisms of energy transfer in order to prevent injuries. In the rest of this chapter, we attempt to do that. It is our contention that most bowel injuries can be avoided with education and relatively simple engineering advances.

In a most simplistic fashion, there are two sites where injury can occur:

1. Within the view of the laparoscope
2. Outside the view of the laparoscope

Injuries within the view of the laparoscope are related to surgical technique and their incidence can be reduced by a better understanding of the energy source.

Electrosurgical injuries outside the view of the scope may occur because of three different types of "stray energy": insulation failure, capacitive coupling, and direct coupling. Although specific documentation of each mechanism is impossible for obvious reasons, unexplained morbidity and deaths have occurred. For the surgical community, emphasis must be placed on biophysics and prevention of injury rather than on current epidemiology; since the potential for injury can be readily demonstrated, the current poorly reported anecdotes will increase as laparoscopic procedures continue to evolve. Furthermore, the potential problems can often be prevented with minimal, if any, increase in cost.

Insulation Failure

The operating surgeon is able to deliver RF energy to the target tissue because of the insulation surrounding the active electrode. There is no standard for insulation of laparoscopic instruments. Several variables are important in evaluating insulation: thickness, dielectric strength (the characteristic of insulating capability), hardness (how readily is it damaged?) and porosity (does it retain moisture?). Insulation defects can be acquired from cannula valve or other mechanical trauma, repeated heating through use or sterilization, manufacturing flaws, or capacitively coupled meltdown. An unrecognized defect in the insulation (i.e., too small to be seen) can deliver 100 percent of the RF energy to a site outside the view of the scope.

The hazard of insulation failure is dependent on the location of the point of failure (Fig. 9-3). Defects in the handle of the electrode (zone 4) are generally a result of poor engineering with exposed metal (particularly trumpet valves) that can burn the surgeon. Zone 1 insulation failure occurs as a result of trauma during insertion through cannula valves and repeated intraoperative use. Insulation breakdown in zone 1 appears to be more common with the hooks and spatulas that have more extensive distal insulation (as opposed to the earlier instruments with exposed metal shoulders). However, most articulating electrodes (scissors and atraumatic grasper-dissectors) have several centimeters of exposed metal that may cause injury or at least "ground out" on nontarget tissue (on the liver during laparoscopic cholecystectomy) with a loss of efficacy at the target tissue.

The zone 2 area represents the shaft of the electrode that is neither within the view of the laparoscope nor inside the cannula. If there is a defect in the insulation of zone 2, there is no clue for the most careful surgeon that insulation failure and thermal injury have occurred.

The signs of insulation failure within zone 3 depend on whether a metal or plastic cannula is used. If a metal cannula is used, there is oftentimes current flow between the metal of the electrode to the metal of the cannula; the resulting arcing of the current creates a lower-frequency current (referred to as a *demodulated frequency)* that can be as low as a few cycles per second. With this lower frequency, there may be neuromuscular stimulation[11] with jerking of the abdominal wall or diaphragm. Almost routinely, there is "lightning artifact" on the video with metal-to-metal arcing that goes unnoticed and unexplained by most practicing surgeons. These indirect signs of insulation failure will suggest to informed surgeons that insulation failure exists. Unfortunately, most surgeons are not knowledgeable about the indirect signs of insulation failure. Furthermore, insulation failure and subsequent bowel burn may occur without any clues before the development of an ileus, infectious complications, or peritonitis. Since there are no clues to insulation failure if the electrode is within a plastic cannula, the need for metal cannulas is apparent. The stray current, once trans-

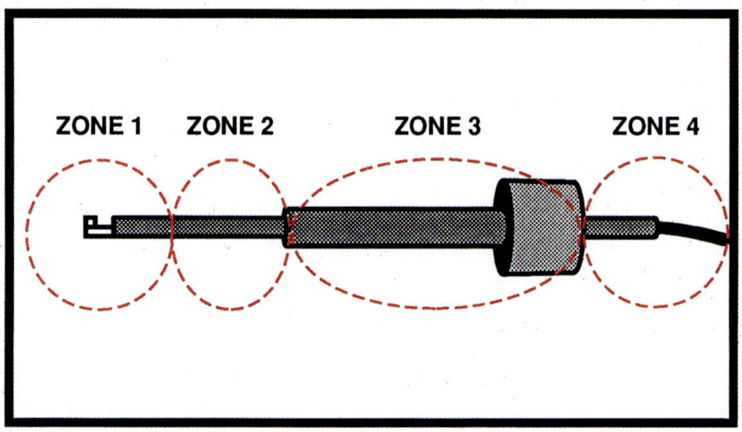

Fig. 9-3. Zones of insulation failure.

ferred to the metal cannula, should be dissipated harmlessly by the broad contact area at the abdominal wall (Eq. 2). Plastic anchoring devices over a metal shaft must be avoided; they will insulate the abdominal wall at the expense of the viscera.

What are the solutions to problems of insulation failure? Superficial logic suggests that disposable instruments might be advantageous. However, the insulation of some disposable instruments is thinner than that of most new, reusable instruments. Additionally, many surgeons consider the patient costs of disposable instruments to be prohibitive.[12,13] All forms of conventional insulation (e.g., plastic, Teflon) are based on a passive system with layers of nonconductors around the electrode. Defects within a passive system may not be detected before injury can occur. A new concept of insulation is based on dynamic monitoring of insulation integrity (Electroscope, Boulder, CO) (Fig. 9-4). The newer electrodes are constructed with a central metal conductor, a layer of insulation, and an outer conductor that is continuously monitored for any electrical current. Continuous monitoring of the active electrode assures the surgeon that energy is being delivered only in zone 1.

Capacitive Coupling

Capacitive coupling is a mechanism whereby electrical current in the electrode (intended) induces a current in nearby conductors (unintended) despite otherwise intact insulation. Some degree of capacitive coupling occurs with all standard monopolar electrosurgical instruments because the electrode is passed either through or near other conductors within the abdomen.[10,14,15] Whether the "stray energy" of capacitive coupling causes any clinical injury depends on (1) the total amount of current that is transferred and (2) the concentration of the current (i.e., the power density) as it makes its way back to the patient return electrode (ground pad).

Typically, 5-mm electrodes are introduced into the abdomen through either 5-mm cannulas or 5-mm reducers within 10-mm cannulas. The cannulas have been constructed with all metal, all plastic, or metal with a plastic abdominal wall anchor. The conductive active electrode within its insulation and the conductive tubular cannula represent a capacitor (capacitor: two conductors separated by a nonconductor). The capacitance of a cylinder within a cylinder is given by the formula

$$C = \frac{2\pi e_0 k L}{\ln (b/a)} \qquad (3)$$

where L is the length of the metal cannula/electrode interface; e_0 is an engineering constant, k is the dielectric constant of the insulation, b is the radius of the trocar cannula, and a is the radius of the active electrode. Thus, the induced current from a surgical electrode to a surrounding cannula is increased in any system in which the length of the surrounding cannula is increased and the distance between the electrode and the surrounding cannula is decreased. The induced

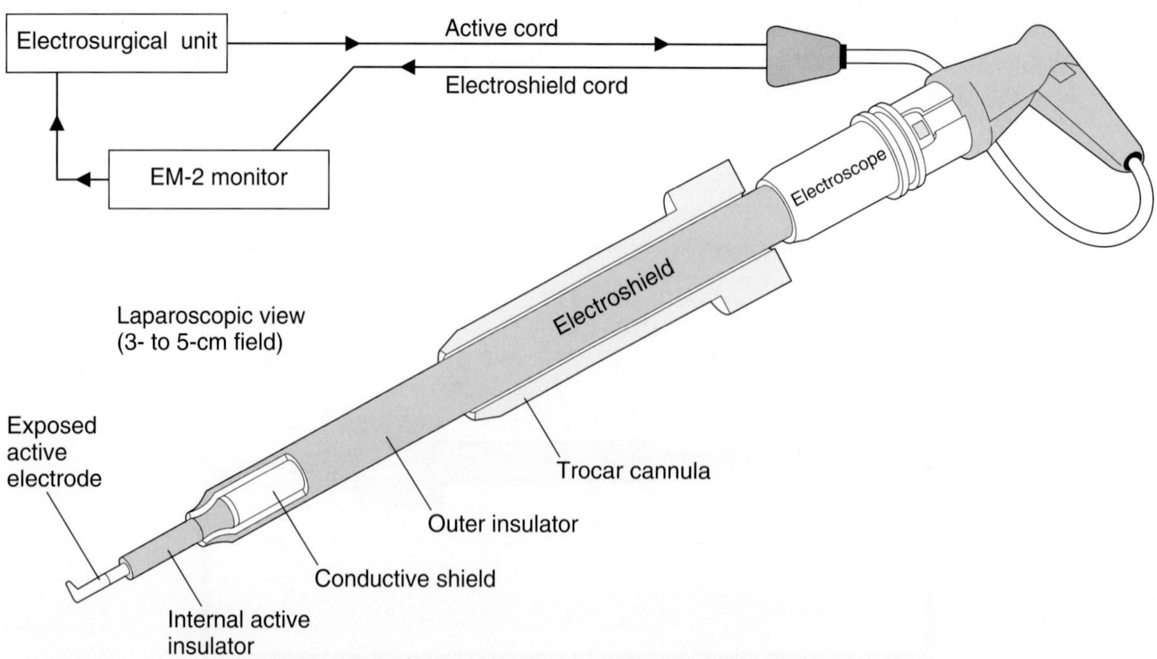

Fig. 9-4. Diagram of the dynamically monitored electrode to guarantee insulation and prevent capacitive coupling to the cannula or biologic tissue.

current occurs in spite of otherwise intact insulation; however, the thin insulation of some disposable electrodes will increase the capacitance of the system. In addition, the 10-mm electrode will transfer more current to a surrounding 10-mm cannula than would a 5-mm electrode. There is also more coupled current when a 5-mm electrode is passed through a 5-mm cannula rather than through a 10-mm cannula.

Capacitive coupling is increased not only by higher wattage but also by generators with higher voltage and frequencies (Table 9-1). The low-voltage "cut" mode exhibits less coupling than the "coag" mode. A low-voltage generator (such as the Valleylab SSE2L) exhibits very little coupling as compared with higher-voltage generators (Force 4B or 40). However, higher-voltage generators are useful because they offer better cutting and desiccation. Surgeons must recognize that open circuit activation (the electrode not touching tissue) dramatically increases the voltage and capacitive coupling.

Cannula selection and design are critical to reduce capacitively coupled injuries.[10–15] If a trocar cannula is employed with a metal sheath and a plastic tissue anchor is used, the abdominal wall may be in contact only with the nonconducting plastic anchor. While this apparatus does hold the cannula in place, it also electrically isolates the metal cannula from the abdominal wall (Fig. 9-5). Therefore, induced current from the cannula could be discharged to an internal organ such as the bowel within close proximity of the isolated metal trocar cannula. A preferable method for fixing the cannula at the abdominal wall is a conductive metal anchor at the skin level, which will distribute the stray current over a large area. (While plastic cannulas will eliminate this component of the "capacitance problem," they will increase the risk in multiple other scenarios.)

Clinically, capacitive coupling can lead to laparoscopic complications. In an experimental model, only 12 W of power from capacitive coupling for 5 seconds can cause full-thickness intestinal injury to the dog.[10] However, documentation in patients is difficult because bowel injury from capacitive coupling occurs outside the view of the laparoscope.

Another potentially dangerous scenario with capacitive coupling can occur with a small electrode that is passed through a metal suction-irrigator.[16] As might be anticipated from Equation 3, the length and proximity of the two conductors promote effective capacitive coupling (almost 70 percent of the intended power is available as stray current). If the device is introduced into the peritoneal cavity through a plastic nonconductive cannula, all of the stray current may be concentrated at a narrow point on the transverse colon. An all-metal cannula at the abdominal wall will "bleed off" the stray current through the abdominal wall, but the use of

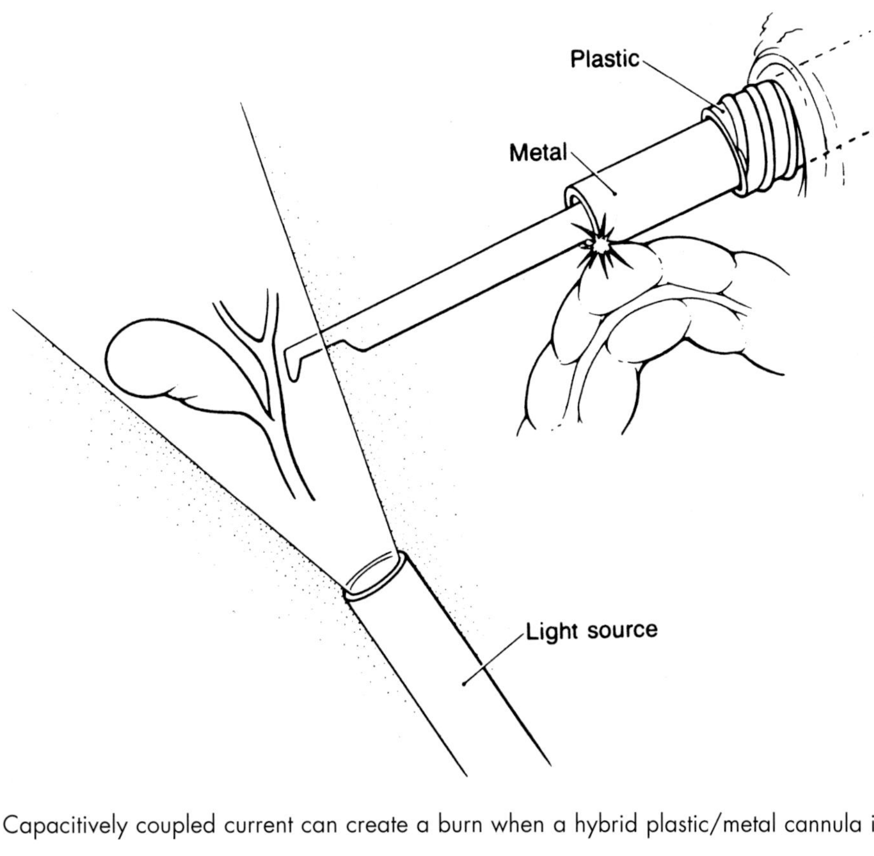

Fig. 9-5. Capacitively coupled current can create a burn when a hybrid plastic/metal cannula is used.

metal also decreases the resistance of the capacitively coupled pathway, and increases the net coupling. High-amperage capacitively coupled currents from the electrode to the metal suction-irrigation sleeve can cause considerable heating to the instrument through "corona heating." Thus, we recommend that most metal-sleeved suction-irrigation electrodes not be used; if they are used, they should be introduced only through a metal trocar or cannula, never a plastic one. Recently developed suction-irrigators have incorporated the safety features of the Electroshield, which "collects and removes" the capacitively coupled current before it can reach the suction-irrigator.

Capacitive coupling is demonstrated quite dramatically when the surgeon receives a burn on the hand from "buzzing" a hemostat during open operations.[17] Surgeons attribute the injury to a hole in their gloves, but few recognize that the hole may have been created by capacitively coupled current. The same energy that can burn a hole in the surgeon's glove can also cause a meltdown of the insulation of some instruments, particularly if the insulation is thin.[7] Fluid, blood, or a bit of tissue on the electrode surface provides the secondary conductor to create an effective capacitor and can melt a hole completely through the insulation. The extremely thin insulation of some instruments decreases the separation of the electrode from the surrounding conductor and increases the capacitance effect (Eq. 3). The problem is further compounded by higher-voltage generators that effectively "drive" the current through intact insulation.

The potential for injury from capacitive coupled currents can be reduced by an understanding of the biophysics and good electrosurgical technique. Hybrid cannulas, suction-irrigation electrodes (with an exposed metal suction-irrigator), and thinly insulated instruments should be avoided. The surgeon should use low-wattage and low-voltage power when possible (use "cut" versus "coag," and minimize open circuit activation). However, higher voltage is essential for effective fulguration, and open circuit activation invariably occurs during electrosurgical dissection. Accordingly, capacitive coupling inevitably occurs when conventional electrosurgical instruments are used. The risks associated with capacitive coupling can be reduced by education but can be eliminated by recently designed electrosurgical instruments that "collect" the stray current, remove it from the surgical site, and monitor (Electroscope) the total amount of current before returning it to the "ground pad." This system confines capacitive coupling to the collecting sheath and monitoring circuit, thereby eliminating transmission to either the cannula or biologic tissues.

Direct Coupling

Direct coupling refers to the condition in which the activated electrode touches other metal instruments (in particular, the laparoscope) within the abdomen, creating a situation whereby the energy can be unknowingly transferred (coupled) to tissue outside the view of the laparoscope (Fig. 9-6). The active electrode is typically within 2 cm of the end of the laparoscope and occasional contact (or close proximity to allow arcing without physical contact) with the laparoscope is a reality.[18] An electrode that has been placed more parallel than perpendicular to the laparoscope may be much closer to the laparoscope than is apparent on the video monitor. When the laparoscope becomes inadvertently acti-

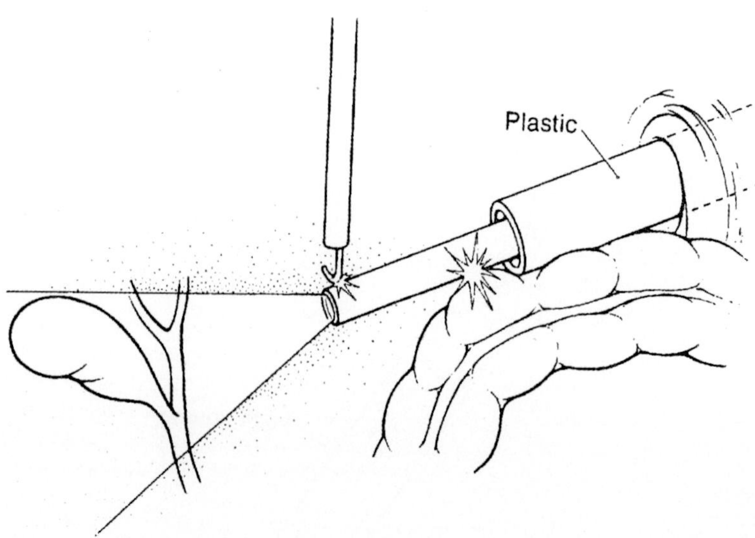

Fig. 9-6. Unrecognized contact between the electrode and the laparoscope may transmit 100 percent of the power to the laparoscope. A plastic cannula increases the risk of bowel burns if this contact occurs.

vated, a metal cannula through which the laparoscope is passed will help disperse the energy at the abdominal wall and markedly reduce the chance for injury. Plastic nonconductive cannulas must be avoided around the laparoscope[7,10,15,19]; they inappropriately insulate the abdominal wall at the expense of the viscera.

CONCLUSION

The primary deficiency of laparoscopic electrosurgery is not technological but rather relates to surgical education regarding the underlying biophysics. The fully developed art of electrosurgery is reflected by the surgeon's ability to manipulate fine electrodes and tissue to achieve results with an appropriate wattage. The informed surgeon understands the relative merit and disadvantages of both high- and low-voltage waveforms; if only cutting is needed, a low-voltage, pure "cut" waveform with a light feathery motion is appropriate. However, high voltage and high wattage are quite useful for deeper desiccation and especially for noncontact superficial arc-fulguration. The safer use of electrosurgery features bursts rather than continuous ESU activation during laparoscopy.

It is impossible to understand safety issues with electrosurgery without a better understanding of biophysics. Injuries related to stray currents (insulation failure, capacitive coupling, and direct coupling) can be reduced and possibly eliminated by using all metal cannulas and recently developed dynamically monitored electrodes. Specific instruments should be avoided: standard metal-sleeved suction-irrigators containing simple electrodes, hybrid cannulas, and thinly insulated electrodes. Finally, the laparoscope should always be introduced through a metal cannula. The recent interest in the art and science of electrosurgery is timely; for informed surgeons, the term *enhanced electrosurgery* seems appropriate.

REFERENCES

1. Voyles CR, Meena AL, Petro AB et al: Electrocautery is superior to laser for laparoscopic cholecystectomy. Am J Surg 160:457, 1990
2. Bordelon BM, Hobday KA, Hunter JG: Laser vs electrosurgery in laparoscopic cholecystectomy. Arch Surg 128:233, 1993
3. Wetter LA, Payne JH, Kirshenbaum G et al: The ultrasonic dissector facilitates laparoscopic cholecystectomy. Arch Surg 127:1195, 1992
4. Deziel DJ, Millikan KW, Economou SG et al: Complications of laparoscopic cholecystectomy: a national survey of 4,292 hospitals and an analysis of 77,604 cases. Am J Surg 165:9, 1993
5. Park YH, Oskanian Z: Obstructive jaundice after laparoscopic cholecystectomy with electrocautery. Am Surg 58:321, 1992
6. Larson GM, Vitale GC, Casey J et al: Multipractice analysis of laparoscopic cholecystectomy in 1,983 patients. Am J Surg 163:221, 1992
7. Voyles CR, Tucker RD: Essentials of Monopolar Electrosurgery for Laparoscopy. Electrosurgical Concepts, Jackson, MS, 1992
8. Pearce JA: Electrosurgery. Chapman & Hall, London, 1986
9. Serway RA: Physics for Scientists and Engineers. WB Saunders, Philadelphia, 1990
10. Voyles CR, Tucker RD: Education and engineering solutions for potential problems with laparoscopic monopolar electrosurgery. Am J Surg 164:57, 1992
11. Tucker RD, Schmitt OH, Sievert CR et al: Demodulated low frequency currents from electrosurgical procedures. Surg Gynecol Obstet 159:39, 1984
12. Voyles CR, Petro AB, Meena AL et al: A practical approach to laparoscopic cholecystectomy. Am J Surg 161:365, 1991
13. Apelgren KN, Blank ML, Slonski CA, Hadjis NS: Reusable instruments are more cost-effective than disposable instruments for laparoscopic cholecystectomy. Surg Endosc 8:32, 1994
14. Tucker RD, Voyles CR, Silvis SE: Capacitive coupled stray currents during laparoscopic and endoscopic electrosurgical procedures. Biomed Instrum Technol 26:303, 1992
15. Barlow DE: Endoscopic applications of electrosurgery: a review of basic principles. Gastrointest Endosc 28:73, 1982
16. Voyles CR, Tucker RD: Unrecognized hazards of surgical electrodes passed through metal suction-irrigation devices. Surg Endosc 8:185, 1994
17. Tucker RD, Fergusson S: Do surgical gloves protect staff during electrosurgical procedures? Surgery 110:892, 1991
18. Soderstrom RM: Letter. JAMA 227:1261, 1974
19. Federal Registry 45:12701, Feb. 26, 1980

Editorial Comment I

Anthony M. Vernava III

Cautery has been employed for millennia by surgeons and physicians to achieve hemostasis. In Egyptian and Roman times, cautery with a hot iron was known to be useful for stopping hemorrhage. Before modern anesthetic techniques, the use of cautery was considered barbaric and cruel because of the pain it elicited; despite its beneficial impact not only on tissue hemostasis but also on wound suppuration. The modern electrocautery device was devised by W. T. Bovie in the 1920s. The successful use of the device by Harvey Cushing to achieve hemostasis during excision of a bloody cranial mass legitimized the device, and over the past 50 plus years, surgeons have increasingly used the device during open surgery. Still, up until very recently, electrocautery was not routinely employed in open operations. The skepticism regarding electrocautery was particularly prominent among "academic" general surgeons. However, surgeons practicing today have had ample experience using electrocautery in "open" operations and have a good understanding of its tissue effects, both beneficial and potentially deleterious.

The application of electrocautery to laparoscopic surgical techniques is important because of the critical need to maintain strict hemostasis in order to visualize proper tissue planes of dissection. Much more so than in open surgery, the surgeon relies almost exclusively on visual landmarks and planes to safely perform the operation. Even a small amount of bleeding can obliterate the visual operative field and render the laparoscopic operation impossible. In addition, even if one controls bleeding that occurs laparoscopically, once the tissue planes have been stained by blood, it can be difficult or impossible to re-identify the correct operative landmarks. Electrocautery dissection is ideally suited to the performance of laparoscopic operations because the cautery effect seals small vessels and keeps the operative field clean and dry. The use of electrocautery in laparoscopic operations is generally safe but does carry with it the risk of unintended intestinal injury.

The chapter by Drs. Voyles and Tucker reviews the physics of electrocautery as it is applied to laparoscopic surgery with a view toward decreasing the already small incidence of injury to the intestine reported to occur during laparoscopic colorectal surgery. They have had a long-standing interest in this topic and have previously published on the issue. Drs. Voyles and Tucker list three general problems as the cause of most injuries:

1. Insulation failure
2. Capacitative coupling
3. Direct coupling

Prevention of these injuries can be accomplished by an improved understanding of how they occur. Relatively simple measures can be taken to prevent injury, including the use of all-metal cannulas and dynamically monitored electrodes. I agree with Drs. Voyles and Tucker that there are specific instruments that should be avoided: hybrid cannulas, thinly insulated electrodes, and standard metal-sleeved suction-irrigators with simple electrodes. I would like to comment on several practical issues related to cautery and safety that Drs. Voyles and Tucker did not specifically address:

1. Smoke should not be allowed to accumulate within the peritoneal cavity because it obscures vision and also promotes spontaneous sparking
2. Ductal-like structures should not be divided with cautery because current flow down these structures may lead to tissue injury at distant sites
3. Care should be taken to avoid using electrocautery adjacent to metal clips or staples
4. Finally, the entire conductive surface of the electrocautery device should be within the visual field during its application to avoid inadvertent injury to nonvisualized structures

Electrocautery is an essential component of laparoscopic surgery. Application of a basic understanding of the physics of electrocautery in laparoscopy (as the authors have provided), coupled with employment of the previously outlined simple safety measures, should continue to improve the safety of this valuable tool.

Editorial Comment II

Steven D. Wexner

Drs. Voyles and Tucker provide an elegant description of the use of monopolar electrosurgery for laparoscopic colon resection. They note in detail not only the relevant principles of physics but also the potential complications that can ensue. Every surgeon who performs laparoscopic colorectal surgery should read this chapter. Regardless of the complications, adherence to the principles outlined within this chapter should allow for safe use of monopolar electrocautery. It is unnecessary to convert to the use of bipolar electrocautery and certainly inappropriate to add laser photocautery to a laparoscopic procedure. Most of the problems from monopolar electrocautery are, as noted by Drs. Voyles and Tucker, completely avoidable if one diligently adheres to the principles of safe surgery. One would certainly not use monopolar electrocautery in the "open" setting without having full comprehension of the structures in the area being cauterized and the potential injuries to those structures, the depth of penetration, and the amount of traction on tissues. The same should be true when performing laparoscopic resections. Therefore, all noninsulated portions of all instruments must be visualized at all times. It is crucial to see, for instance, not only the tips of the scissors but the entire length of both blades as well. This caution is especially true when using the 10-mm-diameter scissors. Furthermore, one must be able to see the exposed metallic portions of all clamps to ensure that spark gaping does not occur. In addition, a capacitance-like reaction can occur when using a metal port. The Ethicon Tristar (Ethicon Endosurgery, Cincinnati, OH) and any other plastic ports should be immune from this complication.

A separate area of concern relates to the depth of penetration. Familiarity with the instruments and techniques should obviate such complications. However, extra caution needs to be taken when dissecting over the iliac vessels, ureters, duodenum, and major colic vessels. When in doubt, sharp dissection without electrocautery can be employed.

10

Operating Room Setup

Garth H. Ballantyne and Dennis G. Begos

Laparoscopy is a high-technology endeavor. As such, it requires equipment and instrumentation that also use advanced technology and that, by their nature, are large and bulky. Laparoscopic colon and rectal surgery is even more sophisticated. In an ideal world, operating rooms would be custom-built to accommodate the needs of the laparoscopic surgeon: they would be large enough to accommodate all the necessary equipment, and would have monitors suspended from the ceiling and freely movable to any required position, remote insufflators and video hardware with small docks or interfaces to minimize clutter and maximize mobility, and fluoroscopy. This list could easily be expanded. However, the facts are that most operating rooms currently in use were built for operations devised in the 18th and 19th centuries. While the ideal laparoscopic surgical environment has yet to be constructed, most operating rooms can be adapted to suit minimally invasive surgery quite nicely. The primary requirement is that they be large enough to accommodate the necessary equipment and that they have sufficient electrical capability.

OPERATING ROOM

The operating room should be large enough to accommodate the necessary equipment. A room traditionally used for major abdominal or thoracic procedures is generally acceptable, although the newer and larger rooms used for cardiovascular surgery are preferable. Endoscopy rooms or small procedure rooms are not sufficient. Electrical capability is also important. Most modern facilities should be set up to handle the loads required by the equipment. If in doubt, or if laparoscopic surgery is being performed for the first time, it is wise to consult with the hospital engineering staff beforehand.

OPERATING TABLE

An electric operating room table, while not absolutely essential, is extremely helpful. Much of the exposure during laparoscopic bowel surgery is dependent on proper patient positioning. The patient is placed into the deep Trendelenburg position to expose the lower portion of the abdomen. There is a critical angle of Trendelenburg positioning at which the small bowel usually slides out of the pelvis past the sacral promontory. If this angle is not reached, the small bowel remains within the pelvis and plagues the surgeon throughout the procedure. Conversely, the patient is elevated into the reverse Trendelenburg position to expose the upper part of the abdomen. This position slides the liver, stomach, and spleen away from the diaphragm, which is essential for inspection of the dome of the liver (Fig. 10-1). An intermediate degree of the reverse Trendelenburg position is helpful for mobilization of the colonic flexures. This position slides the viscera caudad toward the lower abdominal trocar sites, thereby increasing the functional length of the laparoscopic instruments. In addition, this position helps to open the space between the colon and the liver, stomach, and spleen. During dissection of the gutters, the ipsilateral side of the patient is rolled up and the colon retracted away from the lateral abdominal wall. Also, the small bowel slides laterally away from the mesocolon. The ability to move in and out of the Trendelenburg and reverse Trendelenburg positions, rotate the table, and raise and lower the table is absolutely essential. Exposure cannot be obtained without extreme alterations of the patient's position.

PATIENT POSITION

All laparoscopic colon and rectal procedures are performed with the patient in a modified Lloyd-Davies position (Fig. 10-2). The thighs should extend out straight, with no flexion. Any flexion at the hip may interfere with the arcs of the laparoscopic instruments and block their free excursion. Any flexion of the left thigh will severely limit access to the right upper quadrant. Similarly, flexion of the right thigh will retard dis-

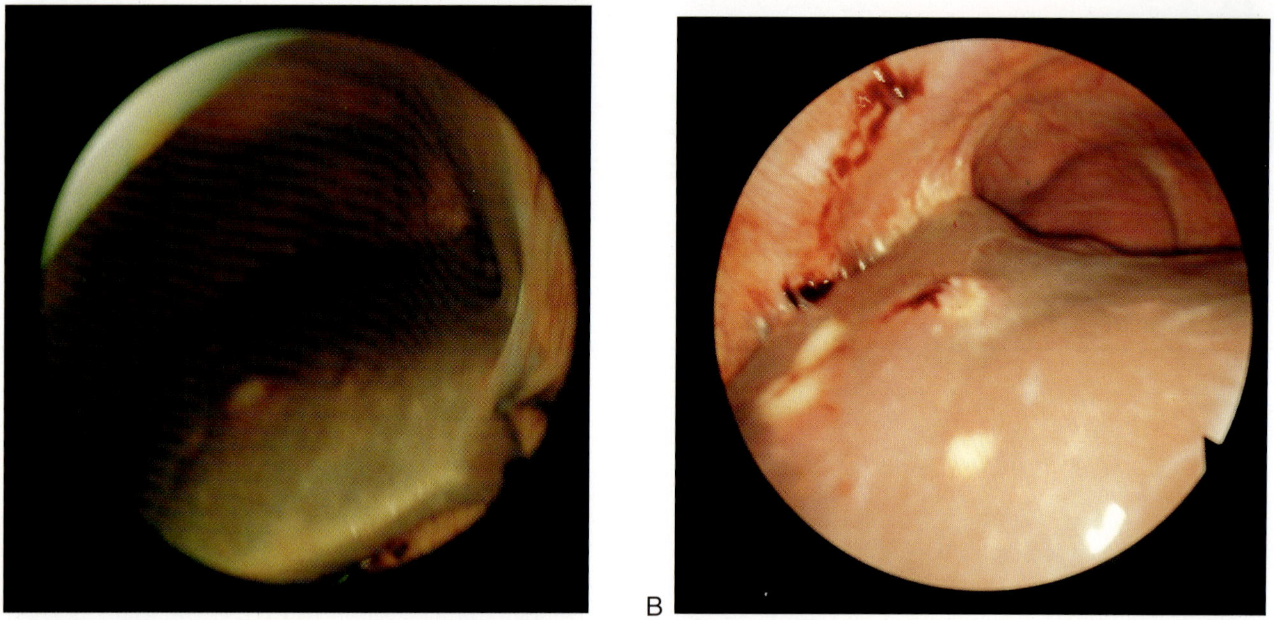

A B

Fig. 10-1. (A) When the patient is in the reverse Trendelenburg position, the domes of the liver drop away from the diaphragm and are easily inspected. This liver appears to be normal. **(B)** Colorectal cancer metastasis on the surface of the right lobe of the liver with adhesions to the abdominal wall is shown.

section in the left upper quadrant. The knees are flexed to protect the structures of the popliteal fossa. This position allows access to the anus for intraoperative colonoscopy as well as insertion of circular stapling devices. Some surgeons displace the rectosigmoid anteriorly and laterally with rigid sigmoidoscopes inserted transanally. In women, retractors can be placed into the vagina to elevate the uterus. This position also allows the surgeon to operate from between the legs of the patient, the so-called French position. This is a convenient stance for upper abdominal dissections such as mobilization of the flexures.

The patient is securely and safely attached to the table to prevent motion or slipping when moved to various positions. Additionally, it is important to adequately pad the legs and ensure that the peroneal nerve is not com-

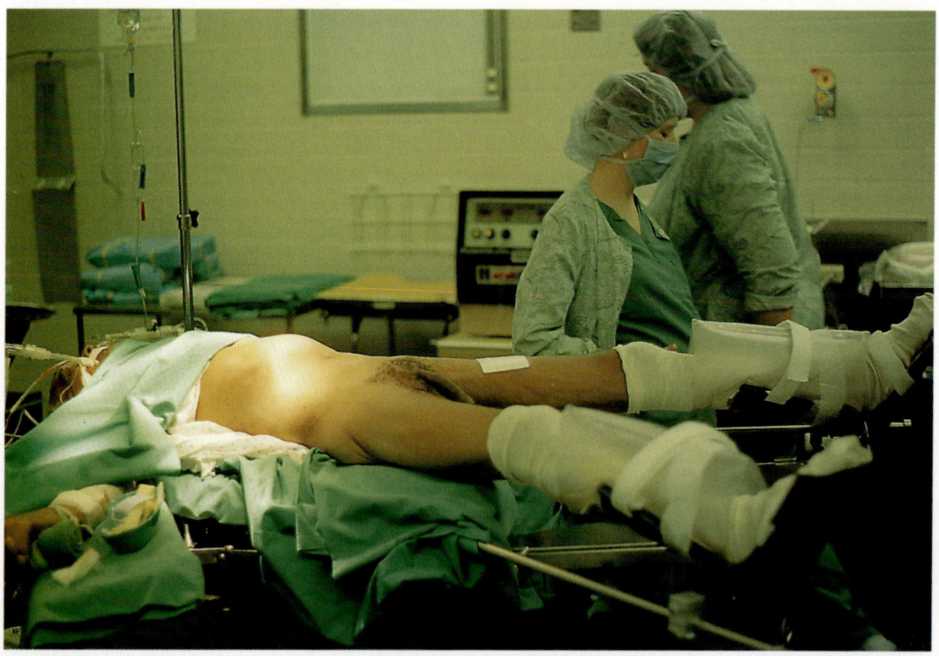

Fig. 10-2. Patient is placed in a modified Lloyd-Davies position with the thighs nearly straight.

pressed by the stirrups. The heads of the fibulas must be easily palpable. Likewise, the ulnar nerve should be padded, and hyperextension of the shoulder should be avoided. Pneumatic compression boots are placed on all patients for prophylaxis against deep venous thrombosis. A nasogastric tube is used to decompress the stomach and a urinary catheter to empty the bladder and monitor urine output. Decompression of the stomach and bladder helps to protect these organs during trocar insertion.

OPERATING ROOM PERSONNEL

A knowledgeable operating room staff is essential; both circulating and scrub nurses should be familiar with all of the laparoscopic instruments required for intestinal surgery because they differ from those used for other laparoscopic procedures. An in-service training session should be undertaken before the first case. Circulating nurses should be thoroughly familiar with all the equipment, including endoscopic apparatus, and should be able to set it up and troubleshoot it.

PATIENT MONITORING

Patients who undergo laparoscopic colorectal procedures are generally elderly and often afflicted with comorbid conditions. The establishment of a carbon dioxide pneumoperitoneum produces specific pulmonary and cardiovascular effects.[1] The anesthesiologist should monitor end-tidal carbon dioxide; ventilation is increased to remove any excess carbon dioxide. In patients with significant restrictive pulmonary disease, arterial blood gases should occasionally be checked. In some patients, end-tidal carbon dioxide may not reliably correlate with serum carbon dioxide partial pressure (PCO_2). The anesthesiologist should expect some increase in peak airway pressures.

Carbon dioxide pneumoperitoneum affects cardiovascular function.[2] The carbon dioxide produces a respiratory-type acidosis that can be controlled at a reasonable level by changes in the ventilation rate. The slight acidosis increases cardiac output because of greater myocardial contractility. The greatest effect on cardiac function comes from position changes of the patient. The deep Trendelenburg position increases venous return and cardiac output. By contrast, the reverse Trendelenburg position decreases venous return and thus, decreases cardiac output. In patients afflicted with significant cardiac or pulmonary diseases, cardiac function can be intraoperatively monitored with transesophageal echocardiography (Fig. 10-3). This apparatus allows continuous monitoring of end-diastolic volume, cardiac ejection fraction, and cardiac output. These measurements suggest that high-risk patients fare very well with laparoscopic colorectal procedures.

INSUFFLATOR

A high-flow insufflator is essential. Laparoscopic colorectal procedures can last 2 to 4 hours. The frequent exchange of instruments through trocars often causes dilation of the fascial defect around the trocar and consequently leaks of carbon dioxide around the trocars. In

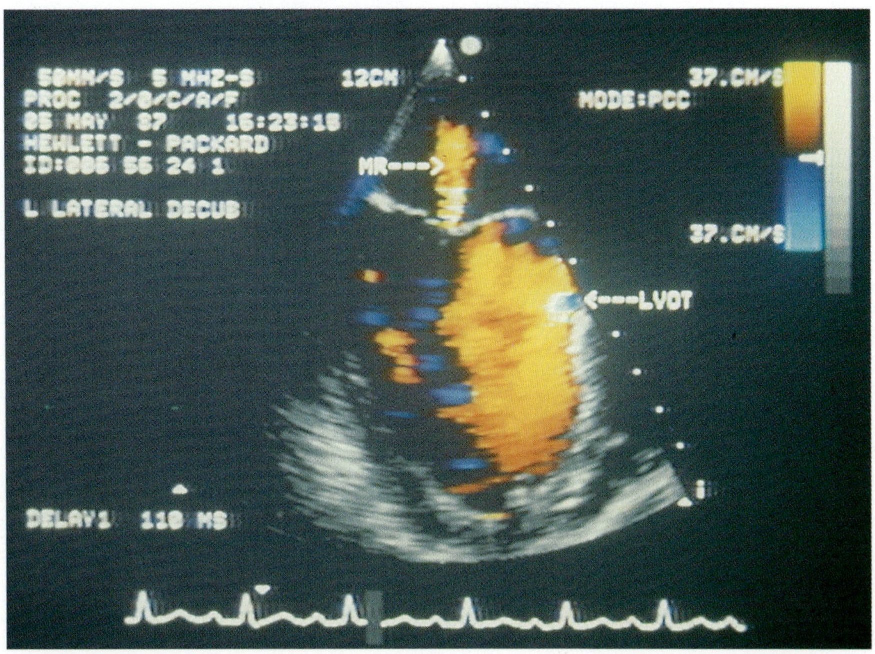

Fig. 10-3. Cardiac function during laparoscopic procedures can be monitored with transesophageal echocardiography. The color Doppler feature of this system allows direct measurement of cardiac output.

addition, the use of irrigation and suctioning devices often expedites exposure in complex procedures. The suctioning devices rapidly sap the pressure of the pneumoperitoneum. The combination of lost pressure around the trocars and through suctioning devices can lead to abysmal exposure and convert an easy laparoscopic procedure into an impossible or dangerous one. These factors may cause a loss of 3 to 5 L/min of gas. An insufflator that can deliver at least 10 L/min may prove necessary to maintain a sufficient pneumoperitoneum (Fig. 10-4). Consequently, an important element in the performance of advanced laparoscopic procedures is the acquisition of high-quality devices. Several companies produce insufflators that generate flow rates of 10, 15, or even 20 L/min of carbon dioxide.

Creative solutions can sometimes overcome the limitations of inadequate equipment. For example, if only older insufflators with flow rates of 6 L/min are available, it is possible to use two of these in tandem. The tubing from each insufflator is attached to separate trocars. Together, these insufflators can achieve rates of 12 L/min.

High-flow rates of carbon dioxide produce two problems. The carbon dioxide is usually used at room temperature. High-flow rates chill the patient and promote fogging of the telescope. Attachment of the tubing from the insufflator to a working port rather than the camera port minimizes the fogging problem to some degree. A better solution, however, is directed toward warming the gas. Some companies are now producing systems that warm the carbon dioxide. As these mechanisms become more available, they should become a standard part of the operating room setup. Until that time, however, surgeons should make every effort to minimize leaks around the trocars and limit the amount of carbon dioxide lost through suctioning.

TELESCOPES

Laparoscopic telescopes have changed little in 30 years. Two types of telescopes should be available for laparoscopic colorectal procedures. The principal camera is the 0-degree, 10-mm-diameter telescope. This front-viewing instrument provides maximum delivery of light down the fiberoptic bundles and offers excellent visualization of most structures. The 0-degree telescope, however, imposes some restrictions of observation under certain circumstances.

The 30-degree, 10-mm-diameter telescope overcomes certain limitations of the 0-degree telescope. As the dissection proceeds deeply into the pelvis, the angle of the telescope and working instruments converges. As a result, the working instruments often obstruct the view of the operative field. In addition, the bulk of the telescopes limits the motions of the operating instruments within the confines of the pelvis. Also, during mobilization of the flexures, the angle of view of the 0-degree telescope becomes tangential to the major anatomic structures. A

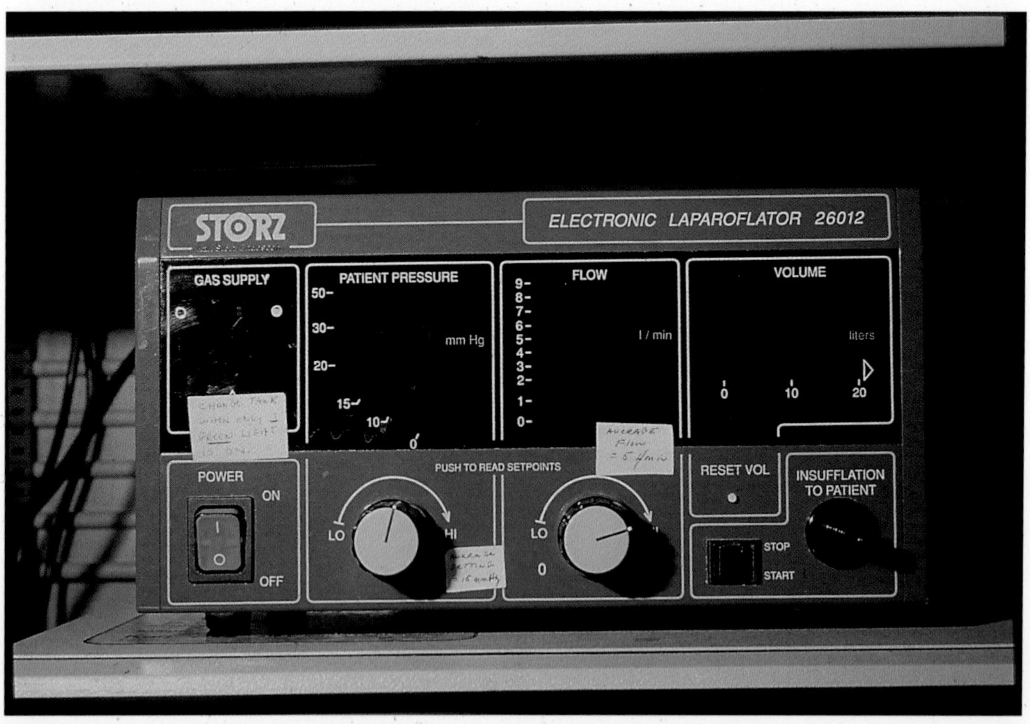

Fig. 10-4. High-flow insufflators (10 L/min or more) are required to maintain the pneumoperitoneum when suction devices are used or when leaks develop around the trocars.

30-degree telescope compensates for the shortcomings of the 0-degree telescope both in the pelvis and at the colonic flexures. In the pelvis, the 30-degree angle allows the telescope to look down on the area of dissection, thus preventing the surgical instruments from obstructing the view of the dissection. In addition, the elevation of the telescope keeps it away from the surgical instruments and prevents it from impeding the excursion arcs of the operating instruments. Similarly, the 30-degree telescope provides a panoramic view of the dissection of the flexures. The duodenum or the hilum of the spleen is easily visualized. Another use for the 30-degree telescope is looking around corners, under structures, or up at the anterior abdominal wall. Rotation of the telescope allows the surgeon to visualize areas that could not be seen with the front-viewing telescope.

The utility of the 30-degree telescope is limited by one shortcoming. The prism that bends the image around the 30-degree angle dissipates a significant quantity of light. As a result, the image through the 30-degree telescope is often much darker than that through the 0-degree telescope.

Simultaneous use of two telescopes is helpful under some circumstances. A second telescope can be used to transilluminate the mesentery for better visualization of mesenteric vessels. During deep pelvic dissections, a second video setup allows the surgeon to see both sides of the instrument when cutting the lateral rectal suspensory ligaments or the mesorectum. This enhanced vision helps avoid injuries to the ureters and eliminates the need for repositioning of a single camera. Also, during complex maneuvers such as construction of intracorporeal anastomoses, the second telescope provides important visual information about the third dimension and may greatly facilitate these steps in the operation.

Flexible telescopes overcome most of the current limitations of the traditional rigid laparoscope (Fig. 10-5). The flexible end allows flexion of the visual field from a front view through any angle up to about 120 degrees. This procedure is achieved without loss of illumination. Consequently, the telescope can be moved to any position within the confines of the abdomen that maximizes visualization of anatomic structures while limiting the telescope's interference with the movement of the operating instruments. In addition, currently available flexible telescopes contain suction and irrigation ports, further increasing the utility of the instruments. In particular, the irrigation attribute facilitates cleaning of the lens.

VIDEO EQUIPMENT

Videolaparoscopy equipment is based on computer technology. As a result, this equipment is undergoing the same rapid rate of evolution as computers. Consequently, the clarity of view in the wide expanse of the abdomen has undergone monumental leaps in improvement in the

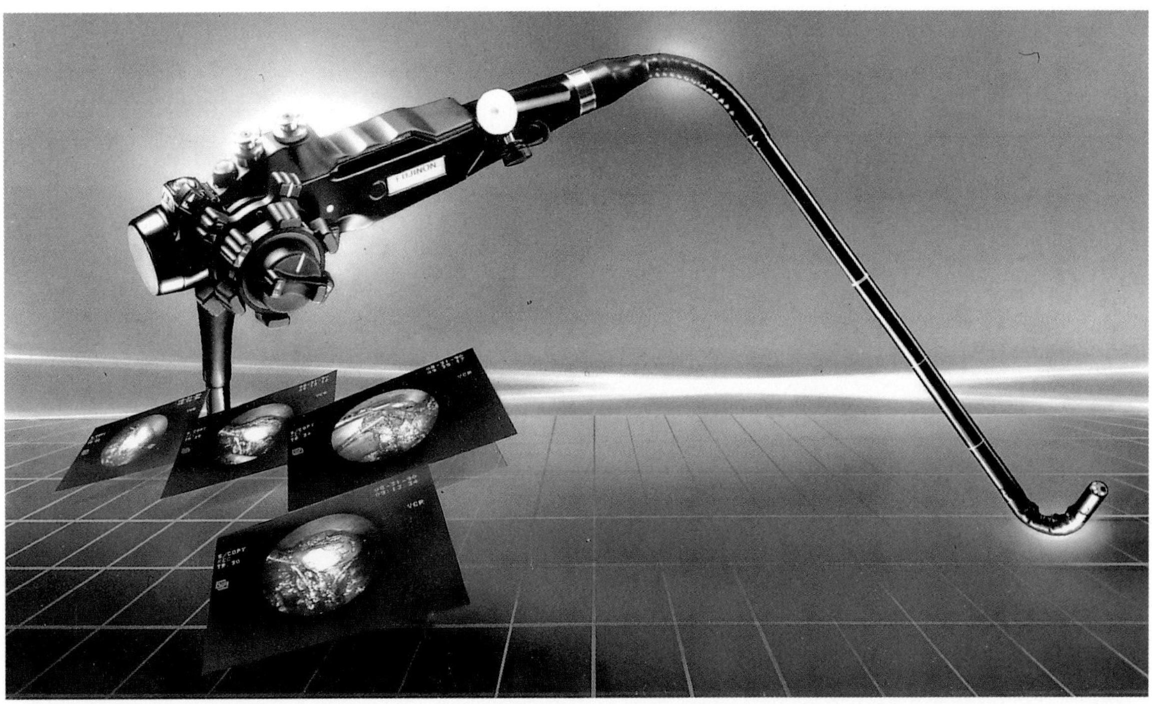

Fig. 10-5. Flexible laparoscopes such as this Fujinon system improve visualization of the domes of the liver and visualization of the colorectum during mobilization of the colonic flexures or during pelvic dissection.

past several years as new generations of computer chips have been introduced. Performance of advanced laparoscopic procedures with equipment purchased just a couple of years ago is significantly more difficult than with current state-of-the-art technology. This trend will continue for the foreseeable future.

The video camera is based on the light-sensitive CCD computer chip. Each chip contains about 300,000 light-sensitive boxes (pixels). The first generation of video cameras relied on a single chip. Groups of three contiguous pixels were covered with color filters for the three primary colors: yellow, blue, and red. These filters allowed each pixel to see only one color. Together the three pixels can produce any color by mixing the three primary colors. This technique, however, reduces the resolution of the chip to only 100,000 pixels. By contrast, the human eye has 100 million rods and cones.

More recently, three-chip video cameras have been introduced. In this system, one CCD chip is used to record one of the primary colors. Together the three can reproduce any color. The functional resolution is increased in this system to 300,000 pixels. Consequently, a three-chip camera provides better clarity than older models.

Three-Dimensional Video Systems

There are new video systems currently available that may prove to be quite valuable. Laparoscopic colorectal procedures are performed in complex three-dimensional zones often bordered by critical anatomic structures. The limited field of view projected by the standard videolaparoscope and its two-dimensional quality limit the clues that serve to orient the surgeon. Consequently, it is very easy for the surgeon to become disoriented as to the position of the surgical instruments within the abdomen and follow the wrong plane of dissection. Furthermore, the two-dimensional image promotes the possibility of past pointing injuries, particularly when electrocautery scissors are used. Three-dimensional videolaparoscopes overcome these limitations of standard laparoscopy systems and greatly facilitate advanced laparoscopic procedures. The advantages of three-dimensional image systems prove most beneficial to laparoscopic surgeons during their early experience with advanced procedures. The greatly enhanced perception of space relations makes orientation much easier to maintain and allows more deliberate and safe movement of instruments. This improved orientation and confidence of movement greatly accelerate the acquisition of skills in the performance of laparoscopic colorectal operations and speed their performance.

Systems such as the 3-D Scope project a true three-dimensional image (Fig. 10-6). Early systems simulated three-dimensional images from a standard two-dimensional laparoscopic image through computer-assisted enhancement. Current systems produce true three-dimensional images with the use of two video cameras. Two CCD chips are positioned at the tip of the videolaparoscope. These cameras are separated so as to provide a stereoscopic view. The images remain separated. Each image is recorded at a rate of 60 frames per second, the same as standard television. The video system

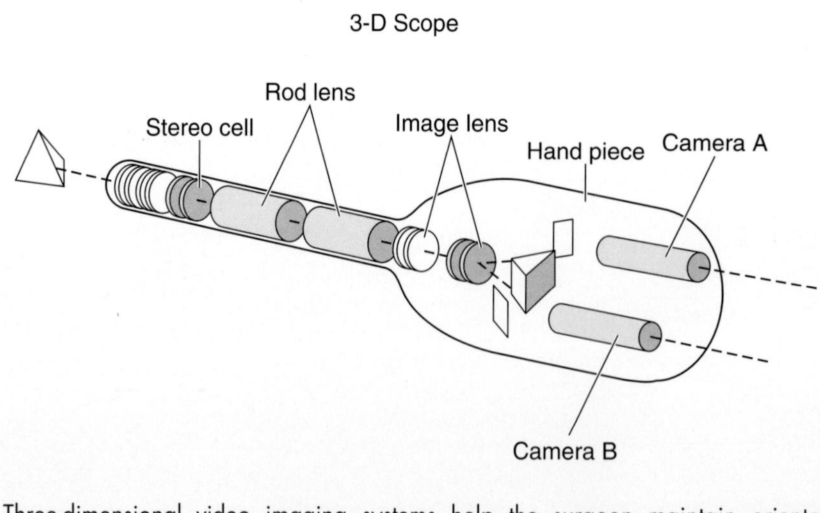

Fig. 10-6. Three-dimensional video imaging systems help the surgeon maintain orientation within the abdomen and promote the ability to perform complex dissections. The 3-D Scope has two video CCD chips within the handle of the laparoscope. These chips obtain a stereoscopic view within the abdomen. The two images are reflected and kept separate from the tip of the telescope through the lens system.

projects alternating frames from each camera on the video monitor at a rate of 120 frames per second (i.e., each image is projected 60 times per second). A circular polarizing filter is mounted on the face of the video monitor. Alternations in current cause the direction of polarization to alternate. The changing polarity of the filter is synchronized with the alternation of the two video images. As a result, the image of the left video camera is always projected through the polarizing filter with one orientation, and the right image is projected through the filter during the opposite orientation. The surgeon wears polarizing sunglasses (Fig. 10-7). The filter on the left eye allows the surgeon to see only the image of the left camera, and the filter on the right eye passes only the image of the right camera. As a result, the brain of the surgeon can synthesize a true stereoscopic, three-dimensional image.

Monitors

The quality of the image that is used for the performance of the operation is determined by several factors. These include the resolution of the video CCD chip, the intensity of the light source, and the resolution of the video monitor. It is important that the quality of the image not be eroded by using a low-resolution monitor. The number of lines of resolution of monitors vary widely. Most standard monitors have approximately 250 lines of horizontal resolution. High-resolution monitors can have 400 or more lines of resolution. Consequently, the resolution of the video system should closely match the resolution of the monitor. The NTSC standard used in the United States and Japan, for example, projects an image with a resolution of 512 × 384 pixels. The PAL standard used in Europe projects an image of 640 × 480. Thus, when using a high-resolution video camera, the surgeon should use a high-resolution monitor to gain the best possible image.

Further improvements in the quality of the video imaging and projection systems have already been introduced. High-definition television (HDTV) is being used on a trial basis in Germany. This system projects an image with 1,000 lines of vertical resolution. It also has a 180-percent larger viewing area and improved color resolution, due to a wider band width that allows color separation. These all combine to provide an estimated 10-fold improvement in resolution over conventional monitors.[3]

Light Sources

Light sources are also undergoing a period of rapid evolution. The initial videolaparoscopic systems available in the late 1980s used halogen light bulbs. Newer systems now use xenon light bulbs, which have vastly increased the delivery of light. The older systems provide an adequate amount of light for the illumination of small areas with a limited depth of field. As a result, these halogen-based systems were adequate for operations such as laparoscopic cholecystectomy, which require limited dissection. By contrast, advanced laparoscopic procedures require wide and deep fields of view. The quantity of light produced by halogen bulbs is adequate for this task (Fig. 10-8). Xenon light sources provide enough light so that complex three-dimensional structures such as the colon can be seen from afar, thus making the task of maintaining orientation within the abdomen much easier.

TROCAR PLACEMENT

The placement of trocars for various laparoscopic colorectal operations has not been standardized. The strategies are important because they determine the tactics of video monitor positioning within the operating room. Each trocar is placed 4 to 5 inches away from any other trocar. This placement minimizes interference with the excursion arcs of instruments passed through the trocar by instruments in other trocars. The trocars are set back at least 5 inches from the area of surgical dissection for which they will be used. If the operation is to be performed only by a surgeon and the camera person, four trocars are required. One port station is used for the camera. The surgeon uses two instruments, one in each hand, through two trocars. The camera person uses one instrument through the fourth port. If an assistant surgeon is available in addition to the camera person, five trocars are used. The camera is inserted through one. The surgeon and assistant both operate using two instruments, one in each hand.

The positioning of the trocars will vary with different colorectal procedures. The trocars are placed so as to facilitate the most difficult part of the anticipated operation. During a right hemicolectomy, the hardest step might be mobilization of the hepatic flexure. In an abdominoperineal resection, the hardest step might be the pelvic dissection. The trocars are positioned around an arc that focuses on the point of expected difficulty (Fig. 10-9). The camera is inserted through a central trocar, such as an umbilical port site. The monitors are then placed so that the operating instruments, the camera, and the surgical team are all pointing toward them (Fig. 10-10). This placement eliminates any difficulty with reversal of images on the monitor and the sensation of operating backward on a mirror (Fig. 10-11). This strategy will facilitate the performance of complex dissections because neither the surgeon nor the assistant surgeon is hindered by reversed motions on the monitor. If the operating team finds itself in a disadvantageous position (Fig. 10-12), time should be taken to move the monitor, allow the team to change position, or to place additional trocars so that the entire team can function at maximum efficiency and safety.

Large trocars should be used for laparoscopic colorectal procedures. Most instruments and most laparo-

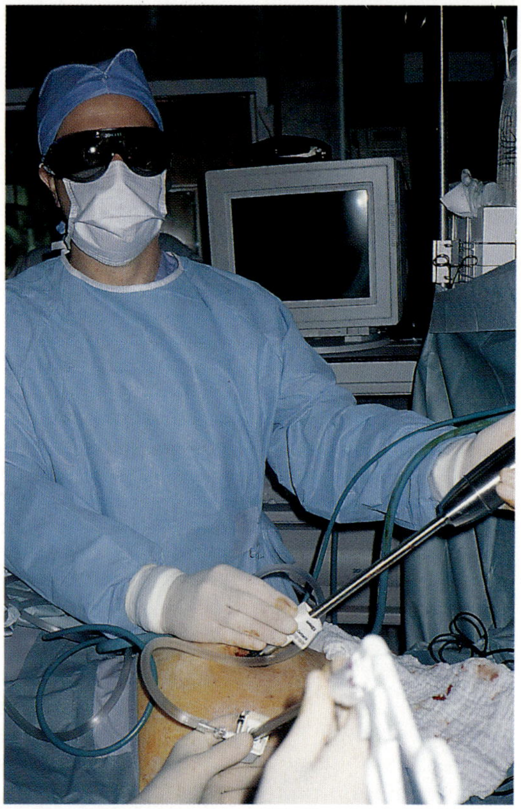

A

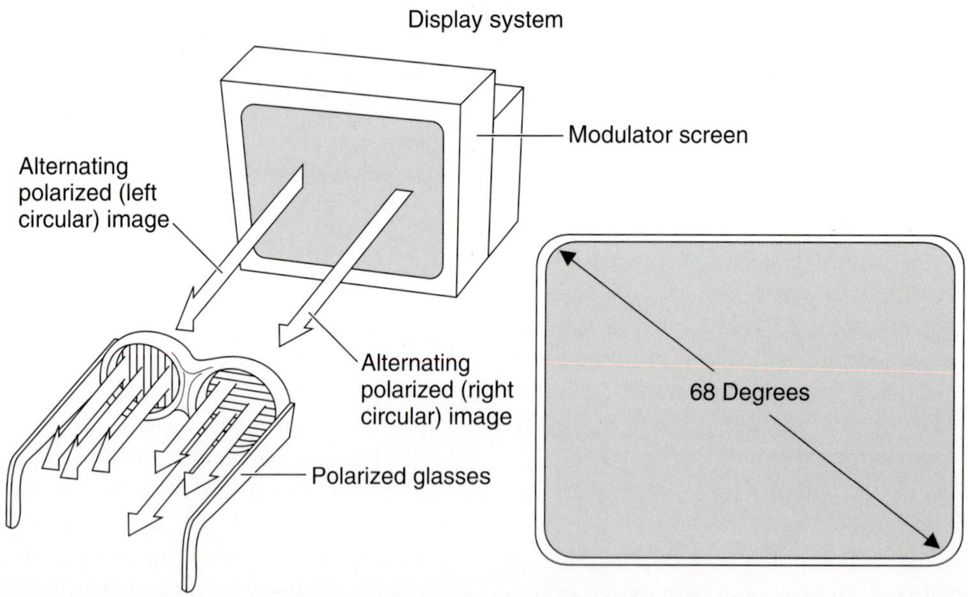

B

Fig. 10-7. (A) 3-D Scope three-dimensional videolaparoscopic system requires the surgeon to wear polarizing sunglasses to separate the two stereoscopic images. **(B)** The polarizing lenses permit each eye to see only one image. Synthesis of these two images generates a true three-dimensional image.

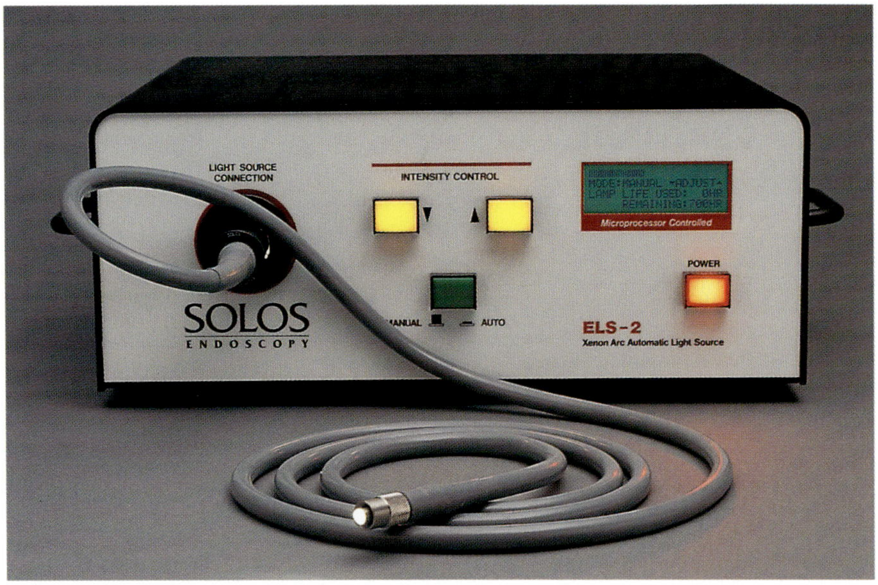

Fig. 10-8. Light sources that use xenon bulbs produce a much greater light intensity than the older systems based on halogen light bulbs. This greater quantity of light allows illumination of large three-dimensional operative fields.

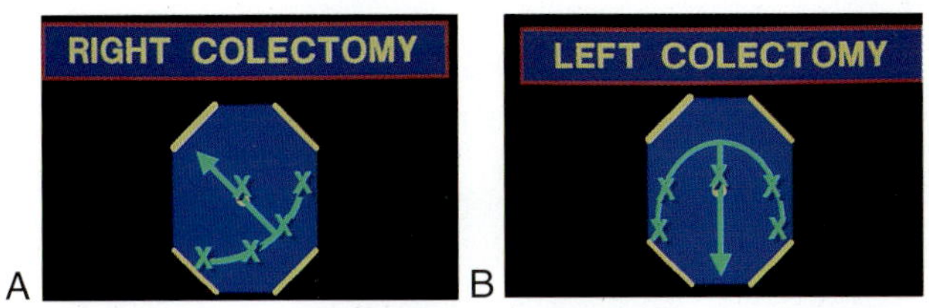

Fig. 10-9. Trocars are placed around an arc that focuses on the planned operative dissection. Ideally, the camera port sits in the middle of the arc generated by the working ports. **(A)** Trocar placement for a right colectomy. **(B)** Trocar placement for an anterior resection.

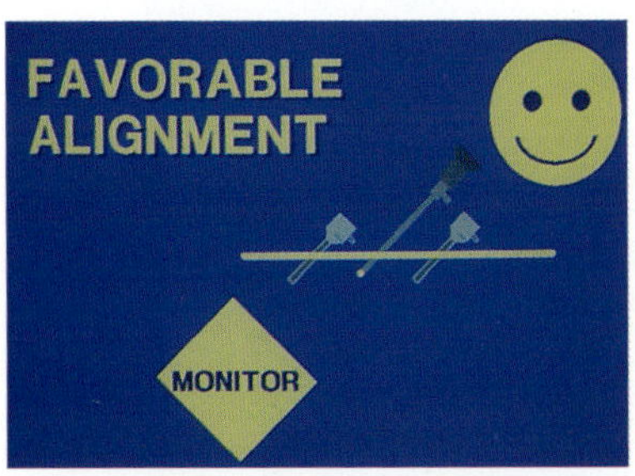

Fig. 10-10. Surgeon, camera, and trocars for the working surgical instruments should all be directed toward the video monitor.

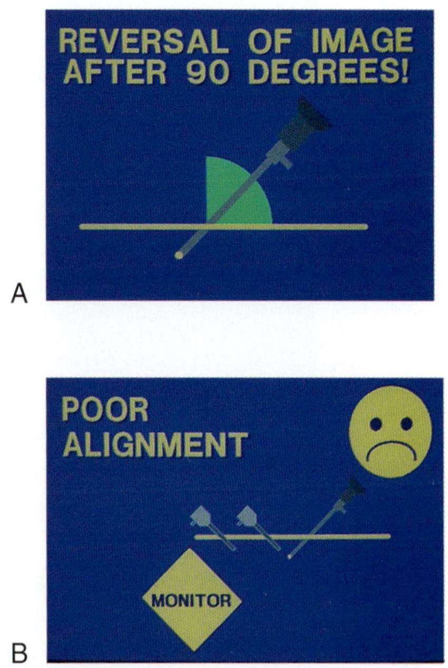

Fig. 10-11. (A) As the orientation between the long axis of the laparoscope and the working surgical instrument passes beyond 90 degrees, movements on the video monitor are reversed. **(B)** Reversal of the image on the monitor hinders movement of the instrument by the surgeon or assistant surgeon.

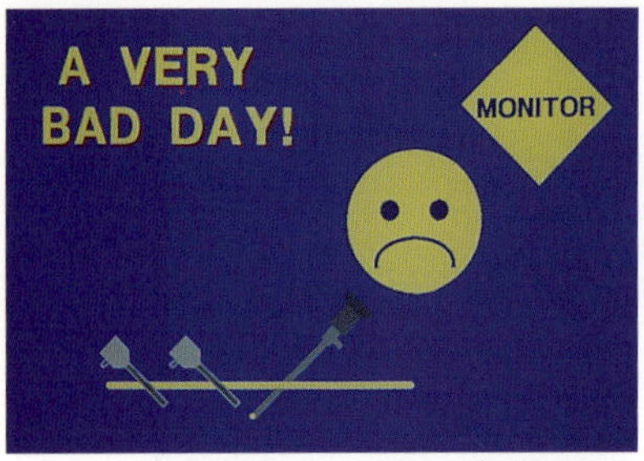

Fig. 10-12. When the position of the monitor or the relative orientation of the laparoscope and surgical instruments is disadvantageous, time should be taken to reposition the laparoscope, instruments, or monitor to a more appropriate position.

scopes are 10 mm in diameter or smaller. As a result, trocars of at least 10 mm in size should be used at *all* trocar sites to allow the insertion of all instruments and the videolaparoscope through any trocar site. Laparoscopic stapling devices require larger trocar diameters. As the surgeon gains experience, the site for a large trocar such as a 15-, 18-, or 33-mm trocar can be selected early in the procedure. Alternatively, 10-mm trocars can be initially used, and when use of the linear stapling device is required, one of the 10-mm trocars can be replaced with a larger trocar.

Newer generations of trocars have overcome many of the problems of older models (Fig. 10-13). Universal

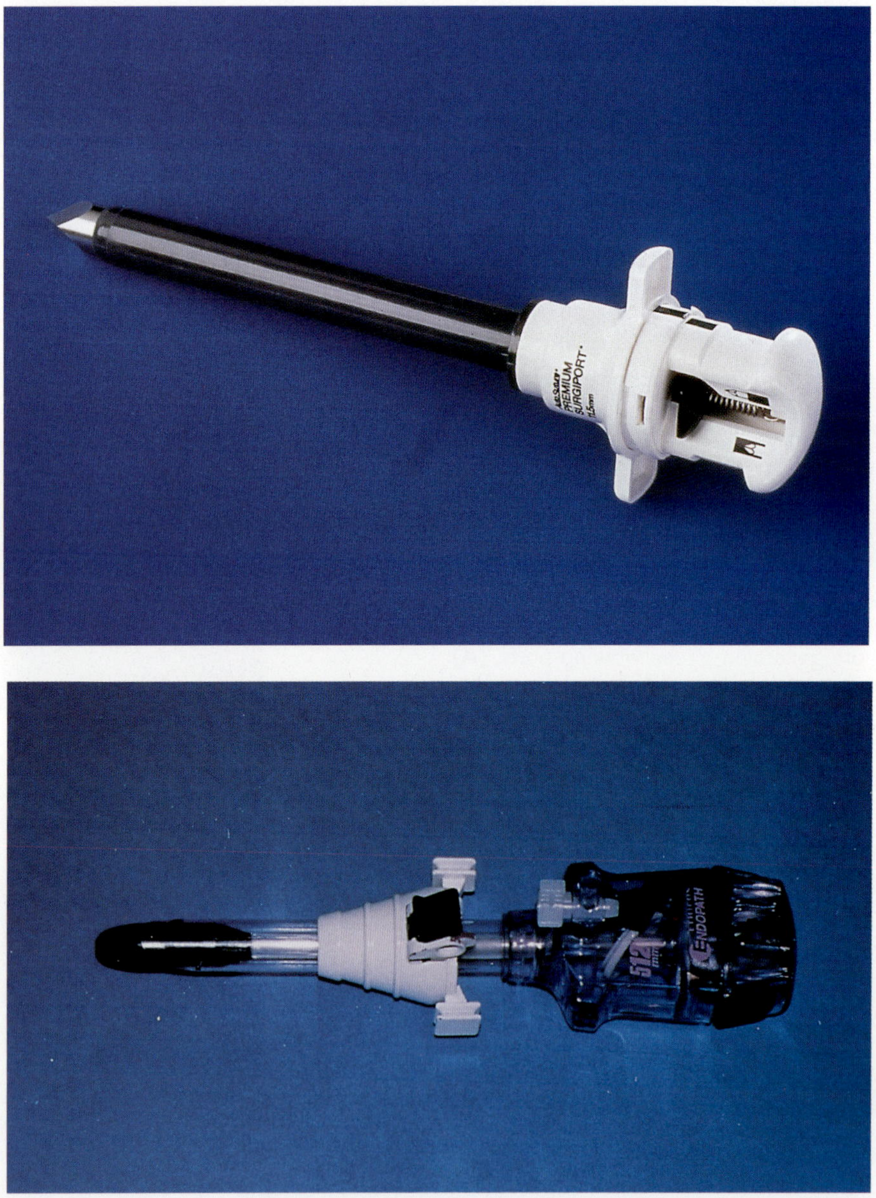

A

B

Fig. 10-13. New generations of trocars now offer adapters for a wide variety of instrument sizes. **(A)** Premium Surgiport (United States Surgical Corporation) allows the insertion of instruments from 5 mm to 12 mm in diameter. **(B)** Ethicon trocar (Ethicon Endosurgery) also permits the insertion of a wide variety of sizes of instruments.

adapters have been developed to allow insertion of a wide variety of instruments through the same trocar. This technique increases flexibility in the performance of difficult operations. In addition, new systems of fixation have largely eliminated problems with leakage of carbon dioxide around the trocars.

Patrick Leahy has found a solution to many of the limitations of currently available instruments. It allows use of the oldest and most versatile of all instruments: the surgeon's hand (Fig. 10-14A). Since an incision is required for retrieval of the specimen during most colectomies, Leahy decided to use it for additional abdominal access for his hand. This access requires making an incision somewhat larger than that used in standard laparoscopic-assisted techniques. An incision 7.5 cm long is used for surgeons with a glove size of 7.5. A plastic sleeve that incorporates a valve, Dexterity (Galileo, Dublin, Ireland), is attached to the incision to maintain the pneumoperitoneum. A wound protector prevents the contamination or seeding of tumor in the wound (Fig. 10-14B). Surgeons use their hand for blunt dissection or retraction of bowel as in open operations. In addition, instruments for open operations, such as roticulating linear stapling devices, can be inserted into the abdomen without loss of the pneumoperitoneum. This system provides an excellent bridge between traditional surgical techniques and newer laparoscopic techniques.

A new trocar system has been introduced that now allows safe access to the lumen of the gastrointestinal tract (Innerdyne). A 5-mm trocar is inserted through the abdominal wall. The bowel is held up by Babcock forceps toward the trocar. The trocar is inserted

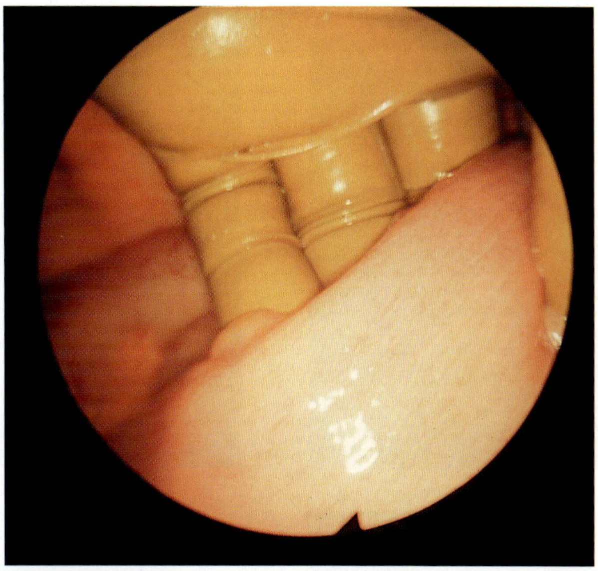

A

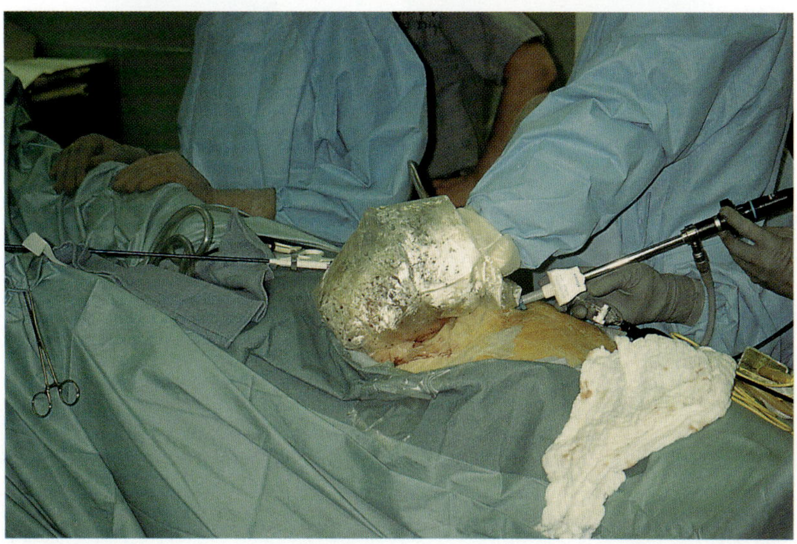

B

Fig. 10-14. **(A)** Dexterity, a new device, allows introduction of the surgeon's hand into the abdomen without loss of the pneumoperitoneum. **(B)** Surgeons inserts their hand into the abdomen through the Dexterity device. A valve maintains the pneumoperitoneum, and a wound protector prevents wound contamination or wound implantation.

through the bowel wall. A balloon cuff is inflated to hold the trocar in place within the bowel lumen and seal the entry site (Fig. 10-15). This technique prevents any spillage of bowel contents and permits access for instruments to perform laparoscopic local excisions of intestinal neoplasms. Flexible endoscopes are used to visualize the intraluminal procedure.

SURGICAL INSTRUMENTS

Laparoscopic colorectal surgery instruments remain in a period of rapid evolution. In the first stage of this evolutionary process, familiar 19th century gastrointestinal surgery instruments were adapted for use during laparoscopy. Typically, long handles were attached to standard instruments such as scissors, forceps, and hemostats. The point of fixation imposed by the trocar, however, limited the degrees of freedom in the movement of this simple instrument. In the next phase of evolution, articulating heads were added to allow a full range of motion (Fig. 10-16). In the current phase, new instruments are being designed to meet specific problems generated by laparoscopic techniques. These include new suturing instruments, pursestring devices, and retractors.

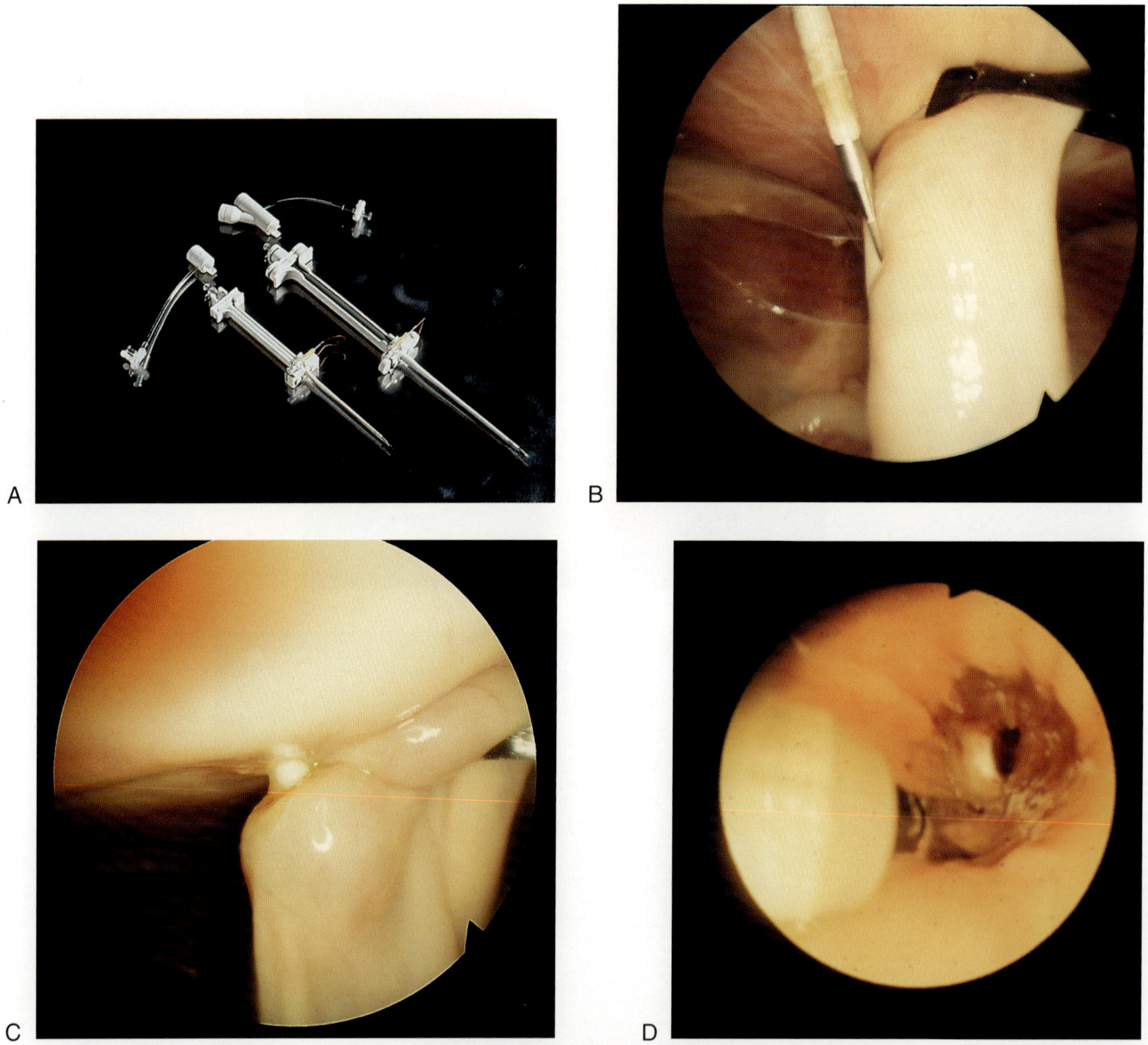

Fig. 10-15. (A) Radially Expanding Dilator (Innerdyne Corporation) trocar system permits transabdominal access into the bowel lumen. **(B)** The needle is used to puncture both the abdominal wall and the bowel wall. **(C)** An inflatable balloon on the catheter tips holds the catheter in place and seals the enterotomy. **(D)** This system allows transabdominal introduction of 5-mm instruments such as electrocautery scissors into the lumen of the bowel.

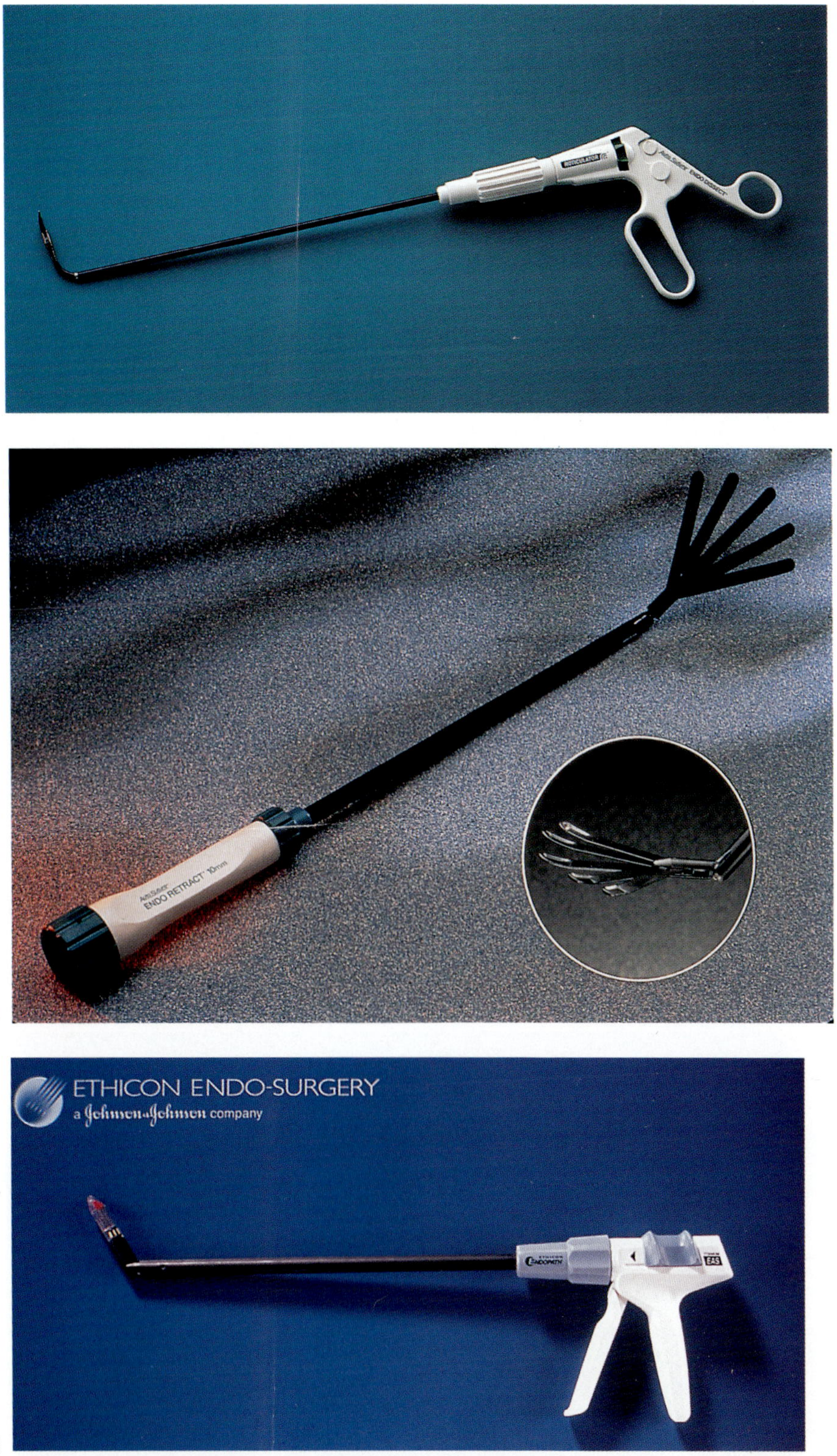

A

B

C

Fig. 10-16. New instruments add multiple joints to the tips of the instruments: **(A)** Roticulating Endo-Dissectors (United States Surgical Corporation); **(B)** Roticulating Five Finger Endoretract; and **(C)** Ethicon stapling device. These instruments allow multiple degrees of freedom for the movement of the instrument's tip. These articulations overcome many of the limitations imposed by the point of fixation when the instrument is inserted through a trocar.

Specific Instruments

Laparoscopic procedures require fewer instruments than do open operations. This results from the tactical constraint that only as many instruments can be used as trocars have been inserted. As a result, the scrub nurse generally requires only a Mayo stand for the laparoscopic instruments. Dissection is accomplished with electrocautery scissors. Under certain circumstances, however, the standard length of laparoscopic scissors proves inadequate. In tall patients, when mobilizing the colonic flexures, or when dissecting below the peritoneal reflection in the pelvis, a long EndoShears (United States Surgical Corporation, Norwalk, CT) greatly facilitates performance of the procedure. If these long instruments are not available, insertion of additional trocars closer to the limits of dissection is required. The surgeon provides the countertraction with a grasping instrument in the nondominant hand. This instrument can be a grasping, dissecting, or Babcock-type instrument. The assistant provides retraction and exposure with two laparoscopic Babcock instruments. Sometimes, such as deep in the pelvis, a fan-type retractor replaces one of the Babcock instruments. An aspiration and irrigation system should be available. Irrigation with heparinized irrigation fluid prevents clot formation and facilitates the aspiration of any blood in the operative field. It is critical to maintain hemostasis, since even small amounts of blood stain the tissues and obscure planes of dissection. Moreover, hemoglobin absorbs light and rapidly darkens the visual field. Most of the procedure is accomplished with these few instruments.

Several additional instruments are used on a limited basis during laparoscopic colorectal operations. A laparoscopic clip applier should be readily available. However, the scalpels of the laparoscopic linear stapling devices cannot cut through these heavy clips. As a result, clips must not be used near planned sites of transection of the mesentery or bowel in cases in which it is anticipated that linear staples will be used. Laparoscopic bulldog clamps can help obtain control of bleeding from major vessels. Availability of these instruments may prevent conversion to an open operation under some circumstances. Laparoscopic bowel clamps prevent leakage of stool during construction of intracorporeal anastomoses. Bowel clamps are also used to occlude the terminal ileum during intraoperative colonoscopy. High-quality laparoscopic needle holders are essential for repair of enterotomies, for suture ligation of vessels, or for construction of intracorporeal anastomoses. The tips should have "diamond tip" jaws. The handle should be of the palm grip type, not the pistol grip type. Both the Jared and Cabot needle holders are excellent. Recently, a new approach has been attempted for the construction of continuous suture lines. A semiautomated suturing device allows the rapid closure of long enterotomies (Fig. 10-17).

Laparoscopic linear stapling devices are essential for all laparoscopic colorectal resections. These stapling devices place multiple rows of staggered staples and divide the tissue between the staple lines with a scalpel. The United States Surgical Corporation instruments place three rows of staples on either side of the incision, and the Ethicon Corporation instruments place two rows on either side. The EndoGIA 30 (United States Surgical

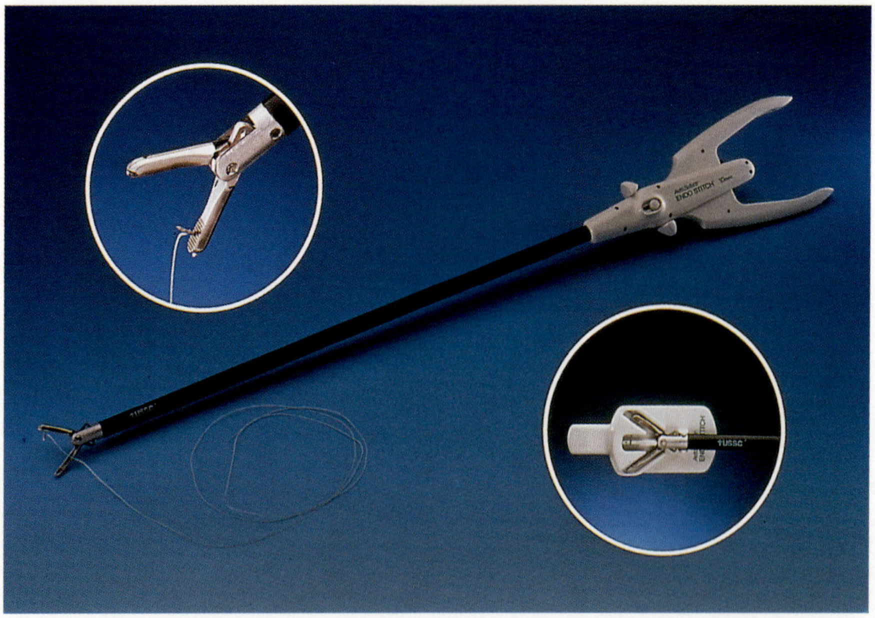

Fig. 10-17. New semiautomated suturing device introduced by the United States Surgical Corporation facilitates the construction of a continuous suture line. The jaws of the instrument pass the needle back and forth.

Corporation) is inserted through a 12-mm trocar whereas the EndoGIA 60 fits through a 15-mm trocar. The Endoscopic Linear Cutter 30 (Ethicon Corporation) requires a 12-mm trocar and the ELC 60, an 18-mm one. These instruments are used to transect the bowel and construct side-to-side, functional end-to-end anastomoses. They can also transect the mesentery. A roticulating linear stapling device has been developed for low anterior anastomoses and should be available for clinical practice in the near future (Fig. 10-18).

Disposable Versus Reusable Laparoscopic Instruments

Disposable and reusable varieties of most instruments are available. Many people argue the benefits of one over the other. Nonetheless, disposable instruments offer the surgeon distinct advantages for advanced laparoscopic procedures. The newer laparoscopic instruments provide movement in all three dimensions. This facility of movement overcomes the limitations of the point of fixation engendered by the trocar. Multiple internal channels and cables within the instruments are required to gain multiple degrees of freedom in motion. These long internal channels and complex hinge systems cannot be cleaned, which is not a problem in disposable instruments. By contrast, this cleaning has proved the greatest limitation for the development of sophisticated reusable instruments. Because of issues of sterilization, makers of reusable instruments are forced to make simple instruments that use traditional, simple metal hinge systems. Complex reusable instruments with articulations that provide motions in all three directions have not been developed because the problem of proper sterilization has not been solved. Other issues have also played a role in this debate. During periods of rapid evolution of technology, disposable instruments offer a distinct advantage. New modifications of instrument design are immediately available for clinical practice since they are phased in simply through resupply of used products.

Cost proves an ambiguous issue. Reusable instruments are expensive. Instruments with cutting edges such as scissors or trocars require frequent sharpening. As laparoscopic reusable instruments have become more complex, their longevity has diminished. The long length of the instruments places extreme leverage on the metal pieces, which leads to rapid fatigue of the metal and ultimately breakage. Moreover, they require skilled cleaning and maintenance. Workers responsible for proper care of the instruments receive high wages, large insurance packages, and pension plans. Reusable instruments carry the risk of transmission of blood-borne infections and associated litigation. Moreover, many of the disposable instruments are not available in reusable equivalents. Resulting cost issues indicate that there is little if any net savings to the hospital by using reusable instruments. Indeed, system-wide cost analysis confirms that in every institution studied, disposable instruments either cost the same as reusable instruments or save the institution money. Because it is difficult to identify any advantages of reusable instruments to the surgeon, it seems difficult to sustain an argument on their behalf.

Display of Disposable Laparoscopic Instruments

The myriad new devices produced by various corporations has led to much confusion. As personnel rotate from operating room to operating room, they often fall behind in knowledge of these instruments. As a result, the duration of advanced laparoscopic procedures is often prolonged by delays in the acquisition of infrequently used instruments from storage rooms. A help-

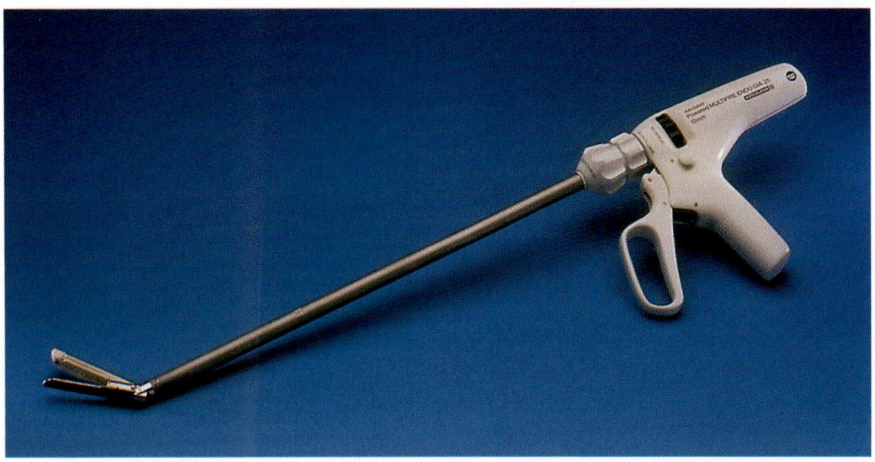

Fig. 10-18. Roticulating EndoGIA 60 allows lower transection of the rectum than can now be accomplished with straight linear stapling instruments.

ful accessory that overcomes many of these problems is a large rack on which the full array of disposable laparoscopic instruments are displayed (Fig. 10-19). With the instruments in clear view, it is easy for the surgeon to point to the desired one instead of having to describe it. This method also facilitates keeping track of the inventory of various instruments.

Traditional Surgical Instruments

All laparoscopic cases may potentially need to be converted to an open procedure, sometimes rapidly and unexpectedly. For this reason, instruments necessary to open the abdomen should be immediately available on a side table. As surgeons gain experience with laparoscopic procedures and gain skills in suturing, obtaining hemostasis, and lysis of adhesions, this precaution may become unnecessary.

INTRAOPERATIVE COLONOSCOPY

Laparoscopy prevents the surgeon from palpating abdominal viscera. Consequently, early colorectal neoplasms are not easily located during initial exploration of the abdomen. Several techniques can be used to determine the location of a colorectal lesion. A preoperative barium enema is adequate if only the general location of the lesion is required. If a right hemicolectomy is planned, the surgeon needs to know only that the lesion is in the right colon. Another useful technique for this purpose is preoperative tattooing of the bowel wall during colonoscopy. The full circumference of the colonic wall should be injected so that the tattoo is not obscured by the mesentery or appendices epiploicae. These methods, however, are not useful in all circumstances.

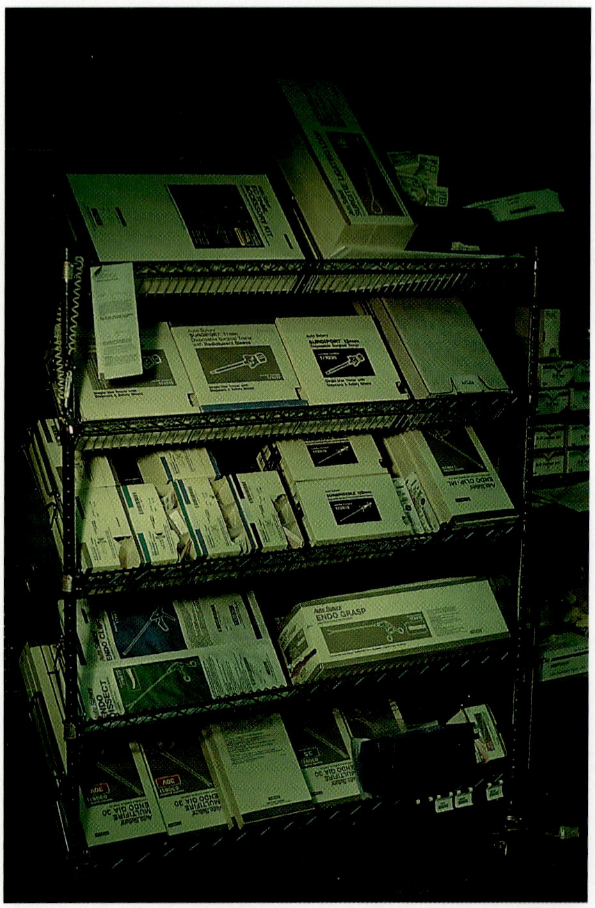

Fig. 10-19. Rack for display of the wide variety of disposable instruments makes these instruments rapidly accessible.

Intraoperative colonoscopy is an important adjunct to laparoscopic colorectal procedures to identify the exact location of lesions, as well as their proximal and distal margins. This information is critical for various types of laparoscopic polypectomies and segmental resections. Similarly, intraoperative endoscopy can ensure that the distal margin of resection is appropriate during anterior and low-anterior resection. Moreover, intraoperative localization of lesions ensures that the specimen will contain a lesion.

The technique is simple, since all patients are already placed in a modified Lloyd-Davies position. After the pneumoperitoneum is established, the terminal ileum is occluded with an atraumatic bowel clamp. The colonoscope is inserted to the level of the lesion. The intensity of the laparoscopic light source is turned down. The light of the colonoscope is easily visible through the wall of the colon or rectum. It should be noted that the light intensity of a flexible endoscope greatly exceeds that of a rigid sigmoidoscope; consequently, a flexible instrument should be used. The laparoscopic surgeon marks the position of the lesion with surgical clips. The colonoscopist directs the application of the clips by observation of the indentation made in the colonic wall by the open jaws of the clip applier. The air within the colon is aspirated as the colonoscope is withdrawn.

LAPAROSCOPIC ULTRASOUND

Surgeons are unable to palpate anatomic structures during laparoscopic procedures. This restriction limits the surgeon's ability to identify intraparenchymal lesions within the liver, detect gallstones within the gallbladder or common bile duct, locate blood vessels, or evaluate lesions. New technologies can replace this lost information: introduction of an ultrasound probe into the abdomen permits accurate detection of hepatic lesions. Indeed, the superiority of intraoperative ultrasound for the detection of liver lesions over computed tomography (CT) or other external imaging modalities is well established.[4] Laparoscopic probes are available from several companies. The Endomedix system uses a "picture in a picture" technology so that the surgeon can follow the movements of the probe and the ultrasound image on the same monitor (Fig. 10-20). The Endomedix probe is coupled with a Doppler system that converts flow rates of blood into sound to facilitate the identification of major vascular structures. The Tetrad probe uses a linear array of ultrasound crystals to provide a high-resolution image (Fig. 10-21). In addition, this company has introduced a flexible laparoscopic ultrasound probe that is particularly helpful in imaging the liver (Fig. 10-22). The probe is easily passed along the surfaces of the hepatic lobes.

Whereas detection of liver lesions and gallstones is well established, other applications remain in a period of development. One promising area is intraoperative staging of colorectal neoplasms. Transluminal ultrasound has been used for many years for the staging of rectal cancers.[5] The ultrasound image reveals the depth of penetration of the lesion, thereby permitting the surgeon to select appropriate treatment for the stage of the patient's disease. Similarly, laparoscopic ultrasound could be used for the intraoperative staging of colonic and proximal rectal lesions. Current probes require enhancement of their near field images and some changes in the focal lengths of the ultrasound probes to provide images of the bowel wall with adequate resolution. Nonetheless, these alterations are relatively minor, and as a result, satisfactory probes should become available in the near future.

Coupling of this technology with a system for the detection of metastatic lesions in lymph nodes or other distant sites will allow accurate intraoperative staging of colorectal neoplasms. The surgeon will be in a position to tailor appropriate treatment modalities to the requirements of a specific lesion in an individual patient. Furthermore, there will be no need for recovery of the specimen in an intact fashion since the intraoperative assessment of the lesion will provide the required information for staging. This advantage will obviate the need for incisions for the recovery of specimens. The specimen will be minced in a bag and aspirated with the suction device.

RADIOIMMUNO-GUIDED SURGERY

Accurate intraoperative staging of colorectal cancers has always been limited by the inability of surgeons to identify metastatic lesions in the mesenteric lymph nodes. Standard staging systems in the late 20th century continue to rely on 19th century staging techniques and histologic examination. Recently, a potentially more sensitive system for the detection of metastatic lesions has been developed. Moreover, this system can be used intraoperatively for the staging of colorectal neoplasms. This system is based on monoclonal antibody binding to antigens on tumor cell surfaces.

Radioimmuno-guided surgery (RIGS) uses radiolabeled monoclonal antibodies that bind tumor cell antigens.[6] Several antibodies are available against tumor-associated antigens such as carcinoembryonic antigen

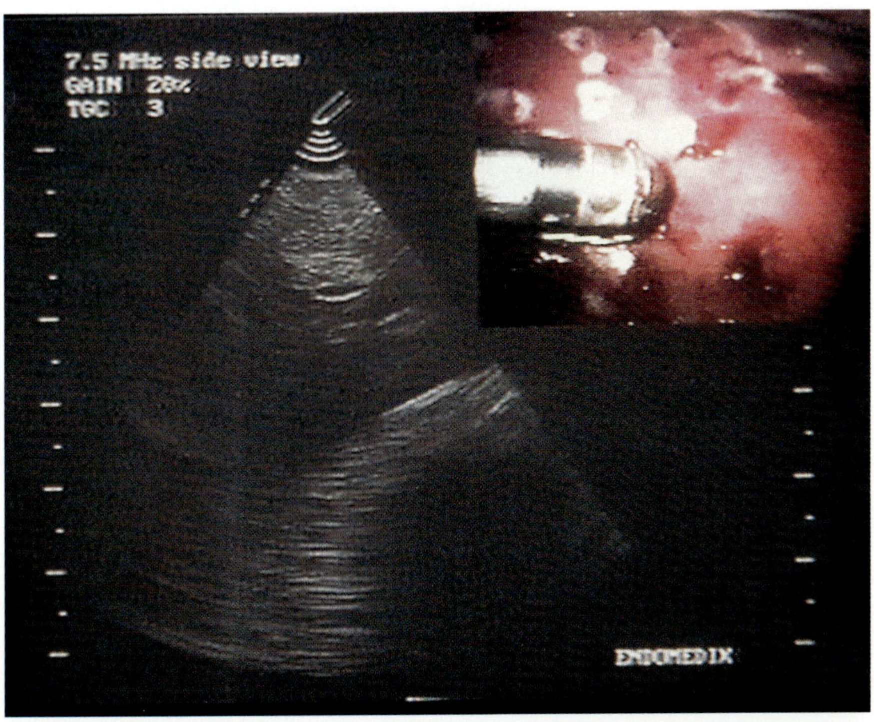

Fig. 10-20. Endomedix laparoscopic ultrasound probe uses "picture within a picture" technology to project both the videolaparoscopic image and the ultrasound image on the same monitor.

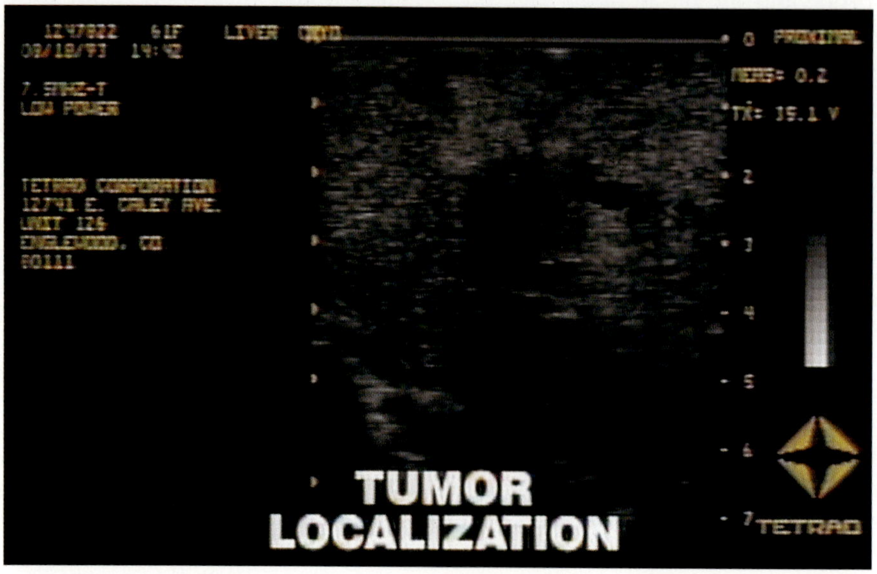

Fig. 10-21. Linear array of ultrasound crystals used in the Tetrad probe provides high-resolution imaging of lesions such as this colorectal cancer metastasis in the liver.

(CEA), 791T/36, B72.3, and CC49. The newest of these, CC49, binds to an antigen expressed by about 95 percent of colorectal cancers. These can be tagged with a γ-emitting isotope iodine 125 (^{125}I), injected intravenously, and detected with a γ-counter. The ^{125}I is used because of its relatively long half-life. The radiolabeled monoclonal antibody is injected intravenously into the patient 2 weeks before the planned operation. The antibody binds to the primary lesion and any metastatic lesions. The 2-week interval allows the radiolabeled antibody to clear from the circulation and diminishes nonspecific binding. The result is decreased background noise and increased sensitivity of the system. Clinical trials have used the handheld γ-detector Neoprobe (Neoprobe Corporation, Columbus, OH) during second look operations for patients suspected of having recurrent colorectal cancer. This system detected unsuspected metastatic lesions in 27 percent of 104 patients with the older B72.3 monoclonal antibody.[7] Recent studies with CC49 suggest that the RIGS system is more sensitive than traditional histologic techniques for the identification of lymph node metastases.

A prototype for a laparoscopic RIGS system has been developed (Fig. 10-23). This system may prove useful for intraoperative localization of the primary colorectal neoplasm as well as for accurate intraoperative staging of metastatic disease. The current probe allows easy scanning of the bowel, mesentery, and potential sites of

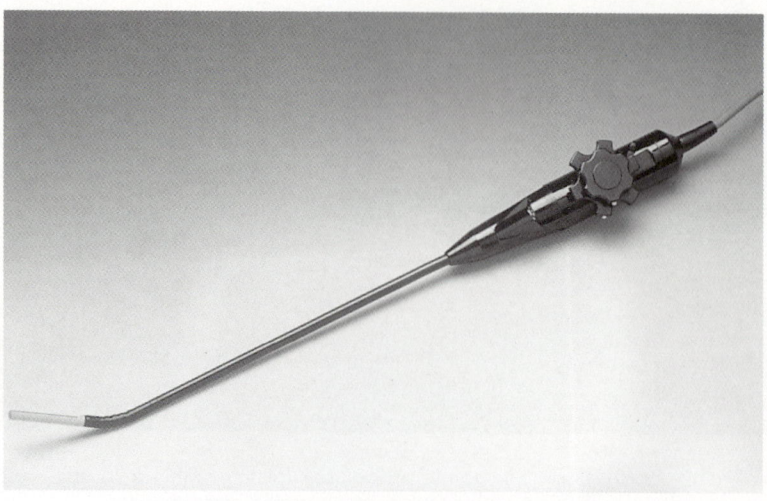

Fig. 10-22. Flexible ultrasound probes (Tetrad Corporation) facilitate imaging of the liver.

distal metastases such as the liver and liver hilum (Fig. 10-24). Clinical trials will be required to confirm the usefulness of this system.

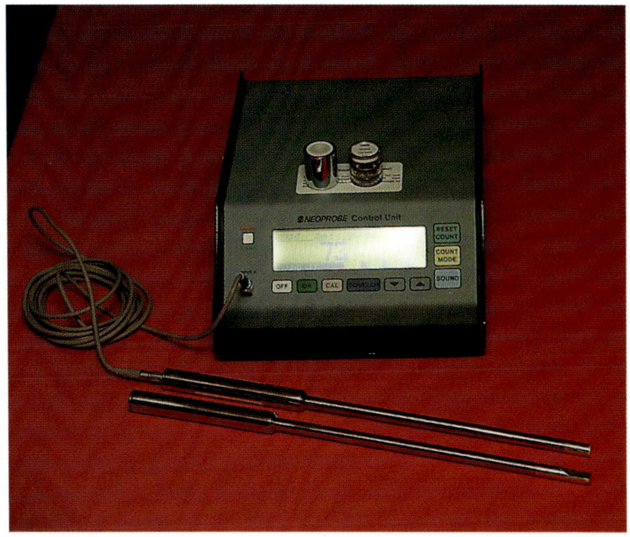

Fig. 10-23. Laparoscopic radioimmuno-guided surgery γ-detector produced by the Neoprobe Corporation allows intraoperative detection of metastases from colorectal cancers.

OPERATING ROOM ORGANIZATION

Advanced laparoscopic surgery requires a wide variety of new technologies. The equipment used for these procedures fills up even the largest operating room suite. Consequently, careful thought and planning must be given to the distribution of equipment around the operating room table. The fundamental strategy is based on positioning the trocars, videolaparoscope, and monitors so that the surgeon is standing comfortably, not operating backward on the screen, and is looking directly at the monitor for most of the procedure. Whenever feasible, electronic equipment is vertically stacked to minimize consumption of floor space. All equipment is placed on carts with wheels or suspended from track systems on the ceiling to allow flexible placement of individual items and easy adjustments during the procedure.

Right Colon Operations

During right colonic operations the surgeon will stand on the patient's left side or between the legs in the so-called French position. The two monitors are placed by the patient's right knee and right shoulder (Fig. 10-25). The monitor by the knee is used during mobilization of the cecum and the monitor by the shoulder for mobilization of the splenic flexure. When used, the colonoscopic video monitor is positioned by the patient's left shoulder. Alternatively, a "picture in a picture" system can be used to insert the colonoscopic image onto the laparoscopic monitors. The scrub nurse stands by the patient's left leg.

Left Colorectal Operations

The surgeon stands on both sides of the patient during various parts of the operation. The most difficult and dangerous parts of the dissection are centered in the pelvis. Consequently, the primary video monitor is positioned between the legs of the patient (Fig. 10-26). If mobilization of the splenic flexure is anticipated, the second monitor is placed by the left shoulder of the patient. If only a pelvic dissection is planned, both monitors can be placed by the patient's feet.

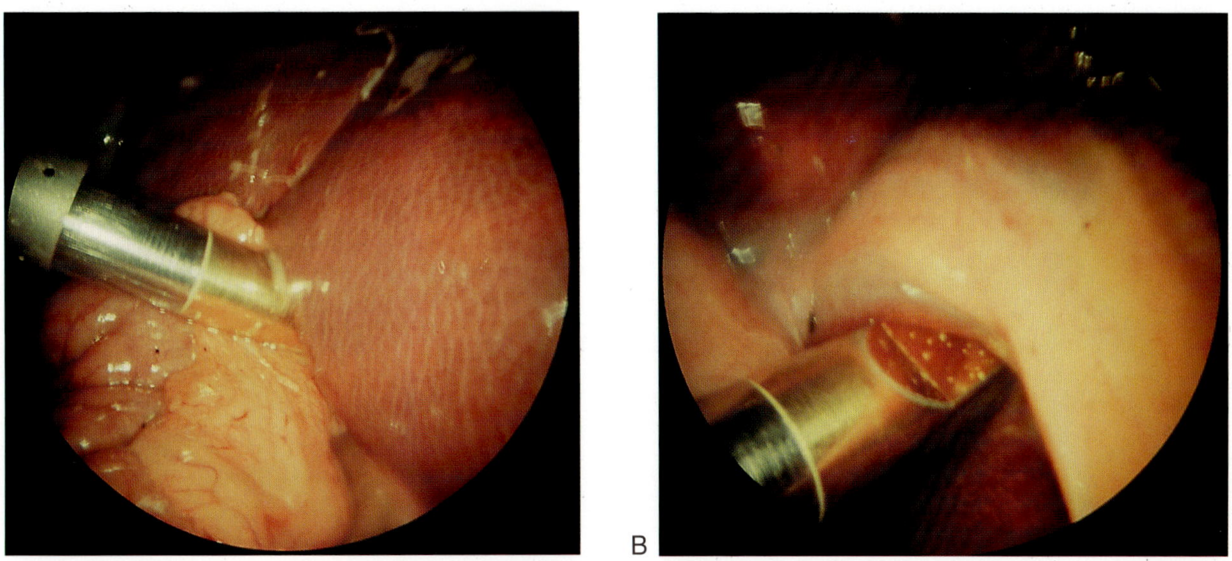

A B

Fig. 10-24. Laparoscopic Neoprobe can detect occult neoplasm through the abdomen such as **(A)** within the liver **(B)** or within the hepatoduodenal ligament.

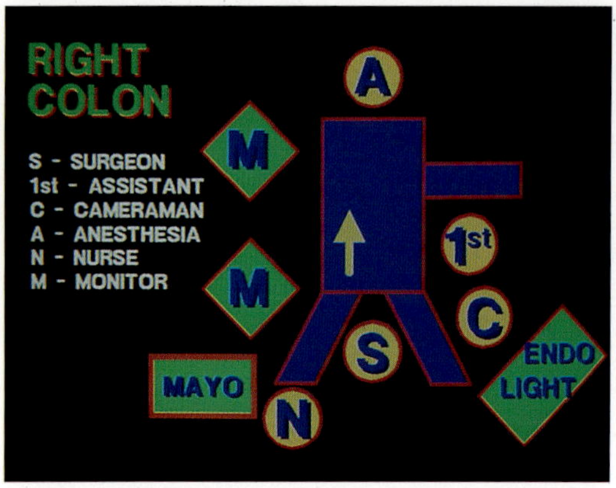

Fig. 10-25. Positioning of equipment and personnel for a right colon operation.

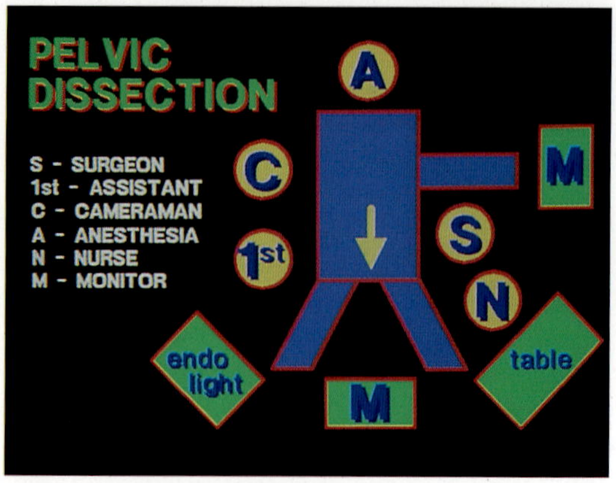

Fig. 10-26. Positioning of personnel and equipment for a pelvic dissection or left colorectal operation.

REFERENCES

1. Svenberg T: Pathophysiology of pneumoperitoneum. p. 61. In Ballantyne GH, Leahy PF, Modlin IM (eds): Laparoscopic Surgery. WB Saunders, Philadelphia, 1994
2. Cunningham AJ: Anesthesia. p. 42. In Ballantyne GH, Leahy PF, Modlin IM (eds): Laparoscopic Surgery. WB Saunders, Philadelphia, 1994
3. Regier H: High-definition video improves quality of laparoscopic images. Gen Surg Laparosc News 14:1, 1993
4. Machi J, Isomoto H, Yamashita Y et al: Intraoperative ultrasonography in screening for liver metastases from colorectal cancer: comparative accuracy with traditional procedures. Surgery 101:678, 1987
5. Milsom JW, Graffner H: Intrarectal ultrasonography in rectal cancer staging and in the evaluation of pelvic disease. Ann Surg 212:602, 1990
6. Lavery IC: Radioimmuno-guided surgery for colon cancer. Semin Colon Rectal Surg 2:54, 1991
7. Sardi A, Agnone CM, Nieroda CA et al: Radioimmunoguided surgery in recurrent colorectal cancer: the role of carcinoembryonic antigen, computerized tomography and physical examination. South Med J 82:1235, 1989

Editorial Comment

Rama M. Jager

Surgeons starting laparoscopic colorectal surgical procedures need to be aware that these advanced endoscopic techniques are more instrument intensive than are laparoscopic cholecystectomies. Laparoscopic colorectal operations require more than one monitor and multiple peritoneal ports. The surgeon needs to shuffle the camera port location and switch sides with the surgical assistant, depending on the field of operation. All these requirements dictate careful planning and attention to details. Drs. Ballantyne and Begos delineate the various aspects of instrumental layout and requirements.

As the authors point out, no hospital can construct special operating rooms for laparoscopic operations. Use of the largest available operating room in the suite is desirable. Surgeons should voice their desires to the hospital administrators regarding the special needs for laparoscopy when new operating rooms are being designed and constructed. Although laparoscopic techniques are far from displacing traditional open laparotomy, the use of therapeutic laparoscopy will certainly increase in the future. Properly designed operating rooms equipped for laparoscopic procedures facilitate wider adaption of the laparoscopic techniques for the purpose of reducing postoperative morbidity.

Some details that I have noticed in conducting laparoscopic colorectal surgery in our hospitals follow. The control switch for the electrical operating table should be accessible to the anesthesiologist, who can then change the table position as needed. Placement of a bean bag under the patient will stabilize the patient more satisfactorily during the extreme degrees of tilting and rotation needed during laparoscopic colonic flexural mobilization. The bean bag should be placed in a way that it does not interfere with intraoperative colonoscopy or transanal insertion of surgical anastomotic staplers. Intraoperative colonoscopy is often necessary during laparoscopic colorectal surgery because the surgeon cannot palpate the lesion. Proper patient positioning should allow intraoperative colonoscopy in any patient needing a laparoscopic colonic resection. The video monitor for the colonoscope can be toward the patient's head to allow a comfortable viewing angle for the colonoscopist. Because of the need for multiple instruments and monitors, the use of two circulating nurses rather than the traditional one circulator during the initial setup will reduce the preparation time. The circulating nurses should be familiar enough with the video equipment to troubleshoot. Otherwise, the task of straightening out video monitor and camera problems distract the surgeon and unduly delay the operation. The hospital clinical engineering department should be available to help the circulating nurses if they cannot solve the video-related difficulties.

Since most laparoscopic colorectal procedures require two monitors, the use of two video instrument carts is helpful. Each cart optimally contains a monitor, a laparoscopic camera, and a carbon dioxide insufflator. The second cart will be helpful as a backup in case one monitor or camera fails. It also allows simultaneous use of a second telescope to transilluminate and provide a panoramic view. The second insufflator also allows maintenance of satisfactory pneumoperitoneum in spite of gas loss during camera exchanges and use of a suction-irrigation system. The carts should be placed so that they can be moved cephalad or caudad without interference from electrical cords or additional equipment on the floor. Various tubes and cords stretch from the operating table to the equipment positioned behind the surgeon and the assistants. The cords include the monopolar and bipolar coagulation cables, the laparoscopic camera cable(s), the cord(s) to light source(s), the tubes for insufflation, and those for suction-irrigation. Proper planning and grouping of electrical cords and tubes are essential to prevent the surgeon or assistant from being boxed in with limited mobility. Multiple cords on the floor also trip the unwary. The surgeon and the assistant often need to exchange their stations during laparoscopic dissection and should be able to do so without disrupting the cable labyrinth. The foot switches for monopolar and bipolar coagulators should be placed on the side where the surgeon stands, preferably on the dominant side. An extra set of foot switches should be placed on the opposite side of the patient. This positioning allows the surgeon to move from the left to the right side of the patient during laparoscopic dissection and use the coagulators without translocating the foot switches. Also, use of small flashlights taped to the foot switches allows their repositioning as needed in the darkened laparoscopy room.

The use of two Mayo trays, one toward the patient's head and other toward the feet, may be helpful in some laparoscopic procedures. The instruments can be distributed over both tables as needed to avoid clutter. Since most laparoscopic colorectal surgical procedures also need a mini-incision for specimen retrieval or extracorporeal anastomosis, one table serves to hold the instruments needed for the mini-incision and the other to hold laparoscopic instruments. Even when a mini-incision is not necessary, the second Mayo table will allow the surgeon to park the laparoscopic instrument during change of a camera to a different port, and so forth.

The use of a three-dimensional laparoscopic camera system is very appealing. The three-dimensional cameras I have used suffered from the problem of decreased illumination as compared with the standard three-chip cameras. Most surgeons trained in videocolonoscopy and two-dimensional videolaparoscopy can realize their surgical objectives without the three-dimensional system. The other practical problem is the logistics of the hospital operating rooms. Unless all the laparoscopic operating rooms have three-dimensional cameras, the surgeon may not be certain whether the three-dimensional camera is available for the planned operation. With improved technology and decreasing prices, it is hoped that three-dimensional cameras will become commonplace.

The technique of using the surgeon's hand through an airtight sleeve (Dexterity) to retrieve the laparoscopically resected specimen and to use stapling devices may be a convolution that adds little to laparoscopic surgery. Many surgeons can accomplish a right hemicolectomy for benign disease through a 7.5-cm incision, and the addition of an airtight sleeve to do the same operation laparoscopically may hinder rather than help. Using various wound edge lifting devices to conduct "gasless" laparoscopic colorectal surgery may be more useful than the airtight sleeve. Further clinical studies are necessary to prove the advantage of this sleeve. Use of a wound protector to prevent bacterial and oncocytic contamination of the wound, by contrast, is unquestionably helpful in laparoscopic colorectal resections.

11

Diagnostic Laparoscopy

Rama M. Jager

Diagnostic laparoscopy as an isolated or initial procedure is often necessary in patients with colorectal disease. Patients with chronic abdominal pain, especially lower quadrant abdominal pain, are often evaluated by gastrointestinal endoscopy followed by imaging studies such as computed tomography (CT) scans and ultrasound examinations. When these studies do not yield the etiologic diagnosis, diagnostic laparoscopy may establish the diagnosis. Even in patients whose abdominal imaging shows abnormalities, laparoscopic inspection, palpation, and biopsy may be necessary to identify the pathologic nature of the lesion. Because of the decreased risk and postoperative morbidity associated with diagnostic laparoscopy in contrast to laparotomy, the former will be more acceptable to the surgeon and the patient.

Every laparoscopic colorectal operation should be preceded by diagnostic evaluation of the intraperitoneal viscera. The laparoscopic surgeon should gain expertise in laparoscopic evaluation of the gastrointestinal system and identification of the abnormalities. The skills learned in diagnostic laparoscopy—including the exposure of various portions of the colorectum, retraction of unwanted small bowel loops along with omentum, and tactile evaluation by remote palpation with a blunt probe—all will be helpful in conduction of therapeutic laparoscopic colorectal procedures.

Some laparoscopies in colorectal surgery may start as diagnostic procedures. Once the diagnosis is established, definitive surgical intervention may be necessary. Also, diagnostic laparoscopy may be needed to determine whether the patient's lesion is amenable to laparoscopic resection or repair. For example, laparoscopic sigmoidectomy may be appropriate for a patient with sigmoid diverticulitis but not for the patient with sigmoid colon cancer associated with malignant involvement of contiguous small bowel or urinary bladder, conditions that unacceptably prolong the operative time and compromise curative cancer resection. Even in patients with established diagnosis of the colorectal lesion, initial diagnostic laparoscopy will help to determine the optimal surgical approach.

Diagnostic laparoscopy is probably the initial laparoscopic procedure undertaken by junior surgical residents and by postgraduate surgeons who have not advanced into therapeutic colorectal laparoscopic surgery. Those surgeons who did not receive training in laparoscopic surgery during their formal surgical residency can benefit from performing diagnostic laparoscopies. This experience helps them to acquire skills to establish and maintain pneumoperitoneum, understand the significance of proper operating room setup and positioning of the patient, recognize gastrointestinal anatomy, and identify abnormalities. Not until novice surgeons have done multiple laparoscopies do they fully understand the pharmacophysiology of pneumoperitoneum and recognize that carbon dioxide pneumoperitoneum is not totally benign but is associated with definite cardiopulmonary stress, a factor that affects the patient selection for prolonged laparoscopic colorectal procedures.

Experience with diagnostic laparoscopy is especially important to postgraduate colorectal surgeons, more so than to general surgeons. General surgeons in North America gain experience in laparoscopy through laparoscopic cholecystectomy. Colorectal surgeons who finished their formal surgical training before 1990 and confine their practice to colorectal surgery fail to get any laparoscopic training. Colorectal surgeons have to extrapolate the animal laboratory training and learn laparoscopic surgical skills during their clinical practice. Diagnostic laparoscopy gives such postgraduate surgeons an opportunity to sharpen their skills in laparoscopic surgery. No amount of inanimate laboratory experience or bench training will be as valuable as learning from one's own patients after proper basic learning. Multiple studies deal with the learning curve phenomenon in laparoscopy and the value of learning from one's own experience.[1–3]

INDICATIONS

Although very few prospective, controlled studies document the advantages of diagnostic laparoscopy for gastrointestinal disease, the clinical benefits from diminished incisional morbidity compared with open laparotomy are observed by most laparoscopic surgeons. It is logical to assume that if laparoscopic evaluation yields diagnostic sensitivity and specificity equivalent or superior to open laparotomy, laparoscopy should supplant exploratory laparotomy whenever feasible. It should be noted, however, that the patient's cardiopulmonary status and disease process also dictate the choice of peritoneal access. Indications for diagnostic laparoscopy in colorectal surgery are expanding with time and accumulation of clinical experience. Some of the current indications are discussed below.

CHRONIC RECURRENT ABDOMINAL PAIN

When a patient presents with chronic, recurrent, nonspecific abdominal pain suggestive of hepatic and colorectal abnormalities, and all intraluminal gastrointestinal endoscopic examinations—along with abdominal imaging studies—fail to yield etiologic diagnosis, diagnostic laparoscopy may be indicated. Excellent laparoscopic exposure of colonic serosal aspects, along with liver surfaces, can be obtained and may help exclude radiographically undetectable Crohn's ileitis, endometriosis of the colon, diverticulitis, and pericolonic adhesions, to name a few elusive diagnoses. Most of the patients can undergo diagnostic laparoscopy on an outpatient basis at a cost not significantly higher than that of abdominal imaging, although the latter is noninvasive and carries less procedural risk. With improving instrumentation and diffusion of skills in diagnostic laparoscopy under local anesthesia, endoscopic evaluation of the peritoneal cavity may become as commonplace as intraluminal gastrointestinal endoscopy.

ABNORMAL ABDOMINAL IMAGING STUDIES

Abdominal imaging can show an intra-abdominal abnormality but rarely is successful in establishing the pathologic diagnosis. CT-guided biopsies can be helpful in some patients. Laparoscopic evaluation to establish the nature of the lesion may become necessary in other patients. For example, hepatic masses identified on CT scans and magnetic resonance imaging (MRI) scans can often be visualized, thus enabling a needle biopsy under direct vision. Any bleeding that ensues from the biopsy site can be controlled by electrocautery or by application of thrombogenic agents under direct vision. In addition to diagnosis and biopsy of intraperitoneal viscera, retroperitoneal masses can often be inspected and biopsied under laparoscopic guidance.

Diagnostic laparoscopy also prevents the need for exploratory laparotomy in a patient who shows pneumoperitoneum following colonoscopic examination. Pneumoperitoneum can be noticed without colonic disruption in some patients and managed well without any exploratory laparotomy if initial diagnostic laparoscopy excludes overt colonic injury. Pneumoperitoneum may need to be established by the open technique in these patients because of the presence of distended colon from recent colonoscopy. If the colon appears free of any overt laceration, microlacerations can be excluded by checking for air leaks after immersing the colon in fluid and insufflating carbon dioxide transanally.

ACUTE ABDOMEN WITH REBOUND TENDERNESS

When a patient presents with acute abdominal pain associated with localized or generalized rebound tenderness, diagnostic laparoscopy may establish the diagnosis and also aid in planning surgical treatment. Some therapeutic procedures, such as appendectomy, can be done at the same time as diagnostic laparoscopy, based on laparoscopic diagnosis. Retrospective studies of patients with acute abdomen have shown a change in the preoperative diagnosis for as much as 19 percent of patients and modification of planned treatment for 13 percent of patients on the basis of laparoscopic data.[4] A study of 120 patients from Dr. Cuschieri's group in the United Kingdom found that treatment plans for intra-abdominal problems were influenced by laparoscopy in 71 percent of patients. Diagnosis or exclusion of intra-abdominal malignancy was achieved in 100 percent of patients.[5]

The acute abdomen is a common diagnostic problem. Diagnostic errors can be minimized and unnecessary laparotomies avoided by judicious use of laparoscopy.[6] Exploratory laparotomy can be preceded and often replaced by diagnostic laparoscopy in many patients. Diagnostic laparoscopy not only helps to determine who can avoid laparotomy but also helps to identify those patients who need laparotomy immediately.[7] For experienced laparoscopists, diagnostic laparoscopy through an umbilicotomy may provide enough information to influence whether a long abdominal incision for further exploration is necessary. It may also reveal the ideal site for the abdominal incision.

DIVERTICULAR DISEASE

Sigmoid diverticulitis is often a clinical diagnosis that can be confirmed by noninvasive abdominal imaging such as CT scanning and colon contrast studies. When the clinical syndrome of repeated attacks of left lower quadrant pain suggests sigmoid diverticulitis and abdominal imaging fails to confirm the diagnosis, diagnostic laparoscopy may be of use in determining the need for surgical treatment of diverticulitis. Complications associated with diverticulitis may need laparoscopic evaluation. Although most colovesical and colovaginal fistulas from sigmoid diverticulitis are evident by history and can be confirmed by radiocontrast studies, laparoscopic examination of the pelvis may be needed in some patients when the fistulas are too minute to be seen radiographically. Laparoscopic identification of thorough, inseparable adherence of urinary bladder, vagina, or uterus to the sigmoid mass may point to the presence of fistulization, a condition that can complicate sigmoid diverticulitis. Patients suspected of solitary cecal diverticulitis or Meckel's diverticulitis leading to acute right lower quadrant pain may also benefit from diagnostic laparoscopy. (The role of diagnostic laparoscopy in acute appendicitis is discussed in Ch. 14.)

ISCHEMIC COLITIS

Diagnostic laparoscopy is helpful in determining the depth of ischemic injury in patients with idiopathic and aneurysmectomy-induced ischemic colitis. When patients with ischemic colitis develop signs of peritoneal irritation (e.g., rebound tenderness), diagnostic laparoscopy enables evaluation of the serosal injury. It further allows the surgeon to check for colonic mural integrity by the technique of transanal carbon dioxide insufflation of the affected colonic segment immersed in saline. In patients with superior mesenteric arterial occlusion, it may be necessary to consider a second look a few days after the initial surgical exploration. Leaving a 24 French Foley catheter through a stab wound at the time of the initial laparotomy (or port entrance site if the initial diagnostic laparoscopy established the diagnosis) will enable initiation of pneumoperitoneum for diagnostic laparoscopy with no need for reopening the abdominal incision. Although this approach is theoretically appealing, the problem of a small intestinal adhesion to the abdominal incision may make visceral visualization less than optimal in some patients.

BLUNT ABDOMINAL TRAUMA AND COLONIC INJURY

Laparoscopy in patients with abdominal trauma has been discussed for the past many decades, but only recently has it gained acceptance. Diagnostic laparoscopy may be effective in selecting patients for conservative management of blunt abdominal trauma. Laparoscopic evaluation for associated occult coloenteric injuries helps the surgeon to decide which patients can be managed conservatively and which patients need laparotomy. In patients with solid organ injury diagnosed on CT scans, laparoscopic diagnosis of associated occult, hollow visceral injury or active bleeding changes the planned conservative, nonoperative management to laparotomy; their exclusion gives assurance that the patient can be managed by clinical observation and conservative management without surgical exploration.

In a prospective study of 15 patients with blunt abdominal trauma and abnormal CT scans, conservative management was employed in the treatment of 8 patients with findings of minor injury and no active bleeding on diagnostic laparoscopy. None of these patients selected on the basis of laparoscopic evaluation failed conservative management, and no complications resulted from laparoscopy.[8] In a second retrospective study, emergency minilaparoscopy in 150 trauma patients accurately identified the need for laparotomy in all but one patient.[9] Laparoscopy is earning a deserved place in the initial diagnostic evaluation of patients with trauma.

DIAGNOSIS OF COLONIC INJURY FROM GUNSHOT AND STAB WOUNDS

Diagnostic laparoscopy can distinguish patients with peritoneal penetration from a gunshot or stab wound and exclude hollow visceral injury from the missile. Laparoscopic exclusion of peritoneal penetration has been proposed to reduce the need for open laparotomy.[10,11] Although diagnostic laparoscopy in trauma patients often requires general anesthesia, the derived information will be more accurate than that acquired from blind peritoneal lavage and other indirect means of detecting intraperitoneal bleeding and hollow visceral disruption.

ACUTE INTESTINAL OBSTRUCTION

In appropriate patients, acute intestinal obstruction, which is often due to intra-abdominal adhesions, may be amenable to laparoscopic diagnosis and resolution by adhesiolysis (Fig. 11-1). Patients with persistent complete intestinal obstruction that does not respond to nasogastric intestinal decompression can be evaluated initially by diagnostic laparoscopy. Placement of peritoneal ports under direct vision is necessary in this group of patients to avoid visceral injury from the Veress needle or from the sharp trocar. When the obstruction is secondary to band adhesions, lysis of the adhesions will resolve the obstruction.[12] Laparoscopy disrupts the peritoneum less than does open laparotomy, and thus it may diminish recurrent adhesion formation more effectively than does the open technique for adhesiolysis.[13] The viability of strangulated small bowel loops can also be evaluated at the time of

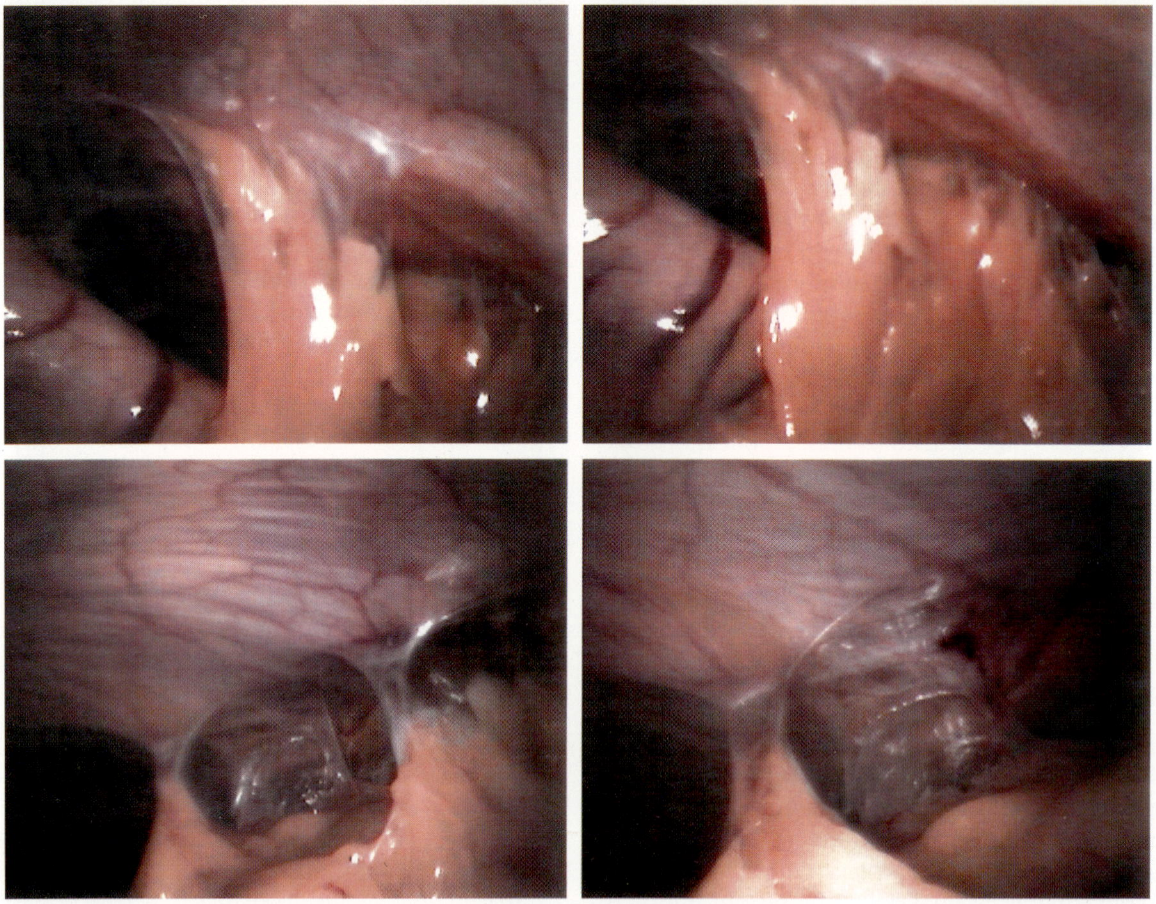

Fig. 11-1. Intra-abdominal adhesions from previous laparotomy.

laparoscopy. In patients with extensive adhesions, however, laparoscopic access may be extremely difficult. An attempt can be made for blunt trocar placement, extending the mini-incision into a formal laparotomy only if laparoscopic access is not feasible because of extensive intraperitoneal adhesions. In patients with extensive intra-abdominal adhesions and multiple sites of obstruction, the time taken for laparoscopic adhesiolysis may be prohibitively prolonged and thus limit the value of laparoscopy to some degree.

When the intestinal obstruction is secondary to incarcerated inguinal or Spigelian hernias rather than intraperitoneal adhesions, laparoscopic approach certainly is ideal to reduce the hernias and to evaluate the incarcerated loops for ischemia. Depending on the patient's clinical status, immediate repair of the inguinal or Spigelian hernias can also be done, or the patient can be brought back to the operating room over the next few days for definitive repair after reduction of the incarceration. The definitive repair, however, should not be unduly postponed because of high incidence of recurrent incarceration.

COLORECTAL CANCER

Abdominal imaging techniques (e.g., ultrasound, CT, and MRI scans) form the initial level of diagnostic evaluation of intra-abdominal malignancy and in determination of the metastatic extent. Diagnostic laparoscopy, however, certainly is more specific and sensitive than the noninvasive imaging studies.[14] Initial laparoscopic evaluation may serve as a basis for avoiding the morbidity of futile laparotomy, evaluating resectability, and planning the surgical approach (Fig. 11-2).

It is yet to be determined whether routine preoperative laparoscopy is helpful in determining the resectability of colorectal cancers in all patients. Although laparoscopy is helpful in preoperative evaluation of patients with esophageal, gastric, and pancreatic carcinomas,[15–18] similar studies have not been conducted in colorectal cancer. Until such studies show the advantages, selective rather than routine use of laparoscopy in patients with colorectal cancer may be more approprate. When imaging studies show extensive extramural invasion of rectal cancer, the surgeon should consider pre-

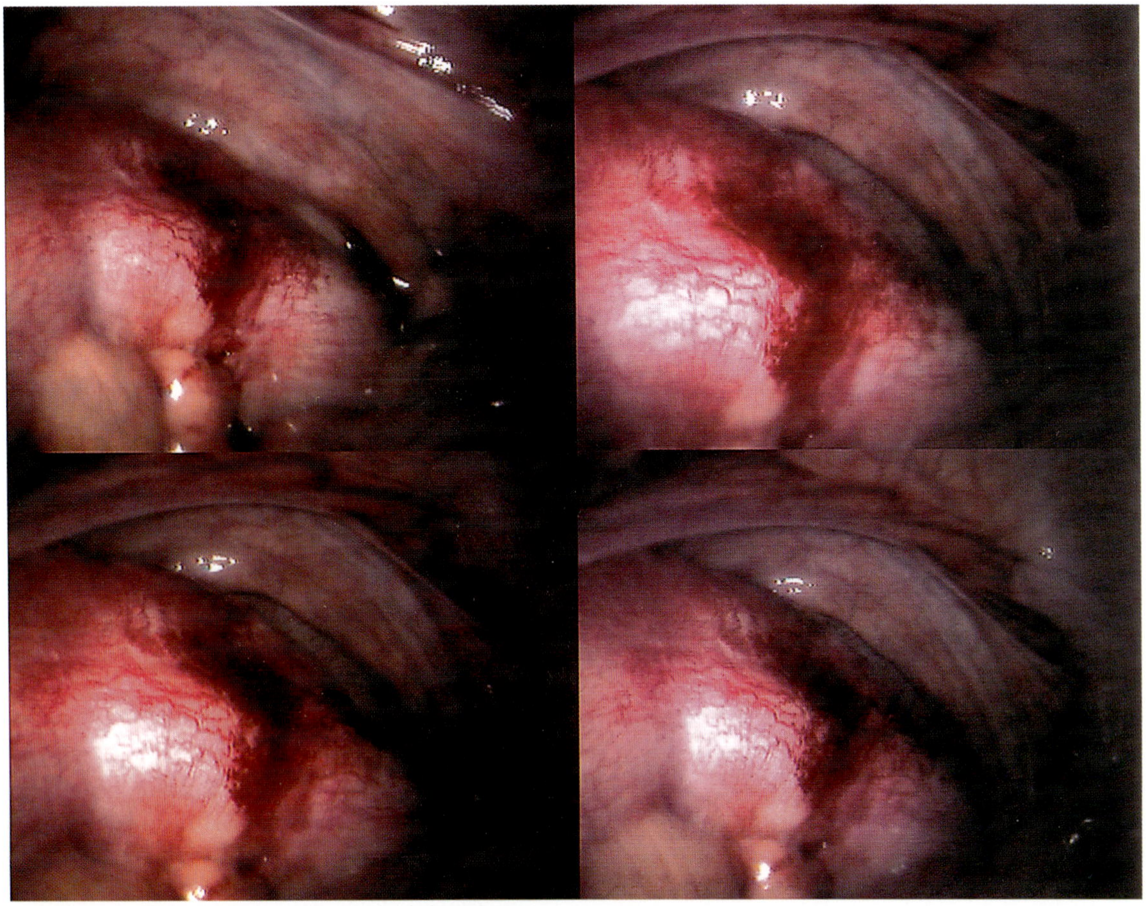

Fig. 11-2. Sigmoid colonic cancer showing serosal invasion. The indurated mass in the sigmoid colon could be palpated with a blunt probe, suggesting the location of cancer.

operative diagnostic staging laparoscopy to determine the resectability and metastatic extent of the lesion. If the surgeon finds intraperitoneal or hepatic metastases not identified by preoperative abdominal imaging, the treatment strategy may change from a radical resection to fecal diversion, followed by chemoradiotherapeutic palliation. Similarly, preoperative diagnostic laparoscopy in a patient with right colonic cancer may change the treatment plan from a radical right hemicolectomy to a segmental laparoscopic colectomy if peritoneal or hepatic metastases are detected. Ability to conduct palliative operations (e.g., segmental resections, fecal diversion, and peritoneal chemotherapeutic port placements) is one benefit from preoperative staging laparoscopy. Whether such benefits justify the additional expenses imposed by the hospital is yet to be answered.[19]

The cost factor should not be ignored. Fiscal cost of laparoscopic equipment is considerable but can be controlled. Criticism of the increased expense may not be valid if nondisposable cannulas and instruments are used for initial laparoscopic evaluation. The biologic cost from diagnostic laparoscopy in cancer patients may be more difficult to address and needs further analysis. The risk of port site malignant implantation from laparoscopy is currently receiving a great deal of attention, not because of the frequency (because the reported incidence is definitely minuscule), but because of the gravity of the problem.[20,21] Advantages gained by laparoscopy should be weighed against risks imposed by pneumoperitoneum-induced complications in patients with cancer.

DETERMINATION OF RESECTABILITY OF HEPATIC METASTASES

Modern techniques of abdominal imaging have improved diagnostic accuracy in management of hepatic metastases of colorectal cancer. However, in 40 to 70 percent of patients with metastatic hepatic malignancies, laparotomy may reveal unresectable disease (Fig. 11-3). Twenty-nine patients underwent staging laparoscopy before a planned laparotomy for resection of a hepatic malignancy that was deemed resectable by

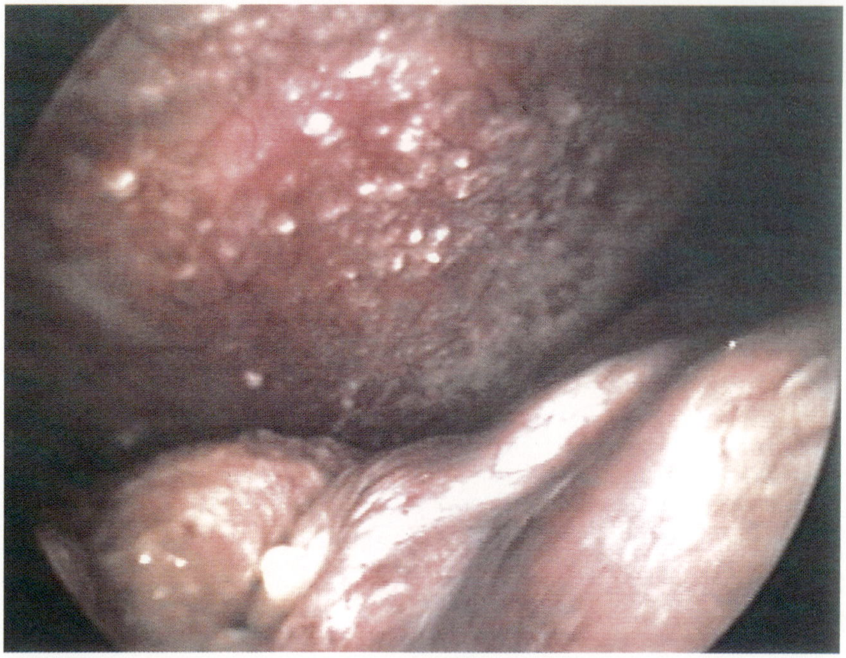

Fig. 11-3. A patient with hepatic metastases also showed extensive peritoneal seeding, thus proving the nonresectability.

CT scan and ultrasonography. Preoperative staging laparoscopy found the hepatic malignancy to be unresectable because of extrahepatic metastatic disease or cirrhosis in 48 percent of 29 patients scheduled for resection based on preoperative CT scans. Because laparoscopy shortened the hospital stay compared with laparotomy in historical controls, diagnostic laparoscopy has been suggested by some authors to precede laparotomy for planned resection of hepatic malignancies.[22]

MALIGNANT ASCITES

Patients with ascites may benefit from diagnostic laparoscopy if a visceral malignancy is suspected. Malignant ascitic fluid is not always exudative, and routine evaluation of the fluid (including peritoneal cytology) may not be conclusive in establishing the diagnosis. Laparoscopy enables parietal peritoneal biopsy and evaluation of visceral and hepatic serosal surfaces for diagnosis and staging of malignancy.[23] At the time of initial diagnostic laparoscopy, an intraperitoneal catheter or port for periodic drainage of ascitic fluid or for intraperitoneal chemotherapy can also be placed. Percutaneous insertion of peritoneal catheter has also been described[24] and can be combined with open laparoscopy technique for managing loculated ascites. Some studies have raised the concern of port site implantation of ovarian carcinoma from laparoscopic evaluation of malignant ascites.[25] The difference in the incidence of wound carcinomatosis following laparoscopy versus following laparotomy is unknown.

ANESTHETIC CONSIDERATIONS

Preoperative Evaluation

The patient's cardiopulmonary, clinical, and laboratory evaluation is necessary (as is the case before any abdominal operation) when the diagnostic laparoscopy is performed on a patient administered general anesthesia. If the surgeon's intentions were to proceed with therapeutic laparoscopy or open laparotomy to repair or resect the lesion, more extensive cardiac evaluation of myocardial ischemia and reserve may be prudent. If the evaluation reveals an unsuspected lesion (which may require unanticipated, prolonged laparoscopic or open abdominal surgery), it is wise to complete the diagnostic laparoscopy and perform the definitive surgical procedure at a later time after conducting further cardiopulmonary workup as needed.

A patient's preoperative cardiac evaluation should take into consideration that carbon dioxide pneumoperitoneum can noticeably elevate the mean arterial pressure and systemic vascular resistance, reducing the cardiac output. The surgeon should realize that laparoscopy can subject the patient to significant hemodynamic stress. Hemodynamic parameters usually return to preoperative levels once pneumoperitoneum is released, contributing to no major perioperative cardiac complications. Often, laparoscopic procedures can be conducted safely even in high-risk patients if aggressive intraoperative monitoring is done.[26]

Patients with chronic pulmonary disease may require careful intraoperative monitoring of arterial blood gases.[27] Hypercarbia with respiratory acidosis is a known complication of laparoscopic procedures, especially in patients with decreased pulmonary flow, limited capacity, and diminished diffusion, all of which increase the likelihood of intraoperative acidosis. Preoperative pulmonary function showing forced expiratory volumes of less than 70 percent and diffusion capacity of less than 80 percent of predicted values can identify those patients at risk of developing intraoperative hypercarbia and acidosis.[28] Those patients, in particular, benefit from arterial blood gas monitoring.

Muscle Relaxation and Anesthetic Agents

Complete muscle relaxation during diagnostic laparoscopy is helpful in establishing and maintaining satisfactory pneumoperitoneum. When patients' abdominal muscles are not totally relaxed, it is difficult to achieve or maintain the intraperitoneal pressure at a satisfactory level to visualize the various intraperitoneal viscera. Some surgeons feel that a taut and nonrelaxed anterior abdominal wall facilitates insertion of laparoscopic trocars. With well-sharpened reusable and modern disposable trocars, however, there is little need for a taut abdominal wall to aid trocar insertion.

There are no specific contraindications for any one anesthetic agent. Nitrous oxide can cause problems with small bowel dilation from its intraluminal diffusion. Nitrous oxide can also diffuse into the peritoneal cavity, increasing the explosion hazard.[29] With the myriad anesthetic agents available, rarely is it imperative for the anesthesiologist to use nitrous oxide for balanced endotracheal anesthesia during laparoscopy. Maintaining open communication with the anesthesiologist is important in achieving safe and satisfactory anesthesia.

BOWEL PREPARATION

Preoperative bowel preparation is helpful to avoid septic complications associated with unplanned bowel injury during laparoscopic evaluations, especially if laparoscopic adhesiolysis is anticipated for satisfactory visceral visualization during diagnostic laparoscopy. Potential for bowel injury exists at several stages of the procedure: (1) insertion of a Veress needle, (2) placement of a fascial pursestring suture in an open insertion by the method of Hasson, (3) laparoscopic adhesiolysis, and (4) capacitive-coupling or conductive electrosurgical visceral injury. Reduction of gastrointestinal bacterial content by preoperative antibiotic and mechanical bowel preparation is optimal and a tolerable inconvenience as it helps to avoid potentially lethal septic complications. (The various mechanical and antibiotic bowel preparations are discussed in Ch. 5.)

OPERATING ROOM SETUP

Proper operating room setup and patient positioning maximize the diagnostic utility of laparoscopy. The dorsolithotomy position and use of cervical catheters may enable moving the uterus to inspect the pelvic fossae. Placing a beanbag under the patient allows safe rotation of the patient to evaluate organs such as splenic and hepatic flexures. Using two monitors (one on either side of the patient) allows inspection of various viscera, adhesiolysis, and organ retraction. (Factors that enter into the ideal room setup are outlined in Ch. 10.)

TECHNIQUE OF PNEUMOPERITONEUM

No one technique is ideal for every patient and for every surgeon. The technique for establishing a pneumoperitoneum and choosing an insertion site for the primary cannula may be influenced by the patient's habitus and previous laparotomies, as well as by the surgeon's experience. (The numerous techniques of pneumoperitoneum are discussed in Ch. 6.) Discussion of a few other topics regarding the technique follows.

Open Versus Closed Technique

Some surgeons prefer establishing a pneumoperitoneum with an atraumatic Veress needle containing a protective spring-loaded obturator. By contrast, open placement of a blunt cannula through a small incision is proposed to reduce most of the complications associated with blind insertion of a Veress needle, such as visceral and vascular injury. In patients who have had multiple previous abdominal surgical procedures, open placement may be less risky than the blind technique. However, it can be more difficult to maintain the pneumoperitoneum when the cannula is placed through the open technique because the carbon dioxide can leak around the cannula in spite of the commonly used olive occluder. A pursestring fascial suture to snug the fascia around the cannula may reduce this leakage problem. This pursestring suture should be placed with great care to avoid injury to subjacent bowel. Bowel injury from the holding stitch intended to secure airtight fascia has been reported.[30] The surgeon should also inspect the initial cannula site by inserting the laparoscope through a secondary port. This technique also excludes visceral injury from the primary cannula insertion or from the pursestring fascial holding suture.[31]

Direct Insertion of Trocars

The technique of direct insertion of a 10-mm trocar has been proposed to save operative time without increasing the risk of visceral and vascular injury.[32] In a randomized prospective study of 200 patients by a group of experienced gynecologic surgeons, direct insertion of a disposable trocar was associated with complications of 0 percent, whereas establishing a pneumoperitoneum with a Veress needle resulted in minor complications of 22 percent.[33] Direct insertion of disposable or reusable trocars, however, may not be appropriate for surgeons lacking extensive laparoscopic experience. The laparoscopic surgeon should also understand that the so-called atraumatic shield of disposable trocars is not totally atraumatic and can lead to unsuspected visceral injury. The safety shield can get caught at the peritoneum, allowing the sharp tip to penetrate the subjacent viscera, especially in patients with adhesions at the site of insertion.

INTRAPERITONEAL LOCAL ANESTHETICS

Postoperative scapular pain from diaphragmatic irritation produced by retained carbon dioxide is a common problem following diagnostic laparoscopy. Exsufflating the carbon dioxide at the end of the operation by abdominal kneading is commonly done to reduce this peritoneal problem. Instillation of intraperitoneal local anesthetic has been proposed to avoid postoperative scapular pain. A French prospective, randomized study[34] has shown that right subphrenic instillation of 0.5 percent lidocaine with epinephrine (320,000 dilution) or 0.125 percent bupivacaine with epinephrine (800,000 dilution) more effectively reduced postoperative shoulder pain than did control instillation of saline. The postoperative need for analgesics was less in the patients who had the intraperitoneal local anesthetics. Intraincisional bupivacaine and intraperitoneal lidocaine instilled into the peritoneal cavity rather than subphrenic space were also found to be effective in reducing postoperative pain.[35] Because the risk from systemic absorption of the local anesthetic is minimal, I routinely use this technique of intraperitoneal instillation of 25 ml of 0.25 percent bupivacaine with epinephrine for my patients undergoing diagnostic laparoscopy.

VERESS NEEDLE INSERTION

Various techniques have been described to facilitate the insertion of a Veress needle. The classical technique of manually pinching, lifting, and tenting the infraumbilical anterior abdominal wall may not be ideal in obese patients, especially if the surgeon weighs significantly less than the patient. An alternate procedure has been proposed: placing two Kocher clamps on the anterior rectus sheath to lift the anterior abdominal wall,[36] tenting the linea alba immediately above the umbilicus, followed by needle insertion through the superior margin of the umbilical ring.[37] The optimal direction of insertion to avoid preperitoneal placement varies depending on abdominal wall obesity. The angle of insertion of the Veress needle or the peritoneal trocar may be closer to 90 degrees in morbidly obese patients.

RISK OF VASCULAR INJURY

The risk of injury to retroperitoneal vessels (e.g., the aorta and the left common iliac vein) that cross the midline should be considered every time the surgeon inserts the Veress needle or a trocar through the umbilicus. The relation of umbilical location to aortic bifurcation and left common iliac vein crossing the midline needs further discussion. In a CT scan study, the mean location of the umbilicus was 0.4 cm caudad to the aortic bifurcation, but it was at or cephalad to the bifurcation in 53 percent of nonobese patients. In obese patients, the umbilicus was located at the bifurcation in 30 percent of patients, and on average, it was 2.4 cm caudal to the bifurcation. In all patients, the umbilicus was cephalad to the point where the left iliac vein crosses the midline. Routine preoperative palpation of aortic pulsation may remind the surgeon of the catastrophic complication of major vessel injury from umbilical needle or trocar insertion.

EVALUATION OF INTRAPERITONEAL VISCERA

Evaluation of the entire peritoneal cavity is the goal of optimal diagnostic laparoscopy. Such an evaluation may require additional cannulas to insert laparoscopic retractors or atraumatic forceps or to lyse intra-abdominal adhesions. Changing the patient's position, using two video monitors (one on either side of the patient), changing the camera port, and having the surgeon move from one side to the other may be necessary to achieve maximal visualization. Using a 30-degree laparoscope and rotating the light cord location without changing the laparoscopic camera orientation will facilitate inspection of the subphrenic intraperitoneal surface of the liver all the way up to its peritoneal attachments to the diaphragm. The transverse colon and mesocolon should be inspected carefully to avoid injury to the full gallbladder by the retractors or holding forceps. Similarly, injury to the sigmoid colonic phlegmon by the grasping forceps is possible in patients with acute sigmoid diverticulitis. Means to move the uterus or vaginal stump by placing a cervical catheter or a sponge forceps may assist in evaluation of true pelvic cavity in female patients. The laparoscopic surgeon lacks tactile ability in evaluating visceral abnormalities. Palpation with a blunt probe placed through a secondary port may be some assistance in some patients. In nonobese patients, inserting a finger through the port entrance wound closest to the lesion, after deflation of the pneumoperitoneum, may grant partial tactile ability to the surgeon.

Collection of peritoneal washing has been suggested in cancers affecting pancreas and stomach. No studies have been done to determine the significance of peritoneal washing in colorectal cancers. Because the amount of operative time spent for collection of peritoneal washing is minimal, it may be advisable to collect peritoneal washing in patients with elevated carcinoembryonic antigen (CEA) who are having diagnostic laparoscopy as a second-look procedure.

INCIDENTAL APPENDECTOMY

Should the surgeon remove an uninflamed appendix if the laparoscopy is done for diagnostic purposes only? When the laparoscopic examination is done to determine the cause of abdominal pain and not for determination of resectability of cancer, incidental appendectomy may be an option. The possible increased risk in abdominal wound infection and possible disruption of the appendiceal stump can be used to argue against this practice. A retrospective review of 100 incidental appendectomies done during diagnostic laparoscopy for gynecologic problems failed to show any significant complications other than umbilical ecchymosis and fever of 24-hour duration. Some surgeons may conduct an incidental appendectomy because of certain potential advantages to patient: avoiding future diagnostic problems if the patient has a similar pain syndrome, eliminating possible future appendicitis, and removing any unsuspected abnormalities in the appendix. The patient's general status, whether the diagnostic laparoscopy is done under general anesthesia or local anesthesia, and the surgeon's laparoscopic expertise all play a role in the decision regarding incidental appendectomy.[38]

LAPAROSCOPY UNDER LOCAL ANESTHESIA

Diagnostic laparoscopy under local anesthesia has been done extensively by European gastroenterologists as an office procedure. Laparoscopy under intravenous sedation supplemented by local anesthesia is proposed as an ideal, minimally invasive technique to detect intraperitoneal disease, sparing some patients extensive laparotomy.[39] Use of nitrous oxide pneumoperitoneum may reduce the operative pain. This approach, however, will not allow conduction of any needed therapeutic laparoscopic procedures. Laparoscopy under local anesthesia is appealing as a purely diagnostic procedure but has not been popular with North American abdominal surgeons. Beck and associates have conducted thousands of diagnostic laparoscopic procedures under local anesthesia and detailed their experience. The reader is referred to their excellent publication.[40]

ADVANTAGES AND DISADVANTAGES

The advantages of diagnostic laparoscopy are obvious. The postoperative incisional morbidity is less than that following laparotomy. Cosmetic results are superior, and the patient can return to productive life sooner than after open laparotomy. Minimal fascial and peritoneal disruption may reduce the risk of intra-abdominal adhesion formation, wound dehiscence, and incisional hernia formation. The magnified view of most of the intra-abdominal viscera is excellent and comparable to that in open laparotomy.

Laparoscopy has some definite disadvantages. Diagnostic laparoscopy may not replace open laparotomy for some time. Portions of the liver cannot be visualized, and most lesions of the liver cannot be palpated. The inherent problem of not being able to palpate a lesion may hinder its universal applicability. Laparoscopy can be time-consuming for most surgeons, and the supporting staff may not be able to set up the laparoscopic equipment in an emergency situation. This problem, however, may be short-lived with increasing use of laparoscopy even in small peripheral hospitals. Added expense from disposable instrumentation and increased operative time should be addressed by every surgeon. As most surgeons gain more experience with laparoscopic procedures and move toward reusable laparoscopic instruments, these disadvantages can be easily overcome. The expense of diagnostic laparoscopy may be partially offset by the avoided, futile, or unnecessary laparotomies and the productive gains from patients' rapid return to work.

FUTURE OF DIAGNOSTIC LAPAROSCOPY

The value of diagnostic laparoscopy may increase in the future by introduction of other noninvasive diagnostic tools such as laparoscopic ultrasound and scintigraphic probes. Ultrasonographic evaluation may enable detection and differentiation of liver lesions in the parenchyma not visible through the laparoscope and not palpable by a blunt probe.[41] Miniature ultrasound probes measuring less than 3 mm in size have been devised. They can be introduced through a therapeutic laparoscope to allow the abdominal surgeon to sonographically palpate tissues lying beneath normal-appearing peritoneum or viscera.[42]

Radioscintigraphic probes in conjunction with radioisotope-tagged monoclonal antibodies may allow diagnosis of occult hepatic metastasis and extracolonic extension of cancer.[43] Pretherapy laparoscopic nodal evaluation (as is possible in pancreatic and esophageal cancers) may become feasible in colorectal cancer.[44] Other innovative techniques, such as use of fluorescein-assisted laparoscopy, may be helpful in evaluating mesenteric ischemia.[45]

Abdominal surgeons are rediscovering the utility of diagnostic laparoscopy. Diagnostic laparoscopy not only provides an excellent magnified view of intraperitoneal viscera and parietal peritoneum but also allows the surgeon to obtain biopsies, conduct palliative surgical procedures (e.g., segmental colectomies), and determine the resectability of colonic malignancy, thus avoiding open laparotomy. Reduction in incisional morbidity and metabolic stress when laparoscopy replaces laparotomy is attractive only if laparoscopy is diagnostically equivalent to open laparotomy. The reported diagnostic accuracy of 99 percent for acute abdominal pain, 70 percent for chronic pain syndromes, 95 percent for focal liver disease, 95 percent for abdominal masses, 97 percent for ascites, and greater than 80 percent for retroperitoneal disease are encouraging. Diagnostic laparoscopy will predictably be used with greater frequency by surgeons, especially when a tissue diagnosis is needed.[46] The sensitivity, specificity, safety, and savings from diagnostic laparoscopy may be comparable to if not superior to open laparotomy.[47]

REFERENCES

1. See WA, Cooper CS, Fisher RJ: Predictors of laparoscopic complications after formal training in laparoscopic surgery. JAMA 270:2689, 1993
2. Guazzoni G, Montorsi F, Bergamaschi F et al: Open surgical revision of laparoscopic pelvic lymphadenectomy for staging of prostate cancer: the impact of laparoscopic learning curve. J Urol 151:930, 1994
3. Stovall TG, Ling FW, Lipscomb GH et al: A model for resident surgical training in laparoscopic sterilization. Obstet Gynecol 83:470, 1994
4. Scott HJ, Rosin RD: The influence of diagnostic and therapeutic laparoscopy on patients presenting with an acute abdomen. J R Soc Med 86:699, 1993
5. Easter DW, Cuschieri A, Nathanson LK et al: The utility of diagnostic laparoscopy for abdominal disorders. Audit of 120 patients. Arch Surg 127:379, 1992
6. Paterson-Brown S: Emergency laparoscopic surgery. Br J Surg 80:279, 1993
7. Paterson-Brown S: The acute abdomen: the role of laparoscopy. Baillieres Clin Gastroenterol 5:691, 1991
8. Townsend MC, Flancbaum L, Choban PS et al: Diagnostic laparoscopy as an adjunct to selective conservative management of solid organ injuries after blunt abdominal trauma. J Trauma 35:647, 1993
9. Berci G: Elective and emergent laparoscopy. World J Surg 17:8, 1993
10. Sosa JL, Markley M, Sleeman D et al: Laparoscopy in abdominal gunshot wounds. Surg Laparosc Endosc 3:417, 1993
11. Sosa JL, Sims D, Martin L et al: Laparoscopic evaluation of tangential abdominal gunshot wounds. Arch Surg 127:109, 1992
12. Adams S, Wilson T, Brown AR: Laparoscopic management of acute small bowel obstruction. Aust NZ J Surg 63:39, 1993
13. Lundorff P, Hahlin M, Kallfelt B et al: Adhesion formation after laparoscopic surgery in tubal pregnancy: a randomized trial versus laparotomy. Fertil Steril 55:911, 1991
14. Walt I, Stewart I, Anderson D et al: Laparoscopy, ultrasound, and computed tomography in cancer of the esophagus and gastric cardia: a prospective comparison for detecting intra-abdominal metastases. Br J Surg 76:1036, 1989
15. Gross E, Bancewicz J, Ingram G: Assessment of gastric carcinoma by laparoscopy. BMJ 28:157, 1988
16. Diagnini G, Caldironi W, Martin G et al: Laparoscopy in abdominal staging of esophageal carcinoma. Gastrointest Endosc 32:400, 1986
17. Warshaw Al, Gu Z, Wittenberg J et al: Preoperative staging and assessment of resectability of pancreatic cancer. Arch Surg 125:230, 1990
18. Kriplani AK, Kapur BM: Laparoscopy for preoperative staging and assessment of operability in gastric carcinoma. Gastrointest Endosc 37:441, 1991
19. Greene FL, Dorsay D: Laparoscopic evaluation of abdominal malignancy. Cancer Pract 1:29, 1993
20. Cava A, Roman J, Quintela AG et al: Subcutaneous metastasis following laparoscopy in gastric adenocarcinoma. Eur J Surg Oncol 16:63, 1990
21. Ramos JM, Gupta S, Anthone GJ et al: Laparoscopy and colon cancer: is the port site at risk? Arch Surg 129:897, 1994
22. Babineau TJ, Lewis WD, Jenkins RL et al: Role of staging laparoscopy in the treatment of hepatic malignancy. Am J Surg 167:151, 1994
23. Desai H: Peritoneoscopy in diagnosis of ascites. J Assoc Physicians India 39:933, 1991
24. Amerling R, Cruz C: A new laparoscopic method for implantation of peritoneal catheters. ASAIO Trans 39:M787, 1993
25. Safran D, Sgambati S, Orlando R III: Laparoscopy in high-risk cardiac patients. Surg Gynecol Obstet 176:548, 1993
26. Gleeson NC, Nicasia SV, Mark JE et al: Abdominal wall metastases from ovarian cancer after laparoscopy. Am J Obstet Gynecol 169:522, 1993
27. Wittgen CM, Andrus CH, Fitzgerald SD et al: Analysis of the hemodynamic and ventilatory effects of laparoscopic cholecystectomy. Arch Surg 126:997, 1991
28. Wittgen CM, Nnheim KS, Andrus CH et al: Preoperative pulmonary function evaluation for laparoscopic cholecystectomy. Arch Surg 128:880, 1993
29. West ST, Haring L: Laparoscopy explosion hazards with nitrous oxide. Anesthesiology 78:875, 1993
30. Sadeghi-Nejad H, Kavoussi LR, Peters CA: Bowel injury in open technique laparoscopic cannula placement. Urology 43:559, 1994
31. Kaali SG, Barad DH: Incidence of bowel injury due to dense adhesions at the sight of direct trocar insertion. J Reprod Med 37:617, 1992
32. Byron JW, Markenson G, Miyazawa K: A randomized comparison of Veress needle and direct trocar insertion for laparoscopy. Surg Gynecol Obstet 177:25, 1993
33. Nezhat FR, Silfen SL, Evans D et al: Comparison of direct insertion of disposable and standard reusable laparoscopic trocars and previous pneumoperitoneum with Veress needle. Obstet Gynecol 78:148, 1991
34. Narchi P, Benhamou D, Fernandez H: Intraperitoneal local anesthetic for shoulder pain after day-case laparoscopy. Lancet 338:1569, 1991
35. Helvacioglu A, Weis R: Operative laparoscopy and postoperative pain relief. Fertil Steril 57:548, 1992
36. Hilgers TW: A simple, safe technique for placement of the Veress needle and trocar in laparoscopy. J Laparoendosc Surg 2:189, 1992
37. Karatassas A, Walsh D, Hamilton DW: A safe, new approach

to establishing a pneumoperitoneum at laparoscopy. Aust NZ J Surg 62:489, 1992
38. Nezhat C, Nezhat F: Incidental appendectomy during videolaseroscopy: one hundred incidental appendectomies were performed in patients undergoing operative laparoscopy (videolaseroscopy) for evaluating and treating various major diseases of the reproductive organs. Am J Obstet Gynecol 165:559, 1991
39. Hatch KD, Surwit EA: Office laparoscopy and biopsy for evaluation of patients with intraperitoneal carcinomatosis using a new optical catheter. Gynecol Oncol 47:337, 1992
40. Beck K: Color Atlas of Laparoscopy. 2nd Ed. WB Saunders, Philadelphia, 1984
41. Fukuda M, Hirata K, Mima S: Preliminary evaluation of sonolaparoscopy in the diagnosis of liver diseases. Endoscopy 24:701, 1992
42. Cohn HE, Barbot D, Gillum DR et al: Sonographically guided laparoscopy and mediastinoscopy using miniature catheter-based transducers. J Ultrasound Med 12:49, 1993
43. Lavery IC: Radioimmuno-guided surgery for colon cancer. Semin Colon Rectal Surg 2:54, 1991
44. LoCicero J III: Laparoscopy/thoracoscopy for staging: pretherapy nodal evaluation in carcinoma of the esophagus. Semin Surg Oncol 9:56, 1993
45. Kam DM, Scheeres DE: Fluorescein-assisted laparoscopy in the identification of arterial mesenteric ischemia. Surg Endosc 7:75, 1993
46. Salky B: Diagnostic laparoscopy. Surg Laparosc Endosc 3:132, 1993
47. Sessions SC, vonRueden D, Uribe A: Diagnostic laparoscopy. J Laparoendosc Surg 1:319, 1991

Editorial Comment I

James Kohn and Philip F. Caushaj

Dr. Jager presents a comprehensive and clear discussion on the utility and pitfalls of diagnostic laparoscopy as well as an overview of the laparoscopic technique. Several issues that Dr. Jager has mentioned in passing deserve further discussion.

Laparoscopic techniques are minimally invasive and associated with new and different complications. These complications have been carefully outlined in this chapter and predominantly include trocar injuries, as well as the physiologic consequences of carbon dioxide pneumoperitoneum. Even though the total complication rate of laparoscopy compared to laparotomy is reduced, there are complications associated with the laparoscopic technique. Moreover, although morbidity may be significantly decreased and diagnosis may be facilitated, the risk/benefit analysis and indications for the procedure have not and should not change. To extend the indications for diagnostic laparoscopy because it appears to be safer than laparotomy may invite a compromise in the preoperative evaluation of the patient and minimize potential complications.

The mortality rate for a diagnostic laparotomy compared to diagnostic laparoscopy is essentially the same. Morbidity is clearly reduced, as discussed in this chapter. Several investigations have been initiated to attempt to clarify the physiologic consequences of laparoscopy, including the measurement of catecholamines, cortisol, interleukins, and other parameters during laparoscopy, as compared to conventional laparotomy. Exposure of the peritoneal cavity to room air, loss of fluid via evaporation, and conventional retraction of the abdominal viscera may be associated with an increased stress response and may possibly account for the differences observed between the techniques. Nevertheless, clinical experience with laparoscopic techniques continues to reaffirm that the length of the incisions or the summation of the length of trocar sites may only be a partial explanation for the diminished postoperative morbidity associated with laparoscopic techniques.

The options for therapeutic intervention and directed treatment during diagnostic laparoscopy are expanding as the technique evolves and new techniques and instrumentation are developed. This is the greatest advantage that diagnostic laparoscopy has to offer. The emphasis on a single procedure yielding increased sensitivity and specificity in establishing a diagnosis while allowing therapeutic intervention has stimulated surgical interest. While imaging studies have increased accuracy and continue to yield increased information that narrows the diagnostic possibilities, the therapeutic capabilities still require open or laparoscopic techniques. Ultimately, cost and clinical outcomes of laparotomy versus laparoscopy would need to be evaluated for certain clinical scenarios (e.g., abdominal pain).

Some discussion is necessary regarding potential limitations of laparoscopy. In postaortic vascular reconstruction, with the possible complication of colonic ischemia, the initial evaluation of the patient must begin with conventional lower gastrointestinal endoscopy. Mucosal changes in the bowel are the earliest recognizable evidence for colonic ischemia, whereas transmural changes are the final pathway. Colonoscopy can be performed in an intensive care unit setting with the patient under sedation to evaluate the colonic viability. If colonic viability is questionable or abnormal on endoscopy, at that juncture, a diagnostic laparoscopy may be performed in association with colonoscopy to ascertain whether full-thickness ischemia is present.

The determination of resectability of malignancy by laparoscopy rarely is disadvantageous. When laparoscopic evaluation is unrewarding, this is apparent to the experienced laparoscopist early in the procedure. This will allow for minimal use of operating room time and costly equipment. As mentioned by Dr. Jager, several advantages to this operative approach in planning as well as the potential for tissue diagnosis favor the laparoscopic technique in this clinical scenario. Furthermore, a nontherapeutic laparotomy in a patient with advanced malignant disease may be a major debilitating variable as well as a major factor in limiting the quality of the patient's life.

In summary, Dr. Jager has offered a scholarly and thorough review of diagnostic laparoscopy that establishes the technical and philosophical basis for this procedure.

Editorial Comment II

Steven D. Wexner

Dr. Jager provides an extremely detailed and comprehensive review of the potential applications of diagnostic laparoscopy. In general, diagnostic laparoscopy should be subdivided into two categories: elective indications and emergent indications. Elective indications are chronic recurrent abdominal pain, diverticular disease, malignant disease, and widely metastatic colorectal carcinoma. These are the patients who can undergo bowel preparation, as discussed by Dr. Jager. These are also the patients who, either because of the minimal nature of the disease or conversely the pervasive nature of their disease, might justifiably undergo a cosmetically superior operation. However, one must bear in mind that tactile sensation is lost. Therefore, evaluation of the liver must proceed using both intraoperative ultrasonography and radioimmuno-guided scanning. Evaluation of the intestine must be by careful, gentle manipulation with clamps.

Dr. Jager discusses "radiographically undetectable Crohn's ileitis." The reader must remember that Crohn's disease begins as a mucosal inflammation, which then eventually is manifested as transmural disease. Therefore, a well-performed enterolysis study should be superior to laparoscopy at detecting early Crohn's disease. More advanced Crohn's disease should be detectable by both approaches. Relative to these specific areas, success at diagnosing radiographically undetectable pathology in patients with chronic recurrent abdominal pain has been universally disappointing. Furthermore, I am unaware of any series in the literature proving the efficacy of laparoscopy in this group of patients.

In terms of the patients with "chronic diverticulitis," laparoscopy does afford the benefit of examining the serosal surface of the colon. However, one must bear in mind that, again, diverticulitis is an intraluminal disease. If serosal inflammation is severe enough to cause a phlegmon, that phlegmon should be detectable by CT scan. Indications for elective resection of diverticulitis include multiple attacks in a patient over the age of 40 to 50 and a single attack in a patient under the age of 40 to 50 (an *attack* is an episode of left lower quadrant pain with pyrexia and leukocytosis responsive to a course of intravenous antibiotics). In this group of patients, one might consider the use of intraoperative colonoscopy and bilateral ureteric catheters. Accordingly, the patient should be positioned as discussed by Dr. Jager.

The last group of patients in the elective category are those unfortunate individuals with widely disseminated colorectal carcinoma. In general, the primary lesion must still be resected in the case of colonic lesions and either resected or diverted as in the case of rectal lesions. However, the issue of port site implantation is of no consequence in this category of patients, because they already have disseminated disease. Accordingly, a patient with widely metastatic carcinoma of the lower third of the rectum who does not wish to undergo an abdominoperineal resection is an excellent candidate for a laparoscopic colostomy creation. Similarly, the patient with a widely disseminated cecal carcinoma is an excellent candidate for a laparoscopic right hemicolectomy. Thus, in the group of patients with chronic diverticulitis, as well as in the group of patients with widely disseminated colorectal carcinoma, the diagnostic laparoscopy should be planned and the patient should be prepared for the procedure to continue to a therapeutic laparoscopy.

The other group of patients in whom diagnostic laparoscopy is potentially applicable are those who require emergent laparoscopy. This group includes those with an acute abdomen, as Dr. Jager suggests, either occurring spontaneously, after blunt trauma, after sharp trauma, after abdominal aortic aneurysm surgery, or as a bowel obstruction. In this group of patients, one must question the cosmetic advantages. Although Dr. Jager mentions that "the cosmetic results are superior," one must recall that this group of patients may have life-threatening injuries, and a cadaver with small puncture wounds represents an inferior result to a live patient with a midline incision. Thus, the surgeon must, as Dr. Jager mentions, select the appropriate patient. The surgeon must be highly skilled, and have the usual assistants, instrumentation, and an entire operating team ready if even contemplating performing laparoscopic surgery in an emergent setting.

Performing laparoscopy in the emergent setting is analogous to performing colonoscopy in Ogilvie syndrome. In the latter instance, one must already be facile at performing colonoscopy in the prepared bowel in the adequately sedated patient. Similarly, the laparoscopic surgeon contemplating emergent laparoscopy must already be adept and facile at the performance of elective diagnostic and therapeutic laparoscopy. Assuming that these qualifications exist and that the patient is hemodynamically stable enough to undergo the procedure, laparoscopy certainly has an advantage in patients with an acute abdomen when acute appendicitis or acute cholecystitis is suspected. In patients with ischemic colitis, it may be far less applicable. First, these patients tend to be highly hemodynamically unstable, and the carbon dioxide shifts induced by pneumoperitoneum may be ill advised. Second, Dr. Jager discusses patients who have recently undergone abdominal aortic aneurysm surgery. This group of patients will undoubtedly be ill suited to emergent laparoscopy because of adhesions and hemodynamic instability. Furthermore, a large recent midline incision already exists, and access requires only removal of the midline suture(s). The only exception in this scenario might be the patient who has undergone a retroperitoneal incision for abdominal aortic aneurysm surgery. In the patient who has undergone either blunt or sharp trauma, laparoscopy may well have advantages. The reader is advised to peruse the trauma literature for an update on the subject.

In patients with acute intestinal obstruction, laparoscopy may, in certain select instances, offer an advantage. However, Dr. Jager mentions that "laparoscopy disrupts the peritoneum less so than open laparotomy, and thus it may diminish recurrent adhesion formation." The reference (ref. 13) cited, however, discusses only adhesions around the fallopian tube. The gynecologic literature is replete with information suggesting the advantages of laparoscopy relative to preservation of reproductive capacity in females. However, little, if any, data are available to suggest that laparoscopy for acute small bowel obstruction is associated with a decreased incidence of either adhesions or the need for a subsequent laparotomy. Although the concept is certainly sound in theory, in practice, it has not yet been proved. Furthermore, again, one must be cautioned that the inherent risks in performance of laparoscopy in the acute setting are formidable. The risk of injury to the small bowel as well as the risk of further hemodynamic insult in a patient who may already have decreased systemic vascular resistance must be considered when planning the approach.

Regardless of the indication, one must remember that Dr. Jager has posed a hypothesis: "if laparoscopic evaluation yields diagnostic sensitivity and specificity equivalent or superior to open laparotomy, laparoscopy should supplant exploratory laparotomy whenever feasible." The word *if* is the chief operative in this sentence. It is important to remember that McDermott et al,[1] Fingerhut(see Ch. 22),[2] Monson et al,[3] Larach et al,[4] and Cohen[5] are only a few of the many surgeons who have reported inappropriate surgery having been performed because of the lack of tactile sensation. One must be very attuned to the fact that when tactile sensation is lost, problems such as failure to localize a synchronous lesion or even the index lesion itself may occur. To counterbalance the loss of tactile sensation, intraoperative colonoscopy should be liberally used. Furthermore, when diagnostic laparoscopy is performed, all the ports should be 10 mm, because it is crucial that the camera can be inserted in each and every port for thorough inspection from all angles. The camera can be either 30 degrees, as Dr. Jager prefers, or 0 degrees, or flexible, as I prefer.

Regardless of the indications and the method, I strongly discourage two techniques discussed in this chapter. First, I believe that incidental appendectomy is unwarranted. Although the incidence of complications in the gynecologic literature may be few, any complication is unacceptable in a patient who would otherwise have an appendix still in place. I also recommend against the use of diagnostic laparoscopy under local anaesthesia. I have had the misfortune of observing several of these procedures when performed by gastroenterologists. The sounds emitted by the patients were reminiscent of those I heard when visiting a reconstructed medieval torture chamber in the basement of an English castle. Clearly, these patients are uncomfortable. Although certain intravenous anaesthetic agents may be used as amnestics and the patient may not remember the experience, certainly, I as the laparoscopist would personally have nightmares about having treated patients in such a barbaric manner. If the indications are so tenuous and dubious, then the procedure should not be done at all. If, conversely, the patient is so unstable that a local anaesthetic agent is the only one permissible, then the patient should be stabilized and the procedure done either as a laparoscopy under general anesthesia or as an emergent laparotomy.

REFERENCES

1. McDermott JP, Devereaux DA, Caushaj PF: Pitfall of laparoscopic colectomy: an unrecognized synchronous cancer. Dis Colon Rectum 37:602, 1994
2. Fingerhut A: Feasibility of laparoscopic colectomy. Presented at the 4th World Congress of Endoscopic Surgery. Kyoto, Japan, June 1994
3. Monson RT, Darzi A, Declan-Carry P, Guillou P: Prospective evaluation of laparoscopic-assisted colectomy in an unselected group of patients. Lancet 340:831, 1992

4. Larach SW, Salomon MC, Williamson PR: Laparoscopic-assisted colectomy: experience during the learning curve. Coloproctology 1:38, 1993

5. Cohen SM, Wexner SD: Laparoscopic colorectal surgery: are we being honest with our patients? Dis Colon Rectum (in press)

12
Laparoscopy and Colonoscopy

David E. Beck

Colonoscopy has proved its benefit in managing many colon and rectal conditions. Laparoscopy, however, remains in a developmental phase. Although increasing numbers of colorectal procedures are being performed with laparoscopic techniques, the precise role of this technology continues to evolve.[1–3] Combining colonoscopy and laparoscopy multiplies their respective advantages, overcomes their respective limitations, and offers significant benefits in several circumstances. This chapter reviews situations in which colonoscopy and laparoscopy can be usefully combined. These situations can be arbitrarily divided into situations in which colonoscopy assists laparoscopic procedures and those in which laparoscopy assists colonoscopic procedures.

COLONOSCOPIC-ASSISTED LAPAROSCOPY

Colonoscopy is helpful in several laparoscopic applications. All patients receive a full mechanical and antibiotic bowel preparation as outpatients. I use a polyethylene glycol (PEG) oral electrolyte lavage, oral metronidazole, and neomycin, as well as intravenous cefotetan. The procedure is performed using general anesthesia with the patient positioned in a modified Lloyd-Davies position with both arms tucked to the side (Fig. 12-1). The patient's hips are placed in less flexure than for a standard open procedure, which allows the endoscopist access to the perineum and provides the laparoscopists adequate room to manipulate their instruments. Significant flexure of the hips would bring the patient's thighs and knees closer to the abdomen and operating field, restricting access and interfering with instrument manipulation. It is also important to secure the patient to the operating room table with tape, shoulder braces, or a beanbag to prevent the patient from slipping off the table when it is tilted to obtain exposure. A Foley catheter and an orogastric tube are placed to decompress the bladder and stomach. A rectal irrigation is performed to ensure that the rectum and left colon are cleaned. The abdomen and perineum are prepared and draped in the usual fashion. A large operating room is helpful to accommodate the required extensive equipment and personnel, which are positioned as described in Figure 12-2. A videoendoscope is especially helpful because it allows the entire operating room team to see what is happening with the colonoscope. Procedures that have been described include assessment of the bowel preparation, colonic lesion location, and removal of specimens.

Preparation Assessment

If an intracorpeal anastomosis is planned, it is essential with current technology to have the bowel lumen as clean as possible. Other procedures usually involve significant bowel manipulation, and some authors prefer to confirm a clean bowel before accomplishing the planned procedure. Currently available bowel occlusion devices are not detachable and occupy a port cannula when in use. Therefore, ensuring that the bowel lumen is clean minimizes the potential for contamination.

Patients are prepared and positioned as described above. After a pneumoperitoneum is established, trocar cannulas are placed. I use all 10/12-mm ports, which allow movement of a 10-mm camera and the full spectrum of bowel instruments to any port, maximizing visualization and operative flexibility.

An exploration with the laparoscopic camera is performed, and an atraumatic bowel clamp is passed through a second port cannula to occlude the ileocecal valve. This procedure prevents excess gas from distending the small bowel, a condition that would limit visibility during the remainder of the procedure. A videocolonoscope is inserted into the anus and passed to the cecum. An effort is made to minimize air insufflation. A colonoscope is used to aspirate any remaining liquid stool as it is

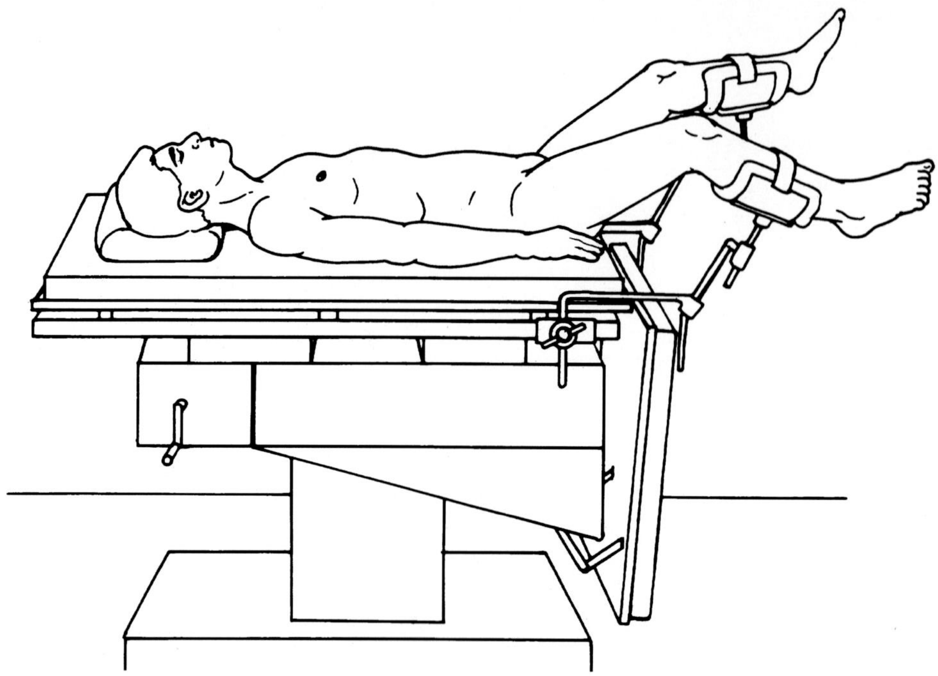

Fig. 12-1. Modified Lloyd-Davies position. Legs with minimal hip flexure are supported by Lloyd-Davies stirrups.

encountered. After reaching the cecum, the scope is withdrawn, and residual fluid and gas are aspirated. The planned procedure can then proceed.

Lesion Location

A severe limitation with laparoscopy is the surgeon's loss of tactile ability. Flat polypoid lesions may be difficult to locate by laparoscopic techniques alone. A colonoscope can identify the location of such a colonic lesion. The ileocecal valve is occluded as described above to limit small bowel distension, and a colonoscope, inserted via the anus, is advanced to the lesion. Movement of the scope tip or the light at the end of the colonoscope can usually be seen via the laparoscope. Additional confirmation can be obtained by gently grasping the bowel just beyond the suspected tip of the colonoscope. The lumenal indentation caused by the clamp can be seen with the colonoscope. After the exact lesion location is identified, the bowel may be marked with a clip applied with a laparoscopic device, a suture, or electrocautery. The planned procedure may then continue.

Lesion or Specimen Removal

Retrieval of a resected specimen with laparoscopy poses a dilemma. Some authors have suggested a transanal extraction of resected specimens. In this technique, the colonic specimen is resected, and the distal rectum is left open. A colonoscope is inserted through the anus and passed through the open end of the rectum into the abdomen. The specimen is located, and a snare passed through the colonoscope is used to grasp the resected specimen. The scope and the secured specimen are then withdrawn out the anus. This maneuver obviates an abdominal wall incision but has several limitations. First, only distal colonic resections are suitable for this technique. Second, the pneumoperitoneum is often lost as the colonoscope is passed through the anal sphincters. Third, the technique is contraindicated in the case of bulky lesions because dilation of the anal sphincter may be necessary to deliver the left colon and its associated mesentery out the anus.[4] Fourth, if the specimen contains a carcinoma, tumor seeding of the anorectum is a risk. In view of these limitations, I do not use transanal specimen removal.

LAPAROSCOPIC-ASSISTED COLONOSCOPY

A small group of patients will have sessile colonic polyps that are too large to safely remove with a colonoscope using traditional techniques. A second group (usually women with a history of previous pelvic surgery) will have polyps or suspicious colonic pathology identified on barium studies, but intra-abdominal adhesions will prevent the colonoscopist from examining the whole colon. Patients with these conditions can potentially benefit from laparoscopic-assisted procedures.

Laparoscopic-Assisted Colonoscopic Polypectomy

Patients suitable for laparoscopic-assisted colonoscopic polypectomy are those with moderate-size polyps

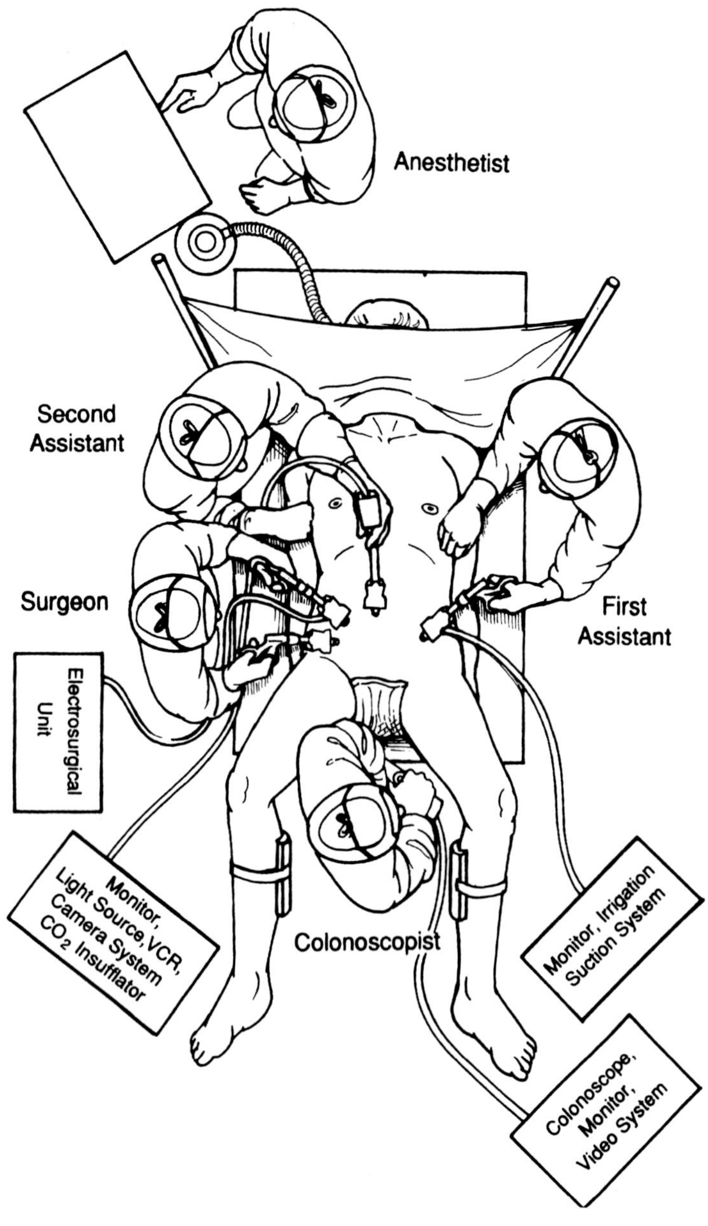

Fig. 12-2. Equipment and personnel positioning for combined laparoscopy and colonoscopy.

that appear to be unsafe to excise with colonoscopy alone[5] (Fig. 12-3). The polyp should not have any of the features associated with invasive cancers (e.g., ulceration, fixation, or hardness). Biopsy of the lesion should demonstrate benign histology, and the patient should also lack other indications for abdominal surgery. Although previous surgery is not an absolute contraindication to laparoscopy, patients with multiple previous operations often have adhesions that restrict the ease with which laparoscopy can be performed. Other relative contraindications include severe chronic obstructive pulmonary disease, inability to tolerate general anesthesia, and the presence of large ventral hernias.

The procedure should be discussed with the patient with special attention given to the possible need for a bowel resection, the potential for bowel injury or leak, and the possibility of incomplete lesion excision. Informed consent for the procedure also includes the developmental nature of laparoscopic procedures and the potential for conversion to an open procedure. The patient receives a full mechanical and antibiotic bowel preparation, as described above, as an outpatient. The procedure is performed using general anesthesia with the patient in the modified Lloyd-Davies position.

In patients with a virgin abdomen, pneumoperitoneum is established using a Veress needle inserted at the umbilicus. A Hasson technique is used in patients

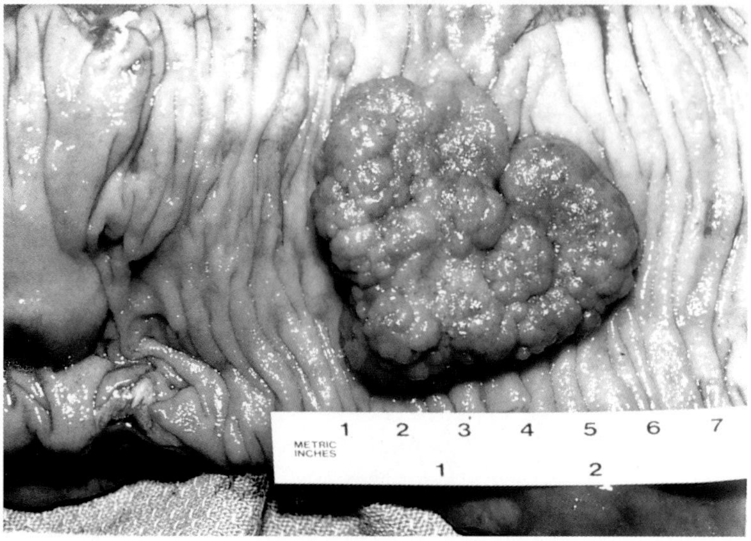

Fig. 12-3. Sessile polyp that would have been suitable for laparoscopic-assisted endoscopic polypectomy. (From Beck and Karulf,[5] with permission.)

with previous surgery. A 10/12-mm trocar is placed at the umbilicus, and a 10-mm, 0 degree camera is inserted. Under direct vision, two or three additional 10/12-mm trocar ports are placed in the abdomen opposite the side of the lesion (Figs. 12-4 and 12-5). I use all 10/12-mm ports to allow movement of the cam-

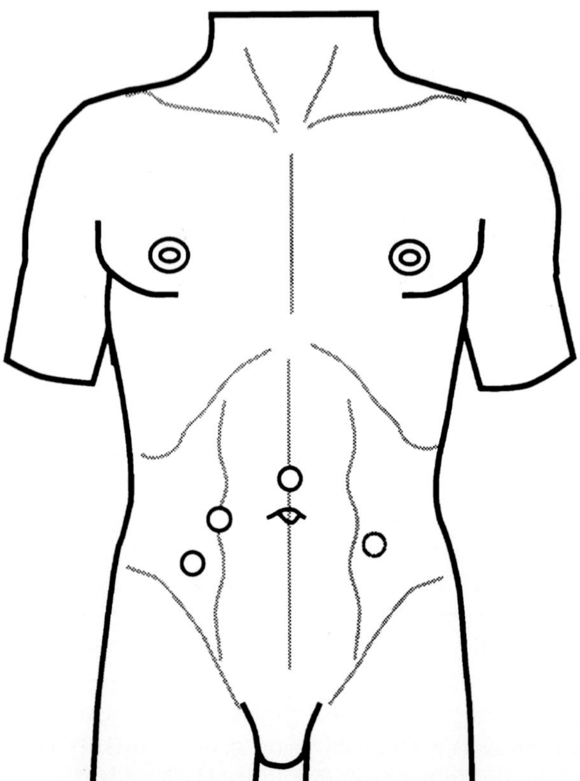

Fig. 12-4. Trocar placement for a sigmoid polyp. If needed, an additional port may be placed in the patient's left upper quadrant (broken circle).

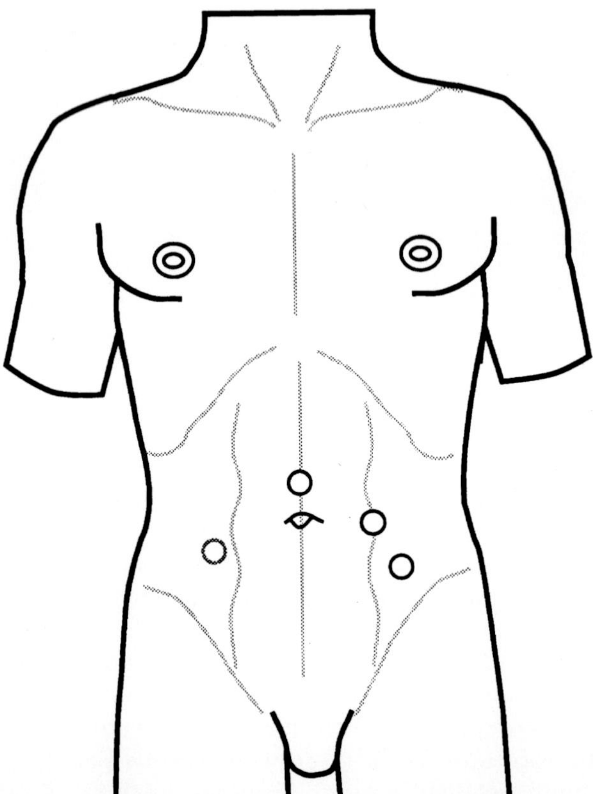

Fig. 12-5. Trocar placement for cecal polyp. If needed, an additional port may be placed in the patient's upper quadrant (broken circle).

era to any port, which maximizes visualizations. Through one of these ports, an atraumatic bowel clamp is used to occlude the colon proximal to the lesion or at the ileocecal valve. As described previously, this procedure prevents excess gas from distending the small bowel, which would limit visibility. The operating room table is tilted to maximally expose the portion of the bowel that contains the lesion.

A videocolonoscope is passed via the anus until the colonic lesion or obstruction is located. Once the lesion is identified, it is grasped with biopsy forceps or an electrocautery snare passed through the colonoscope. Retracting this instrument allows the exact location of the lesion to be identified with the laparoscopic camera. If the dimpled area in the colon is not accessible, the colon may be mobilized (dividing the colonic reflections with traction and cautery scissors) to produce a free surface over the lesion. If adhesions prevent insertion of the colonoscope to the colonic lesion, the adhesions may be divided with scissors or cautery inserted through additional ports (Figs. 12-4 and 12-5). If the colonic mesentery overlies the polyp, a resection may be indicated.

Once the lesion is accessible, an electrocautery snare is passed through the colonoscope and used to grasp the polyp. If the colon is not dimpled after closure of the snare, a polypectomy is performed with laparoscopic observation. If the colon is dimpled by the snare, several options are available. The technique of saline-assisted polypectomy or mucosal stripping may be used.[6–8] This technique involves injection of 2 to 5 ml of saline or an epinephrine and saline solution (1:100,000) into the submucosal plane with a sclerotherapy needle passed through the biopsy port of the colonoscope. This fluid distends the submucosal layer and elevates the polyp from the surrounding tissue. This cushion increases the distance between the mucosa and the serosal surface of the bowel and reduces the chances of a full-thickness perforation. After injection of the distention solution, the area of injection is inspected with the laparoscopic camera as the snare is retightened. If the area is no longer dimpled, the snare polypectomy proceeds under direct vision. If dimpling remains, other maneuvers may be used.

One of these maneuvers is to invert the unopened colon over the polyp, changing a sessile lesion to one that appears pedunculated. The maneuver can be accomplished by oversewing the dimpled area using laparoscopic techniques. I have used running or interrupted sutures of 4-0 Ethibond (Ethicon, Inc., Somerville, NJ) with extracorporeally tied knots (Fig. 12-6).

Following inversion of the lesion, the electrocautery snare is used to perform a full-thickness polypectomy of the inverted bowel by using cutting and coagulation current. Use of a bipolar snare may increase the safety

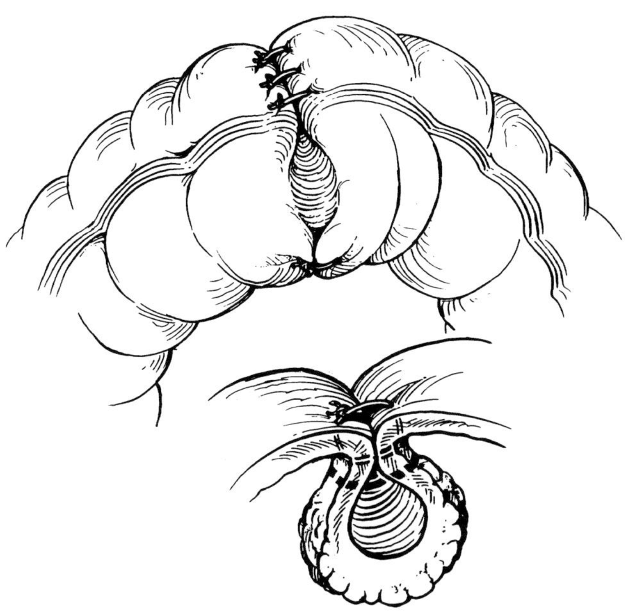

Fig. 12-6. Inversion of polyp with sutures. Inset illustrates a cross-section of a lesion inversion. Dotted line identifies the plane of snare excision.

of this technique.[9] After the lesion is detached from the bowel wall, the excision site is inspected, and air insufflation is used to confirm the integrity of the remaining bowel. Dripping a small amount of saline over the distended suture line allows ready identification of any leaks. Any leak or defect is repaired with additional sutures.

After bowel integrity is ensured, the specimen is removed with the colonoscope and submitted for pathologic review. If invasive cancer or incomplete margins are identified, a resection can be performed.

The trocar sites are closed by approximating the anterior fascia with 2-0 Vicryl (Ethicon) sutures, and the skin is closed with 4-0 Vicryl sutures and Steri-strips (3-M, St. Paul, MN).

If the colon is not opened, the patient may be discharged later the same day. If the colon requires oversewing, the patient is observed as an inpatient. Discharge occurs when the patient can tolerate a regular diet. Follow-up recommendations include a repeat colonoscopy at 3 months after surgery.

Laparoscopic-assisted colonoscopic polypectomy allows complete excision of moderate-size sessile polyps and may spare selected patients a colonic resection. However, with current adjuvant therapies, a laparoscopic-assisted colonoscopic polypectomy is not suited for malignant lesions. If pathologic evaluation of the removed lesion identifies an invasive malignancy, an adequate bowel resection is indicated. This may be performed with open or laparoscopic technique at the time of the polypectomy or a later date.

Diagnostic Colonoscopy

Occasionally, patients are encountered with suspected colonic lesions (e.g., from a barium enema or computed tomography scan), making it impossible to perform a complete colonoscopy. Inability to complete the colonoscopy may be due to intra-abdominal adhesions from previous surgery or a very redundant colon. Previously, an exploratory laparotomy would have been necessary. In selected patients, laparoscopic techniques may be used to divide the adhesions that limited complete colonoscopy.

LIMITATIONS

Limitations to the greater use of laparoscopic techniques combined with colonoscopy include deficiencies in equipment, the associated length of operating time, and cost. The costs associated with these procedures include the operating room, general anesthesia, endoscopy, and the laparoscopy equipment. These costs must be balanced against those associated with a major laparotomy or colonic resection. Successful use of the techniques described in this chapter may eliminate the need to open the patient's bowel, thus sparing the patient the morbidity associated with a major resection.

I have limited my use of laparoscopy to situations in which this new technology appears to offer significant patient advantages. The techniques described above can safely remove large polypoid lesions and divide adhesions that restrict colonoscopy. A major limitation of combining these two techniques is the cost. It is estimated that a successful laparoscopic-assisted polypectomy costs three to four times that of a routine polypectomy but less than a major surgical resection.[4]

Laparoscopy and colonoscopy can be combined to maximize patient benefit. Evaluation of the advantages and disadvantages of these technologies—along with additional experience—will define their appropriate role in patient management.

REFERENCES

1. Fall PM, Thorson AU, Beart RW et al: Laparoscopic colectomy: a critical appraisal. Dis Colon Rectum 36:28, 1993
2. Wexner SD, Johansen OB, Nogueras JJ et al: Laparoscopic total abdominal colectomy. A prospective trial. Dis Colon Rectum 25:651, 1992
3. Wexner SD: Laparoscopic colectomy. p. 2434. In Keighley MEB, Williams NS (eds): Surgery of the Anus, Rectum and Colon. WB Saunders, London, 1993
4. Beck DE: Laparoscopic-assisted colonoscopic polypectomy. Surg Oncol Clin North Am 3:679, 1994
5. Beck DE, Karulf RE: Laparoscopic-assisted full-thickness endoscopic polypectomy. Dis Colon Rectum 36:693, 1993
6. Williams CB: Colonoscopy and polypectomy. p. 130. In Fielding LP, Goldberg SO (eds): Rob and Smith's Operative Surgery—Surgery of the Colon, Rectum and Anus. 5th Ed. Butterworth-Heinemann, Oxford, 1993
7. Waye JD: Saline-assisted polypectomy, the cushion technique. A new method to increase safety of colonic sessile polypectomy. Gastrointest Endosc 39:259, 1993
8. Karita M, Tada M, Okita K et al: Endoscopic therapy for early colon cancer: the strip biopsy resection technique. Gastrointest Endosc 37:128, 1991
9. Tucker RD, Platz CE, Sievert CE et al: In vivo evaluation of monopolar versus bipolar electrosurgical polypectomy snares. Am J Gastroenterol 85:1386, 1991

Editorial Comment I

Kenneth A. Forde

The periodic need to inspect the lumen of the gastrointestinal tract at the time of celiotomy in both elective and emergent situations has been satisfied as well as enhanced with the development of flexible fiberoptics and, subsequently, videoendoscopy. Dr. Beck is to be commended for addressing several important questions that need to be answered and for enunciating that flexible and rigid endoscopy and intraluminal and intracavitary examination show promise of complimenting each other. The use of flexible endoscopy and laparoscopic surgery is a natural development, and the major indications should be at least the same as those developed for traditional open procedures. However, as Dr. Beck has carefully noted, with the inherent inability to manually palpate the viscera during laparoscopic surgery, the indication "localization of nonpalpable lesions" becomes more prominent. Conceptually, then, colonoscopy is potentially adjunctive to laparoscopy as intraoperative colonoscopy has been to celiotomy. One wonders how much of this chapter is theoretical and how much is confirmed by actual experience, however.

PREPARATION ASSESSMENT

Assessment of preparation is one of the constant benefits of intraoperative colonoscopy. The surgeon should be careful in handling a lesion with significant stenosis of the bowel. The colonoscopist could insufflate the bowel proximal to the lesion, creating an undesirable and unsafe situation without achieving the goal of assessment of preparation. All who have performed intraoperative colonoscopy to any significant extent are aware of the difficulty in avoiding bowing of the colon in segments that are redundant and unfixed. These include the sigmoid and transverse colon. No matter how careful and experienced the endoscopist is at intraoperative colonoscopy, it is often necessary for the operating surgeon to assist in bowel decompression before removing the instrument.

There is concern among many who undertake laparoscopic colectomy that more manipulation of tumor may be necessary with current techniques than is oncologically desirable. Because intraoperative colonoscopic examination involves even further manipulation, it might be useful to advise that tumoricidal agents be used just before bowel anastomosis to at least reduce some potential for suture line recurrence, recognizing that this is only one factor in the genesis of tumor implantation and growth.

LESION LOCALIZATION

Lesion localization is, of course, one of the major current indications for intraoperative colonoscopy—seeing the lesion that cannot be felt. Location of the polypectomy sites in patients subsequently deemed candidates for colonic resection is another appropriate indication for intraoperative colonoscopy.

LESION REMOVAL

Dr. Beck is to be commended for pointing out the limitations of current laparoscopic transanal specimen removal techniques, especially the potential for sphincter injury and contamination with both bacteria and tumor cells. As he notes, the technique he describes does not obviate these problems.

LAPAROSCOPIC-ASSISTED COLONOSCOPY

The problem with sessile polyps is not necessarily the size of the lesion but its geography. For example, if there is carpeting of the mucosa, the adenomatous tissue may be completely and safely removed only by resection. Laparoscopic-assisted colectomy is attractive in situations in which routine colonoscopy of an otherwise manageable situation has been frustrated by adhesions. Adhesions may be so dense, however, that laparoscopic and even open surgical attempts at their lysis may not be adequate to allow colonoscopic polypectomy.

The description of laparoscopic-assisted colonoscopic polypectomy may be a rationalization. Because no pathognomonic features allow reassurance that a large sessile polyp is benign, every polypectomy has to be seen as an excisional biopsy. Total sampling is necessary before one can be assured that the lesion is entirely benign. Such total sampling is best done by total excision; in the case of a sessile lesion, a resection as for cancer should be performed. If laparoscopic colon resection is to achieve the same oncologic goals as the open method, this consistency would have to be maintained until tools have been developed that might replace current imaging and histologic techniques in determining the extent of neoplasia and predictability of biologic behavior. The technique described as laparoscopic-assisted colonoscopic polypectomy is purely mechanical and reveals no consideration of pathology or the potential for seeding lymphatics with tumor cells, according to current concepts. The techniques of saline-assisted polypectomy and mucosal stripping have been described but hardly established.

I am aware of no evidence that confirms the idea that inadequate cancer excision followed by resection is an optimal and safe technique. Repeat colonoscopy will only discover the cancer recurrence when it is mucosal. Unfortunately, recurrence may often be extramucosal and not necessarily local-regional but also distant.

LIMITATIONS

Could some of the costs of laparoscopy and colonoscopy be decreased by preoperative colonoscopy in an endoscopy suite rather than the operating room, perhaps by techniques of localization such as fluoroscopy or endoscopic tattooing? What about the cost of removing a polyp, finding it is an invasive cancer, and then having to perform still another lengthy procedure? What time delay is necessary under such circumstance? When is it safe to proceed with the second operation, and are any special precautions to be taken? Figure 12-3 could easily have been an invasive carcinoma on final histologic examination. These are judgments we are still unable to make with certainty on endoscopic examination. This chapter is at least provocative but at most potentially dangerous. Although much in this work is daring (e.g., the implicit challenges to standard accepted oncologic surgical technique), most is so far conjectural. I believe it is appropriate to (1) challenge some of the adages of previous generations and (2) recognize that there are other changes in the management of surgical patients that allow for speedier recovery and less invasiveness. However, to do so without confirmatory information will mislead less insightful practitioners who may believe that they are behind by not being involved with the new surgery.

I hope that my detailed comments have shown that much in this chapter is logical and acceptable, but far too much is still in evolution and should not yet be put forth as doctrine. The practicing surgeon can incorporate the established benefit of intraoperative colonoscopy into the evolving techniques of laparoscopic colon surgery. The discerning surgeon will, it is hoped, discover the limitations of colonoscopy under laparoscopic guidance before inappropriately attempting to incorporate some of Dr. Beck's ideas into current practice.

Editorial Comment II

Rama M. Jager

Intraoperative colonoscopy is not only useful but also at times indispensable in laparoscopic colorectal surgery. Dr. Beck carefully details his technique of colonoscopic polypectomy under laparoscopic guidance and laparoscopic polypectomy under colonoscopic guidance. Judicious concurrent use of both endoscopic procedures avoids the need for an open laparotomy in properly selected patients.

Any discussion on the advantages of laparoscopic procedures compared with open laparotomy invariably and rightfully includes a statement that these advantages are not proven, but only "theoretical." Application of laparoscopic techniques in colorectal surgery, and for that matter in all gastrointestinal surgery, is in evolution. Both the advantages and disadvantages from this new technique are currently being evaluated both by systematic collection of retrospective clinical data that can be compared with historical controls and by randomized comparative clinical trials.

No one doubts that caution in application of laparoscopic colorectal surgery is prudent. It is a demonstration of one's surgical maturity to remember that therapeutic laparoscopic techniques in colorectal surgery are unproven and untested. Feasibility studies such as detailed by Dr. Beck are extremely important to promote the surgical innovation in our constant attempt to reduce patients' morbidity from surgical maneuvers. After all, surgery is a paradoxical craft. Surgeons treat by inducing trauma, however selective and specific. We should not harm our patients by trying untested techniques. By contrast, we should remember that most of our conventional surgical wisdom is untested. All of us operate under the cloud of medical uncertainty and therapeutic ambiguity every day of our surgical lives. A progressive surgeon not only avoids undesirable zeal, but stays clear of undue caution.

Proper and safe conduction of any laparoscopic procedure requires attention to details in preoperative preparation and operating room setup (an indispensable requirement for laparoscopic colectomy) and tolerance of frustration. The laparoscopic techniques are instrument intensive. All precautions taken to position the patient properly, as discussed by Dr. Beck, are essential. These precautions avert intraoperative problems that prolong the operative time and, at times, lead to abandonment of laparoscopic procedure. Measures such as protection of neurovascular prominences from positional injury, proper thigh flexion during lithotomy to avoid interference of thighs with movement of laparoscope, and use of the largest operating room available for laparoscopic procedures facilitate a safe, smooth, and swift operation.

Positioning of the monitor for the colonoscopist is as important as the positioning of laparoscopic monitors. Figure 12-2 depicts the operating room setup used by Dr. Beck. If the operating room layout permits, it is more convenient and ergonomic to have the colonoscopic monitor toward the patient's head so that the colonoscopist does not have to look back at the monitor while inserting the colonoscope or resecting the polyp. This layout of the monitors, also requires that the video processor for the colonoscope be at a separate location than its monitor.

As Dr. Forde indicates in his comments, sigmoid and transverse colonic redundancy may affect the colonoscopic advancement. The usual maneuvers, such as transabdominal counterpressure during the regular colonoscopy, obviously are not feasible during the intraoperative colonoscopy. Measures to stabilize the redundant segments using atraumatic endoscopic bowel clamps may enable completion of colonoscopy. Care is necessary to ensure that the colonic wall or the mesocolon is not injured during these maneuvers to stabilize the flexures. The degree of difficulty in intraoperative colonoscopic maneuvering could be anticipated, since the intraoperative colonoscopist has most probably done the preoperative colonoscopy.

The problem of colonic dilation proximal to an obstructive lesion from insufflation during intraoperative colonoscopy is a concern. Colonoscopy, however, is rarely necessary to identify an obstructive colonic lesion. In fact, obstructive lesions with consequent inadequate bowel preparation are a relative contraindication to laparoscopic resection. Such lesions are more appropriately resected by the conventional open techniques.

Does colonoscopic insufflation distend the colon so much that it interferes with laparoscopic dissection? Although it is a valid concern, I rarely found it a problem as long as small intestinal insufflation is prevented as discussed in this chapter. One technical modification may obviate these problems with unwanted colonic or enteric dilation from insufflation. Most colonoscopes are equipped for carbon dioxide insufflation as well as air insufflation. Use of carbon dioxide rather than air to insufflate the colon will allow rapid resorption of carbon dioxide, and resolution of colonic distension during laparoscopic mobilization. Even if carbon dioxide escapes into the small intestine, the dilated loops of small intestine return to normal status within a few minutes, allowing further laparoscopic dissection.

It is tempting to consider transanal removal of the resected colonic segment. This maneuver avoids need for a separate incision. The disadvantage of passing a nonsterilized colonoscope anally and insufflating room air into the peritoneal cavity contraindicate such a maneuver. In addition, there is the problem of difficulty with anal dilation needed to remove a bulky specimen.

When the lesion cannot be resected colonoscopically under laparoscopic guidance, the technique of pseudodiverticulization may be a treatment option. The colon wall overlying the polyp is retracted with a grasping forceps, and the polyp containing segment of the colon is transected by an endoscopic stapler. The danger of compromising colonic lumen makes this approach useful only when the polyp is present in the mobile or well-mobilized right colon with adequate lumen to spare even after excision of the polyp. The resected specimen can be easily removed through a 12-mm cannula.

When a polyp near the ileocecal valve cannot be resected by laparoscopic assisted colonoscopy, a 3- to 4-cm muscle splitting incision to exteriorize the cecum for extracorporeal segmental resection is expeditious and safe. This incision also avoids the problem of compromising the ileocecal valve lumen by the endoscopic stapler. In a similar fashion, when the surgeon is not certain that totally laparoscopic excision of the polyp under colonoscopic guidance is safe or feasible, laparoscopic mobilization followed by segmental resection after exteriorization through a small muscle splitting incision is an option.

Some may argue that if a polyp cannot be excised colonoscopically, it should be removed by standard segmental resection rather than by convoluted attempts by concurrent use of colonoscopy and laparoscopy. This strategy is too rigid. While malignant foci in a polypoid lesion cannot be excluded with certainty, an experienced endoscopist can estimate whether the chances of malignant transformation are high. Those lesions with high probability of malignant transformation should be handled much like any other colon cancer. Those with least likelihood of harboring malignant foci may be amenable to colonoscopic resection under laparoscopic guidance or laparoscopic resection under colonoscopic guidance. The resected specimen can be evaluated for the presence, differentiation, and muscularis mucosa penetration of malignant foci, which may determine the need for further resection.

In his comments, Dr. Forde questions the propriety and validity of such strategy. If a colonoscopic resection (under laparoscopic guidance) of a colonic polyp potentially harboring a malignancy is counter to currently accepted oncosurgical dogma, the standard colonoscopic resection (without laparoscopic guidance) of any sessile polyp is also inappropriate. This is not so. Thousands of gastroenterologists remove polypoid lesions endoscopically and refer the patient to the surgeon if the endoscopically resected lesion shows malignant foci upon histologic examination. I concede that a common practice is not necessarily the right practice. Ample evidence speaks for this practice. The published data support the current practice of colonoscopic resection of sessile polyps. The natural course of colonoscopically resected polypoid lesions containing malignant foci and the treatment strategy in managing these patients by further surgery has been studied extensively. The reader is referred to multiple previous publications dealing with this issue of colonoscopic resection of polyps that may potentially harbor a malignant focus.[1–4]

Surgeons, by nature and training, are cautious and conservative. Our traditional caution is appropriate in application of the techniques outlined by Dr. Beck in this chapter. Individual surgeon's laparoscopic and colonoscopic skills and the nature and geography of the polypoid lesion decide the optimum mode of resection of colonoscopically nonresectable polyps. The available options include the colonoscopic resection with laparoscopic guidance, the laparoscopic resection with or without colonoscopic guidance, the segmental resection, and the standard colonic and lymph nodal resection. No one technique is optimal for all the patients and their variety of lesions.

REFERENCES

1. Geraghty JM, Williams CB, Talbot IC et al: Malignant colorectal polyps: venous invasion and successful treatment by endoscopic polypectomy. Gut 32:774, 1991
2. Morson BC, Whiteway JE, Jones EA et al: Histopathology and prognosis of malignant colorectal polyps treated by endoscopic polypectomy. Gut 25:437, 1984
3. Nivatvongs S, Rojanasakul A, Reiman HM et al: The risk of lymph node metastasis in colorectal polyps with invasive adenocarcinoma. Dis Colon Rectum 34:323, 1991
4. Decosse JJ: Malignant colorectal polyp. Gut 25:433, 1984

13 Laparoscopic Enterostomy

Rama M. Jager

Surgical creation of colostomy and ileostomy as an isolated surgical procedure for fecal diversion is not uncommon. A separate abdominal incision is often necessary to mobilize the ileal or colonic loop and to bring out the loop as a stoma. The laparoscopic approach to stomal establishment avoids the need for separate abdominal incision, reducing the incisional morbidity and, thus, easing a rapid return of the patient to functional status. Absence of a separate abdominal incision enables rapid initiation of postoperative chemotherapy and radiotherapy. This approach is an advantage for those patients with obstructive left colon or rectal cancer who need colostomy as a temporary fecal diversion procedure. A report of my experience with 10 patients who had laparoscopic enterostomy showing its safety and feasibility follows.

EXPERIENCE

Indications

Enterostomy with no associated bowel resection is most often done for a temporary fecal diversion when severe inflammatory bowel disease fails to respond to medical treatment. Patients with a nonresectable obstructive rectal or sigmoid colonic carcinoma often need a temporary left colostomy to provide a fecal outlet. Radiotherapy of a semiobstructed left colon cancer can lead to edema and inflammation, which further compromise the colonic lumen. In these patients, the fecal diversion facilitates postoperative radiotherapy. The common indications for enterostomy as an isolated intraperitoneal procedure are listed below.

1. Severe inflammatory bowel disease not responding to medical treatment
2. Colonic pseudo-obstruction
3. Idiopathic colonic inertia

(Continues)

4. Neurogenic colonic hypomotility (associated with paraplegia)
5. Anal incontinence
6. Fecal diversion before recurrent recto-vaginal fistula repair
7. Fecal diversion for radiation proctitis or radiation-induced rectourethral fistula
8. Nonresectable rectal cancer

Surgical Technique

Preoperative Evaluation and Operating Room Setup

Cardiopulmonary evaluation and estimate of surgical risk are done preoperatively as in conventional open colostomy. Preoperative measures include both mechanical and antibiotic bowel preparation. Mechanical bowel preparation understandably is not feasible in patients with obstructed left colon cancers. Preoperative marking of the stoma site reduces problems with inappropriate stomal placement and consequent stomal care difficulties.

The patient is placed in the supine position. General anesthesia with complete muscle relaxation is essential. Avoiding nitrous oxide prevents dilated small bowel loops. The surgeon stands contralateral to the side of stomal location. Two monitors, one on either side of the patient, are optimal, although the procedure can be done with a single monitor because minimal intraperitoneal dissection and retraction are necessary.

Pneumoperitoneum

Under general anesthesia, a pneumoperitoneum raising the intraperitoneal pressure to 15 mm Hg can be established with a Veress needle. The inferior rim of the umbilicus serves as the access site for most patients. A 10-mm umbilical port is placed into the peritoneal cavity to insert the videolaparoscope. The peritoneal cavity is carefully evaluated for metastatic disease if the stoma is being conducted for a malignant lesion. Under direct vision, a 5-mm suprapubic port is placed to serve as a dissecting port. The right-handed surgeon places the dissecting port superior to the umbilical port when standing at the patient's left side while doing an ileostomy. The dissecting port is placed inferior to the umbilical port when a right-handed surgeon is doing a sigmoidostomy and is standing on the patient's right side. Through the preoperatively marked site, a surgical stomal exit wound is created by removing a circular disc of skin and subcutaneous tissue; the anterior rectus sheath is then incised. The rectus muscle is split, taking care to prevent injury to the inferior epigastric vessels. In some patients, it is easier to identify and ligate the inferior epigastric vessels than it is to try to obtain hemostasis after injuring the vessels during the fasciotomy. The posterior rectus sheath is left intact. A 10-mm port is placed through the posterior rectus sheath under direct vision, visualizing entrance of the trocar with a videolaparoscope.

If a blind puncture with the Veress needle is not possible, a small fasciotomy at the potential stomal site allows open technique for peritoneal cannula placement. In patients who have had previous abdominal surgical procedures and thus have subperitoneal intra-abdominal adhesions, the open approach to cannula placement may be more appropriate. The problem of carbon dioxide leakage around the cannula is more common with the open placement of the cannula. This leakage makes maintenance of a pneumoperitoneum frustrating and cools the laparoscope, promoting fogging of the lens. A pursestring fascial suture around the peritoneal cannula may prevent leakage of carbon dioxide and hypothermic problems. The pursestring suture should be placed with care to avoid bowel injury.[1] Any adhesions at the site of cannula placement can be digitally lysed or cleared by sharp dissection.

Laparoscopic Dissection

Care and gentleness in enteric mobilization are essential. Using an endoscopic Babcock forceps through the 10-mm port at the stomal site, the portion of the intestinal loop (sigmoid colon or ileum) to be exteriorized is grasped. Endoscopic Babcock forceps can be traumatic and can injure the intestinal segment. An electrosurgical scissors introduced through the suprapubic 5-mm port enables mobilization of the intestinal loop. Ileal mobilization is rarely difficult. Patients who have had previous appendectomy may have extensive adhesions, hampering the distal ileal mobilization. Some patients have congenital adhesions around the ileocecal region and the appendix. These adhesions need lysis.

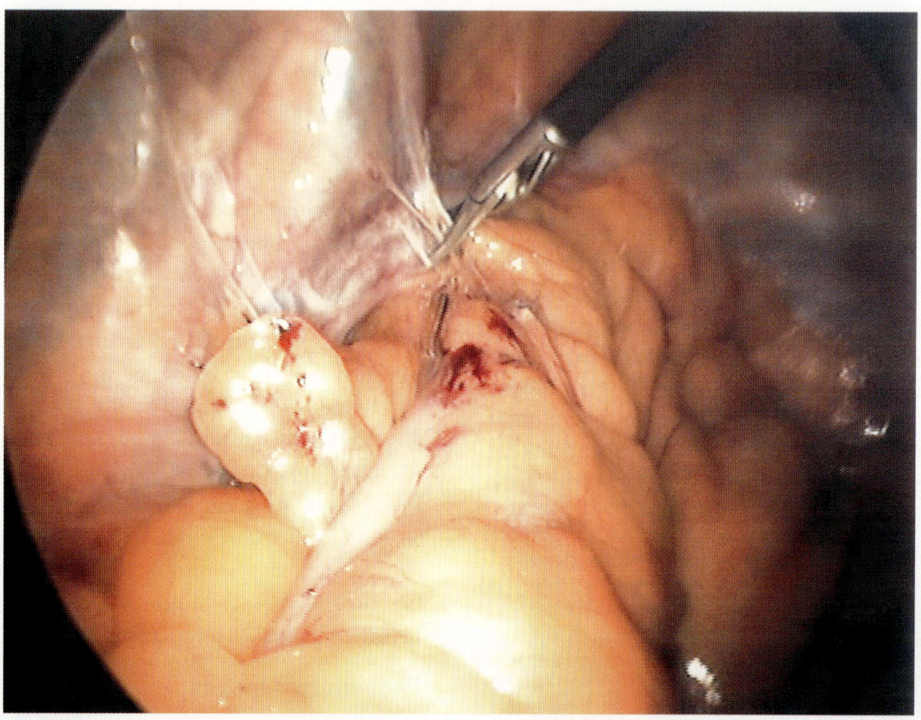

Fig. 13-1. Electrodissection and mobilization of sigmoid colon to facilitate its delivery through the colostomy site.

Sigmoid mobilization may involve left paracolic dissection (Fig. 13-1). Care should be taken to avoid electrocoagulation around the left ureter, which can lead to thermal injury-induced ureteral stenosis. When the cancer involves the sigmoid colon, mobilization of descending colon and splenic flexure (Fig. 13-2) will enable a descending colostomy, a better option than a transverse colostomy for left colonic obstruction. Splenic flexure mobilization may require a second 10-mm left upper quadrant cannula for a second Babcock forceps to retract the splenic flexure inferiorly and medially. Shifting the videolaparoscope to the left upper quadrant port and using the umbilical port for dissecting instruments may be necessary in obese patients.

Although transverse colostomy can also be done laparoscopically, rarely is it necessary to use laparoscopic mobilization because the circular trephine wound made for the stoma is often adequate to identify the mobile greater omentum and transverse colon and to exteriorize the loop. Also, transverse colostomy is difficult to manage postoperatively and better avoided.

After satisfactory mobilization of the intestinal loop, the loop is brought close to the posterior abdominal wall fascia by the endoscopic Babcock forceps (Figs. 13-3 and 13-4). Partially deflating the pneumoperitoneum helps the loop exteriorization. After ensuring that the loop can be exteriorized, the surgeon completely deflates the pneumoperitoneum. The posterior fascia is incised on either side of the 10-mm port. The fascial defect is dilated to two fingerbreadths, and the intestinal loop is delivered out of the peritoneal cavity (Fig. 13-5). The exteriorized loop is grasped with a regular Babcock forceps, replacing the endoscopic Babcock forceps, and is anchored to the fascia with multiple absorbable serosal interrupted sutures. These sutures are not obligatory. The laparoscopic portion of the stomal creation is now complete, and all the cannulas are removed (Fig. 13-6). I do not place a supporting rod but rely on serosal and mucocutaneous sutures to hold the stoma in place and prevent retraction.

All the umbilical fascial defects are repaired with interrupted absorbable sutures, and the skin wounds are completely closed before the stoma is matured. The stoma is matured by using multiple interrupted absorbable sutures, establishing a primary mucocutaneous junction. Eversion of the proximal limb and closure of the distal limb as needed are similar to the open technique of ileostomy. If an end-on stoma is obligatory, the loop is transected with a stapler and the distal end is buried in the subcutaneous tissue.

Patient Data

Ten of my patients had laparoscopic enterostomy as an isolated surgical procedure, five having had ileostomies and the other five, colostomies. Three of the five patients who had colostomies had a fecal diversion to treat an

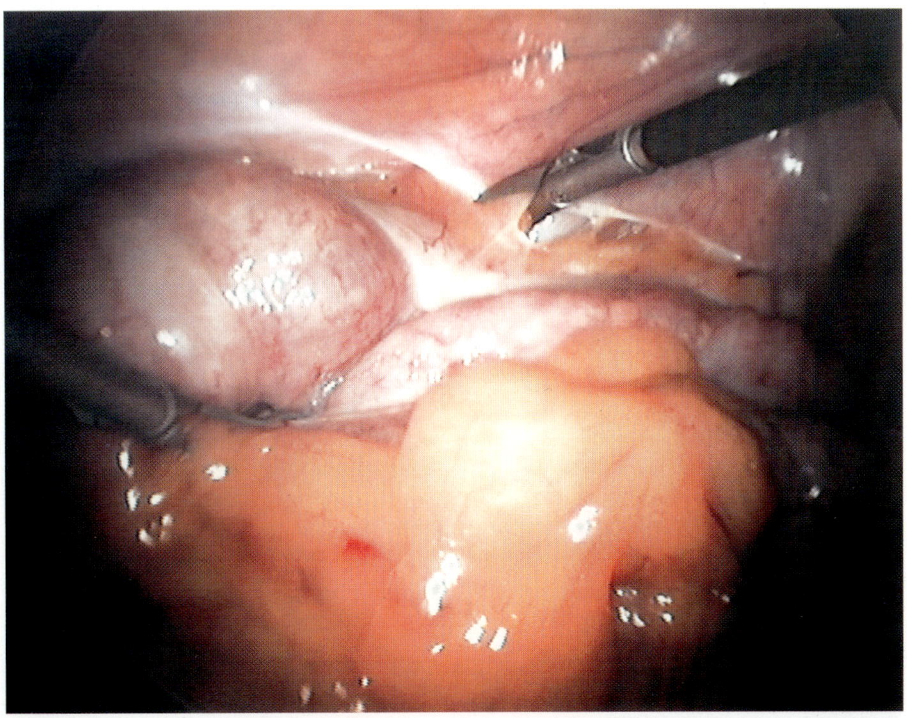

Fig. 13-2. Mobilization of descending colon may be necessary to enable left colonic delivery.

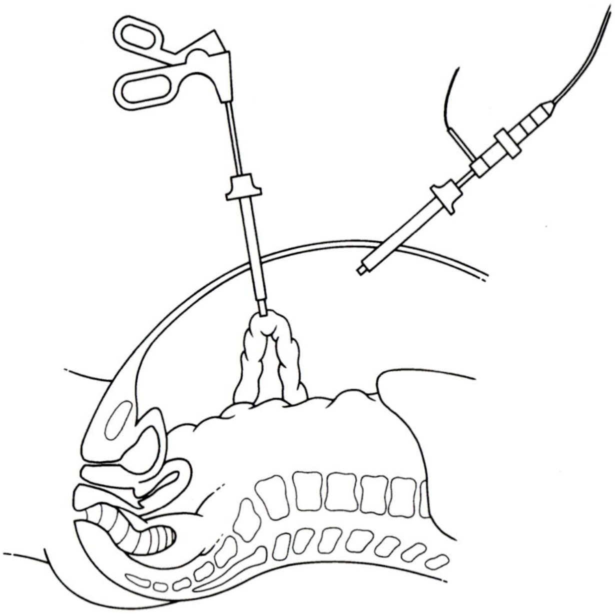

Fig. 13-3. Diagram of laparoscopic ileostomy with two ports.

obstructive or inoperable rectal carcinoma. One patient had severe constipation produced by pelvic outlet dysfunction secondary to paraplegia, and one had intractable bleeding from radiation proctitis needing repeated blood transfusions. Two ileostomies were done to treat intractable Crohn's disease by temporary fecal diversion. Two patients had a temporary ileostomy after a resection of large rectal villous adenomas through a trans-sphincteric approach. The average operative time for the enterostomal surgical procedure was 1 hour and 10 minutes (40 to 114 minutes), and the average duration of postoperative ileus was 1 day (1 to 2 days). The postoperative surgical complications included colostomy prolapse that required colostomy revision. Also, immediate postoperative obstruction developed at the ileostomy site in two patients, needing drainage of the afferent limb by insertion of a Levine tube. The stomal obstruction resolved within 2 days of the intubation. (The patient data are presented in Table 13-1.)

Conclusion

Laparoscopic techniques have a role in management of colorectal disease.[2] Colostomy or ileostomy as an isolated surgical procedure without a bowel resection lends itself well to this approach. A colostomy or an ileostomy does not need extensive laparoscopic mobilization. The laparoscopic identification of ileal or sigmoid anatomy is not difficult. Thus, the laparoscopic enterostomy may be the entry operation into the arena of laparoscopic colorectal surgery for those surgeons with minimal laparoscopic experience. Novice laparoscopic surgeons may not be experienced in blind puncture technique of pneumoperitoneum. Because the abdominal wall fascial defect is necessary for exteriorization of the intestinal segment, the fascial defect serves to establish a pneumoperitoneum, using the

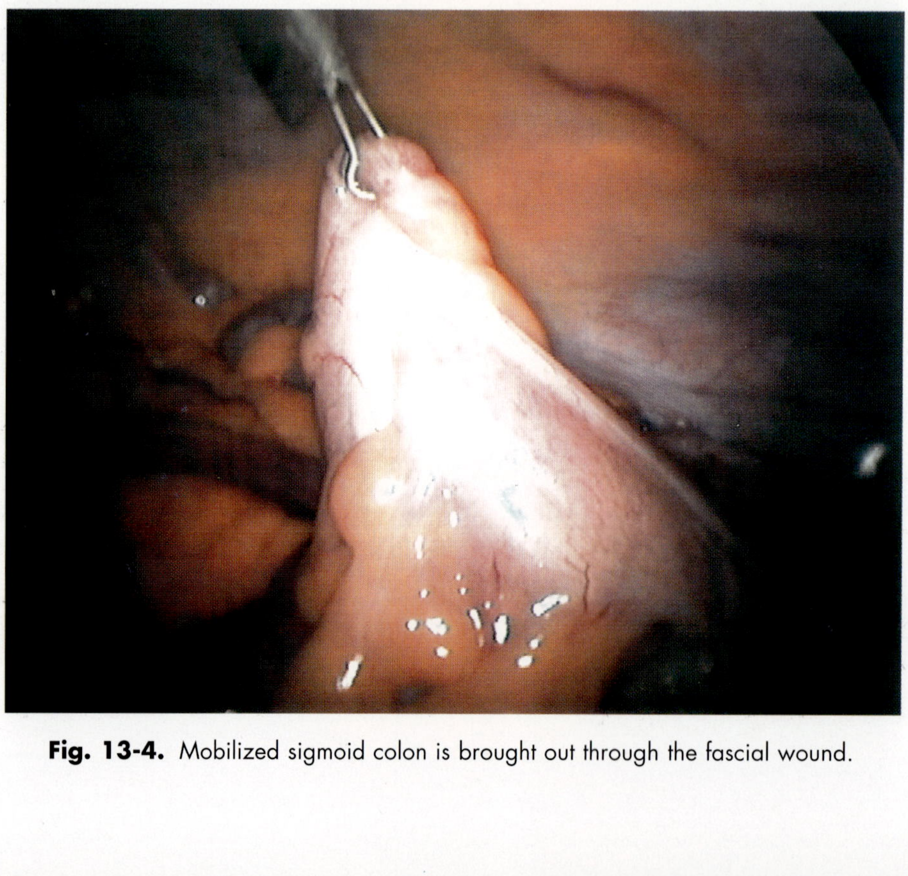

Fig. 13-4. Mobilized sigmoid colon is brought out through the fascial wound.

Table 13-1. Patient Data on Laparoscopic Enterostomy

Patient Number	Age	Sex	Indication	Stoma Type	Operative Time (min)	Duration of Postoperative Ileus (days)	Complications
1	35	F	Intractable Crohn's colitis	Ileostomy	68	1	—
2	42	M	Intractable Crohn's colitis	Ileostomy	47	2	Temporary obstruction at stoma
3	42	M	Intractable Crohn's colitis	Ileostomy	54	1	Temporary obstruction at stoma
4	61	M	Temporary fecal diversion following trans-sphincteric excision of rectal mass	Ileostomy	60	1	—
5	69	M	Obstructive rectal carcinoma	Sigmoid colostomy	40	1	Colostomy prolapse
6	46	M	Intractable constipation	Sigmoid colostomy	114	1	—
7	71	M	Radiation proctitis	Sigmoid colostomy	65	1	—
8	62	F	Obstructive rectal carcinoma	Sigmoid colostomy	64	2	—
9	66	M	Obstructive rectal carcinoma	Sigmoid colostomy	98	2	—
10	56	M	Obstructive rectal carcinoma	Sigmoid colostomy	80	1	—

open technique. This open technique of peritoneal access avoids the most common laparoscopic complications that are secondary to the use of a Veress needle and the blind trocar insertion.

NECESSITY OF LAPAROSCOPIC GUIDANCE IN CONDUCTION OF ENTEROSTOMY

Loop or end-on transverse colostomies often could be established via the initial trephine wound without laparoscopy or a separate abdominal incision.[3–8] Although a laparoscopic approach to transverse colostomy has been reported,[3] laparoscopy is often not necessary for this operation. The easily identifiable and reachable greater omentum and mobile intraperitoneal transverse colon can be exteriorized with least difficulty through the initial trephine wound.

By contrast, sigmoidostomy and ileostomy often require a separate abdominal incision other than the

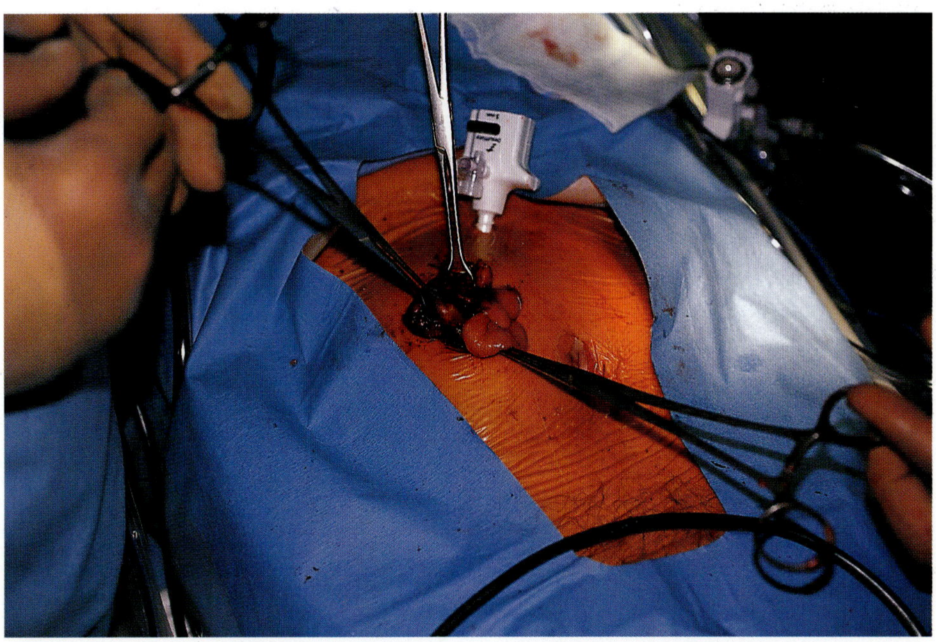

Fig. 13-5. Exteriorization of the sigmoid loop.

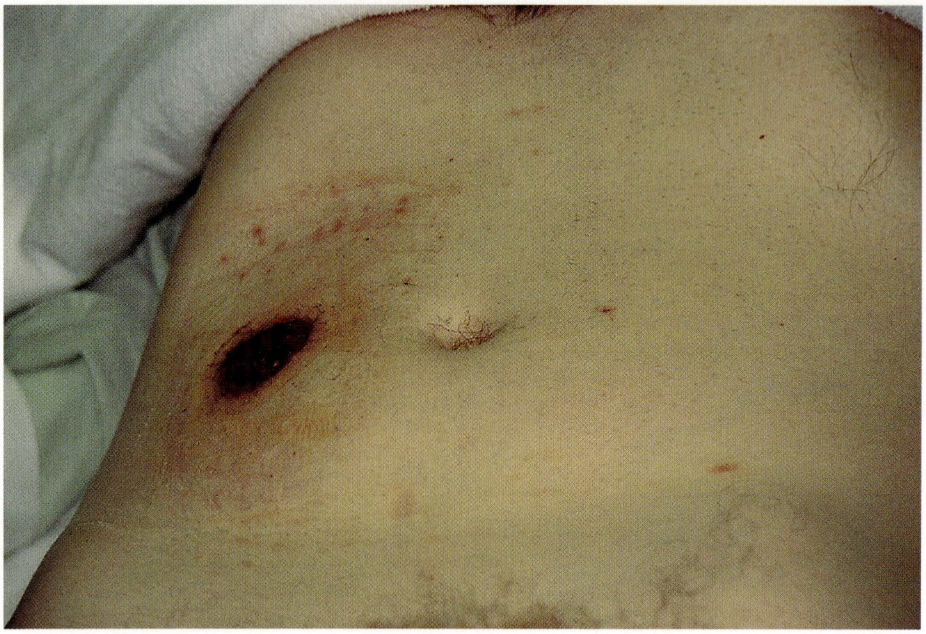

Fig. 13-6. Laparoscopic ileostomy in a patient with intractable Crohn's disease.

circular wound for the stomal exit. Many patients have either some congenital or postoperative surgical adhesions around the bowel loops (Fig. 13-7) from previous gynecologic surgery, appendectomy, and the like. Often, it is difficult to mobilize and deliver the sigmoid colonic and ileal segments in morbidly obese patients. Some patients have a short, adipose sigmoid mesocolon or scarred ileal mesentery that is difficult to mobilize and exteriorize without making a substantial abdominal incision. The laparoscopic approach to identification, mobilization, and delivery of an intestinal loop out of the peritoneal cavity through the abdominal wall is a less traumatic way of establishing enterostomies.[4–6]

Obstructive sigmoid and rectosigmoid colonic cancers are optimally resected during the initial surgical exploration, even in obstructed causes. Intraoperative gut lavage can simplify primary anastomosis, avoiding the need for a temporary fecal diversion because of an

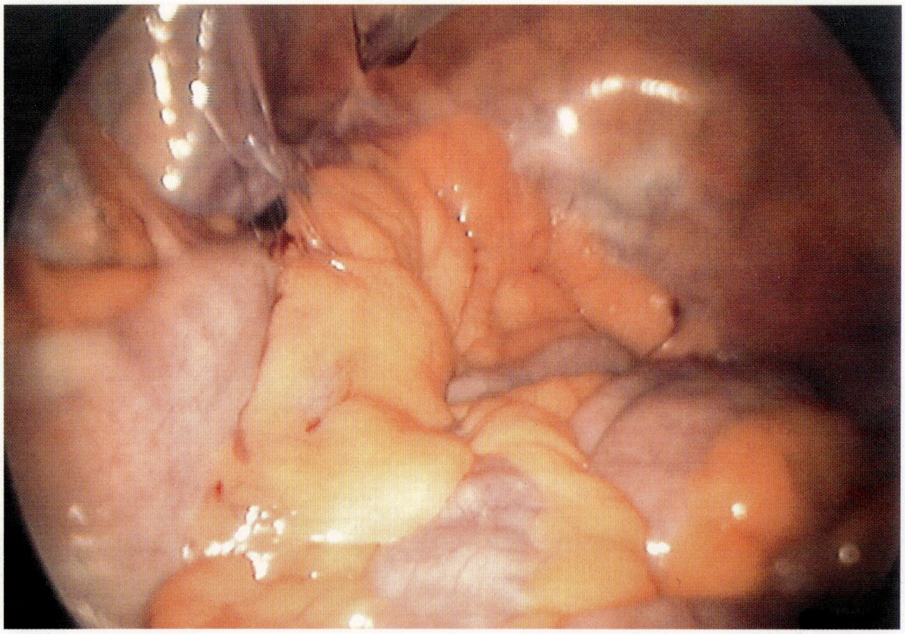

Fig. 13-7. Adherence of sigmoid colon to the left lateral parietes.

inability to conduct preoperative mechanical bowel preparation. In patients who are poor surgical risks or when the malignant invasion of adjoining organs demands preoperative radiotherapy, primary resection and anastomosis may not be feasible. In this group of patients, radiotherapy may further compromise partially occluded colonic lumen. A temporary fecal diversion may ease safe continuation of radiotherapy before a curative cancer resection is attempted.

When a primary resection of obstructive sigmoid and rectosigmoid cancers is not feasible, various options for a fecal diversion exist. A diverting sigmoid colostomy may not be desirable because of the proximity to the lesion. Transverse colostomy provides a satisfactory temporary fecal diversion but may lead to postoperative stomal care problems. Also, transverse colostomy may necessitate an extended left hemicolectomy when the patient is brought back for a curative cancer resection. A descending colostomy is appropriate, but mobilization of splenic flexure of the colon may require a long abdominal incision. Mobilization of the entire left colon, including splenic flexure, can be done well laparoscopically, enabling exteriorization of the mobilized descending colon, avoiding the need for a separate abdominal incision.

Obesity poses a relative contraindication to most laparoscopic colorectal surgical procedures. In contrast to other colorectal operations, a laparoscopic approach to enterostomy is preferred to the open approach even in obese patients. Pneumoperitoneum and satisfactory muscle relaxation will lift the anterior abdominal wall away from the intestinal loop that needs to be delivered out of the peritoneal cavity and eases mobilization even in obese patients. Laparoscopic adhesiolysis will allow laparoscopic enterostomal creation in some patients even with multiple intra-abdominal adhesions, as long as the initial peritoneal access can be established.

Loop colostomies as well as end-on colostomies (by transecting and burying the efferent limb in the subcutaneous tissue) could be accomplished well under laparoscopic guidance. If a patient requires enterostomy for more than 4 to 6 weeks, an end-on stoma may be less commonly associated with a postoperative prolapse. The intestinal loop is delivered out of the peritoneal cavity under laparoscopic guidance, and the transection is done outside the abdominal wall under direct vision.

The laparoscopic approach for an enterostomy has multiple potential advantages. The incisional morbidity from a long abdominal incision may be reduced. Consequently, patients may return to work sooner, and the postoperative pain is less. Patients with cancer start chemotherapy and radiotherapy sooner following the establishment of stoma because there is no abdominal incision.

Operative time is not unduly prolonged compared with the open technique; the use of reusable trocars and instruments will not increase the exposure of the operation. Care of the stoma after laparoscopic enterostomy may be easier than care after open enterostomies, which necessitate a separate abdominal incision in the proximity. The problem of infection of the abdominal access incision from stomal contamination is also avoided in patients with laparoscopic enterostomy.

The complication of obstruction at the stomal site should be kept in mind during laparoscopic enterostomy. A laparoscopically mobilized intestinal loop can be delivered through a fascial defect smaller than what is required during open enterostomy. The postoperative intestinal wall edema at the stomal site can lead to obstruction at the fascial defect if the defect is smaller than two fingerbreadths wide. This obstruction can be prevented by two-finger dilation of the fascial defect around the endoscopic Babcock forceps, holding the loop before bringing it out through the fascial defect. If obstruction develops in spite of satisfactory fascial incision, gentle intubation of the afferent limb and suction for a few days may be all that is needed to resolve the obstruction. Revision of the stoma is necessary only if afferent limb intubation and decompression fail.

Most surgeons place a supporting rod or a silicone drain[7] through the mesentery or mesocolon. Sutures approximating the serosa to the anterior abdominal fascia and the mucosa to the skin are adequate in preventing stomal retraction. The stomal edema produced by the operation also helps prevention of stomal retraction. In more than 100 enterostomies using the conventional open technique, I have not used a supporting rod and have never encountered stomal retraction. Stomal prolapse rather than stomal retraction is a problem with the enterostomies; use of a supporting rod, therefore, is not necessary. Other advantages from avoidance of a supporting rod or silicone drain include ease of postoperative stomal care and prevention of mesenteric or mesocolic hematoma from rod insertion.

Other local stomal complications (e.g., mucocutaneous stomal necrosis and infections) have been proposed to be secondary to use of multifilament Vicryl (Ethicon, Inc., Somerville, NJ) instead of monofilament sutures such as Maxon (Davis & Geck, Pearl River, NY).[9] I have not noticed any similar problems in the experience reported, although all the stomas were sutured with Vicryl. With increasing experience, laparoscopic approach to enterostomy can be conducted with minimal complications.

SUMMARY

The laparoscopic approach is uniquely suited for creation of an enterostomy as an isolated procedure to provide temporary or permanent fecal diversion.

Avoidance of a separate abdominal incision other than the stomal site reduces postoperative incisional morbidity and allows rapid initiation of postoperative chemotherapy or radiotherapy in patients with non-resectable obstructive colorectal cancers. The technical ease of laparoscopic enterostomy permits its use by all the abdominal surgeons now entering the field of laparoscopic colorectal surgery.

REFERENCES

1. Sadeghi-nejad H, Kavousse LR, Peters CA: Bowel injury in open technique laparoscopic cannula placement. Urology 43:559, 1994
2. Falk PM, Beart R, Wexner SD: Laparoscopic colectomy: a critical appraisal. Dis Colon Rectum 36:28, 1992
3. Duh Q, Way LW: Diagnostic laparoscopy and laparoscopic cecostomy for colonic pseudo-obstruction. Dis Colon Rectum 36:65, 1993
4. Fuhrman GM, Ota DM: Laparoscopic intestinal stomas. Dis Colon Rectum 37:444, 1994
5. Lange V, Meyer G, Schardey HM et al: Laparoscopic creation of a loop colostomy. J Laparoendosc Surg 1:307, 1991
6. Lyerly HK, Mault JR: Laparoscopic ileostomy and colostomy. Ann Surg 219:317, 1994
7. Jess P, Christiansen J: Laparoscopic loop ileostomy for fecal diversion. Dis Colon Rectum 37:721, 1994
8. Khoo RD, Montrey J, Cohen MM: Laparoscopic loop ileostomy for temporary fecal diversion. Dis Colon Rectum 36:966, 1993
9. Bagi P, Jendresen M, Kirkegaard P: Early local stoma complications in relation to the applied suture material: comparison between monofilament and multifilament sutures. Dis Colon Rectum 35:739, 1992

Editorial Comment

Steven D. Wexner

Although Dr. Jager bases his conclusions for this chapter on experience with 10 patients, the conclusions seem quite universal. Some skeptics may suggest that a trephine stoma is less expensive and possibly more rapid than is laparoscopic creation of a stoma. I would strongly argue that point. As Dr. Jager notes, even the most obese patient is often an excellent candidate for laparoscopic creation of a stoma. The only situation that has made stoma creation difficult and has caused my colleagues and I to convert 1 of our 20 stoma creations to open technique was extensive adhesions. In the other 19 cases, we were successful; the mean time for stoma creation fell from 90 minutes to approximately 30 minutes. This time includes the initial Veress needle placement to placement of the appliance over the completed stoma. Thus, the procedure can be performed quickly and safely. Furthermore, the procedure can often be performed very rapidly. For example, a thin patient with advanced perianal Crohn's disease who does not desire a total proctocolectomy but wishes to try out a temporary loop ileostomy can generally have that stoma created within a matter of 10 to 15 minutes. The major advantage of a laparoscopic loop or end stoma creation as compared to a trephine loop or end stoma is direct visualization. There is never any confusion about the delivery of the appropriate end of bowel in the appropriate nonrotated position.

Although Dr. Jager and I agree in principle as to the creation of stomas, my technique varies to a degree. I do not re-review all of the technique but direct the reader to three publications describing the techniques of port placement and the technique of stoma creation.[2–4] In short, I have found that preoperative stomal marking should be done in the same fashion as it would be for open stoma creation. The second port, used for the camera, is placed in the midline, midway between the umbilicus and the xiphoid. I have found that the standard umbilical position is too close to the iliac fossa port and interferes with adequate visualization of proximal and distal limbs when creating a loop ileostomy or an end sigmoidostomy. For the sake of cosmesis and satisfactory ergonometrics, the optional second port is also marked by the stoma therapist in a relatively contralateral position. However, that optional second port is placed *lateral* to the rectus muscle and preferably *within* a skin fold or previous scar. If such folds or scars are not available, then the stoma therapist will search out Langer's lines and use these as a guide. There is no role for creation of a loop sigmoidostomy, a loop transverse colostomy, or any form of ascending colostomy or cecostomy in any situation either laparoscopically or open. All four of these stomas are too difficult for the patient to manage, have high incidences of prolapse, and in the latter two situations have a high-volume malodorous output. Thus, the three stomal alternatives are end sigmoid or descending colostomy or end or loop ileostomy. Formation of any of these stomas is exactly the same in that all three of the aforementioned ports are 10/12-mm ports. The stoma site port is exchanged in the Seldinger manner for an 18-mm port at the time of stoma formation. In all cases, adequate mobilization should be accomplished such that extracorporeal bowel division can be undertaken for conversion of a loop to an end stoma if desired. The efferent end can either be left in the subcutaneous space, returned to the abdominal cavity, or, in the manner described by Pearl and Abcarian, converted to a minimal mucous fistula at the same site as the stoma.[4]

The creation of a stoma is an excellent method by which to enhance one's laparoscopic skills. As such, I strongly recommend that early during one's experience one should perform laparoscopic fecal diversion in any patient who requires fecal diversion.

REFERENCES

1. Teoh TA, Reissman P, Verzaro P et al: Enhancing cosmesis in laparoscopic colorectal surgery. Dis Colon Rectum 38:213, 1995
2. Teoh TA, Reissman P, Cohen SM et al: Laparoscopic loop ileostomy, letter. Dis Colon Rectum 37:514, 1994
3. Wexner SD, Taranow D, Johansen OB et al: Loop ileostomy for fecal diversion. Dis Colon Rectum 36:349, 1993
4. Pearl RK, Abcarian H: Diverting stomas. p. 107. In Mackeigan JM, Cataldo PA (eds): Intestinal Stomas. Quality Medical Publishing, St. Louis, 1993

14

Laparoscopic Appendectomy

Cheng-Kiong Kum and Peter M. Y. Goh

Acute appendicitis is the most common surgical emergency in the world. In 1889, McBurney[1] published his first series of acute appendicitis. Since then, appendectomy through a right lower quadrant incision has evolved to be the standard treatment for acute appendicitis for more than 100 years. In 1983, Semm[2] reported the first case of laparoscopic appendectomy in which a noninflamed appendix was removed. It was not until 1987 that the first case of an inflamed appendix removed by laparoscopic means was reported.[3]

WHY DO IT LAPAROSCOPICALLY

Why should one bother to remove the appendix laparoscopically when most surgeons claim that they can remove the appendix through a cosmetic incision within a short time, with minimal complications, and a short hospital stay? Despite being the most common surgical emergency, the management of acute appendicitis has not been satisfactory. Three significant problems remain: misdiagnosis, early morbidity from wound infection, and late morbidity from postoperative adhesions.

Worldwide, the misdiagnosis and associated normal appendectomy rate in most surgical units is 15 to 30 percent.[4] Studies on women in the reproductive age group reported rates as high as 45 percent.[5,6] Surely, in the present state of the art of medicine, with the diverse diagnostic tools available, one cannot accept such a high misdiagnosis rate in any surgical pathology. In addition, normal appendectomies are not harmless, as often claimed, but have been associated with significant morbidity and mortality.[5]

Infection of the wound is the main cause of postoperative morbidity and prolonged hospitalization after appendectomy.[7] The wound infection rate for nonperforated acute appendicitis despite wide-spectrum antibiotic coverage (metronidazole plus another antibiotic) ranges from 4 to 7 percent, a significant percentage for a common condition. Certainly, the rate rises to 10 to 25 percent for perforated appendices, when antibiotic prophylaxis was inadequate, or when the surgery was performed in district hospitals. Wound infection predisposes to wound dehiscence and incisional hernia. Postappendectomy adhesions, especially between the bowel and the abdominal wall at the site of the incision, are estimated to occur in 80 to 90 percent of patients, with 2 to 5 percent developing significant problems of intestinal obstruction.[8,9] The significance of laparoscopic appendectomy is that it provides solutions to all three problems. The laparoscope is an effective and practical diagnostic tool; the technique of laparoscopic appendectomy can reduce wound infection to almost zero; and evidence shows that adhesions are minimal after laparoscopic appendectomy.

PATIENT SELECTION

Six categories of patients confront the laparoscopist:

1. Patients with equivocal signs and symptoms, such that the diagnosis of acute appendicitis cannot be confirmed
2. Patients with acute appendicitis
3. Patients with perforated appendicitis and localized peritonitis
4. Patients with perforated appendicitis and generalized peritonitis
5. Patients with appendiceal masses
6. Patients with additional problems such as pregnancy, coagulopathy, and adhesions from previous laparotomy

The first group is important because it forms the main source of misdiagnosis. In these cases, the diagnostic part of laparoscopy is the more important procedure. The decision for diagnostic laparoscopy is clinical. It is indicated in patients with persistent right iliac fossa pain and tenderness. The abdominal pain starts in the epigastrium or periumbilical region and then localizes in the right iliac fossa. Anorexia, pyrexia, and leukocytosis are not predictive, but they often influence the decision of the surgeon to operate. Simple tests such as microscopic examination of urine and human chorionic gonadotropin assay should be routine, especially in women. As a general rule, patients should not undergo laparoscopy unless their symptoms and signs would have warranted surgery in the days when laparoscopy was not available. Laparoscopy, although a simple procedure, requires general anesthesia and carries a definite risk of bowel and vessel injury. If a radiologist skilled in ultrasonography of the appendix is available, ultrasonography is a good alternative to aid in diagnosing acute appendicitis.[10] Unfortunately, in most centers, the expertise is not available, and laparoscopy remains the only practical method of avoiding misdiagnosis.[11] Patients with acute appendicitis form the largest group requiring the procedure. It must be emphasized to the patient that conversion to a laparotomy (less than 5 percent) may be necessary, and consent for laparotomy must always be taken.

Perforated appendices with localized peritonitis can be safely dealt with laparoscopically. All necrotic tissues must be removed, and the pelvis, right paracolic gutter, and subhepatic and subphrenic regions must be thoroughly washed with at least 2 L of saline. It is definitely worthwhile for the surgeon to spend 15 minutes just washing the above areas, adjusting the position of the patient as necessary to achieve good access. Postoperatively, the patient must be given 5 days of antibiotics. Drains are usually not necessary. Meticulous technique and adequate antibiotic therapy are essential to prevent intra-abdominal abscesses.

The laparoscopic approach to appendectomy is contraindicated for perforated appendices with generalized peritonitis. The distended bowels from the ileus make laparoscopy difficult and dangerous. Patients with appendiceal masses should be treated conservatively with intravenous antibiotics and their progress monitored. Laparoscopic appendectomy can be electively performed in patients who respond to the conservative management. Computed tomography and colonoscopy may be required to differentiate appendicitis from cecal tumors in suspected cases. Open surgery is necessary for those individuals who do not respond to the conservative regimen. Laparoscopy in these cases is very difficult, because bleeding and obscure anatomy make the operation unsafe.

General contraindications of laparoscopy apply, such as coagulopathy and significant cardiorespiratory impairment. Obesity does not preclude the procedure; in fact, obese patients are the ones who probably benefit the most because long incisions, required just to access the peritoneal cavity, are avoided. Previous lower abdominal operation requires open introduction of the first port, followed by feasibility assessment for laparoscopic resection. In pregnant women, laparoscopic appendectomy can be performed at up to 20 weeks of gestation.[12,13] Thereafter, the lack of intraperitoneal space makes the procedure difficult. Laparoscopy is especially advantageous in locating the exact position of the appendix in the pregnant woman. The effect of carbon dioxide pneumoperitoneum on the fetus has not been thoroughly studied; thus, the fetal heart beat should be monitored continuously during the operation.

PREOPERATIVE PREPARATION

The patient is assessed for risk of general anesthesia. The proposed sites of port placement are explained to the patient, and the possibility of conversion to a laparotomy should also be emphasized. The abdomen is depilated from just above the umbilicus to about 4 cm below the pubic hairline and laterally to the anterior superior iliac spines. For acute appendicitis, urinary catheterization is not required if the patient's bladder was evacuated within the last hour before surgery. If not, an in and out catheterization is performed to prevent disturbance of visual exploration of the pelvis by the bladder. If a perforated appendix is expected, it is better to have an indwelling catheter, because the operation may be prolonged. The balloon in the urinary catheter need not be filled with more than 5 ml of saline; a large balloon can be a hindrance. Prophylactic antibiotics (intravenous gentamicin and metronidazole) are given at induction.

Patient Position

The patient is in a supine position with a 15 percent Trendelenburg's tilt. This is a safe position to introduce the Veress needle and obtain an adequate initial inspection of the lower abdomen. Further Trendelenburg's and left tilt may be required for retrocecal appendices. The skin is disinfected from the xiphisternum to the midthigh (with special attention to the umbilicus) and draped to expose the umbilicus, pubic bone, and the anterior superior iliac spines.

Instrumentation

The following instruments are required:

1. One monitor on the right side of the patient, in the center: one monitor is sufficient; if a second is available, it is placed at the foot for the convenience of the scrub nurse
2. Video camera in the same position as the monitor: a one-chip camera is adequate for this procedure
3. Light source: also in the same position
4. Carbon dioxide insufflator near the head on the right side: pressure limit set to 14 mm Hg
5. Monopolar or bipolar diathermy machine near the patient's head on the right side
6. Suction and irrigation devices at the foot: 1 L of saline prepared with another liter available
7. 0-degree 10-mm diameter laparoscope introduced through the umbilical port
8. One 10/11-mm trocar for the laparoscope in the umbilicus position; one 10/11-mm trocar in the left suprapubic region as the main working port and one 5-mm trocar in the right suprapubic region as the assisting port; one 10- to 5-mm converter for the main port
9. One 9-mm dissecting forceps with diathermy capability, to be used through the main port
10. 5-mm bowel grasping forceps for the edematous appendix (or a 5-mm toothed grasping forceps) to be used through the assisting port
11. 5-mm endoscopic scissors with diathermy capability to be used through the main port
12. 10-mm endoscopic clip applicator and 10 clips (rarely is there need to use more than 10 clips)
13. One catgut Roeder loop with applicator (and one more immediately available)
14. 10-mm grasper for removal of the appendix
15. Endoscopic pouch device if the appendix is too big for the main port

(Continues)

16. 5-mm suction-irrigation device
17. Veress needle
18. Tubes and cables for carbon dioxide, light, diathermy, suction and irrigation
19. 2-0 absorbable suture for approximating the fascia of the 10-mm trocar sites at the end of the procedure
20. Skin suture
21. 20 ml of 1 percent bupivacaine for local infiltration around the port sites at the end of the procedure (optional)

If possible, a 30- or 35-mm endoscopic stapler, together with the appropriate trocar for its usage, should be available in the operating room, in case the base of the appendix is necrotic and not safe for the use of a Roeder loop. Alternatively, laparoscopic suturing equipment should be available. A laparotomy set should be available in all cases.

OPERATIVE TECHNIQUE

One cameraman and one scrub nurse are needed. If a cameraman is not available, the nurse can perform these duties. The staff is ergonomically positioned as shown in Figure 14-1. A 10-mm incision is made in the lower part of the umbilicus through the skin and subcutaneous tissues. The Veress needle is tested to ensure that the spring mechanism is intact and it is flushed through with saline to establish patency. It is inserted with a slight tilt toward the pelvis to avoid the danger of damaging the aorta, which bifurcates about 4 cm caudad to the umbilicus. A distinct give is felt as the needle penetrates the fascia, often followed by another give as it penetrates the peritoneum into the peritoneal cavity.

The needle should be felt to be moving freely in all directions. Aspiration and hanging drop tests are performed with a syringe filled with 5 ml of saline. When connected to the carbon dioxide insufflator at low flow (not more than 2 L/min initially), the pressure reading should not be more than 7 mm Hg; usually, it should be less than 5 mm Hg. If the pressure reading is high, the needle may be retracted slightly and jiggled to displace the omentum in which the needle tip may be embedded. If that fails to bring the pressure down immediately, the needle must be removed and another puncture attempted. Failure to achieve safe pneumoperitoneum via the closed method after 3 to 4 attempts warrants open introduction.

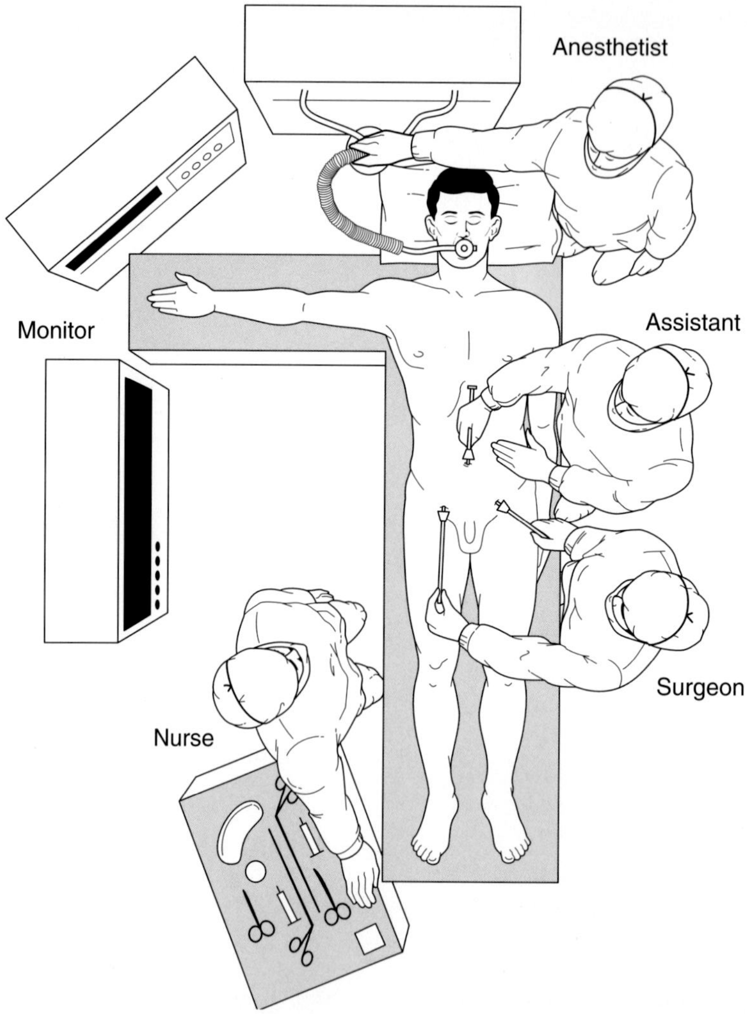

Fig. 14-1. Position of staff and equipment for laparoscopic appendectomy.

When the intra-abdominal pressure reaches 14 mm Hg, the abdomen is palpated to confirm that the abdominal wall is under good tension, and thus it is safe to insert the 10/11-mm trocar. The trocar is inserted in the same direction as the Veress needle, avoiding the aorta and vena cava. The laparoscope, with its tip warmed in hot water, is then inserted in the same direction as the previous two punctures to exclude iatrogenic intra-abdominal injury, followed by a general visual inspection of the whole peritoneal cavity to exclude any obvious second pathology. Often, tell-tale signs of inflammation around the cecum can be seen at this stage.

Another 10/11-mm incision is made in the left suprapubic region at or just above the pubic hairline (Fig. 14-2). The skin should be illuminated by the laparoscope to identify and, thus, avoid the inferior epigastric vessels. The trocar is aimed toward the cecum; the insertion must be completely under vision, avoiding damage to the bladder, bowel, and common iliac vessels. The peritoneum is loose at this region and may be lifted away from the muscle layer, making penetration difficult. However, this problem can always be overcome by gentle manipulation. A converter is placed on the trocar, and a nontraumatic forceps is introduced to locate the appendix and confirm the diagnosis (Fig. 14-3). With the advanced imaging equipment and instruments presently available, the appendix is easily located. If the appendix appears normal, a thorough examination of the abdomen must be made. Special attention is paid to the pelvic organs in women, colon (especially the cecum, ascending and sigmoid), small bowel (at least the distal 100 cm), gallbladder, liver, and duodenum.

Once the diagnosis of acute appendicitis is confirmed, another 5-mm trocar is inserted in the right suprapubic region to be the assisting port. It is again placed just above the hairline, avoiding the inferior epigastric vessels, under direct vision, and in the direction of the appendix. A 5-mm bowel-grasping forceps is introduced to grasp the appendix. Forceps of this type

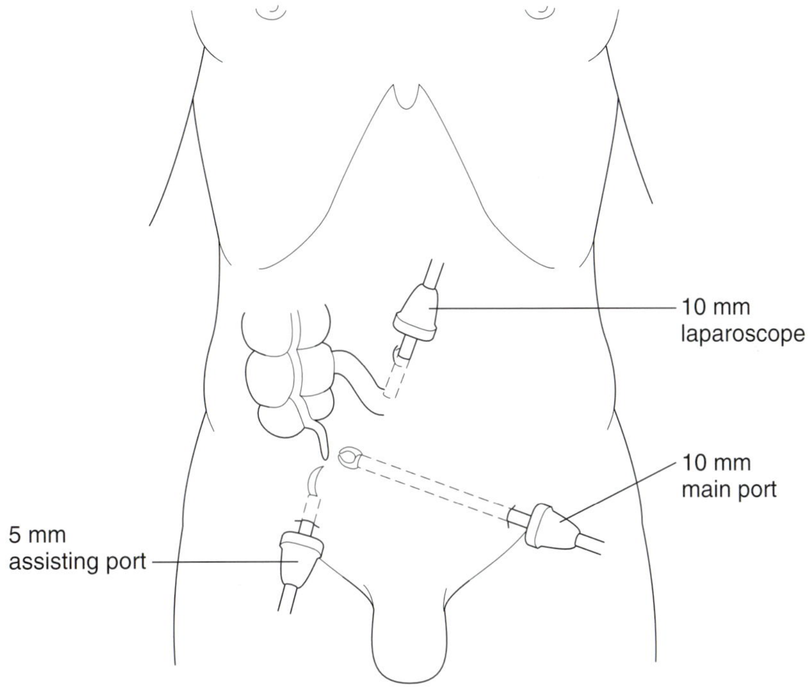

Fig. 14-2. Position of ports for the two-handed technique of laparoscopic appendectomy.

are most appropriate because they are relatively atraumatic and allow a good grip. A secure grip on the appendix is essential to stretch the mesoappendix. Once this maneuver is achieved, ligating the appendicular artery will be easy. Often, the appendix may be adherent to the peritoneal wall or behind the cecum. In these cases, a 5-mm dissecting forceps is used to gently free the appendix by blunt dissection, aided by the

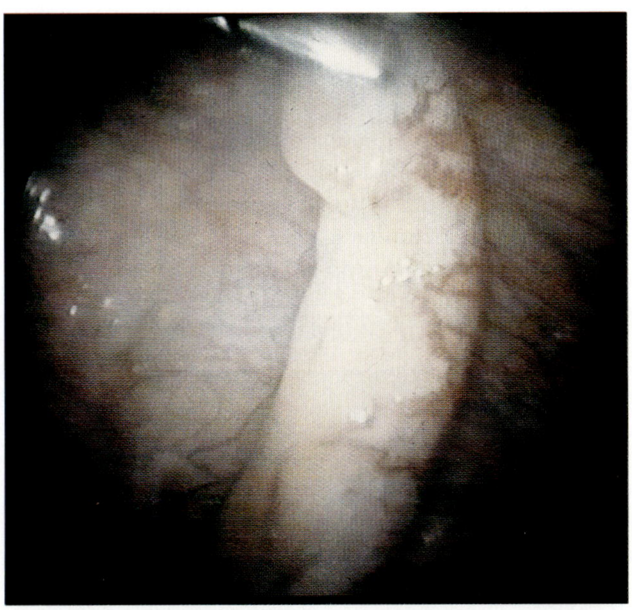

Fig. 14-3. Laparoscopic view of an inflamed appendix.

forceps in the assisting port. Throughout the operation, the surgeon uses both hands: the right hand for instruments in the main port and the left hand for assisting. The tip and base of the appendix are the two key points that must be identified to avoid leaving behind necrotic appendicular tissue that may predispose the patient to intra-abdominal abscess formation. The bowel forceps grip either the tip or middle of the appendix, whichever gives the better stretch on the mesoappendix. If the bowel forceps is not available, a pair of toothed forceps is necessary to hold the edematous appendix. Ordinary forceps cannot hold the inflamed appendix effectively.

The thickness of the mesoappendix is assessed. Often, endoscopic clips can be applied directly. If the mesoappendix is too thick, diathermy is performed on the peritoneum over it with the dissecting forceps, and the peritoneum is stripped to identify the appendicular artery, which is then clipped. The appendicular artery does not need to be dissected completely. Two clips, 3 to 4 mm apart, are placed on the mesoappendix near the appendix (Fig. 14-4). A pair of scissors, applied through the main port, is used to transect the clipped portion of the mesoappendix distal to both clips (Fig. 14-5). Minor bleeding may be encountered from the distal end of the cut mesoappendix; the bleeding will stop, because the appendicular artery is an end artery. The purpose is to leave little mesoappendix with no clips so that extraction of the appendix through the 10/11-mm port will be successful. The process of clipping and cutting is repeated

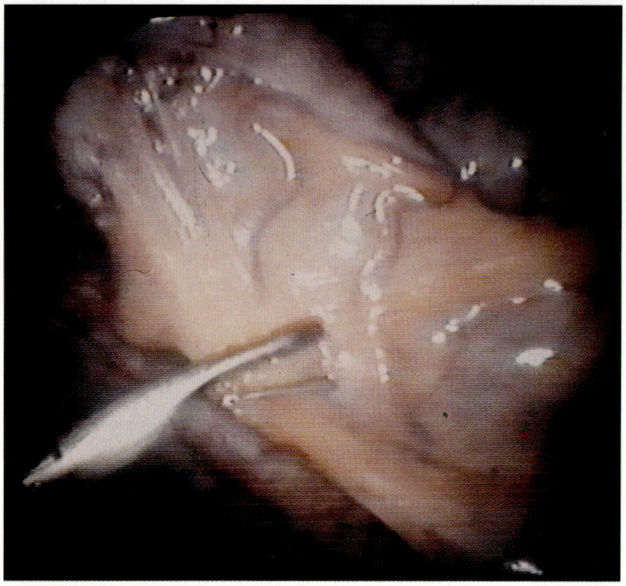

Fig. 14-4. Placement of two clips to secure the appendicular artery.

until the clean healthy base of the appendix is exposed (Fig. 14-6). A Roeder loop of catgut is then applied through the main port and tied securely around the base (Fig. 14-7). A healthy, nonedematous base requires only one tie. However, if the base is edematous, two ties should be employed 3 to 4 mm apart. If the base is also necrotic from the inflammatory process, endoscopic staplers may be needed to transect across part of the cecum. (This procedure is discussed later in the chapter.)

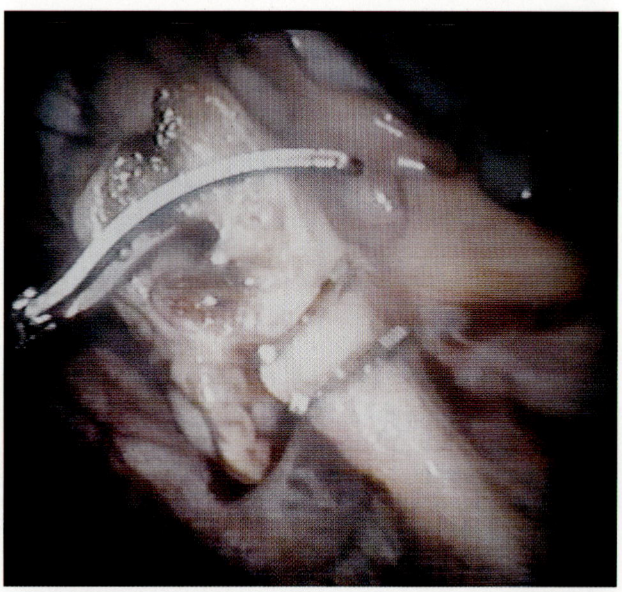

Fig. 14-5. Mesoappendix cut distal to applied clips.

A clip is applied about 10 mm from the tie to minimize spillage of appendiceal contents when cut. The appendix is then transected about 6 to 7 mm from the last tie to prevent slippage of the tie (Fig. 14-8). The stump is briefly coagulated to seal and sterilize it. Invagination is not necessary.[16] A 10-mm grasper is used to grasp the cut end of the appendix, which is then extracted through the main port. If dissection was kept close to the appendix, 80 to 90 percent of inflamed appendices can be extracted through the port (Figs. 14-9 and 14-10). During extraction, the valve on the port must be depressed to keep it open so that the appendix does not become lodged in the port. In this way, the appendix does not contaminate the wound. If the appendix is too thick to be extracted through the port, by no means should the surgeon be tempted to remove the port with the appendix half dangling from one end. This will compromise the principle of noncontamination of the wound. Two methods can be employed. The appendix can be removed piecemeal by forceful pulling of chunks of the organ through the port. This is a quick and effective, but messy method. Alternatively, an endoscopic pouch (or the thumb of a size-8 glove or a sterile condom) can be inserted through the main port and the appendix maneuvered into it. The pouch is closed and extracted together with the port at the end of the procedure. Rarely is there a need to change to a larger size port.

The operative site, pelvis, and right paracolic gutter are washed with saline. The wash often accumulates in the right subphrenic space, which should also be aspirated. Hemostasis of the mesoappendix and the stump is checked. The operating table is replaced to the normal position, excess saline is aspirated, and the ports are removed under vision. As much gas as possible should be evacuated from the abdomen before the last port is removed. Herniation of bowel or omentum through the port sites should also be prevented. The fascia at the 10-mm port sites are closed with 2-0 absorbable sutures, followed by skin sutures. A long-acting local anesthetic agent (e.g., 1 percent bupivacaine) is infiltrated around the port sites. The urinary catheter, if any, is also removed at the end of the operation.

A summary of the steps in laparoscopic appendectomy is shown below.

Technique of Laparoscopic Appendectomy

1. Confirm the diagnosis
2. Conduct a general laparoscopic examination

(Continues)

3. Identify the tip and base of the appendix
4. Ligate the mesoappendix close to the appendix and dissect until a clean healthy base is exposed
5. Secure the base with one or two Roeder loops of catgut; place a clip distally to minimize spillage
6. Transect the appendix 6 to 7 mm from the tie; briefly coagulate the stump
7. Extract the appendix without wound contamination
8. Irrigate the operative site, pelvis, and right paracolic gutter with saline

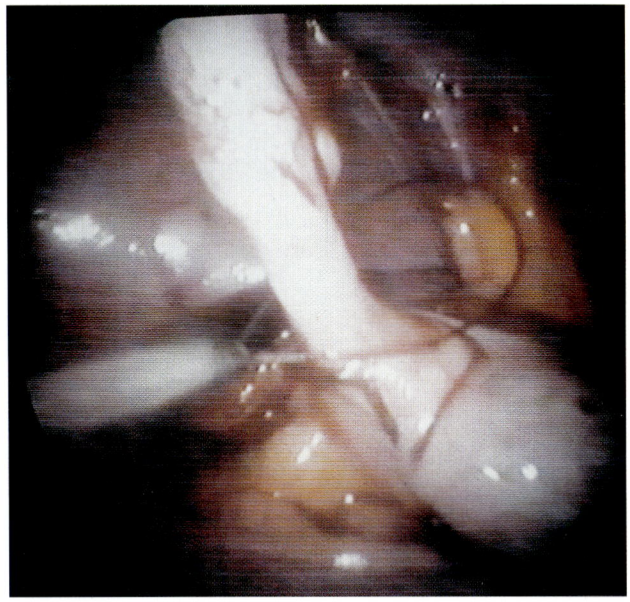

Fig. 14-7. Loop of catgut placed around the base of the appendix.

POSTOPERATIVE CARE

Two more doses of antibiotics are given to patients with acute appendicitis; these are continued for 72 hours after gangrenous appendicitis and for 5 days after perforated appendicitis. The patient is prescribed intramuscular meperidine at 1 mg/kg every 4 hours together with intramuscular metoclopromide at 10 mg every 4 hours. Fluids are given after 6 to 12 hours. If oral fluids are tolerated, oral naproxen sodium 550 mg bid is prescribed for pain relief. A diet is often served after 24 to 48 hours. Patients are discharged when the diet is tolerated well and fever has subsided. Patients are reviewed in the outpatient clinic at 1 to 2 weeks, at which time the wound is assessed for infection and activity status is monitored.

DIFFICULT CASES

Difficulty may be encountered in the form of a retrocecal appendix, an appendix with a necrotic base, or a per-

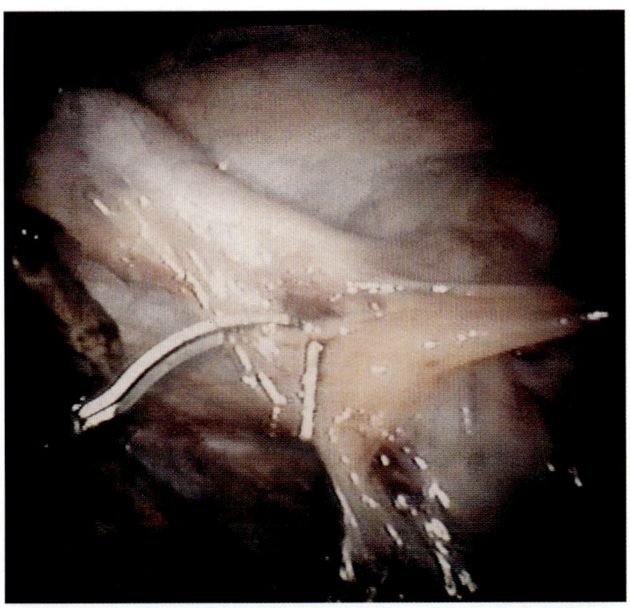

Fig. 14-6. Dissection until a clean healthy base is defined.

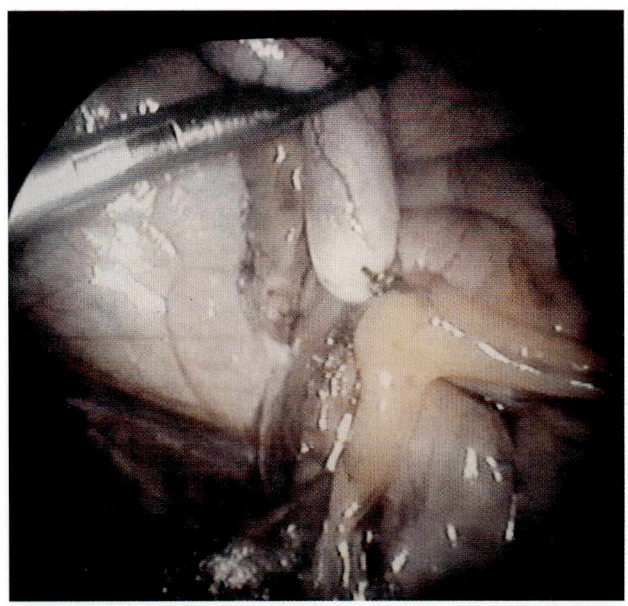

Fig. 14-8. Clip placed about 15 mm from the Roeder loop to prevent spillage of appendiceal contents.

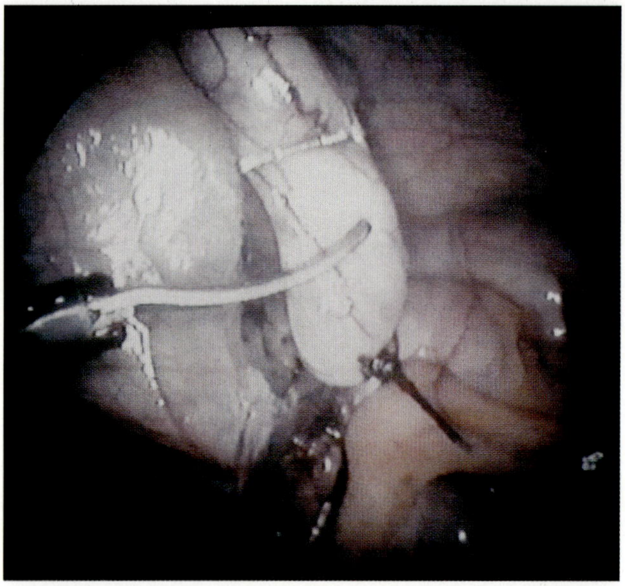

Fig. 14-9. Appendix transected 6 to 7 mm from the tie.

forated appendix. These appendices can be handled without the need to change the port positions. The inexperienced surgeon must not hesitate to convert to laparotomy if difficulties become insurmountable.

Retrocecal Appendix

Up to one-half of the appendices may be retrocecal in position. However, most are held in position only by thin peritoneal adhesions and can be easily manipulated free by a combination of blunt and sharp dissection. Better exposure is attained by putting the patient in the deep Trendelenburg position and tilted to the left. Rarely, another 5-mm port may be necessary in the right hypochondrium to raise the cecum. In the case of the immobile cecum, simple dissection of the peritoneal reflection of the cecum in the paracolic gutter will effectively free the cecum and improve the exposure tremendously. As mentioned above, the key is to identify the base and tip of the appendix. In these cases, the difficulty lies in visualizing the tip. By dissecting close to the appendix and by palpating with the forceps, the tip position can be ascertained. Once the tip is seen, it is held with a strong grasper, and the dissection proceeds as normal, with the branches of the appendicular artery secured with clips.

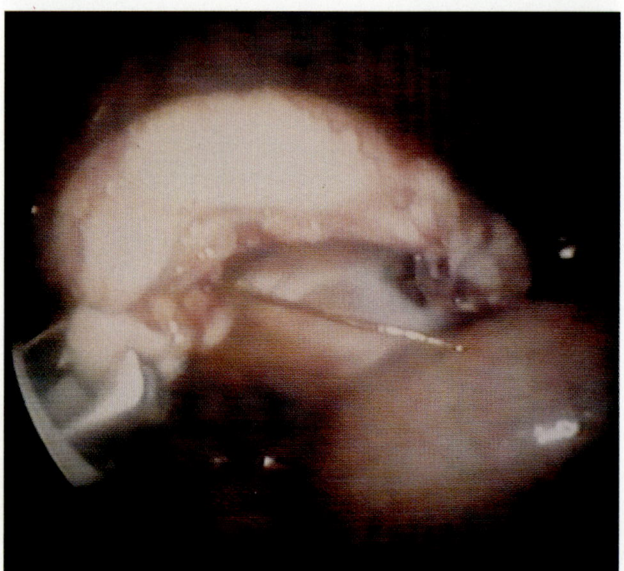

Fig. 14-10. Extraction of the appendix through the 10/11-mm left suprapubic port.

Cecal mobilization makes retrograde appendectomy a technique seldom used. Retrograde appendectomy entails clearing the mesoappendix, by coagulation and blunt dissection, from 1 to 2 cm of the base. Two clips are applied 1 cm apart at the base; the appendix is transected in between. The distal end is held by a grasper, and dissection proceeds distally till the tip is free. After the appendix is extracted, the stump is reinforced with a Roeder loop. Careful inspection must be done, after washing, to avoid leaving remnants of the appendix behind. The extracted specimen should also be examined to ensure that it is complete.

Unhealthy Base

Rarely, the base may be involved significantly in the inflammatory process and appear necrotic; Roeder loops alone are not safe, because the base may slough. This problem can be managed in two ways. The base, after application of the loop, may be laparoscopically invaginated with a Z-stitch using 3-0 catgut. The surgeon must be proficient in laparoscopic suturing. Alternatively, a 30- or 35-mm endoscopic stapler can be inserted through a 12-mm port and applied across the healthy part of the cecum (Figs. 14-11 and 14-12). Care must be taken not to compromise the ileocecal valve.

Perforated Appendix

The clinical impression of perforation is often confirmed on introduction of the laparoscope, when free pus may be seen in the pelvis or paracolic gutter. The main port is inserted, and the pus is aspirated, followed by appendectomy in the usual manner. Adherent omentum can be easily teased away. The appendix is often friable and may break on traction. Pieces of the appendix are extracted, making sure all necrotic tissues are removed. A fecolith, frequently present, must be looked for and removed if it has dropped into the peritoneal cavity. Two Roeder loops should be applied in perforated cases, because the base is

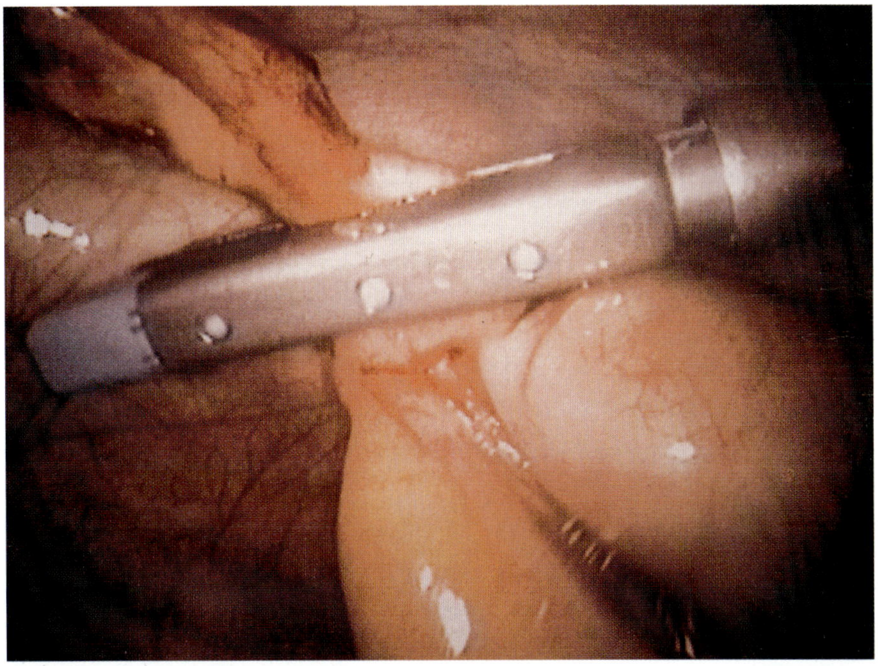

Fig. 14-11. Application of a 30-mm EndoGIA stapler across the base of the appendix.

usually edematous. Thorough washing of the pelvis, paracolic gutter, subhepatic space, subphrenic space, and the small bowel is an important part of the procedure. At least 2 L of saline is required for effective cleansing. Drains are usually not necessary. Antibiotics must be continued for 5 days.

RESULTS

Several case series of laparoscopic appendectomy have been reported since 1987.[3,15–17] All of them report laparoscopic appendectomy to be safe. It provides patients with improved cosmesis, a decrease in morbidity, reduced wound pain, shorter hospitalization, and a quicker return to normal activities. Recently, two prospective but nonrandomized trials were published, both of which found significantly less wound infection and shorter hospital stays in the laparoscopic group.[18,19] Biases were inherent in these trials, however, and a randomized controlled trial was needed to ascertain whether laparoscopic appendectomy is truly superior to open appendectomy.

RANDOMIZED CONTROLLED TRIAL

We conducted a randomized controlled trial to compare the operative results and postoperative recovery of laparoscopic and open appendectomy. Between February and August 1992, all patients above the age of 12 years and diagnosed to have acute appendicitis were randomized to either open or laparoscopic appendectomy. Seventy-two patients were randomized to the open group and 65 to the laparoscopy group. The two groups were comparable for age, gender, and weight (Table 14-1). Almost all patients were of the American Society of Anesthesiologists (ASA) I category. All patients had intravenous gentamicin and metronidazole before the surgery. The open technique was performed through a

Table 14-1. Patient Characteristics and Histology of Appendices

	Open Group	Laparoscopic Group	*t*-Test *(P)*
Total no.	72	65	
Age (mean ± SD)	30.7 (± 7.3)	33.1 (1± 4.9)	NS
Sex (M/F)	0.4:1.0	0.5:1.0	
Weight (kg) (mean ± SD)	57.1 (± 6.2)	57.4 (± 4.3)	NS
Histology			
Normal	11 (15%)	9 (14%)	NS[a]
Perforated	4 (6%)	3 (5%)	
Acute	57 (79%)	53 (81%)	

Abbreviations: NS, not significant; SD, standard deviation.
[a]Fisher's exact test.

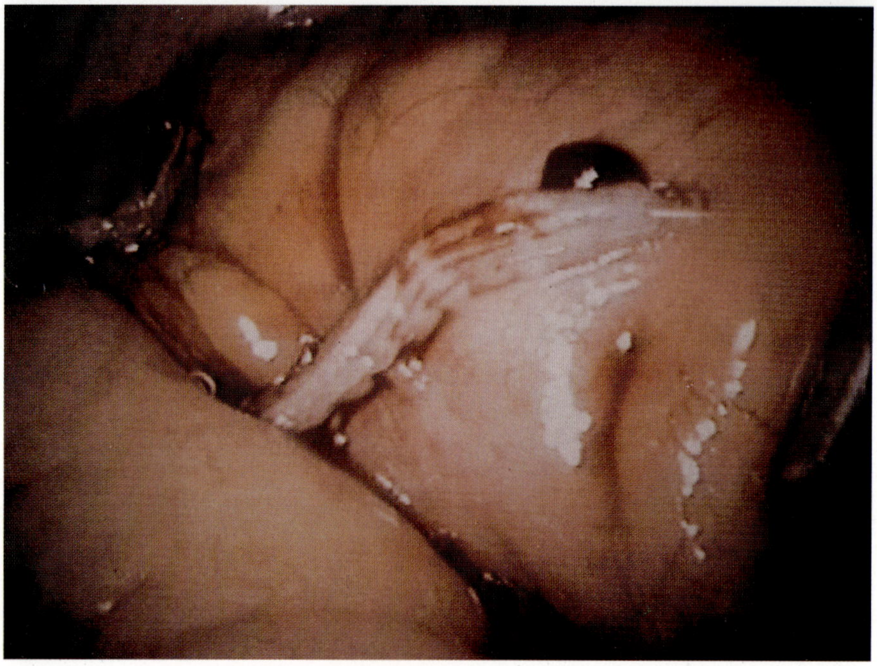

Fig. 14-12. A secure stapled base of the appendix.

standard right lower quadrant incision, with precautions to avoid unnecessary wound contamination, by registrars or residents with at least 6 months' experience. Seventy-five percent (50 of 65) of the laparoscopic appendectomies were done by one laparoscopically trained registrar and the rest by two laparoscopically trained consultants. Only surgeons who have performed more than 15 of either operation in the respective groups were allowed to participate in the study.

The technique described above was used. Monopolar diathermy was used sparingly in all cases for dissection and hemostasis. Successful removal of the intact appendix through the cannula was achieved in 57 patients (87 percent). In 9 patients (13 percent), the appendix was too big for the cannula and was placed in the thumb of a size-8 glove and extracted without contamination. No conversions to an open procedure were made.

Histopathology Findings

The definition of acute appendicitis was based on the histologic findings of a significant number of polymorphonuclear neutrophils in the mucosa or the presence of these cells in the muscle layer of the appendix. In each group, about 15 percent were normal appendices and 6 percent were perforated appendices (Table 14-1).

Operation Time

The duration of surgery was defined as the time from skin incision to the time the wound was completely dressed. The mean duration in the laparoscopic group was 43 (SD 17) minutes compared to 40 (SD 15) minutes in the open group. The difference was not statistically significant.

Postoperative Analgesia Requirements

Postoperatively, intramuscular meperidine at 1 mg/kg every 4 hours was given on demand. Oral naproxen sodium was given as 550 mg bid on demand when patients were able to take liquids. The number of doses given was recorded. There was no difference in the number of pethidine doses requested by the two groups (Table 14-2). But when it came to oral analgesia, the open group required more doses compared with the laparoscopy group. Although the difference between 2.8 and 5.0 doses was statistically significant, the clinical significance is doubtful.

Postoperative Recovery

Fluids were prescribed on the return of active bowel sounds. Diet was resumed when the patients tolerated fluids well. Patients were discharged when diet was tolerated well and they were afebrile. No significant difference was found in the return of bowel sounds and commencement of fluids and diet intake (Table 14-2). Although patients with open surgery stayed, on the average, 1 day longer, this was not statistically significant.

Wound Infection

The patients were reviewed after 1 week at the outpatient clinic. Wound infection was defined as purulent discharge from the wound site. In the open group,

Table 14-2. Results of the Randomized Controlled Trial

	Open Group	Laparoscopic Group	*t*-Test *(P)*
Duration of operation (min) (mean ± SD)	40.1 (± 15.5)	43.4 (± 17.1)	NS
Meperidine (1 mg/kg) (mean ± SD)	1.3 (± 0.3)	1.0 (± 0.3)	NS
Oral analgesics (naproxen 550 mg) (dose) (mean ± SD)	5.0 (± 1.2)	2.8 (± 1.0)	<0.05
Feeding (days) (mean ± SD)	1.2 (± 0.4)	0.9 (± 0.2)	NS
Diet (days) (mean ± SD)	1.8 (± 0.5)	1.8 (± 0.2)	NS
Hospital stay (days) (mean ± SD)	4.2 (± 1.0)	3.2 (± 0.6)	NS
Wound infection	7 (9.7%)	0	0.014[a]

[a]Fisher's exact test.

seven (9.7 percent) patients had wound infections, but in the laparoscopy group, none had wound infections ($P = 0.014$ Fisher's exact test). No complications resulted from the laparoscopic technique, and no postoperative intra-abdominal abscess occurred in either group.

Return to Normal Activities

The patients were interviewed at 1 month to determine the period of debility before returning to full activities. For those who had not returned to full activities by 1 month, a second interview was held 2 weeks later. It was not possible to analyze the delay before return to full work because the wide diversity of occupations between the two groups made them incomparable. The range of home activities (cooking, gardening, child care) and social activities (school, shopping, movie going) were, however, similar in both groups. Return to full activity (i.e., able to pursue activity at a level of intensity, duration, and frequency similar to that before the operation) took about 2 weeks longer in the open group compared with patients in the laparoscopy group ($P < 0.01$ and $P < 0.05$ for home and social activities, respectively).

CONCLUSION

The effectiveness of laparoscopy as a diagnostic tool was determined in a previous prospective trial in which two cohorts of 102 (study group) and 248 (control group) patients admitted with acute right iliac fossa pain were studied.[11] Twenty-eight patients with equivocal but persistent pain in the study group were subjected to diagnostic laparoscopy before laparotomy. In this group, the laparoscopist was able to differentiate the inflamed appendices from normal ones, resulting in a zero normal appendectomy rate. By contrast, the 61 patients in the control group with persistent pain after 8 to 12 hours of observation underwent laparotomy, yielding a normal appendectomy rate of 15.7 percent; the difference was statistically significant. Although it is now widely accepted that laparoscopy is a useful and practical diagnostic tool, the popularity of its therapeutic counterpart, laparoscopic appendectomy, has been limited. This limitation can be traced to several misconceptions about the procedure itself.

The critics were not convinced about the benefits of removing the appendix laparoscopically. They thought that it took much longer and considered it too costly.[20] The advantages of laparoscopic appendectomy are summarized below.

Advantages of Laparoscopic Appendectomy

- Confirms the diagnosis
- Allows visualization of pelvic organs and other organs if the appendix is normal
- Reduces postoperative pain
- Shortens hospitalization by 1 day
- Reduces wound infection
- Allows earlier return to normal activities
- Minimizes scars
- Offers good training
- May reduce postoperative adhesions

Several large series and trials mentioned above have shown that laparoscopy is safe and can be performed routinely with minimal morbidity. Laparoscopy allows excellent visualization of the pelvic organs, the main causes of confusion in diagnosis, and the rest of the abdomen. Acute cholecystitis and perforated duodenal ulcers mimicking appendicitis have been diagnosed through the laparoscope, facilitating well-placed incisions. Moderate reduction in postoperative analgesic requirements has been reported,[20] probably as a result of the smaller wounds. Hospitalization stay has also been reduced in most studies. However, the two most important advantages are the drastic reduction in wound infection and the ability to return to activities earlier than usual. These reduce the overall health and economic cost of acute appendicitis.

Superior cosmesis can be attained in laparoscopic appendectomy because the umbilical incision is well camouflaged and the two suprapubic ports lie below the bikini line. Laparoscopic appendectomy is also good training for surgeons starting laparoscopic surgery, being easier and safer than laparoscopic cholecystectomy. Furthermore, some preliminary evidence suggests that removal of the appendix laparoscopically may result in fewer adhesions[9]—an important cause of long-term morbidity such as adhesion colic, intestinal obstruction, and infertility.

The misconception that laparoscopic appendectomy takes longer has been dispelled by results of studies[15–18] that have shown the procedure to be as fast as the open method after the learning curve has been surpassed. The cost can be reduced with reusable instruments and is definitely more than compensated by the reduction in wound infection, shorter stay, and earlier return to work.

Finally, laparoscopic appendectomy is not simply a laparoscopic procedure looking for an indication but a procedure that is definitely superior to open surgery and has tangible benefits to the patients. Its ability to almost eradicate wound infection and perhaps reduce adhesions will undoubtedly have an impact on the overall prognosis of acute appendicitis.

REFERENCES

1. McBurney C: Experience with early operative intervention in cases of disease of the vermiform appendix. NY Med J 50:676, 1889
2. Semm K: Endoscopic appendectomy. Endoscopy 15:59, 1983
3. Schreiber J: Early experience with laparoscopic appendectomy in women. Surg Endosc 1:211, 1987
4. Thomas E, Mueller B: Appendectomy. Diagnostic criteria and hospital performance. Hosp Pract 4:72, 1969
5. Chang F, Hogle H, Welling D: The fate of negative appendix. Am J Surg 126:752, 1973
6. Woodward A, Hemingway D, Greany M et al: Which patients should undergo laparoscopy? BMJ 296:1740, 1988
7. Krukowski Z, Irwin S, Denholm S et al: Preventing wound infection after appendectomy: a review. Br J Surg 75:1023, 1988
8. Pieper R, Kager L, Nasman P: Acute appendicitis: a clinical study of 1018 cases of emergency appendectomy. Acta Chir Scand 148:51, 1982
9. DeWilde R: Goodbye to late bowel obstruction after appendectomy. Lancet 338:1012, 1991
10. Puylaert J: Acute appendicitis: ultrasound evaluation using graded compression. Radiology 158:355, 1988
11. Kum C, Sim E, Goh P et al: Diagnostic laparoscopy: reducing the number of normal appendectomies. Dis Colon Rectum 36:763, 1993
12. Schreiber JH: Laparoscopic appendectomy in pregnancy. Surg Endosc 4:100, 1990
13. Schreiber JH: Results of outpatient laparoscopic appendectomy in women. Endoscopy 26:292, 1994
14. Engstrom L, Fenyo G: Assessment of stump invagination: a prospective and randomized trial. Br J Surg 72:971, 1985
15. Pier A, Gotz F, Bacher C: Laparoscopic appendectomy in 625 cases: from innovation to routine. Surg Endosc Laparosc 1:8, 1991
16. Saye W, Rives D, Cochran E: Laparoscopic appendectomy: three years' experience. Surg Endosc Laparosc 2:109, 1991
17. Valla J, Limmone B, Valla V et al: Laparoscopic appendectomy in children: report of 465 cases. Surg Laparosc Endosc 1:166, 1991
18. McAnena O, Austin O, Hederman W et al: Laparoscopic versus open appendectomy. Lancet 338:693, 1991
19. Tate J, Chung S, Dawson J et al: Conventional versus laparoscopic surgery for acute appendicitis. Br J Surg 80:761, 1993
20. Loh A, Taylor R: Laparoscopic appendectomy. Br J Surg 79:289, 1992

Editorial Comment I

Joaquim Gama-Rodrigues and Afonso H. S. e Sousa, Jr.

Appendectomy by a laparoscopic approach is not yet very popular, but multiple studies have been published. This randomized clinical trial with 140 patients by Drs. Kum and Goh is welcome. Although both treatment groups in their trial are very similar, the randomization may not have completely abolished the selection bias. The surgical team who conducted the conventional appendectomy is clearly less experienced than the one using the laparoscopic approach.

There are many justifications for performing laparoscopic appendectomy. Drs. Kum and Goh present the available data from the literature supporting the advantages of laparoscopy in diagnosing acute appendicitis accurately and in reducing the incidence of infection. Currently, no data confirm that fewer adhesions result (with or without clinical repercussions) from laparoscopic appendectomy or that it reduces the expenses.

Undeniably, the laparoscopic technique offers conditions to do appendectomy more safely and completely than does the conventional approach. The appendix is identified and mobilized by digital palpation during the open technique. The laparoscopic view of the appendix and adjacent viscera is superior to that obtained through a right lower quadrant incision. The laparoscopic identification, dissection, and liberation are carried out under direct vision—the desired aim in all surgical procedures. We find that the use of angled lenses provides better visualization of the structures. This is especially true in patients with many intra-abdominal adhesions or when the appendix is subserosal or retrocecal. In some patients, however, we prefer early conversion of laparoscopy to laparotomy, if the number of dilated intestinal loops prevents proper visualization. Dilated intestinal loops are not uncommon in patients with acute peritonitis from ruptured appendix and may contraindicate laparoscopy.

The laparoscopic approach may be useful in some patients with acute peritonitis from appendicitis. For example, the peritoneal cavity, including purulent pockets between the subhepatic and subphrenic loops, must be thoroughly cleansed, a procedure more readily done laparoscopically. These areas would be difficult to reach through a conventional appendectomy incision. In our series of 32 cases, 3 patients presented with severe peritonitis with various purulent collections. We drained these pockets with the laparoscopic method without converting the laparoscopic technique to a laparotomy. (Conversion rate of the series is approximately 6 percent.) Postoperatively, these patients with peritonitis had a prolonged ileus. The subphrenic and subhepatic abscesses required no supplemental therapy, and the patients did not develop abdominal wall infections.

In almost half of our series (13 cases), we employed a technical modification that does not require ligation of the appendiceal artery. The top of the appendix is grasped, and the mesoappendix is dissected very close to the appendix. The appendiceal artery is left intact. Hemostasis is accomplished by electrocautery of the branches of the appendiceal artery. With this technique, the anatomic elements remain more evident and the treatment of the appendiceal base is simplified. A 90-degree rotation of the appendix from one side to the other eases the dissection and provides the necessary tension for electrocoagulation. Little by little, the appendix is introduced into the trocar of the right iliac fossa, exteriorizing the mobilized appendix. In two patients, we had to change the 10-mm trocar to a wider one to accommodate a thick appendix. The appendiceal stump can be treated extracorporeally because the cecum can be exteriorized through the trocar incision site after desufflation of the pneumoperitoneum.

We note with interest the data supporting rapid recovery of patients treated by laparoscopic appendectomy. Open appendectomy involves use of a small muscle-splitting incision. Patients recover rapidly. Laparoscopic appendectomy reduces the incision size still further and disrupts the peritoneum even less than does the open technique, fostering the rapid convalescence.

In conclusion, we believe that this study provides data supporting the superiority of laparoscopic appendectomy over the conventional open appendectomy. These data should encourage those who do not currently perform laparoscopic appendectomy to reassess their opinions. More clinical data can thus be accumulated with increasing clinical experience, and subsequently the role of laparoscopic appendectomy can be better appraised.

Editorial Comment II

Rama M. Jager

The standard technique of open appendectomy through a right quadrant incision suffers from the problem of incisional morbidity, limited ability to explore the abdomen, and long-term complications from intra-abdominal adhesions caused by peritoneal disruption. These disadvantages are magnified if the patient with right lower quadrant abdominal pain is found to have no appendicitis on exploration. The surgeon has to weigh the morbidity from the operation against the risk of appendiceal perforation. The gravity of appendiceal perforation from delayed diagnosis forces the surgeon to favor surgical exploration. The surgeon may have avoided an unnecessary exploration, if a diagnostic alternative less invasive than exploratory laparotomy were available.

LAPAROSCOPY COMES TO THE RESCUE

Laparoscopic appendectomy is, from a historical point of view, the older procedure. The first laparoscopic appendectomy was done by Kurt Semm in 1982. That is at least 5 years before the first laparoscopic cholecystectomy. For some unknown reason, it never ignited the interest of the surgical community as much as did the laparoscopic cholecystectomy. Interest in laparoscopic surgery grew explosively with laparoscopic cholecystectomy, which led to application of laparoscopic technique to treatment of appendicitis.

Other studies,[1–4] including Drs. Kum and Goh's data from their prospective study in this chapter, support the advantages of the laparoscopic approach to management of patients with right lower quadrant abdominal pain and with the clinical diagnosis of acute appendicitis. The potential advantages include (1) the ability to identify the appendix in all anatomic locations, (2) diagnostic accuracy comparable to the open technique, and (3) the facility to examine the intraperitoneal viscera for nonappendiceal causes of acute abdomen. The laparoscopic surgeon either removes the appendix through the cannula or enclosed in a plastic bag. Similar precautions during the extraction of the resected appendix through an open incision may avoid the high rate of wound infection faced by Drs. Kum and Goh. The lack of a plastic protector during their open appendectomies might explain the differences in wound infection rate in the described trial. Because the peritoneal disruption is less with the laparoscopic approach than with the open technique, it is reasonable to assume that the degree of intra-abdominal adhesions (and the long-term problems such as intestinal obstruction and infertility) may be less severe with the laparoscopic technique. Long-term follow-up patients in Drs. Kum and Goh's clinical trial may provide the needed proof for this putative advantage.

Long-term studies are also needed to conclusively prove the superiority of laparoscopic appendectomy over the open technique. Given the current data, the laparoscopic approach may be equivalent to the open technique in its therapeutic efficacy. It may also decrease the rate of avoidable laparotomies without compromising the rate of perforation when the diagnosis of appendicitis is equivocal.

The disadvantages of cost and prolonged operative time prevent some surgeons from adapting the less invasive approach to appendectomy. The unfamiliarity of operating room personnel with laparoscopic equipment, especially when the operation is done in the early morning hours, probably contributes to the surgeon's reluctance to remove the appendix laparoscopically. Problems of prolonged operative time from technical inexpertise and the logistics of laparoscopy at late hours disappears as experience increases. The high cost of laparoscopy is offset somewhat by reduced length of hospital stay and rapid return to work after the operation. Also, the cost stems mostly from the use of disposable trocars and dissecting instruments and can mount up to $2,000 per patient.[5,6] The solution is obvious. Use of reusable trocars and dissecting instruments avoids the problem of increased cost of laparoscopic technique.

The minimally invasive nature of laparoscopy may increase its use in patients with right lower quadrant abdominal pain when noninvasive clinical and ultrasonographic diagnoses are inconclusive. The tendency to laparoscope every patient with right lower quadrant abdominal pain should be tempered. Proper clinical examination enhances the diagnostic accuracy without increasing the rate of perforated appendicitis. One study reported a reduction of the negative appendectomy rate of 20 percent to 11.3 percent by using a clinical scoring system.[7] Use of ultrasonography may also avoid the rate of negative laparoscopies, although most radiologists still have to develop the needed expertise.

When the probability of appendicitis is high, diagnostic laparoscopy is preferred to exploratory laparotomy. Even surgeons who are still learning laparoscopic appendectomy can place a trocar through a 1-cm incision in the right lower quadrant for diagnostic laparoscopy. With improved optics and illumination, even a 5-mm laparoscope may provide the needed view. Exclusion of appendicitis and other causes of acute peritonitis complete the operation. If the appendix is inflamed, it can be mobilized, resected, and retrieved through an enlarged trocar wound. This approach reduces the incisional morbidity and peritoneal disruption compared with the open McBurney incision.

A FEW TECHNICAL VARIATIONS AND PROBLEMS

Drs. Kum and Goh suggest that a Foley catheter need not be placed preoperatively. Because it is difficult to predict the duration of the operation and the intraperitoneal abnormalities, the surgeon should insert a Foley catheter in all patients undergoing diagnostic laparoscopy for right lower quadrant abdominal pain. Morbidity from a Foley catheter that resides for a few hours is small. Retrieval of the resected appendix sometimes requires a larger cannula. A sterile sigmoidoscope can be inserted through the enlarged 10-mm trocar site and the specimen retrieved through the scope without contaminating the wound. In appropriate patients, an endoscopic clip can be applied to occlude the appendiceal stump, although placement of a loop ligature (EndoLoop) is as convenient and fast as the clip.[8]

A rare complication following laparoscopic appendectomy is the syndrome of cecal dysmotility. This condition may be secondary to high-frequency electrocoagulation around the base of the appendix and during the transection of the appendix.[9] Proper precautions with electrosurgical instruments to avoid cecal thermal injury around the appendiceal base may reduce the severity of this problem.

The laparoscopic surgeon should also be aware of completely removing the appendix by careful dissection of the base of the appendix. Recurrent appendicitis from incomplete laparoscopic removal of the appendix has been described,[10] although it is difficult to explain how a surgeon cannot visualize and transect the junction of the appendix and the cecum. Overzealous excision of the cecum should also be avoided to reduce operative morbidity. Like its open counterpart, careful and meticulous dissection and complete excision of the appendix are important in laparoscopic appendectomy.

REFERENCES

1. Lathrop JC, Lloyd LR, Boccaccio JE et al: Laparoscopic appendectomy for acute appendicitis: is there really any benefit? Am Surg 59:541, 1993
2. Rothenbuhler JM, Linder P: Laparoscopic versus conventional appendectomy: a comparison. Helv Chir Acta 59:567, 1993
3. Hill AD, Murphy PG, Thornton J: A prospective randomized trial of laparoscopic versus open appendectomy. Surgery 112:497, 1992
4. Richards W, Watson D, Lynch G et al: A review of the results of laparoscopic versus open appendectomy. Surg Gynecol Obstet 177:473, 1993
5. Lathrop JC, Lloyd LR, Boccaccio JE et al: Laparoscopic appendectomy for acute appendicitis: is there really any benefit? Am Surg 59:541, 1993
6. Gilchrist BF, Lobe TE, Schropp KP et al: Is there a role for laparoscopic appendectomy in pediatric surgery? J Pediatr Surg 27:209, 1992
7. Lehmann K, Villiger P, Jenny M: Negative appendectomies can be decreased by improved clinical assessment alone. Helv Chir Acta 58:837, 1992
8. Cristalli B, Chiche R, Izard V et al: Pelvic pain in women. Evaluation of a celioscopic intraperitoneal appendectomy technique. The appendix stump was closed with a clip applicator. Ann Chir 45:529, 1991
9. Waleczek H, Recknagel S, Hegelmaier C et al: Temperature range in bipolar high frequency coagulation of the appendiceal stump. Chirurg 64:1036, 1993
10. Devereaux DA, McDermott JP, Caushaj PF: Recurrent appendicitis following laparoscopic appendectomy. Dis Colon Rectum 37:719, 1994

15

Laparoscopic Rectopexy for Rectal Prolapse

Ara Darzi and John R. T. Monson

The widespread success of laparoscopic cholecystectomy has led to the development of a wide range of laparoscopic surgical procedures such as hernia repair,[1,2] vagotomy,[3] hysterectomy,[4] and Nissen fundoplication.[5] The most recent addition to the list of procedures that can be undertaken by a minimally invasive approach is laparoscopic colectomy.[6] Procedures for treating rectal prolapse may constitute some of the best applications for colorectal laparoscopic techniques. Although the condition is benign, rectal prolapse is often debilitating. Furthermore, many patients are elderly or medically unfit, or both. A technique of laparoscopic rectopexy performed using the EndoStapler (EndoHernia, United States Surgical Corporation, Norwalk, CT) is described.

PATIENT PREPARATION

For all patients, consent is obtained for possible conversion to an open procedure, and routine antithrombotic precautions are taken with heparin and thromboembolic disease (TED) support stockings because of the increased operative time. Routine bowel preparation is employed, and all patients receive standard antibiotic prophylaxis.

INSTRUMENTATION

Full videoendoscopy facilities are required. For routine laparoscopic colonic surgery, the following instruments are required: two Babcock-type bowel-grasping instruments (P.C.I. Instrument, Liptingen, Germany), EndoShears, a disposable endoscopic scissors, and EndoSciz (United States Surgical Corporation), another endoscopic scissors that has the advantage of holding tissues away from potentially important structures before cutting with diathermy. An EndoStapler is used to staple the Marlex mesh to the sacrum.

OPERATIVE TECHNIQUE

A nasogastric tube and urinary catheter are passed when the patient is anesthetized. All procedures are performed with the patient in the Lloyd-Davies position. Pneumoperitoneum is created using a standard technique for insufflation with a Veress needle and is maintained at 12 to 16 mm Hg by an automatic carbon dioxide insufflator. A 10-mm 0-degree telescope is inserted through a subumbilical port, and initial laparoscopy is performed.

The operator stands on the left side of the patient; two video screens are positioned on either side of the knee. Three 12-mm trocars are introduced into the abdomen to facilitate use of the EndoStapler laparoscopic stapling instruments. In all ports, SurgiGrips (United States Surgical Corporation) are essential to prevent air leaks and to maintain an efficient pneumoperitoneum throughout the operation.

The camera is inserted into the right iliac fossa port; the Babcock instrument is passed through the left iliac fossa port holding the rectosigmoid junction upward and to the left. The second Babcock grasping instrument is passed suprapubically to elevate the middle third of the rectum. This maneuver provides tension on the peritoneal reflection on the right side of the rectosigmoid junction. The peritoneal reflection is divided, using an EndoSciz and by careful dissection (Fig. 15-1), the avascular plane between the fascial capsule of the rectum anteriorly and the fascia of Waldeyer posteriorly are bluntly dissected with the laparoscope.

Division of the lateral ligaments is easily performed under direct vision. Posteriorly, the pelvic nerves are identified and preserved. Close and magnified views of the mesorectum ensure the correct planes of dissection with minimal bleeding. In a woman, retraction of the

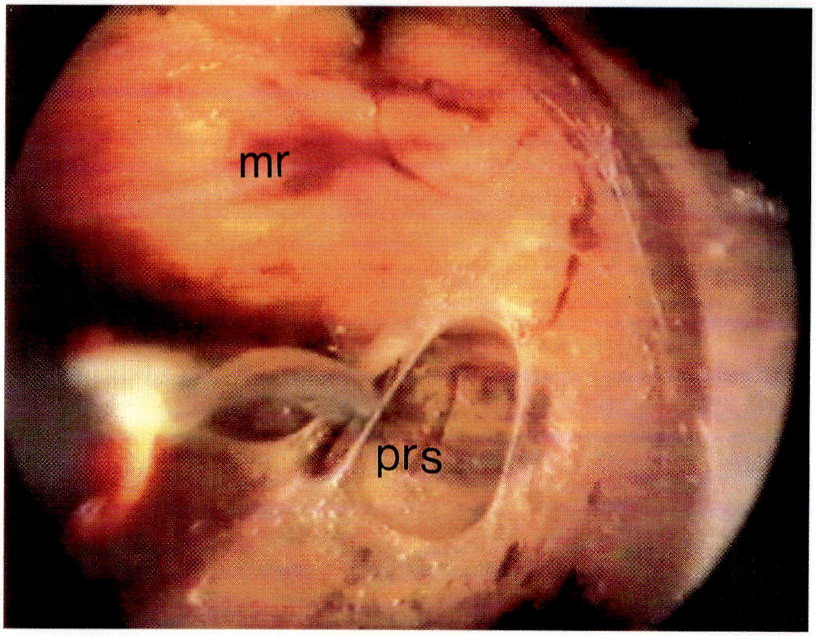

Fig. 15-1. Dissection in the presacral avascular space. mr, midrectum; prs, presacral space.

pouch of Douglas is facilitated by holding the cervix upward with a blunt Hulka cervical forceps (Rockett Ltd., Watford, UK) held through the vagina by an assistant. This maneuver elevates the cervix and body of the uterus. As mobilization proceeds toward the pelvic floor, an assistant's finger in the vagina aids elevation of the vagina and thus dissection of the rectum from the vagina. In a man, the urinary bladder neck and the prostate can be elevated by using a rigid cystoscope.

At this point, a triangular strip of polypropylene mesh (Surgipro Mesh, United States Surgical Corporation) approximately 10 by 6 cm is rolled and introduced into the abdomen through the subumbilical port for placement in the presacral space. The EndoStapler is then introduced into the right iliac fossa port, and the mesh is stapled to the sacrum. On average, three to four staples are used to staple the mesh to the sacrum (Fig. 15-2). After fixation of the mesh, the

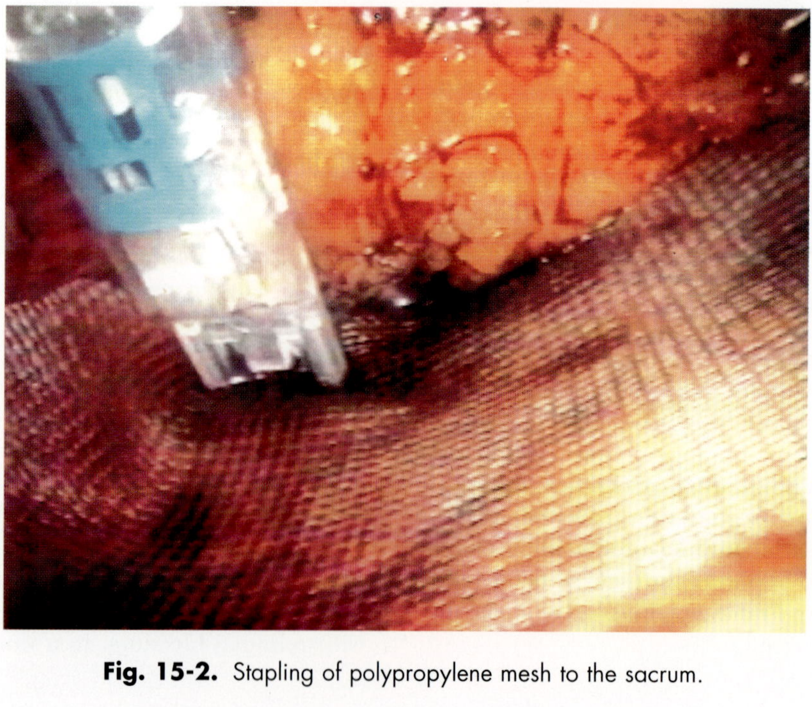

Fig. 15-2. Stapling of polypropylene mesh to the sacrum.

rectum is held on light tension, using the laparoscopic Babcock forceps. The right limb of the mesh is positioned and secured to the adventitial tissue of the rectum using the stapler. Staples are placed only along the superior and inferior mesh edges. The rectum is then retracted to the right, and the left limb of the mesh is brought around the rectum and secured to the rectal adventitia in similar fashion at the upper and lower mesh edges.

The laparoscopic ports are then removed, followed by closure of the defects. Perioperative antibiotics are employed.

RESULTS

The postoperative course has been uneventful, with rapid resumption of normal bowel function. Our mean hospital stay has been 5 days with early mobility being a marked feature in these patients.

CONCLUSION

Laparoscopic surgery has had an enormous impact on the practice of general surgery. Laparoscopic cholecystectomy has been undeniably successful.[1]

Laparoscopic colonic surgery has the same potential benefits as laparoscopic cholecystectomy with potentially a shorter postoperative stay and less postoperative pain.[6] Laparoscopic colonic surgery has been embraced with a combination of enthusiasm and circumspection by colon and rectal surgeons. Increasing availability of appropriate instrumentation and increasing technical facility have expanded the applications of these techniques. The recent introduction of a commercially available EndoHernia stapler for use in laparoscopic hernia repair has provided the tool necessary for laparoscopic rectopexy, in order to avoid suturing and knot tying, both of which are tedious and time consuming.

Morbidity appears to be reduced, particularly with regard to septic complications. Our preliminary experience leads us to suggest that, as laparoscopic technology advances and surgical expertise is gained, this minimally invasive approach will soon have a major impact on the practice of colorectal surgery. The benefit of such a minimally invasive approach to rectal prolapse becomes especially obvious in the elderly or physiologically disabled patient with prolapse. Because many patients presenting with rectal prolapse are old and infirm, surgeons tend to favor low-morbidity, local operations on the anal canal.[7] Such local procedures include the Thiersch wire or a Silastic sling around the anal canal.[8] Some advocate radical operations such as rectosigmoidectomy[9] or combined abdominoperineal pelvic floor repair[10,11] for those patients who are fit to undergo major procedures. However, these operations have, in addition to their morbidity and mortality, a high recurrence rate.

Others have advocated rectal fixation or rectopexy. Graham[12] was the first to mobilize the rectum down to the levator muscles. This approach is still considered the most important step, indicating the importance of mobilizing the rectum to the pelvic floor. The currently preferred operative technique represents a modification in which fixation procedures of the entire mobilized rectum are used. These operations rely on a polyvinyl-alcohol sponge[13] inserted in the presacral space to fix the rectum to the sacrum or, on suturing an inert sling, to fix the mobilized rectum to the sacral promontory. The irritant properties of a polyvinyl-alcohol sponge help to fix the rectum firmly but also predispose it to infection or rejection. The inert polypropylene mesh fixation in front of the rectum (Ripstein repair) has been associated with acute kinking of the bowel or, if too tight, with intestinal obstruction.[14] Early experience with these complications led us to adopt a modification of the procedure whereby the inert polypropylene mesh is inserted behind the rectum to the sacrum to achieve posterior fixation.

Patients with normal bowel habit (or diarrhea) and no history of constipation or obstructed defecation are probably ideal candidates for laparoscopic rectopexy without resection, especially in the absence of significant redundancy of the sigmoid colon. In patients with massive procidentia, the presence of a large mesorectum and redundant sigmoid will more likely mandate a resective procedure.

Increasing familiarity among colon and rectal surgeons with laparoscopic procedures and the current availability of laparoscopic hernia staplers make laparoscopic abdominal rectopexy an attractive and minimally invasive option for patients with the rectal prolapse who might not be fit for an open abdominal procedure.

REFERENCES

1. Myers WC, Branaum GD, Farouk M et al: A prospective analysis of 1518 laparoscopic cholecystectomies. N Engl J Med 324:1073, 1991
2. Paget GW: Laparoscopic repair of inguinal hernia. Med J Aust 156:508, 1992
3. Katkhouda N, Mouiel J: A new technique of surgical treatment of chronic duodenal ulcer without laparotomy by videocelioscopy. Am J Surg 161:361, 1991
4. Nezhat CR, Burrell MO, Nezhat FR et al: Laparoscopic radical hysterectomy with para-aortic and pelvic node dissection. Am J Obstet Gynecol 166:864, 1992
5. Cuschieri A, Shimi S, Nathanson LK: Laparoscopic reduction, crural repair, and fundoplication of large hiatal hernia. Am J Surg 163:425, 1992
6. Monson JRT, Darzi A, Carey PD et al: Prospective evaluation of laparoscopic-assisted colectomy in an unselected group of patients. Lancet 340:831, 1992
7. Goligher JC: Surgery of the Colon, Anus and Rectum. 4th Ed. Bailliere Tindall, London, 1980

8. Hopkinson BR, Hardman J: Silicone rubber perianal suture for rectal prolapse. Proc R Soc Med 66:1095, 1973
9. Porter NH: Collective results of operations for rectal prolapse. Ann R Coll Surg Engl 62:386, 1980
10. Goligher JC: The treatment of complete prolapse of the rectum by the Roscoe Graham operation. Br J Surg 45:323, 1957
11. Hughes ESR, Gleadell LW: Abdominoperineal repair of complete prolapse of the rectum. Proc R Soc Med 55:177, 1962
12. Henry MM: Rectal prolapse. J Hosp Med 24:302, 1980
13. Wells CA: Polyvinyl-alcohol sponge. An inert plastic for use as a prosthesis in the repair of large hernias. Br J Surg 42:618, 1955
14. Miller RL: Ripstein procedure for rectal prolapse. Am Surg 45:531, 1979

Editorial Comment I

Irwin R. Berman

Drs. Darzi and Monson have appropriately identified repair of rectal prolapse as a reasonable target for laparoscopic approaches. In my view, correction of rectal prolapse may afford one of the best applications for laparoscopic procedures by colorectal surgeons. Laparoscopic proctopexy provides a minimally invasive option for operations that are otherwise of significant physiologic impact, particularly in the elderly and those with multiple systems problems. Moreover, excellent visibility afforded by laparoscopic magnification makes the technique equally attractive for younger patients who require abdominal correction of rectal prolapse, especially when impotence or infertility may be a complication from extensive pelvic dissection.

The technique described by Drs. Darzi and Monson is essentially equivalent to that of open abdominal mesh rectopexy, largely paralleling the guidelines of my June 1992 publication on this subject.[1] Twelve-millimeter ports, Babcock forceps, and coagulating scissors are mainstays of instrumentation. I have personally used an umbilical tape around the sigmoid for retraction during dissection. This technique affords excellent sigmoid retraction in virtually any direction during mobilization of the rectum, simply by grasping the umbilical tape tether. Dissection of the rectum from the presacral space and from the vagina are quite straightforward. Blunt and sharp dissection allow complete circumferential mobilization of the rectum all the way to the levators. The entire procedure is performed with the patient in Trendelenburg's position, using appropriate shoulder supports.

Anteriorly, dissection in the rectovaginal plane is enhanced by insertion of a large (60-ml) syringe casing or other obturator into the vagina. Magnification by the laparoscopic camera provides excellent visualization during all phases of this dissection and may help to minimize the adverse effects of pelvic dissection in men. Posteriorly, the ureters and hypogastric nerves are identified and avoided. Division of the lateral rectal stalks may or may not be performed, depending on the elected procedure. If sigmoid resection is not performed with rectopexy, lateral stalk division may be unnecessary. Constipated patients and those in whom rectopexy may produce untoward angulation of a redundant sigmoid on the rectum may need sigmoid resection in addition to rectopexy as the more appropriate procedure, a combination of operations that may also be performed laparoscopically. Naturally, a mesh prosthesis is best avoided when sigmoid resection is performed, because the mesh prosthesis may increase the hazard of infection with foreign body material.

Our original description of this procedure details the use of a rectangular mesh strip secured to the sacrum with a 7-mm long titanium surgical thumbtack; derived from a hemorrhage-occular pin.[2] Sacral attachment with staples may not be uniform or predictable. Often, multiple staples are required, increasing the hazard of presacral bleeding. Use of the flanged sacral thumbtack is both predictable and secure; the tack is delivered into a seated position below the sacral promontory using a weighted sleeve on the laparoscopic tack driver.

The initial laparoscopic driver provided for this purpose was straight, making suprapubic insertion imperfect for tack placement below the promontory, the optimum location for sacral attachment. My co-workers and I therefore described transvaginal insertion of the tacker, which afforded excellent placement of the tack squarely below the sacral promontory. Because most patients with rectal prolapse are women and many have had a hysterectomy, this can be a clean and straightforward maneuver, greatly facilitated by insertion of a 12-mm trocar directly through the bacteriologically prepared vaginal vault. Using the vaginal port, pneumoperitoneum is retained as the tack is placed in its proper position below the sacral promontory. The vaginal defect is later repaired by a single laparoscopic suture. All trocar defects are closed by suture as the procedure is completed.

In our initial report,[1] the double-headed sacral tack was used to secure a horizontally placed mesh as a posterior cradle for the rectum. The mesh was then tacked to the adventitia of the rectum precisely as Drs. Darzi and Monson have now quoted from our report. More recently, an articulated tack delivery system is evolving; its angled tip should afford more predictable presacral attachment through a suprapubic insertion port. This approach will have the beneficial effect of avoiding vaginal entry, especially in patients with an intact uterus.

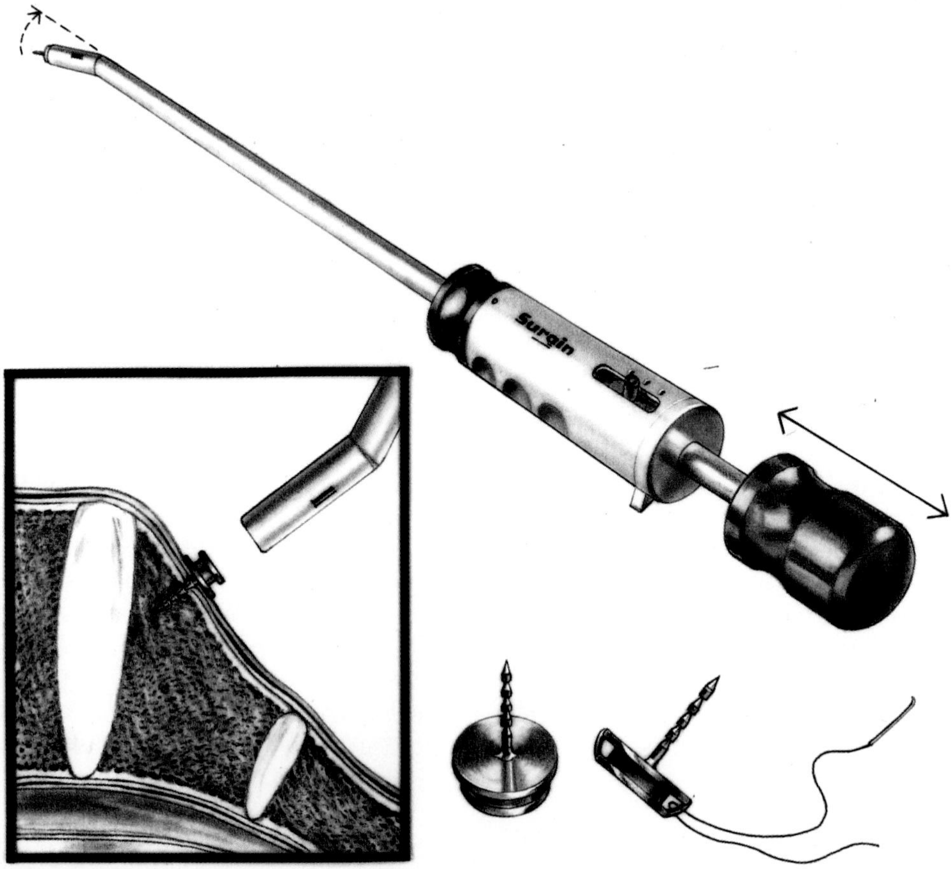

Fig. 15-3. Laparoscopic sacral suspension device showing a tacker with articulated tip for suprapubic insertion. Inset illustrates the ideal position of a flanged two-headed tack below the sacral promontory. The conventional tack (for mesh attachment) and a modification incorporating two suture loops are also illustrated. (Courtesy of Surgin Surgical Instrumentation Inc., Tustin, CA.)

The suprapubic port and the articulated tack delivery system also provide a more predictable access for men requiring abdominal rectopexy (Fig. 15-3).

Since our initial description of this procedure, I have continued to be enthusiastic regarding thumbtack applications for laparoscopic sacral suspension. However, it is a fact that a relatively small number of patients with rectal prolapse are ideally suited to mesh rectopexy. Moreover, a definite subset of patients with rectal prolapse will require sigmoid resection at the time of rectopexy, a setting in which use of foreign body material is usually contraindicated. Therefore, a further modification of the tack itself has been developed, allowing *suture* attachment to the tack for lateral rectal stalk fixation when mesh is not appropriate (Fig. 15-3). Constipated patients and those with very redundant sigmoid or massive procidentia will often require sigmoidectomy. Suture fixation to the sacrum, rather than mesh fixation, is appropriate for such patients.

Operations for combined pelvic prolapse (rectum *and* vagina) may also be appropriate for laparoscopic presacral tacking, restoring suspension of prolapsing rectum and vagina with a single laparoscopic procedure. Dissection of the enterocele thus becomes an integral part of the anterior rectal dissection between the rectum and vagina. Assuming that sigmoid resection will not be required, a vertical mesh strip may then be inserted between the rectum and vagina and tacked at its upper end to the sacrum using the laparoscopic tack driver. Both the rectum and vagina may then be secured to the vertical mesh suspender, as described by Sullivan et al.[3] Polypropylene mesh for this purpose is possibly ideal because it allows fibroblastic ingrowth and fixation of the mesh in its rectovaginal position, essentially obliterating the enterocele as healing occurs. The uppermost portion of the mesh strip may optimally be covered by peritoneum or sigmoid, tacked over the exposed mesh. Several companies are currently developing mesh laminates that may eventually eliminate the debate as to whether reperitonealization is necessary in this application.

I am pleased that Drs. Darzi and Monson have selected my laparoscopic fixation technique as a launching point for their contribution to this book.

Although details regarding continence, impotence, and recurrence are not reported, I have every expectation that results from laparoscopic rectopexy will be equivalent to open proctopexy operations in comparable patients, assuming equivalent dissection and assuming that staple fixation to the sacrum will have reasonable surgical longevity.

ACKNOWLEDGMENTS

Dr. Berman has participated in the design, development, and commercialization of laparoscopic sacral tacking devices (Surgin Surgical Instrumentation Inc., Tustin, CA).

REFERENCES

1. Berman IR: Sutureless laparoscopic rectopexy for procidentia: technique and implications. Dis Colon Rectum 35:689, 1992
2. Stolfi VM, Milsom JW, Lavery IC et al: Newly designed occluder pin for presacral hemorrhage. Dis Colon Rectum 35:166, 1992
3. Sullivan ES, Stranburg CO, Sandoz IL et al: Repair of total pelvic prolapse: an overview. Perspect Colon Rectal Surg 3:119, 1990

Editorial Comment II

Rama M. Jager

Proctopexy is uniquely suited for a laparoscopic approach because of excellent visualization of the presacral space and ease of dissection. Drs. Darzi and Monson described their technique in detail in this chapter. My discussion elaborates on some of the technical modifications.

Proper mechanical and antibacterial bowel preparation is obligatory for all patients undergoing proctopexy. Although the colorectal lumen is not entered during the routine laparoscopic proctopexy, the possibility of the sutures or staples penetrating the mucosa should be considered. It may also be necessary to resect the sigmoid colon when the sigmoid colon is redundant and the risk of sigmoid volvulus is high because of mesocolic anatomy. Patients with chronic constipation may also benefit from a sigmoid and low anterior resection, along with proctopexy to treat the rectal prolapse.

While the 0-degree laparoscope is quite satisfactory for most laparoscopic proctopexy operations, use of the 30-degree scope helps difficult dissections by enabling different fields of view. Some surgeons routinely use 30-degree scopes for most laparoscopic operations. It does take some time to get used to the 30-degree scope before the surgeon can take advantage of various viewing angles.

Proper positioning of the patient before draping is obligatory, not only to reduce position-related neurovascular complications, but also to facilitate swift operative technique. When a uterine cervical mobilization or cystoscopy is considered, appropriate vaginal and pubic preparation and placement of instruments are simple predraping maneuvers that reduce operative impediments.

Presacral dissection should be confined close to the midline to avoid presacral venous plexuses. The farther the surgeon moves away from the midline, the closer one is to the thin-walled internal iliac vessels, the source of major bleeding during presacral dissection. If presacral venous bleeding is encountered, the laparoscopic maneuver described by Drs. Darzi and Monson, of using an EndoStapler to occlude the bleeding vessel, may prove helpful.

Numerous operations are currently popular to repair the full-thickness rectal prolapse. Selection of the best surgical procedure for the treatment of the complete rectal prolapse is difficult amid the myriad techniques. The choice of the operation depends not only on the surgeon's experience but also on the general health of the patient and the degree of surgical risk. Some suggest that the perineal repair of the rectal prolapse is less risky than transabdominal repair for elderly and debilitated patients.[1] Surgical techniques that include rectal mobilization and fixation result in a recurrence rate of up to 4 percent.[2]

New techniques should lower the rate of recurrence and complications without increasing the surgical risk significantly. No single technique suits all patients and all surgeons. The technique described by Drs. Darzi and Monson will be a welcome addition to the current approaches to treatment of this debilitating disease. Long-term clinical follow-up is necessary to show that the stapling to anchor the mesh is free of complications such as staple migration into the rectal lumen. The technique of not encircling the rectum with the mesh but anchoring the centerfold to the presacral fascia may avoid the common postoperative constipation following proctopexy. Some manometric and volumetric studies in patients with open proctopexy have suggested that extensive presacral dissection and transection of lateral stalks can increase rectal sensory thresholds, producing postoperative dyschezia.[3] Whether a similar phenomenon occurs with meticulous laparoscopic presacral dissection is unknown.

REFERENCES

1. Bosmans L, Storms P, Gruwez JA: Perineal repair of procidentia recti with a silastic sling. Acta Chir Belg 93:268, 1993
2. Kuijpers HC: Treatment of complete rectal prolapse: to narrow, to wrap, to suspend, to fix, to encircle, to plicate or to resect? World J Surg 16:826, 1992
3. Ribero F, Delaini GG, Canino V et al: The functional and manometric-volumetric results following abdominal rectopexy for total rectal prolapse. Chir Ital 44:257, 1992

16

Laparoscopic Sigmoid Colectomy

John R. T. Monson and Ara Darzi

Laparoscopic surgery has made a major impact on surgical practice, recently including colonic surgery. In practice, most operations are performed using a technique of laparoscopic assistance whereby some components of the operation are performed in a conventional fashion following initial laparoscopic mobilization of the bowel. A major reason for this approach is that in most instances laparoscopic techniques do not allow for easy delivery of resected colonic segments. In addition, current technology is not adequate for a safe, reliable, and timely intracorporeal reanastomosis. Consequently, these elements of the operation are usually performed extracorporeally in a traditional manner, although through a much smaller abdominal incision.[1] Resection of the rectum and sigmoid colon, however, lends itself to a totally intracorporeal technique. Delivery of the resected specimen may be via a transanal route, and by continuing laparoscopic and transanal placement of stapling instruments, it is possible to construct a reliable anastomosis.

PATIENT PREPARATION AND SELECTION OF CARE

Preoperative preparation should include documentation of the site of the lesion with contrast radiology because of the inaccuracy of colonoscopy in providing information concerning the site of the pathology. In some cases, injection of India ink or methylene blue into the lesion at the time of colonoscopy may aid subsequent identification at laparoscopy. It is vital to have accurate localization of the lesion in patients with polypoid lesions where serosal abnormalities are unlikely at laparoscopy and tactile confirmation of location is unavailable. Preparation is otherwise as for traditional colonic surgery with particular attention paid toward meticulous bowel preparation.

OPERATIVE TECHNIQUE

A nasogastric tube and urinary catheter are passed when the patient is anesthetized. The procedure is performed with the patient in the Lloyd-Davies position with the legs flat to avoid interfering with the insertion of instruments into ports (Fig. 16-1). Pneumoperitoneum is created using a standard technique. A 10-mm 0-degree telescope is inserted through a subumbilical port, and initial laparoscopy is performed.

We use 10- or 12-mm endoscopic ports throughout, one subumbilically and potentially one in each of the four quadrants (Fig. 16-2). In all ports, SurgiGrips (United States Surgical Corporation, Norwalk, CT) are essential to prevent air leaks and to maintain an efficient pneumoperitoneum throughout the operation, which may be jeopardized by frequent insertion and removal of dissecting instruments. An additional 12-mm port is inserted suprapubically to allow use of a linear stapler (EndoGIA, United States Surgical Corporation) for intracorporeal mesenteric and bowel division. Following initial laparoscopy, the lesion to be resected is identified, and mobilization of the portion of colon to be resected is commenced.

Retraction of the left side of the colon is achieved by grasping the bowel with a Babcock instrument passed via the trocar in the right hypochondrium, which holds the descending colon cephalad and toward the midline. The second Babcock instrument is passed via the right iliac fossa port and holds the sigmoid colon in a caudal direction and toward the midline. Judicious use of tilting of the operation table can facilitate retraction of the colon and exposure of the paracolic gutter. In addition, it aids in rolling the small bowel away from the operative field, which would otherwise be at risk of inadvertent damage. Dissection and mobilization are

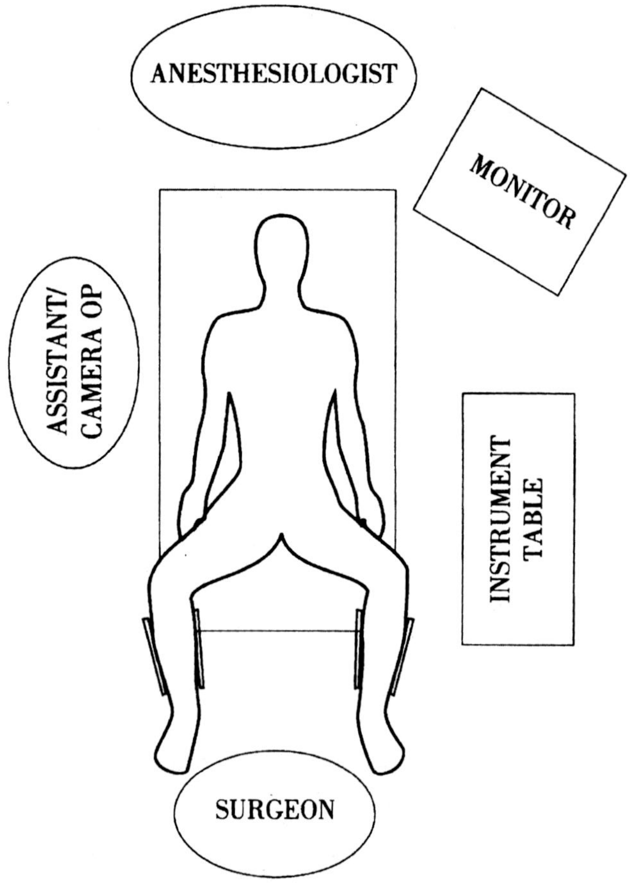

Fig. 16-1. Theater setup.

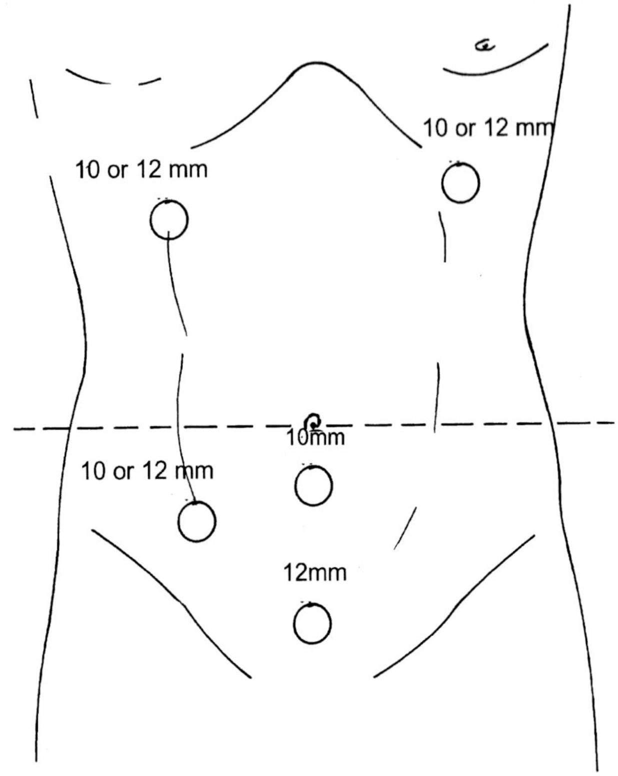

Fig. 16-2. Port placement.

performed using a combination of sharp scissors dissection and hook diathermy. These instruments are inserted via the port in the left iliac fossa.

The dissection is started by dividing the congenital adhesions commonly seen between the sigmoid colon and the abdominal wall. Identification and preservation of the ureter and gonadal vessels are established at this early stage. Mobilization of the bowel is continued proximally toward the splenic flexure. For mobilization of the splenic flexure, the bowel should be grasped on the midtransverse colon and tension applied downward and to the right via the right upper quadrant port. A second grasping instrument should be applied to the descending colon via the right iliac fossa port with tension applied downward and toward the midline. Dissection is via the left iliac fossa port and may require the use of especially long scissors to reach the further limit of dissection. If desired, the inferior mesenteric vessels may be isolated and divided using a linear stapler as an initial step before mobilization of the bowel. This approach facilitates subsequent resection and mobilization of the bowel. Alternatively, vessel division may be delayed until bowel mobilization is completed.

For a left colonic resection, the bowel is divided at the level of sacral promontory using a 30- or 60-mm linear stapler (EndoGIA), introduced through a 12- or 15-mm suprapubic laparoscopic port. The mesentery is then divided proximally up to the level of the proximal resection margin using a combination of diathermy, clips, and linear stapling. The proximal colon is then divided, and consequently, at this stage, the specimen is free in the peritoneal cavity.

The triple stapled end-to-end anastomosis is then commenced as follows; the anvil and shaft of a 28-mm circular stapler (Premium EEA, United States Surgical Corporation) is passed transanally after rectal washout using cytotoxic agent. The anvil is then delivered into the peritoneal cavity after the staple line has been divided along the top of the rectum. Next, the anvil is detached from the stapler and delivered to the peritoneal cavity. A 2-0 Vicryl suture (Ethicon, Inc., Somerville, NJ) on a curved needle is tied through a hole in the shaft of the anvil before the insertion of the stapler. The anvil of the circular stapler head is inserted completely into the proximal descending colon after the staple line has been opened. Noncrushing bowel clamps may be placed over the proximal colon to prevent spillage of fecal material. The needle is then passed through the bowel wall 2 to 3 cm proximal to the free border of the colon and left intact (Fig. 16-3). The proximal colon is then closed once more using a 30- or 60-mm linear stapler. The end of the

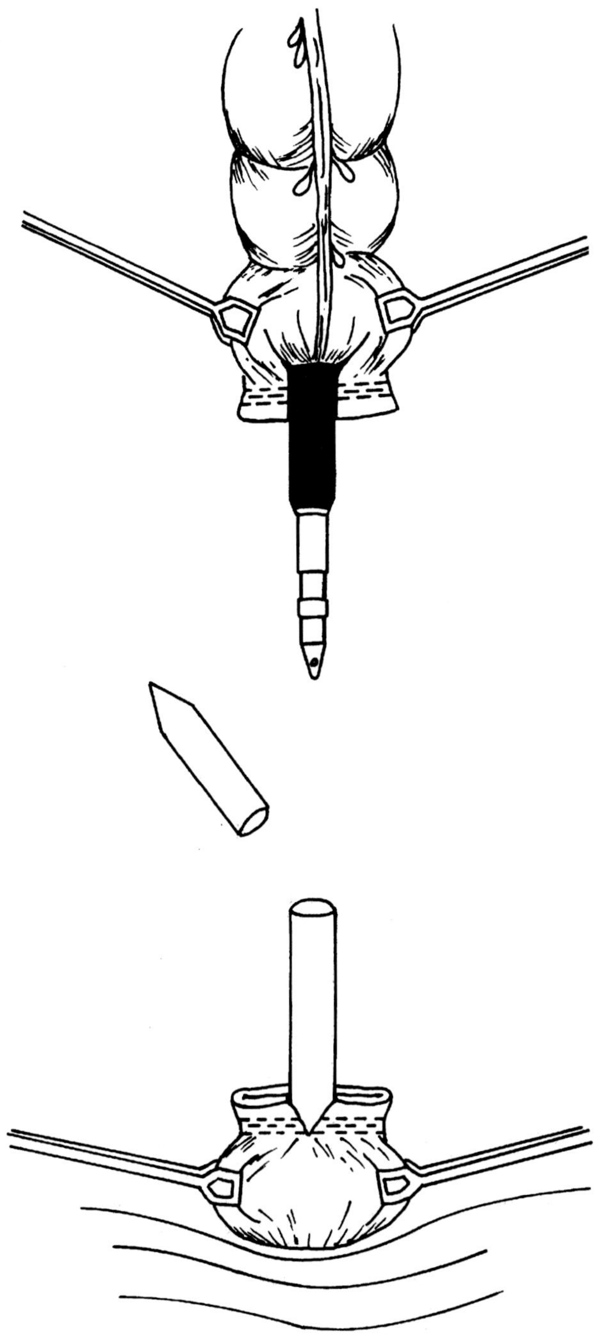

Fig. 16-3. Spike removed from CEEA circular stapler.

suture provides a pulley mechanism to retrieve the anvil and shaft of the stapler head. Tension on the exposed suture pulls the shaft up against the wall of the bowel. A small enterotomy is then made over the tented serosa, which is then pulled through the bowel wall ready for subsequent anastomosis.

The edges of the open distal rectum are grasped with two Babcock forceps, and the specimen is pushed through the rectum and delivered transanally. An operating sigmoidoscope may aid in grasping and subsequent delivery of the specimen. Particular care is taken to ensure easy passage of the resected colon in order to avoid damage to the rectal wall or sphincter mechanism. The rectum is then closed using a linear stapler passed through the suprapubic laparoscopic port.

The circular stapling instrument is then passed transanally to the level of the staple line in the rectum. The central spike is advanced through the stump of the rectum adjacent to the transverse staple line and then removed and delivered through one of the 12-mm ports (Fig. 16-4). The shaft of the instrument head is grasped by an endoscopic 10-mm Babcock clamp and reconnected to the stapler trocar. The instrument is closed and fired to give a circular triple stapled end-to-end anastomosis. The stapler is removed transanally and inspected for two complete doughnuts of tissue around the shaft.

CONCLUSION

Increasing availability of appropriate instrumentation and increasing technical facility have expanded the applications of these techniques. For the most part, recent reports of laparoscopic colectomy have concen-

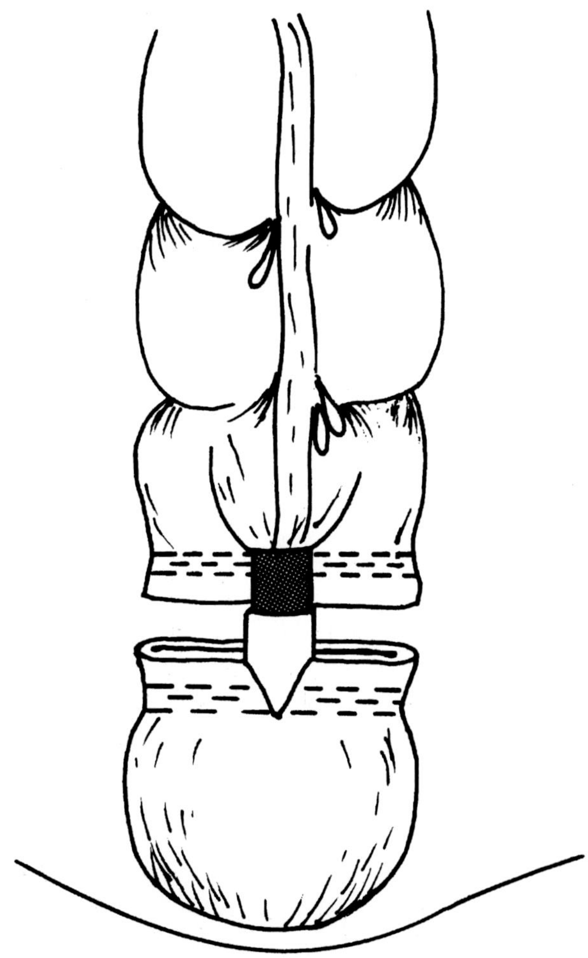

Fig. 16-4. Two ends of bowel approximated and the circular stapling device fired.

trated on laparoscopic assistance where the colon is mobilized laparoscopically, allowing the mesenteric vessels and bowel to be divided intracorporeally or extracorporeally.[1,2] A small incision is made where the specimen is delivered and the bowel is anastomosed extracorporeally. The technique reported here employs a total laparoscopic approach. As with all laparoscopic colonic procedures, it is essential that the dissection be carried out with the minimum of blood loss to prevent light absorption by hemoglobin and consequent loss of picture quality. Traditionally, this meticulous technique uses a considerable amount of coagulation diathermy. Recently, however, we have been concerned about anecdotal reports of ureteric injuries following laparoscopic colonic resection despite apparently successful identification at the time of surgery. We believe that ureteric injuries may be diathermy-related in the same way that the common bile duct may be at risk during cholecystectomy. Consequently, during the identification of the ureter, we use minimal diathermy to reduce the possibility of thermal injury.

Although technically attractive, the totally laparoscopic approach is really suitable for a minority of cases, such as diverticulitis, prolapse, or polyps. The role of this procedure in cases of malignancy must remain under evaluation. The potential for tumor implantation following transanal passage of the resected specimen must be a concern, especially in operations for curative resection. However, some patients with widespread metastatic disease and a small primary lesion in the left colon may benefit from such a procedure. Another question must concern the passage of bulky specimens through the rectum, whether benign or malignant, where this may lead to unnecessary long term-damage to sphincter function or, indeed, splitting of the rectal wall. At present, the ability to deliver the specimen in this way can only be finally assessed when delivery is actually attempted. Should this prove difficult because of the size of the lesion, it is currently our policy to abandon transanal delivery and remove the specimen through a small suprapubic abdominal incision. Despite these concerns, technical developments (e.g., protective sleeves) may resolve some of these issues, allowing the indications for this procedure to be extended.

REFERENCES

1. Monson JRT, Darzi A, Carey PD et al: Feasibility and preliminary results of laparoscopic-assisted colectomy in a prospective unselected groups of patients. Lancet 340:831, 1992
2. Schlinkert RT: Laparoscopic-assisted right hemicolectomy. Dis Colon Rectum 34:1030, 1991

Editorial Comment

Rama M. Jager

Sigmoid colectomy, either for benign disease such as a diverticular stricture or for a carcinoma, is a common operation in colorectal surgery. The laparoscopic approach is suitable not only to mobilize the sigmoid colon and mesocolon but also to resect and anastomose. Although right colonic anastomosis following laparoscopic resection is commonly done extracorporeally, left colonic anastomosis after laparoscopic resection can be done intracorporeally with the end-to-end circular anastomotic stapler.

Attention to details is essential. Positioning of the patient is important to use gravity-aided displacement of small bowel loops away from the sigmoid colon, mesocolon, and rectum. The patient can be positioned on a beanbag and rotated during the operation to displace the small loops to the right. The lower extremities should be positioned with minimal or no thigh flexion, avoiding locking of knees. Excessive thigh flexion may limit the freedom of instruments inserted through the lower quadrant ports.

Use of two monitors is optimal in a laparoscopic sigmoid colectomy. The left-sided monitor should be initially at knee level during the sigmoid dissection and moved cephalad during the dissection of the splenic flexure. This positioning avoids the problem of paradoxical movement during laparoscopic dissection. Space should be sufficient for a third monitor to view the colonoscopic image. The monitor for videocolonoscope is optimally placed to the left of the patient's shoulders for the right-handed colonoscopist. Use of the largest available operating room for laparoscopic procedures is helpful to fit multiple monitors.

It is imperative that the surgeon identify the location of the sigmoid lesion. Careful palpation with two endoscopic Babcock forceps (Fig. 16-5) at times locates the sigmoid mass. Small and soft sigmoid masses (villous adenomas and small cancers) cannot be palpated with this approach. Intraoperative colonoscopy may be necessary to locate the lesion to be resected.

The left ureter is the most vulnerable structure in the left lower quadrant of the abdomen that needs protection during laparoscopic sigmoid colectomy. Early identification of the left ureter and its protection against mechanical or electrical injury during laparoscopic mobilization

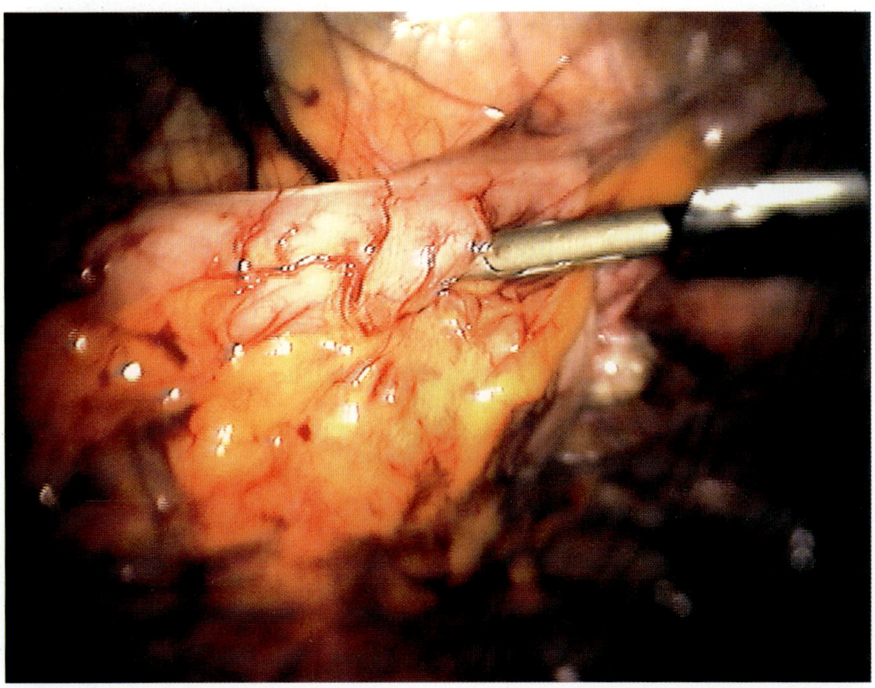

Fig. 16-5. Laparoscopic palpation of the sigmoid colon with two endoscopic Babcock forceps.

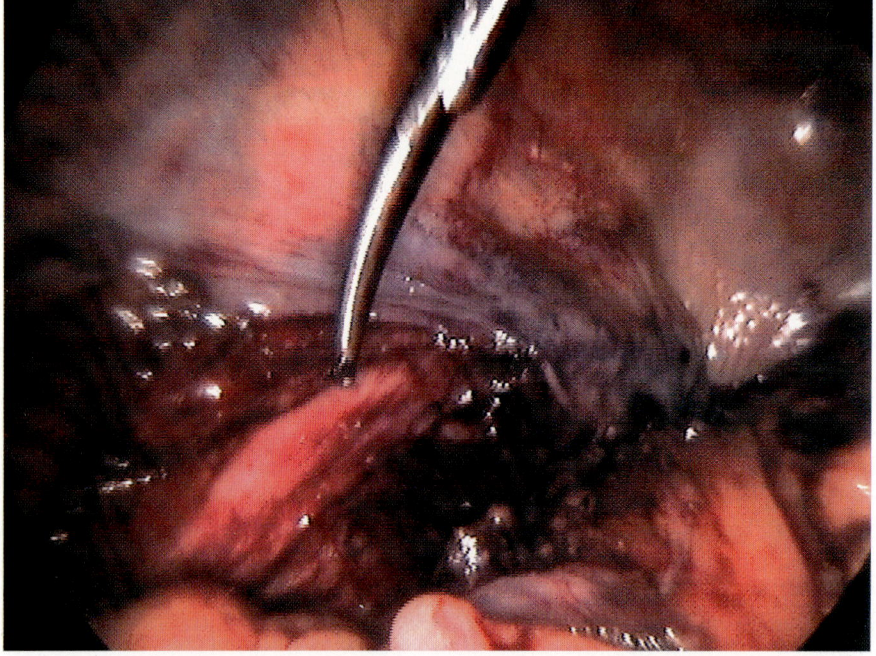

Fig. 16-6. Laparoscopic identification of left ureter.

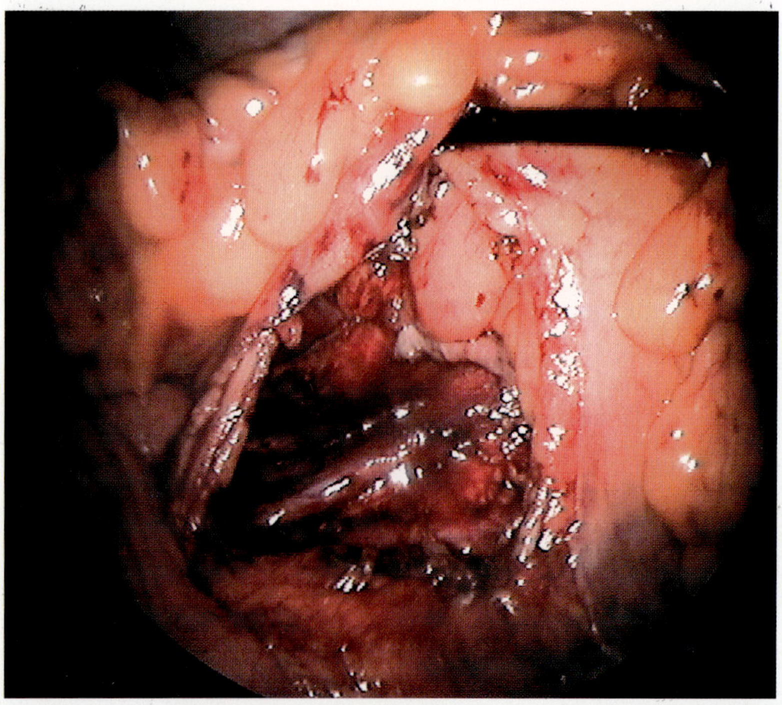

Fig. 16-7. Left ureter placed in direct view during sigmoid mobilization.

are essential (Fig. 16-6). The laparoscopic surgeon does not have the advantage of palpating the ureter or the ureterovesical junction to confirm ureteral identification. The surgeon has to rely on the anatomic location and ureteral peristalsis to locate and protect the ureter. The dissection around the ureter should be done with the least amount of monopolar electrosurgery possible to avoid electrical tissue injury to the ureter, which may manifest postoperatively as a ureteral stricture. The bipolar electrocoagulation is preferred to monopolar electrosurgical instruments to coagulate any bleeding in the ureteral vicinity. The placement of ureteral stents, illuminated or nonilluminated, is not necessary unless the patient has diverticular phlegmon or colovesical fistula, which may make ureteral dissection bloody and ureteral protection difficult. The left ureter should be visualized periodically during the sigmoid mesocolic dissection to avoid injury (Fig. 16-7).

The dissection to the left of the sigmoid colon is initially limited to identification and exposure of the left ureter. Although the camera and dissecting instruments are poised for left paracolic and left pararectal dissection, an extensive initial dissection to the left of sigmoid colon and mesocolon may create problems with bleeding. This bleeding can interfere with further dissection of the right leaf of mesocolon and mesorectum. Liberal use of suction-irrigation with heparin-containing (1,000 U/L) solutions is necessary to ensure proper identification of tissue planes if the right-sided mesocolic or mesorectal dissection produces more than the usual amount of bleeding. Using the 30-degree rather than 0-degree laparoscope may be helpful in some patients. By rotating the laparoscope axially and keeping the same camera orientation, the surgeon can view the operative field from different angles and choose the optimum view for safe dissection.

The sacral promontory serves as a laparoscopically palpable landmark during the pararectal dissection. This landmark also helps to decide the optimal distal margin of resection. As it is with the open resection of sigmoid diverticulitis, rectal transection should be at or below the sacral promontory to reduce the problem of recurrent diverticulitis.

As Drs. Monson and Darzi point out, the surgeon should be aware of the problems of tumor seeding and anal sphincteric dilation during transanal specimen retrieval. The placement of the resected specimen in a plastic bag helps reduce the problem of seeding. Whether the specimen is retrieved transanally or through a small muscle-splitting, suprapubic, or left lower quadrant abdominal incision depends on the size of the surgical specimen. When in doubt, a small abdominal incision enables safe specimen retrieval. A 4-cm abdominal wall incision will also help anchoring of the anvil in the descending colon and permit specimen retrieval. Although it is attractive to conduct sigmoid colectomy totally laparoscopically, a small abdominal incision may facilitate a swift and safe operation without adding significantly to the postoperative morbidity.

17

Laparoscopic Abdominoperineal Proctosigmoidectomy

John R. T. Monson and Ara Darzi

The widespread success of laparoscopic cholecystectomy has led to the development of a wide range of laparoscopic surgical procedures such as hernia repair,[1,2] vagotomy,[3] hysterectomy,[4] and Nissen fundoplication.[5] The most recent addition to the list of procedures that can be undertaken by a minimally invasive approach is laparoscopic colectomy.[6,7] The development of endoscopic procedures for malignant disease not only involves considerable technical refinement but ultimately must also be accompanied by the facility to remove a malignant tumor in a surgically acceptable fashion in comparison with standard open colectomy.

We report our experience of a laparoscopic-guided abdominoperineal resection of the rectum.

OPERATIVE TECHNIQUE

The surgeon stands on the left side of the patient; two video screens are positioned on either side of the knees (Fig. 17-1). Three 12-mm trocars are introduced into the abdomen to facilitate use of the laparoscopic stapling instruments (Fig. 17-2).

Retraction

Initially, the camera is placed through the umbilical port. A Babcock forceps is passed through the left iliac fossa port, pulling the sigmoid colon in a cephalad direction and to the left. After identifying the ureter, the peritoneum on the right side of the sigmoid mesentery is divided; two windows are created in the sigmoid mesentery on either side of the mesenteric vessels to facilitate division of the mesenteric vessels with the linear stapler. Care must be taken to ensure that no additional structures are included in the jaws of this instrument at the time of division.

Mobilization

After the inferior mesenteric vessels have been divided, the camera is moved to the right iliac fossa port, and the Babcock forceps is passed through the left iliac fossa port, holding the rectosigmoid junction upward and to the left. A second Babcock grasping instrument is passed suprapubically to elevate the middle third of the rectum, providing tension on the peritoneal reflection on the right side of the rectosigmoid junction. The peritoneal reflection is divided by using EndoSciz hook scissors (United States Surgical Corporation, Norwalk, CT). By careful dissection, the avascular plane between the fascial capsule of the rectum anteriorly and the fascia of Waldeyer posteriorly is exposed.

Division of the lateral ligaments is easily performed under direct vision using simple diathermy or between titanium clips. Posteriorly, the pelvic nerves are identified and preserved, and the mesorectum is completely excised. Close and magnified views of the mesorectum ensure the correct planes of dissection with minimal bleeding. In a woman, dissection in the pouch of Douglas is facilitated by holding the cervix upward with a blunt Hulka cervical forceps (Rockett Ltd., Watford, UK) or by an assistant's fingers held through the vagina. This elevates the cervix and body of the uterus. As mobilization proceeds toward the pelvic floor, an assistant's finger in the vagina aids elevation of the vagina and thus dissection of the rectum from the vagina. Most of the rectal mobilization is completed from this right-sided approach, starting on the right lateral aspect around posteriorly and up to the left side. This leaves a small amount of dissection to be completed on the left pelvic wall, which is approached directly from the left side of the rectum.

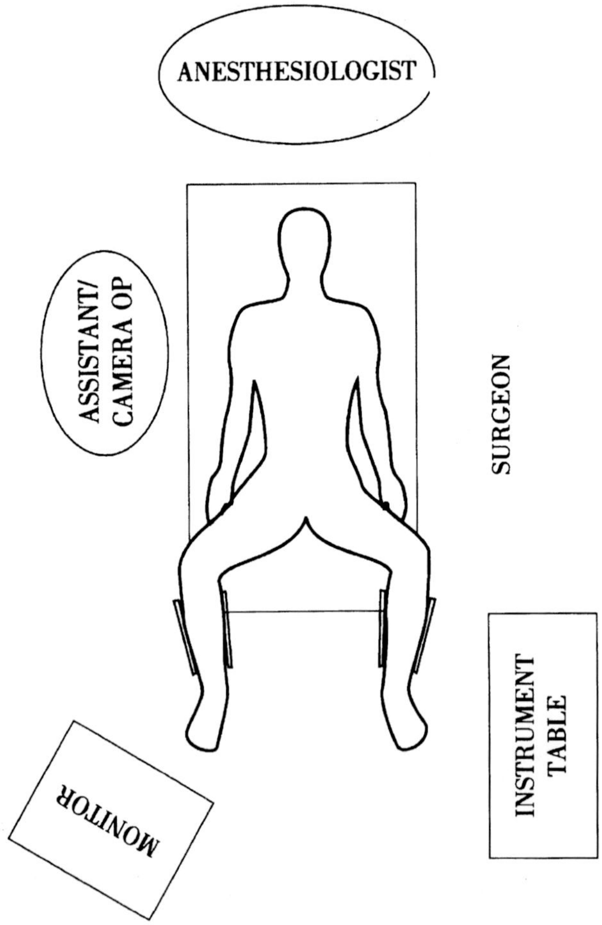

Fig. 17-1. Theater setup.

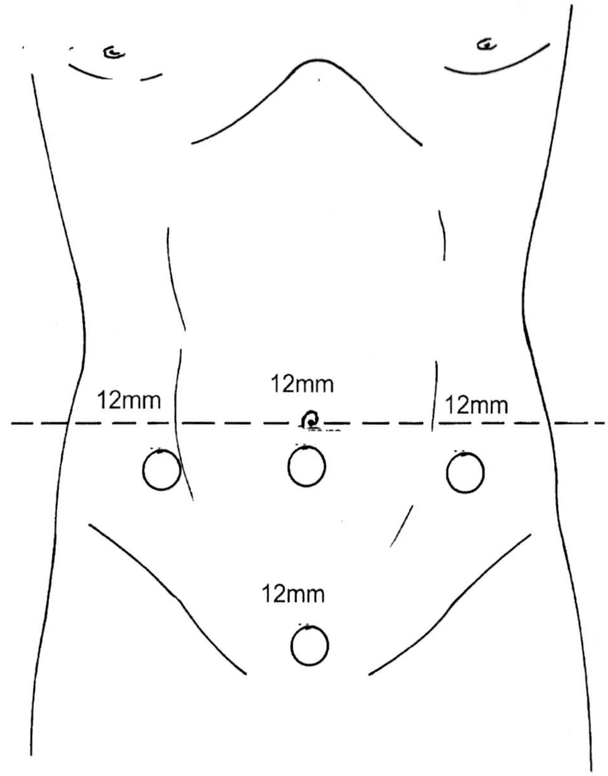

Fig. 17-2. Port positioning.

Perineal Phase

Having completed most of the dissection laparoscopically, the perineal phase of the operation is commenced in a standard manner. Division of the skin and subcutaneous fat allows a window to be made posteriorly in Waldeyer's fascia by laparoscopically cutting down under direct vision onto the perineal operators fingers. The finger is left in place to maintain pneumoperitoneum, while the left colon is transected by using a linear stapler in preparation for removal of the specimen. The remainder of the perineal dissection is completed, and the specimen is delivered through the perineal wound. An end colostomy is fashioned by bringing the colon out through the left iliac fossa trocar site. Two suction drains are inserted through the perineum, and the perineal incision is closed in layers.

CONCLUSION

Laparoscopic surgery has already revolutionized the practice of biliary surgery and seems likely to have an increasing impact on surgical techniques.[8] As instrumentation becomes more readily available and increasingly sophisticated, the range of procedures attempted will inevitably increase.

Our initial experience in laparoscopic colectomy confirms that this operation is technically feasible in most patients. The considerable reduction in postoperative pain has led to rapid patient recovery with an attendant decrease in complications such as chest and, particularly, wound infections. However, for most colorectal excisions, the technique of laparoscope assistance is employed with delivery of the resected specimen through a greatly reduced abdominal incision.

In abdominoperineal resection of the rectum, an abdominal incision is completely avoided. The resulting left iliac fossa colostomy is brought out through a 12-mm trocar site. Consequently, the procedure can be termed truly laparoscopic.

Although long-term follow-up is required to address the issue of local cancer recurrence, we believe that the view provided in the pelvis by laparoscopy is significantly better than at laparotomy and allows excellent anatomic definition and meticulous dissection. This would suggest that the ability to perform a radical clearance of tumor in cases of malignancy is surgeon-dependent rather than a factor of the surgical approach. However, we emphasize that longer follow-up is required before this contention could be substantiated.

The view suggested by Wickham et al,[9] "as iatrogenic trauma declines so therapeutic success increases," has clearly been demonstrated in this case with early mobilization and reduced postoperative discomfort. We believe that, as laparoscopic technology advances and surgical expertise is gained, this minimally invasive approach will soon have a major impact on the practice of colon surgery.

REFERENCES

1. Nyhus LM: Laparoscopic hernia repair: a point of view. Arch Surg 127:137, 1992
2. Paget GW: Laparoscopic repair of inguinal hernia. Med J Aust 156:508, 1992
3. Katkhouda N, Mouiel J: A new technique of surgical treatment of chronic duodenal ulcer without laparotomy by videocelioscopy. Am J Surg 161:361, 1991
4. Nezhat CR, Burrell MO, Nezhat FR et al: Laparoscopic radical hysterectomy with para-aortic and pelvic node dissection. Am J Obstet Gynecol 166:864, 1992
5. Cuschieri A, Shimi S, Nathanson LK: Laparoscopic reduction, crural repair, and fundoplication of large hiatal hernia. Am J Surg 163:425, 1992
6. Schlinkert RT: Laparoscopic-assisted right hemicolectomy. Dis Colon Rectum 34:1030, 1991
7. Monson JRT, Darzi A, Carey PD et al: Prospective evaluation of laparoscopic-assisted colectomy in an unselected group of patients. Lancet 340:831, 1992
8. Tompkins RK: Laparoscopic cholecystectomy: threat or opportunity? Arch Surg 125:1245, 1990
9. Wickham JEA: Minimally invasive therapy, editorial. 1:1, 1991

Editorial Comment I

Ferdinand Koeckerling

In recent years, abdominoperineal excision of the rectum for rectal carcinoma has increasingly been replaced by sphincter-preserving techniques. The use of the circular stapler has now made it possible to create reliable anastomoses in the region of the pelvic floor. The technique of intersphincteric rectal resection with transanal anastomosis permits the treatment of a carcinoma located at a distance of 4 to 5 cm from the anal verge and not invading the perirectal tissue while preserving the sphincter. By complying with certain selection criteria, it is possible to treat early-stage (pT1, pT2 inner layer of the muscularis propria) rectal carcinomas curatively by transanal full-thickness excision, while preserving the sphincter. By employing this differential therapeutic approach, the rate of abdominoperineal excisions of the rectum for low rectal carcinomas has been reduced to 10 to 15 percent.

In curative surgery of rectal carcinoma, including all resections performed above and below the peritoneal reflection, the incidence of metastasis to the lymph nodes along the trunk of the inferior mesenteric artery is 3 percent of all patients and 6.5 percent of all patients with confirmed lymph node metastasis. In view of this fact, since 1980, in many centers, the inferior mesenteric artery is routinely ligated before resection of the sigmoid or rectum, or rectal amputation. We, with Drs. Monson and Darzi, consider routine division of the inferior mesenteric artery trunk to be a necessary prior step in the laparoscopic abdominoperineal excision of the rectum. On the basis of our experience to date, we believe that this procedure can be reliably performed using laparoscopic linear cutters or PDS clips.

As is the case with extended lymph node dissection, pelvic dissection and the creation of a colostomy can also readily be carried out as a laparoscopic procedure. The frequently expressed oncologic reservations about laparoscopic colorectal procedures are less relevant to abdominoperineal excision of the rectum, because the essential part of the oncologic operation is done in the standard manner via a perineal access. The strict selection criteria for rectal excision (i.e., exclusively for very low malignant lesions) means that the laparoscopic pelvic dissection is carried out largely above the level of the tumor. Like Drs. Monson and Darzi, we also find that the view low down in the pelvis is even better with the laparoscope than with conventional surgery and that the relevant anatomic planes and structures can be more accurately dissected in the fascial planes. With appropriate experience, mobilization of the rectum in the relevant anatomic planes can be effected down to the floor of the pelvis. Improvements in technique and further development of the instrumentation will help facilitate these demanding surgical steps.

Technical feasibility, however, tells us little about the oncologic quality of the operation. We also emphasize the need for clinical studies on the long-term results of laparoscopic abdominoperineal excision of the rectum to treat low rectal carcinoma. In prospective, randomized multicenter studies, the technical feasibility, postoperative course, and long-term results of the laparoscopic excision of the rectum should be compared with those achieved with the standard surgical procedure for low carcinomas. American and European multicenter studies aimed at providing answers to these questions are presently being designed and conducted.

Editorial Comment II

Rama M. Jager

The laparoscopic approach is especially suitable for abdominoperineal resection because the perineal incision serves to remove the resected surgical specimen. Laparoscopic visualization of presacral space is superior to that obtained during the open technique. Oncosurgical equivalency or superiority of the laparoscopic technique over the conventional open technique is yet to be proved, although many surgeons (including Drs. Monson and Darzi) submit its feasibility and probable equivalency to the open technique.

Like every other laparoscopic procedure, positioning of the patient is an important technical detail. The patient can usually be placed in a modified dorsolithotomy Trendelenburg's position, with little to no thigh flexion. A beanbag under the table stabilizes the patient and allows a steep Trendelenburg's position. The beanbag should not extend below the patient's coccyx so that the perineal dissection can be done with little interference.

There is no single optimal port placement for the laparoscopic abdominoperineal resection. This chapter enunciates the usual principles of port placement (also detailed in Ch. 8). A few suggestions follow. One port should be placed at the site of colostomy to avoid an extra incision. The surgeon should keep a satisfactory distance between the ports to avert intraperitoneal or external interference during dissection. The angle between the axis of the camera port and the dissecting instrument port should be reduced to prevent paradoxical movement from reversal of video images. Until the surgeon establishes an optimal port pattern, use of 12-mm ports at all sites enables use of an endoscopic stapler through all the port sites. The surgeon should not hesitate to exchange sides with the assistant and to shuffle the camera to different ports as needed. The 30-degree scope allows different views of the operating field so that the surgeon can choose the optimal view.

Identification of the left ureter is essential before any further laparoscopic dissection (Fig. 17-3). As Drs. Monson and Darzi appropriately point out, use of monopolar coagulation in the ureteral vicinity should be limited to reduce electrical injury and consequent

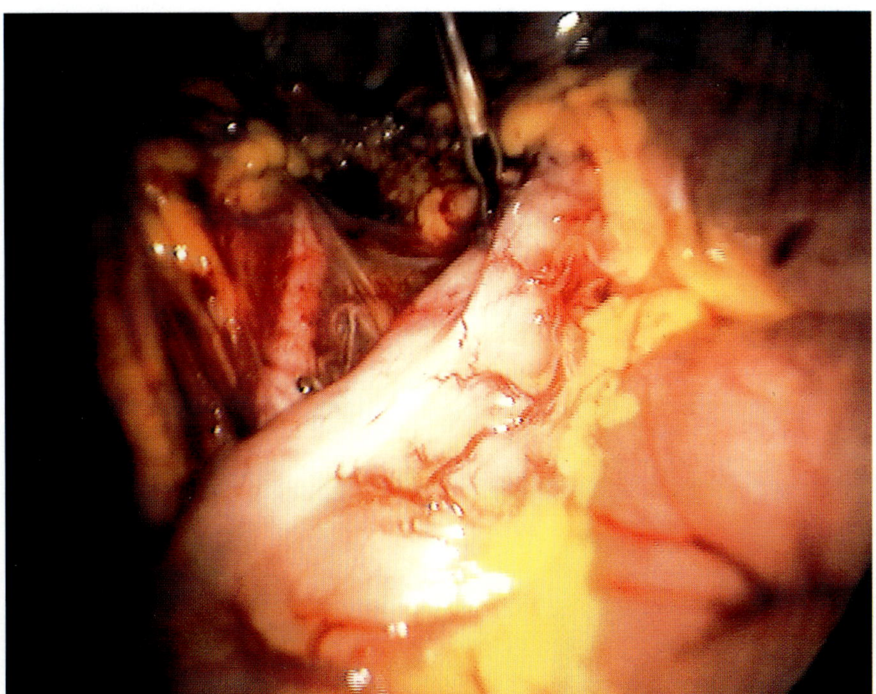

Fig. 17-3. Forceps medially retracting the sigmoid colon and exposing the left ureter.

ureteral stenosis. Bipolar coagulation can be useful if the surgeon encounters bleeding near the left ureter. The right ureter can be identified more easily than the left ureter and rarely suffers from the same vulnerability because of its anatomic location.

The other vital structures near the sacral promontory that are vulnerable to injury during laparoscopic dissection include the left common iliac vein. In a steep Trendelenburg's position, the vein may not be prominent for easy identification. In a thin patient, careful reflexion of the peritoneum medial to and covering the iliac vessels prevents venous laceration. Having a second instrument table containing the instruments for laparotomy and vascular repair may be helpful in the uncommon event of left iliac vascular injury during laparoscopic dissection.

The right pararectal dissection can be done well even with the patient tilted to the right. The surgeon should dissect the right side of the mesorectum and the right lateral stalk initially before embarking on dissection of the left side. This technique prevents problems with bleeding from left pararectal dissection gravitating to the right side, interfering with the dissection when the patient is tilted to the right. Similarly, the dissection should be started as far inferior as possible and continued craniad to avoid problems with pooled blood in the pelvis.

The perineal phase of the operation may need adjustment of the lithotomy position by increasing the thigh flexion. It is difficult to do perineal dissection with little or no thigh flexion. I place my patients in a supine position initially, changing the posture to lithotomy after completion of the laparoscopic dissection, sigmoid transection, and colostomy. The ports can be left in, the patient's position changed to lithotomy, and the abdomen redraped. This allows proper positioning of the patient for rapid perineal dissection. With this approach, the surgeon can prevent prolonged lithotomy positioning with its resultant complications and also allow laparoscopic visualization while the perineal surgeon is operating. The laparoscope-guided illumination of the pelvis will help the perineal surgeon to control bleeding in deep pelvic fossa during the perineal dissection.

The laparoscopic approach does not replace the conventional approach to an abdominoperineal resection. Obesity is a relative contraindication because of the prohibitively prolonged operating times for laparoscopic dissection. When rectal cancer invades adjacent viscera such as the levatores ani, proper delineation of the invasion is not laparoscopically feasible. In these patients, the tactile limitations render a safe and satisfactory laparoscopic dissection difficult and tedious. By contrast, initial diagnostic laparoscopy to determine the laparoscopic resectability can be done in all patients with minimal risk and expenditure of time. Diagnostic laparoscopy is converted to therapeutic laparoscopic abdominoperineal resection, in appropriate patients, depending on the operative findings.

18

Laparoscopic Restorative Proctocolectomy

Stephen M. Cohen and Steven D. Wexner

The laparoscope has evolved from a simple tool used by the gynecologist for the evaluation of pelvic disorders to a leading instrument applied to therapeutic intervention in all fields of surgery. Much of the demand for minimally invasive surgery has been both patient as well as market driven. The claims of less pain, shorter hospitalization, and improved long-term cosmetic result may obfuscate the patient's concern with cure of disease. As this patient demand increases, the natural progression is to evaluate more complex intra-abdominal conditions in which the laparoscope can be effectively used.

Several surgical alternatives are available for the patient with either mucosal ulcerative colitis or familial polyposis.[1] The most popular continence-preserving option is the ileoanal reservoir procedure (IAR). The procedure consists of a total abdominal colectomy, proctectomy with or without a mucosectomy, and creation of an ileal reservoir with ileal pouch–anal anastomosis. Since its introduction, the IAR has increased in popularity and has become the most common definitive operation for mucosal ulcerative colitis.[2] Because most of these patients are young, cosmesis may play a significant role in their willingness to undergo surgery.

TECHNIQUE

Preoperative preparation is similar to that used for an open procedure.[3] Consent is obtained from all patients for a formal laparotomy. Patients are given a mechanical bowel preparation with both parenteral and oral antibiotics before the operation. After the induction of general endotracheal anesthesia, a nasogastric tube and an in-dwelling bladder catheter are placed to minimize the risk of trocar injury to the stomach and bladder, respectively. The patient is placed in the supine modified lithotomy position in Allen stirrups (Allen Medical, Bedford Heights, OH). The hips and knees should each be flexed no more than 15 percent; greater flexion will hamper instrument movement. This position allows more flexibility for the surgeon, assistant, and camera operator.

The abdomen is prepared and draped in the standard fashion to provide wide exposure. The patient is then placed in a steep Trendelenburg's position, and a 1-cm transverse incision is made above or below the umbilicus. The Veress needle is introduced, and correct placement is verified in four ways. First, the surgeon should have a manual tactile sense that the needle has entered the peritoneal cavity. Second, an audible noise should be appreciated as the needle enters the abdominal cavity. Third, a few milliliters of sterile water are placed on top of the vertically held needle conus. By lifting the anterior abdominal wall, the surgeon creates negative intra-abdominal pressure, and the liquid is drawn into the abdominal cavity. Finally, high-flow insufflation should result in a gradual rise in the intra-abdominal pressure. A rapid rise in pressure or the appearance of subcutaneous crepitus indicates preperitoneal needle placement. After pneumoperitoneum is established with carbon dioxide to a pressure of 15 mm Hg, the Veress needle is removed and a 10/12-mm trocar is placed through this infraumbilical port site. The camera is then introduced through the port, and all subsequent work is undertaken under direct endoscopic visualization.

The selection of port sites depends on both the patient's body habitus and the type of resection. An example of standard port site placement is shown in Figure 18-1. In general, it is important that ports be close enough to one another so that instruments can reach the operative field with ease and aid in traction,

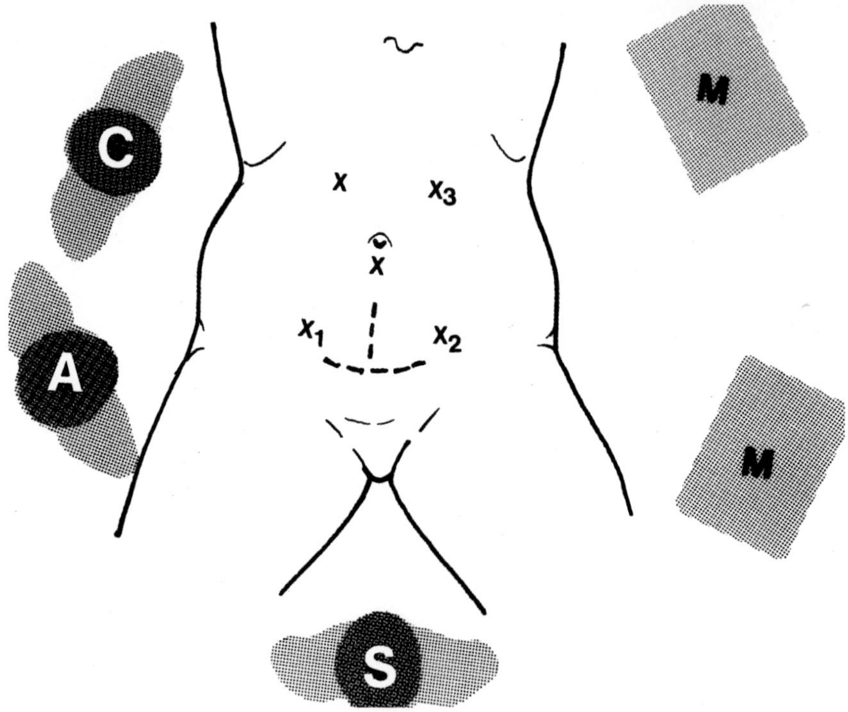

Fig. 18-1. Standard port site placement. (From Wexner et al,[9] with permission.)

yet not so close as to cause interference of the instruments with each other. If future incisions are planned, such as for a drain or stoma, an attempt should be made to place the ports in these locations. Similarly, ports can be situated at such positions to allow substitution of a larger port or creation of a small incision for specimen removal. Alternatively, ports can be placed on either side of what will eventually be the incision. Thus, many factors affect port site placement, including ease of dissection, creation of anastomosis, specimen retrieval, and the need for stomas or drains. It is important to note that all ports should be at least 10 mm in diameter for laparoscopic intestinal surgery for two reasons. First, unlike the gallbladder, the target organ is not fixed or localized, and thus, the camera and all instruments must be able to be used in all ports. In laparoscopic intestinal surgery, both the camera and the instruments frequently need to be repositioned to ensure adequate visualization around the colon and rectum. Hence, the use of all 10-mm ports ensures maximal flexibility. Second, to markedly decrease the size of a Kocher cholecystectomy incision, the ports used for laparoscopic cholecystectomy must be as few in number and as small in diameter as possible. This feature is critical because a Kocher incision is often only 8 to 10 cm in length. However, an appreciable reduction from a standard 25- to 30-cm midline incision can be realized even after the introduction of five or more 10/12-mm ports.

Before attempting mobilization, a thorough and complete inspection of the abdominal cavity should be performed as in open surgery. All abdominal wall adhesions are lysed to allow safe placement of subsequent trocars. Adhesiolysis is best accomplished by a combination of traction and division with sharp dissection and electrocautery. There are many advantages of the monopolar cautery as compared with laser for laparoscopic colectomy, including greater operator familiarity with cautery, much lower overall costs, and less equipment in an already crowded operating suite. Furthermore, the potential for inadvertent injury resulting from uncontrolled depth of penetration is a major disadvantage of the laser.

It is of paramount importance to remember that table positioning can facilitate the retraction of loops of bowel from the operative field. For example, when mobilizing the sigmoid colon, placing the table in Trendelenburg's position with a tilt to the right can help to keep the small bowel loops away from the pelvis. Similarly, when mobilizing the hepatic flexure, the reverse Trendelenburg position and a table tilt to the left can be most helpful. If further retraction is needed, an assistant can insert a laparoscopic retractor through one of the previously placed ports. It also may be necessary to add additional ports to aid retraction. We prefer a fluid state of port introduction rather than synchronous placement of a set number of ports. Differences in patient anatomy and disease status make this situation analogous to enlargement of a laparotomy incision during an open case.

Mobilization of the colon from the retroperitoneum is accomplished by grasping the colon with specially designed noncrushing intestinal clamps and retracting in a medial direction, thus exposing the white line of Toldt. This avascular plane can then be divided with a combination of blunt and sharp dissection; electrocautery is used for both dissection and hemostasis. If larger vessels are encountered at the flexures, ligation is with either surgical clips or endoloops.

After the colon has been mobilized as completely and as safely as possible, the abdomen can be opened through a true Pfannenstiel incision, incorporating the two lowest port sites. The colon can be delivered through the incision and the mesentery divided (Fig. 18-2). The remainder of the procedure (proctectomy, formation of ileal J-pouch, and ileal pouch–anal anastomosis) is performed under direct vision in the standard fashion. The loop ileostomy can be delivered through the right iliac fossa port. The pelvic drain is brought either through the paraumbilical or the left iliac fossa port. The immediate and final postoperative appearances are shown in Figures 18-3 and 18-4, respectively.

RESULTS

Schmitt and co-workers[4] reported on 22 patients who underwent laparoscopic-assisted ileal pouch–anal anastomosis (LAC). The diagnosis in these 22 patients included mucosal ulcerative colitis (MUC) in 16, familial adenomatous polyposis (FAP) in 5, and juvenile polyposis in 1. These patients were compared with 20 age-, sex-, and diagnosis-matched controls (SC) who underwent restorative proctocolectomy using a standard midline incision. The length of ileus was similar in both groups. The mean time to resolution of ileus was 4.3 days (range 4 to 11 days) in the LAC group and 3.3 days (range 2 to 5 days) in the SC group. The mean time until oral intake was 3.6 days (range 0 to 7 days) in the LAC group and 4.3 days (range 3 to 8 days) in the SC group. In analyzing the length of hospitalization, again, the groups were similar. The mean length of hospitalization was 8.7 days (range 7 to 13 days) in the LAC group and 8.9 days (range 6 to 18 days) in the SC group (Table 18-1). However, a difference was noted between the two groups with respect to the length of the operation. The mean length of operation in the LAC group was 4 hours (range 2 to 5.5 hours), while the mean length in the SC group was 2 hours (range 2 to 5 hours). It is interesting that the ranges, however, were basically identical, highlighting that the surgeon is apt to encounter both easy and difficult cases regardless of the surgical modality used. Intraoperative or postoperative transfusion was required in 16 of the LAC patients (73 percent) and in only 7 of the SC patients (35 percent) ($P<0.05$). However, the mean number of transfusions in each group was 2 (LAC, range 1 to 15, and SC, range 2 to 5). These patients were not stratified for either preoperative hemoglobin or steroid dose. This result mirrors that reported by Peters and Bartels.[5] Their group measured both preoperative and 24-hour postoperative hemoglobin levels as an indirect indicator of operative blood loss. They demonstrated no statistically significant difference between the two groups, although they observed a trend toward a greater fall in the laparoscopic group (more intraoperative blood loss

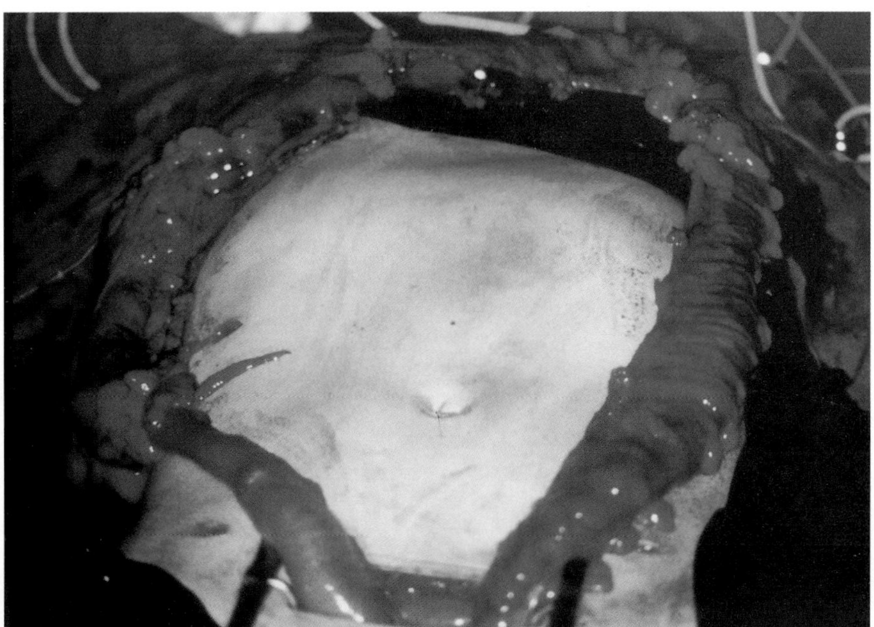

Fig. 18-2. Colon delivered through the incision and the mesentery divided. (From Schmitt et al,[4] with permission.)

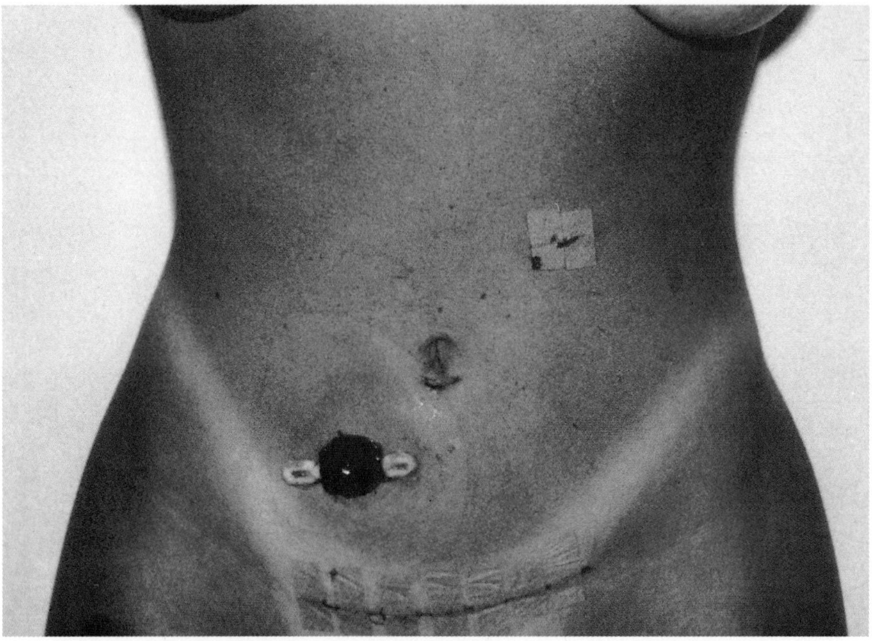

Fig. 18-3. Immediate postoperative appearance.

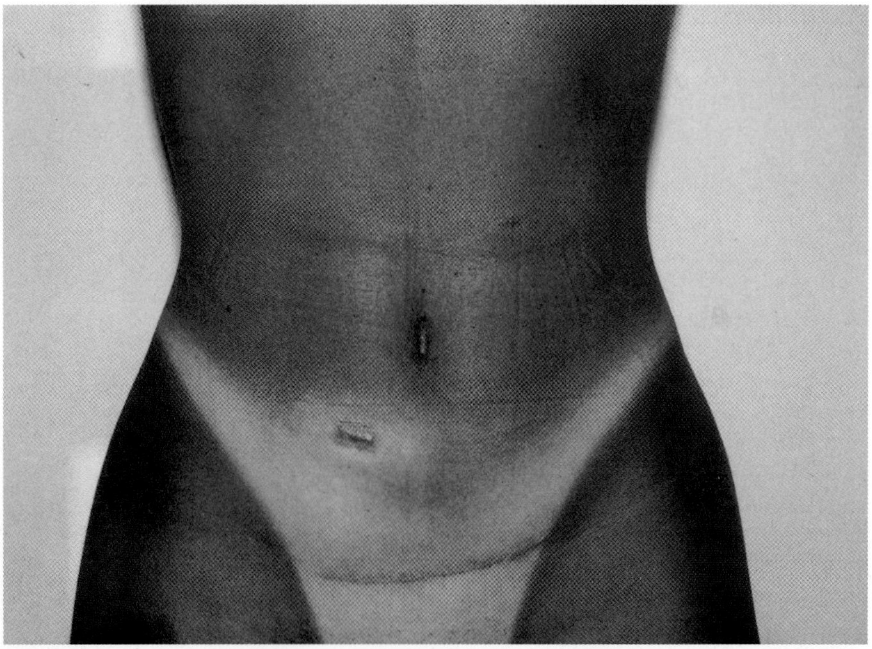

Fig. 18-4. Final postoperative appearance. (From Schmitt et al,[4] with permission.)

Table 18-1. Comparison of Time Parameters[a]

	Laparoscopic-Assisted (N = 22)		Standard Open Procedure (N = 20)	
Mean length of ileus (days)	4.2	(4–11)	3.3	(2–5)
Mean time until oral intake (days)	3.6	(0–7)	4.3	(3–8)
Mean length of hospitalization (days)	8.7	(7–13)	8.9	(6–18)

[a]Numbers in parentheses are the range.

Table 18-2. Comparison of Postoperative Morbidity and Mortality[a]

	Laparoscopic-Assisted (N = 22)	Standard Open Procedure (N = 20)
Morbidity		
Ileus	7 (32)	4 (20)
Urinary infection	2 (9)	0
Wound infection	3 (14)	1 (5)
Deep venous thrombosis	0	1 (5)
Arrhythmia	0	1 (5)
Line sepsis	2 (9)	0
Reoperation	1 (5)	0
Total	15 (69)	7 (35)
Mortality	0	0

[a]Numbers in parentheses are the percentage.

using the laparoscope). Thus, the only two studies that have quantified blood loss have documented a higher loss with laparoscopic than with open surgery. These data refute the subjective claims made by the others.[6]

Although no postoperative mortality occurred, 12 of the 22 (55 percent) LAC patients and 6 of the 20 (30 percent) SC patients experienced postoperative morbidity (Table 18-2) ($P < 0.05$). The two most common complications were ileus and wound infection. One patient in the LAC group required reoperation in the immediate postoperative period because of intra-abdominal hemorrhage. This incidence of complications is much higher than that seen in patients who have undergone segmental colectomy.[7,8]

In our first published prospective comparison of laparoscopic restorative proctocolectomy with standard controls, we found no significant differences in the length of ileus, time until oral intake, or time to hospital discharge.[9]

As more experience is gained with the use of the laparoscope, surgeons will continue to attempt larger and more complicated procedures. However, enthusiasm must be tempered with reality. Specifically, failure to adhere to basic proven surgical tenets to facilitate inadequate or cumbersome technology is unacceptable. We must continue to evaluate the parameters in a meaningful prospective fashion to perform the necessary statistical evaluations needed to decide what role laparoscopic colon surgery will have in our future armamentarium.

REFERENCES

1. Gemlo BT, Goldberg SM: Choice of surgical procedure for chronic ulcerative colitis. In Telander RL, Nyhus LM (eds): Problems in General Surgery. JB Lippincott, Philadelphia, 1993
2. Kelly KA: Anal sphincter saving operations for chronic ulcerative colitis. Am J Surg 163:5, 1992
3. Wexner SD, Beck DE: Sepsis prevention in colorectal surgery. p. 41. In Fielding LP, Goldberg SM (eds): Operative Surgery: Colon, Rectum, and Anus. 5th Ed. Butterworth Heinemann, London, 1993
4. Schmitt SL, Cohen SM, Wexner SD et al: Does laparoscopic-assisted ileal pouch anal anastomosis reduce the length of hospitalization? Int J Colorectal Dis 9:134, 1994
5. Peters WR, Bartels TL: Minimally invasive colectomy: are the potential benefits realized? Dis Colon Rectum 36:751, 1993
6. Senagore AJ, Luchtefeld MA, Macheigan JM et al: Open colectomy versus laparoscopic colectomy: are there differences? Am Surg 59:549, 1993
7. Reissman P, Wexner SD, Cohen SM et al: Complications of laparoscopic colorectal surgery, abstracted. Surg Endosc 8:562, 1994
8. Wexner SD, Cohen SM, Johansen OB et al: Laparoscopic colorectal surgery: a prospective assessment and current perspective. Br J Surg 80:1602, 1993
9. Wexner SD, Johansen OB, Nogueras JJ, Jagelman DG: Laparoscopic total abdominal colectomy: a prospective trial. Dis Colon Rectum 35:651, 1992

Editorial Comment

Rama M. Jager

Proper positioning promotes rapid and safe laparoscopic dissection by displacing small bowel loops away from the colon and the mesocolon. Because the dissection involves various segments of the colon, the operating table may be placed in steep Trendelenburg's and reverse Trendelenburg's positions, depending on the flexure being dissected. Also, "airplaning" to the left or right is also helpful. Beanbag placement under the patient will stabilize the patient during these positional changes. A beanbag should be positioned in a way that does not interfere with the perineal portion of the operation.

As Drs. Cohen and Wexner point out, there is no single optimal pattern for port placement. Ports larger than 10 mm permit interchangeable use of all the ports for camera, dissecting instrument, and stapler use. All the ports need not be large. A 5-mm port a few centimeters above and a second 5-mm port below the umbilical camera port are useful to introduce the electrosurgical scissors for mobilization of the colonic flexures. In contrast to the usual dictum to keep ports apart to prevent fencing, these 5-mm ports for dissection can be close to the umbilical camera port. The dissecting instrument usually travels parallel to the camera port and rarely at an acute angle. A dissecting port on either side of the camera port is optimal for dissection because the surgeon has to change sides depending on the flexure being mobilized.

Whether the laparoscopic approach to restorative proctocolectomy is superior to the standard open technique is unknown. Drs. Cohen and Wexner's experience with their laparoscopic technique shows no specific advantage with the new approach compared with their historical controls. Further randomized clinical trials—as well as retrospective comparative clinical observation using the age-, sex-, body habitus-, and disease-matched historical controls—will help us understand whether the laparoscopic approach is the treatment of choice or another approach to total abdominoperineal restorative proctocolectomy.

The laparoscopic approach to proctocolectomy requires a separate abdominal incision for specimen retrieval, mesocolic transection, and pouch construction. The length and type of this incision dictate the degree of postoperative morbidity. One surgeon may resect the colon, free the rectum, and construct the pouch through a 6-cm incision. A different surgeon or the same surgeon in a different patient may need a 12-cm incision to accomplish the same objective. The patient's body habitus affects the choice and advantages of different methods of peritoneal access. For example, an extremely obese patient may need a long extension of the midline incision toward the xiphisternum to free the splenic flexure when the operation is done through the standard open approach. On the other hand, laparoscopic splenic flexure mobilization is safe and swift, requiring no supraumbilical extension of the incision even in obese patients. The reader should take all these factors into consideration in deciding the best peritoneal access for restorative proctocolectomy.

Avoiding the supraumbilical extension of the abdominal incision by laparoscopic mobilization of the splenic (Fig. 18-5) and hepatic flexures (Fig. 18-6)—even if the rest of the operation is done by the open technique—is intuitively appealing. I notice that the laparoscopic mobilization of the splenic flexure is easier than the open technique in obese patients. Some find fault with the laparoscopic technique because of the time and cost factors. The criticism that the laparoscopic technique increases operative time and expense may vanish once the surgeon gains more experience and uses disposable ports and dissecting instruments. In spite of all these intuitively apparent advantages, the superiority of laparoscopic approach is yet to be proved. Currently, available data, including the data cited in this chapter, do not dispel the potential advantages of the laparoscopic approach. The surgeon's goal is not to replace the conventional technique with the new laparoscopic approach. Our aim is to reduce the incisional morbidity and still realize the same surgical benefit.

There are multiple appropriate indicators for postoperative morbidity. They not only include the duration of ileus and hospital stay, as evaluated in Drs. Cohen and Wexner's study, but also the postoperative analgesia needed, the duration of time away from productive work, the risk of postoperative incisional hernias, and finally, the complications from intra-abdominal adhesions. Further long-term studies will help to properly compare the laparoscopic technique with the conventional open operation.

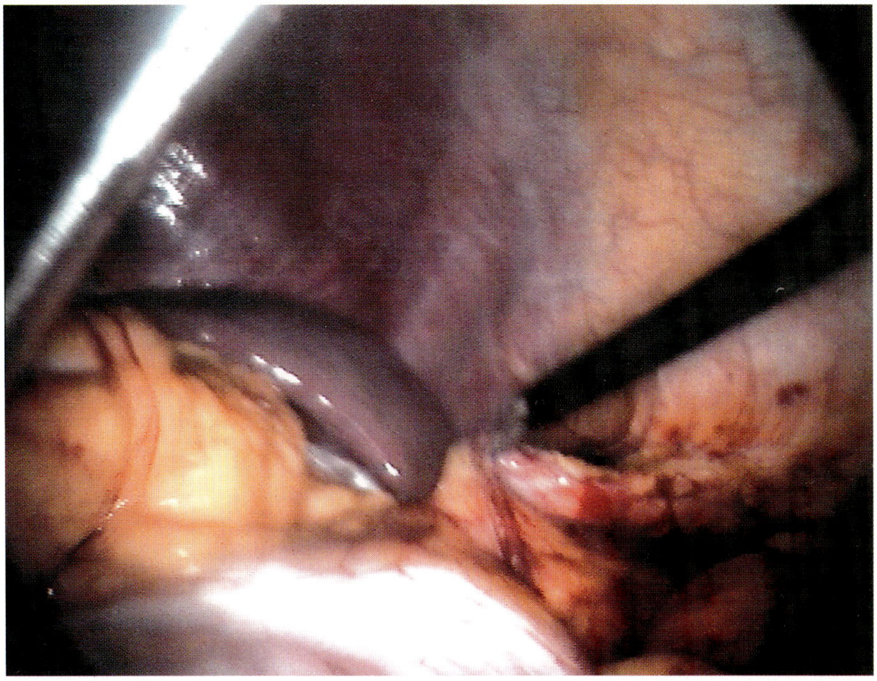

Fig. 18-5. Laparoscopic mobilization of splenic flexure.

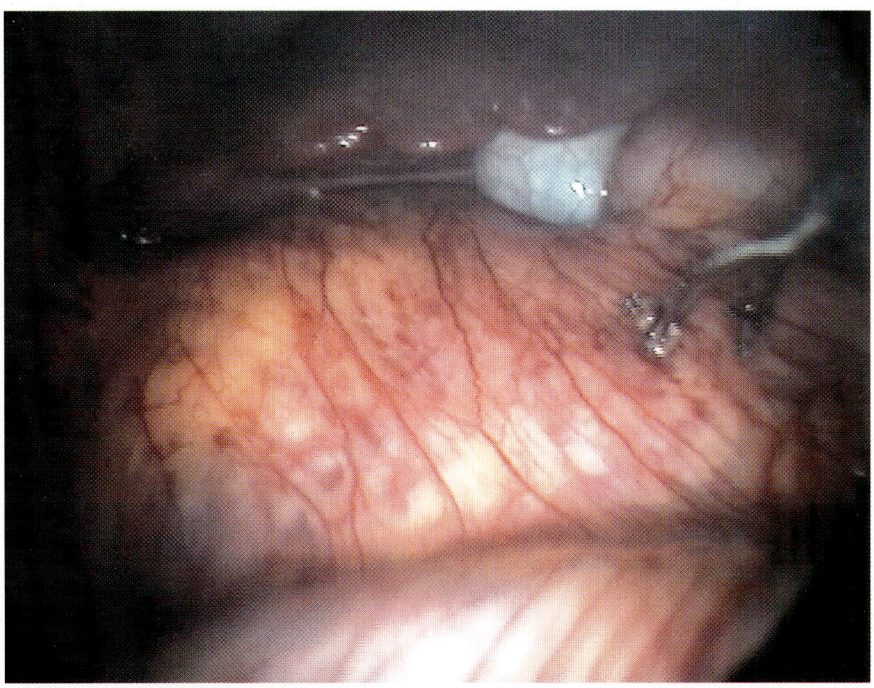

Fig. 18-6. Laparoscopic mobilization of hepatic flexure.

19

Anastomosis With Laparoscopic Pursestring Suture Clamp

Ferdinand Koeckerling, Ignaz Schneider, Ingo Gastinger, Bernd Schneider, and Franz P. Gall

One of the main problems in laparoscopic colorectal surgery is the anastomosis, which has led to the development of laparoscopic-assisted colorectal resections.[1] The necessity of a more or less large minilaparotomy limits the clear advantages of laparoscopic-assisted colorectal operations as compared with conventional procedures. A further limitation is, in our opinion, the possibility of tumor seeding by the unprotected retrieval of a tumor-infested bowel section through a minilaparotomy. The safest way seems to be a purely intracorporeal resection with placement of the resected specimen into a cell- and water-impermeable endopouch and retrieval through a 33-mm trocar. We believe that transanal retrieval over an open rectal stump[2] can lead to technical and oncologic problems. In intracorporeal resection, we therefore preferred the completely closed technique in which we double-staple the proximal and distal bowel lumen using linear cutters. We were then faced with the problem of preparing the proximally stapled bowel for circular anastomosis. However, the necessary technology was missing. We were able to show experimentally that the triple-stapling anastomosis technique had good results, but a broad clinical application failed because of the difficulty of introducing the anvil into the proximal bowel end.

To overcome this problem, we developed a laparoscopic pursestring suture clamp that permits preparation of the bowel end for circular anastomosis following complete intracorporeal and closed colorectal resection.

INSTRUMENTS

Our pursestring suture clamp is a reusable steel instrument based on the conventional pursestring suture clamp that has been adapted to meet the specific needs of laparoscopic surgery (Fig. 19-1A). The laparoscopic pursestring suture clamp consists of the suture clamp for placement of the pursestring suture and a longer shaft. The suture clamp and the shaft are constructed so that they can be inserted into the abdomen through a 12-mm trocar. At the end of the shaft, there is a rotating mechanism over which the suture clamp can be opened and closed (Fig. 19-1B). In the anterior and posterior section of the suture clamp, there are two drill conduits for the introduction of conventional pursestring sutures. Using this laparoscopic pursestring suture clamp, we are able to place laparoscopic pursestring sutures rapidly. The anastomosing techniques used in conventional colorectal surgery can be transferred to laparoscopic colorectal surgery.

INDICATIONS

The boxed list gives our indications for laparoscopic sigmoid resection with modified triple-stapling anastomosis using the pursestring suture clamp. The clamp enables use of laparoscopic triple-stapling anastomosis technique in a broader spectrum of clinical applications, such as stenosis from sigmoid diverticulitis.

TECHNIQUE

The clinical case presented involved a malignant sigmoid polyp that was incompletely removed and required a second operation in the form of a sigmoid resection. A laparoscopic assessment of the tiny lesion was not possible; therefore, after placing the patient on the rectal table and inserting the working trocars, we performed an intraoperative colonoscopy[3] (Fig. 19-2A). The gastroenterologist, who had previously removed

Indications for Laparoscopic Sigmoid Colectomy

Benign disease
- Diverticulitis
- Adenoma
- Extensive iatrogenic perforation
- Endometriosis
- Crohn's disease

Malignant disease
- Palliative resections (segmental resection)
- Adenocarcinoma pT1 (segmental resection)
- Adenocarcinoma pT2 (extended resection with high ligation of inferior mesenteric artery)
- Adenocarcinoma pT3 (extended resection with high ligation of inferior mesenteric artery)

the malignant polyp, was then able to precisely locate the lesion. We then marked it with clips (Fig. 19-2B). Because the patient had an elongated sigmoid and a carcinoma in early stages, a simple sigmoid resection was indicated. The resection line on the sigmoid mesentery was marked using an electrocautery hook (Fig. 19-2C). We then identified the left ureter—a routine step in all laparoscopic colorectal procedures. Within the already marked area, the sigmoid mesentery was opened in preparation for distal and proximal transection with the linear cutter (Fig. 19-2D).

Following this, the colon and the attached mesocolon were divided proximally and distally with the 60-mm linear cutter (Fig. 19-3). This approach has two advantages: (1) not only the proximal but also the distal ends are sealed, preventing spillage of bowel contents; and (2) the cancer-containing bowel sections are stapled on both ends, in keeping with our goal of preventing cancer seeding. Thus, this technique appears to be a desirable one from both an oncologic standpoint and from the standpoint of preventing fecal spillage.

The next step consists of specimen retrieval. A water- and cell-impermeable endopouch is inserted into the abdomen (Fig. 19-4A), opened, and the specimen placed inside the pouch (Fig. 19-4B). The pouch is then removed through the 33-mm trocar up to the abdominal wall, opened outside the abdomen, and the contents are removed lengthwise with a grasping forceps (Fig. 19-4C). An adequate margin of clearance to all sides of the tumor specimen can be appreciated (Fig. 19-4D & E).

The next step is the preparation of the proximal bowel end for the insertion of the anvil. We introduce the laparoscopic pursestring suture clamp through a 12-mm trocar and open it (Fig. 19-5A). The pursestring suture clamp is placed across in an antimesenteric direction so that the junction of the colonic wall and the mesocolon are displaced from the suture site (Fig. 19-5B). This method avoids problems arising in the junctional area of the colonic wall and mesocolon during later creation of the circular anastomosis. We have encountered some technical problems in laparoscopic triple-stapling anastomosis. Following the placement of the pursestring suture clamp, the conventional pursestring suture is laid in the abdomen through a separate trocar containing a needle holder and placed through the distal drill conduits (Fig. 19-5C). The suture is introduced into the pursestring suture clamp until the point of the needle emerges (Fig. 19-5D). The needles are pulled toward the pursestring suture clamp and pulled through a trocar.

Once the pursestring suture is placed (Fig. 19-6A), the proximal bowel end, which has been clamped from the antimesocolic side, can be opened (Fig. 19-6B). Optical magnification helps to maintain a correct tissue distance while creating a pursestring suture (Fig. 19-6C). The pursestring suture clamp is then removed, and the bowel lumen is opened with a grasping forceps (Fig. 19-6D). Placement of the pursestring suture using the pursestring suture clamp requires a maximum of 2 to 3 minutes. The anvil of the gas-tight circular stapler is inserted into the abdomen over the 33-mm trocar and placed into the open lumen of the proximal bowel end (Fig. 19-6E).

The knots on the pursestring suture are placed using normal surgical knots and a knot pusher (Fig. 19-7A). Following this, the anvil can be disconnected from the circular stapler with swabs on sticks (Fig. 19-7B). Preparations for the anastomosis are thus completed. The circular stapler is inserted transanally; the central pin is pushed through the fat-free area of the rectal stump, and the instrument is reconnected (Fig. 19-7C). After closure and firing of the stapler as well as reopening with three half-turns, the instrument is carefully removed from the bowel lumen. Once this step is completed, the fine anastomosis line created by the stapler can be seen (Fig. 19-7D). The two complete and plump stapler doughnuts confirm a perfect anastomosis (Fig. 19-7E).

(Text continues on page 224)

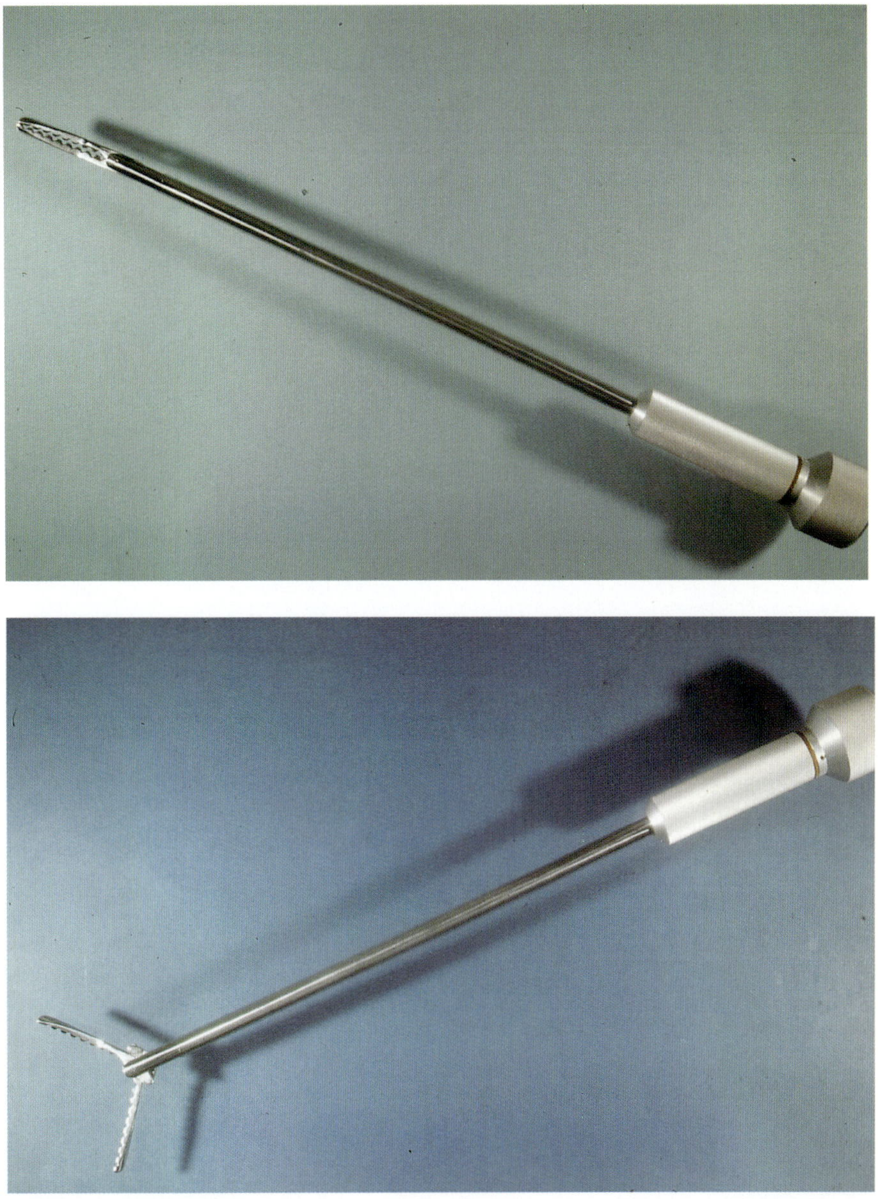

A

B

Fig. 19-1. (A) Laparoscopic pursestring suture clamp (Ethicon, Inc., Somerville, NJ). **(B)** A rotating mechanism at the end of the shaft opens and closes the suture clamp.

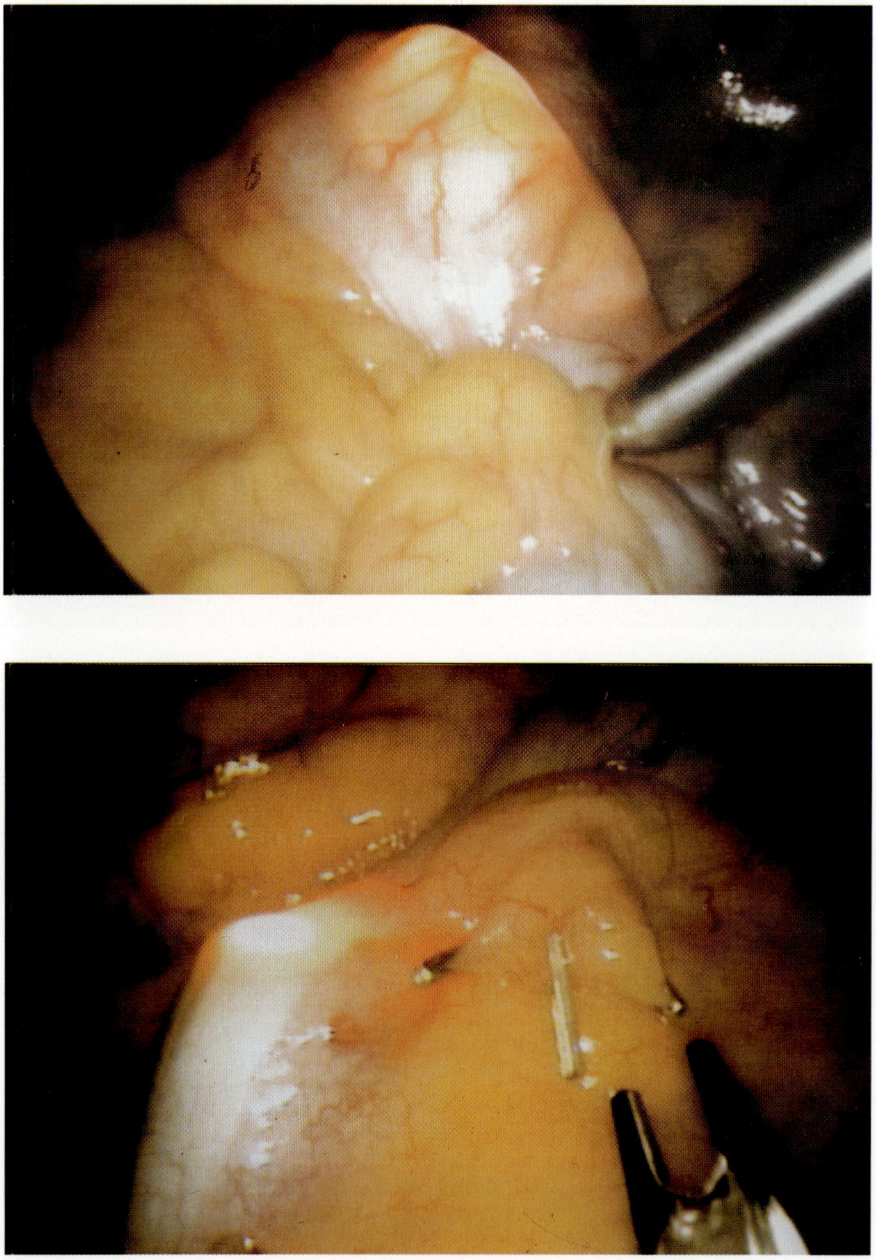

Fig. 19-2. (A) Intraoperative colonoscopy for marking of the tiny lesion. **(B)** The gastroenterologist precisely locates the lesion, and it is marked with clips. *(Figure continues.)*

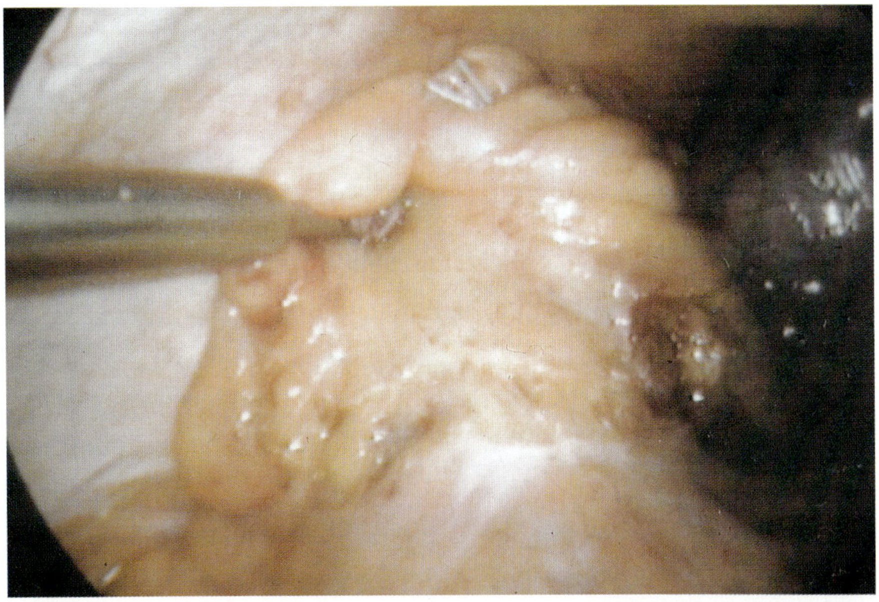

C

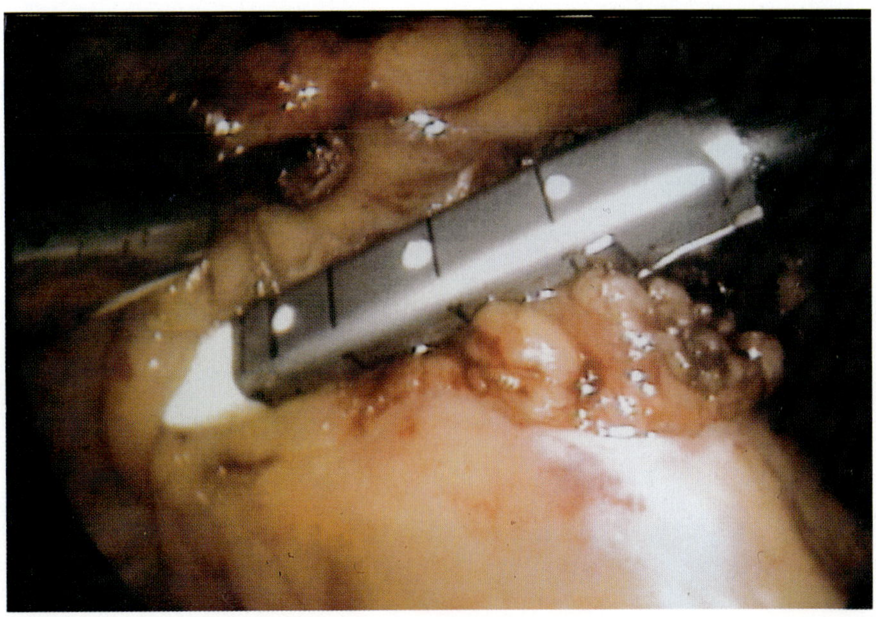

D

Fig. 19-2 *(Continued).* **(C)** The resection line on the sigmoid mesentery is marked using an electrocautery hook. **(D)** Transection of sigmoid mesentery with linear cutter.

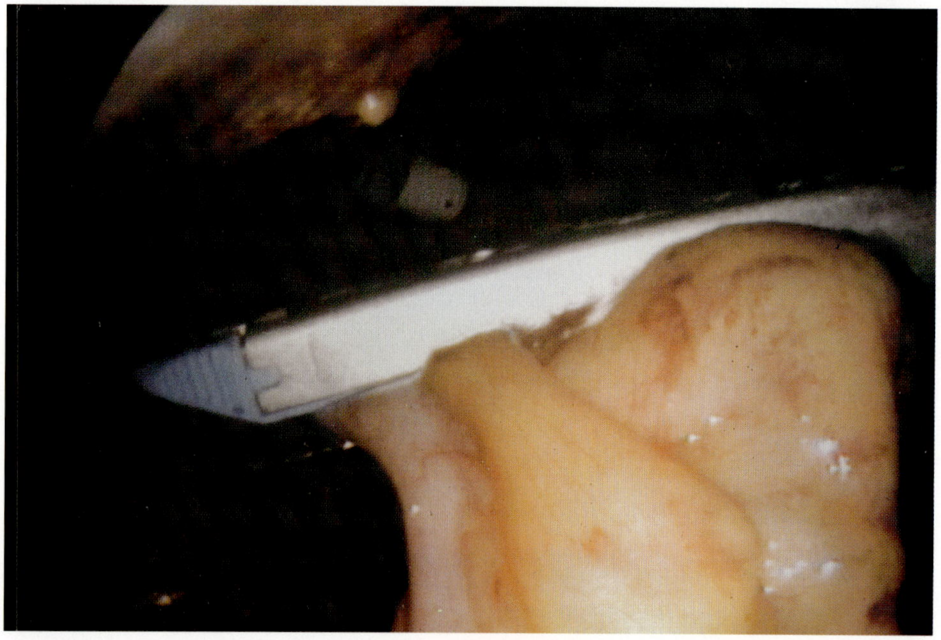

A

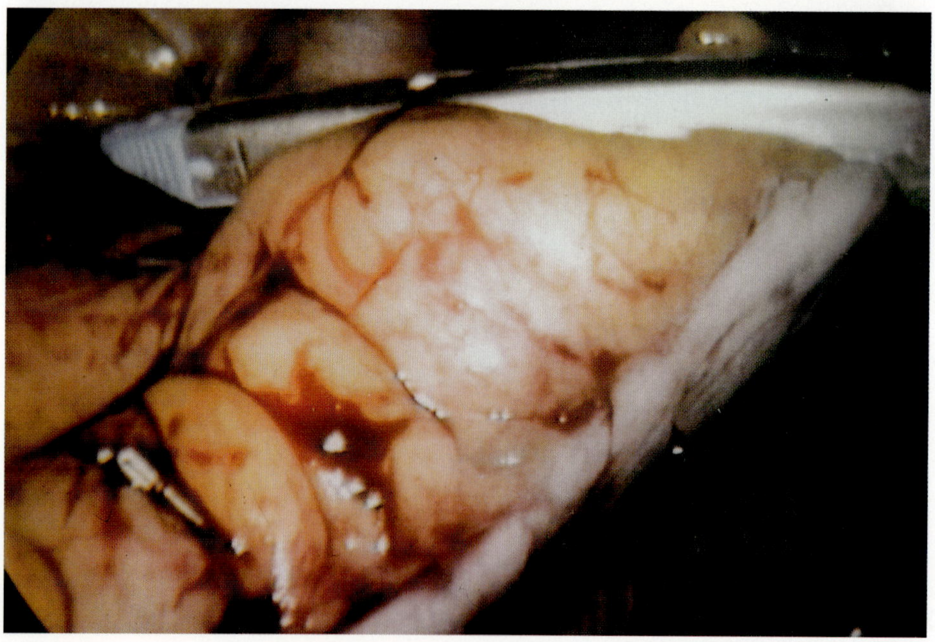

B

Fig. 19-3. (A) Proximal division of the colon and attached mesocolon with the 60-mm linear cutter. **(B)** Distal division of colon and mesocolon using 60-mm linear cutter.

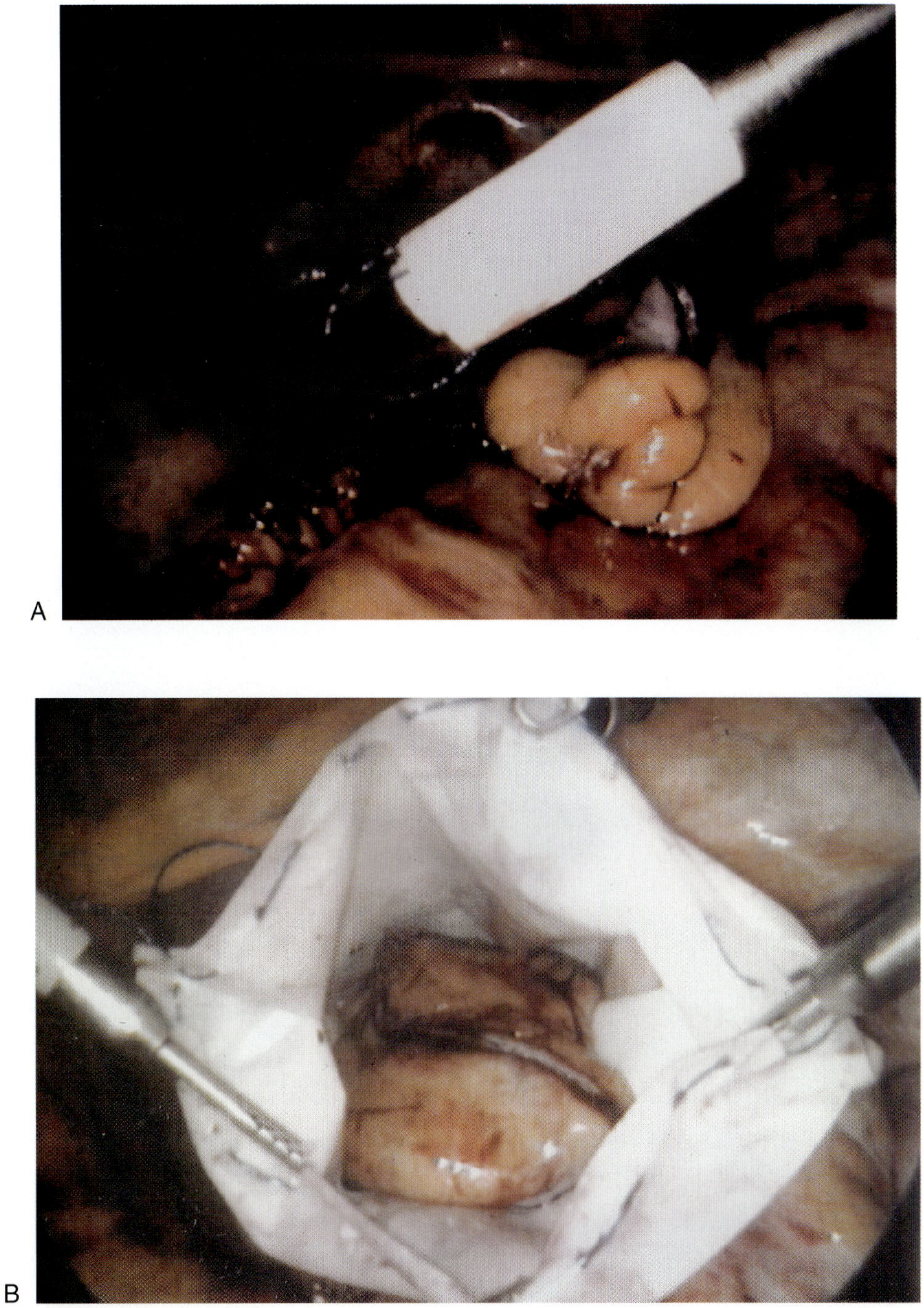

Fig. 19-4. (A) Insertion of a cell- and water-impermeable endopouch. **(B)** Specimen placement inside the pouch. *(Figure continues.)*

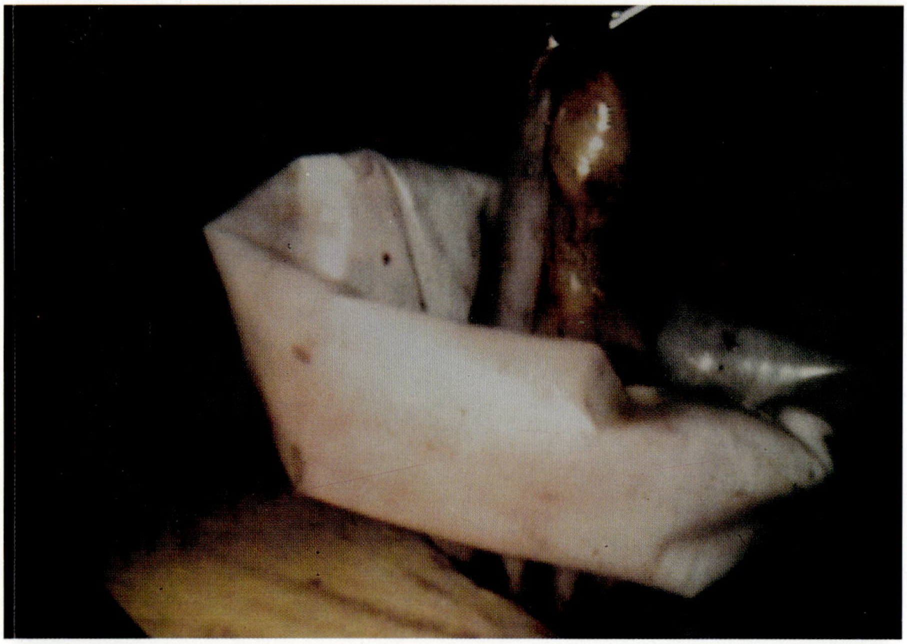

C

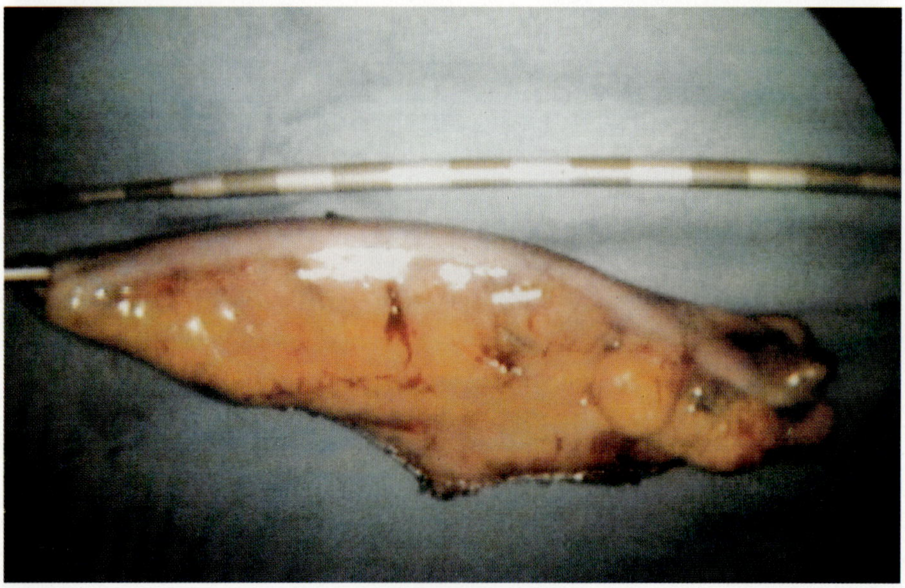

D

Fig. 19-4 *(Continued).* **(C)** The pouch is removed through a 33-mm trocar up to the abdominal wall, opened outside the abdomen and the specimen removed lengthwise with grasping forceps. **(D)** Sigmoid specimen with attached mesentery. *(Figure continues.)*

E
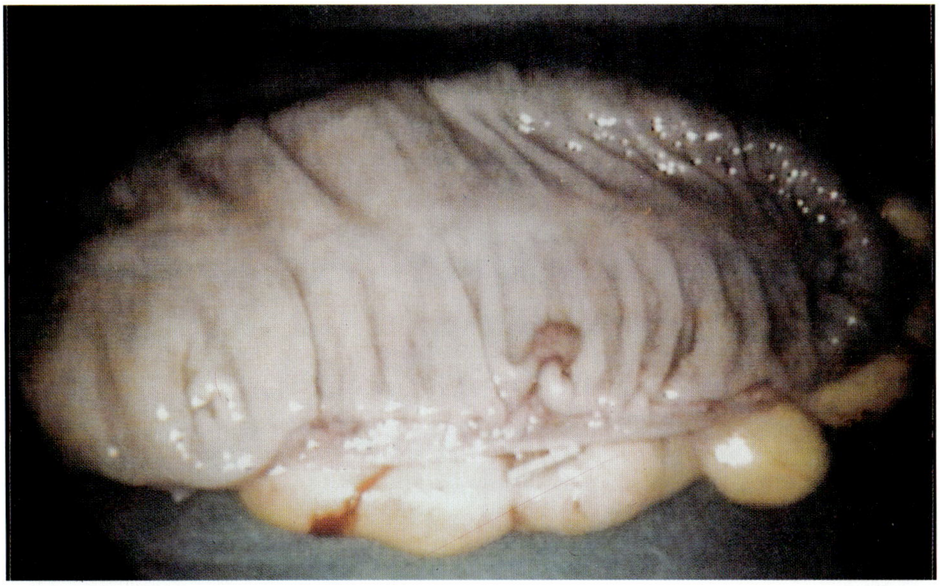

Fig. 19-4 *(Continued).* **(E)** An adequate margin of clearance to all sides of the tumor specimen can be appreciated.

A
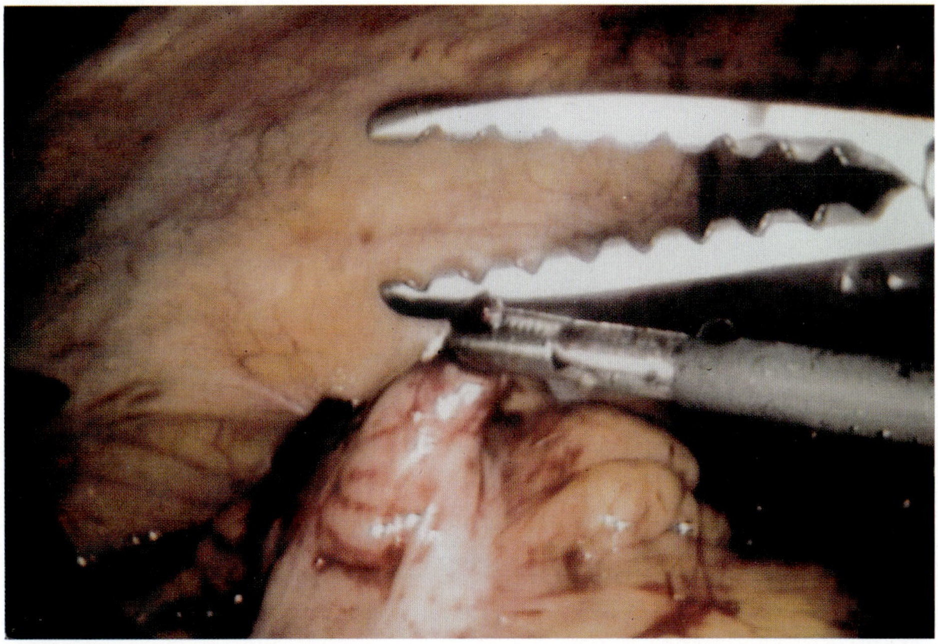

Fig. 19-5. **(A)** Introduction and opening of the laparoscopic pursestring suture clamp. *(Figure continues.)*

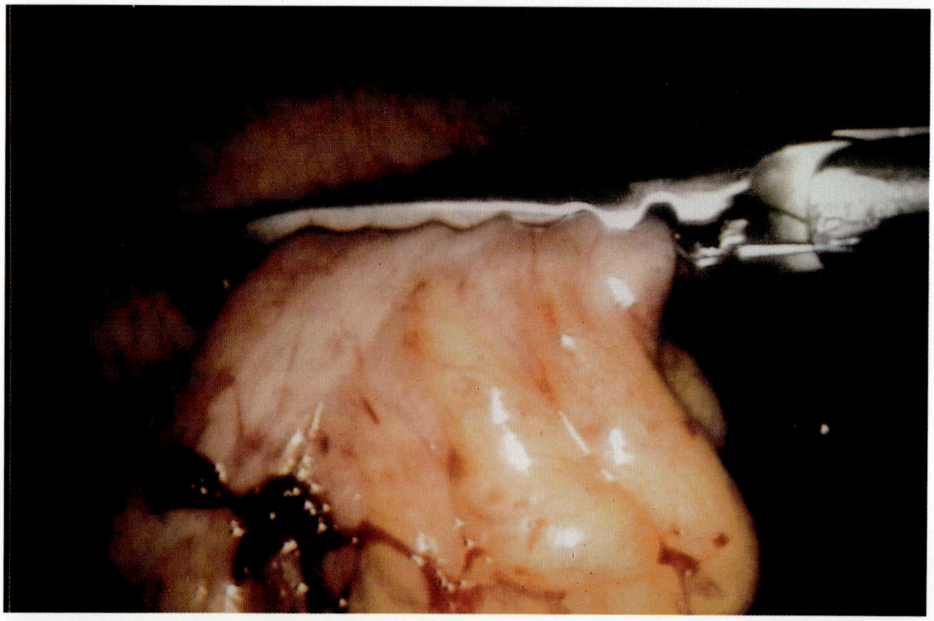

B

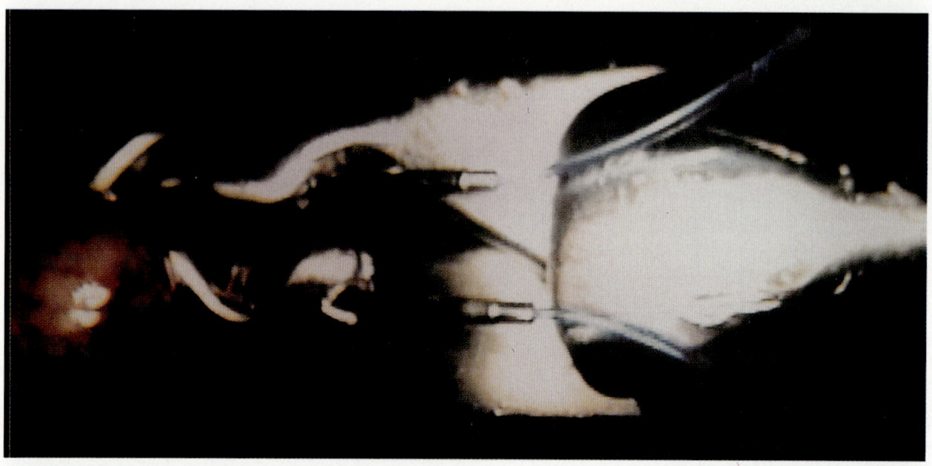

C

Fig. 19-5 *(Continued).* **(B)** The pursestring suture clamp is placed across in an antimesenteric direction so that the juncture of the colonic wall and the mesentery are displaced from the suture site. **(C)** Placement of the pursestring suture through the distal drill conduits. *(Figure continues.)*

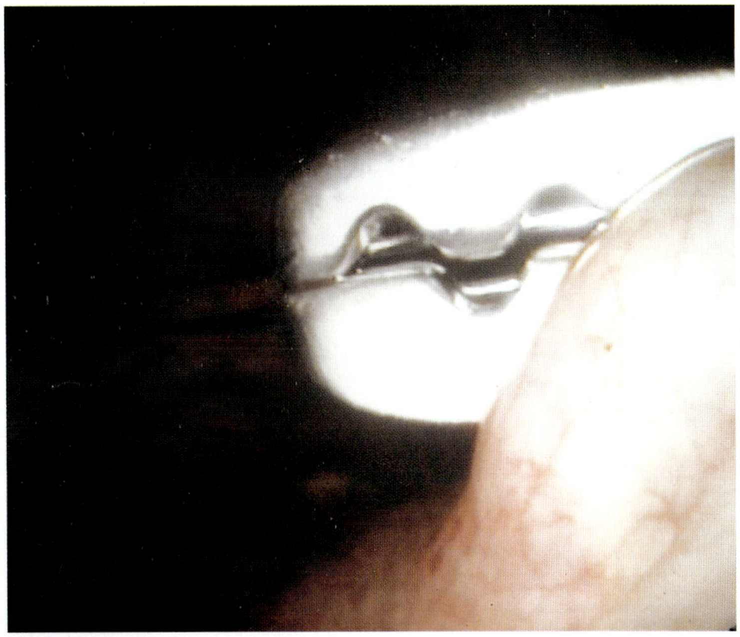

D

Fig. 19-5 *(Continued).* **(D)** The suture is introduced into the pursestring suture clamp until the point of the needle emerges.

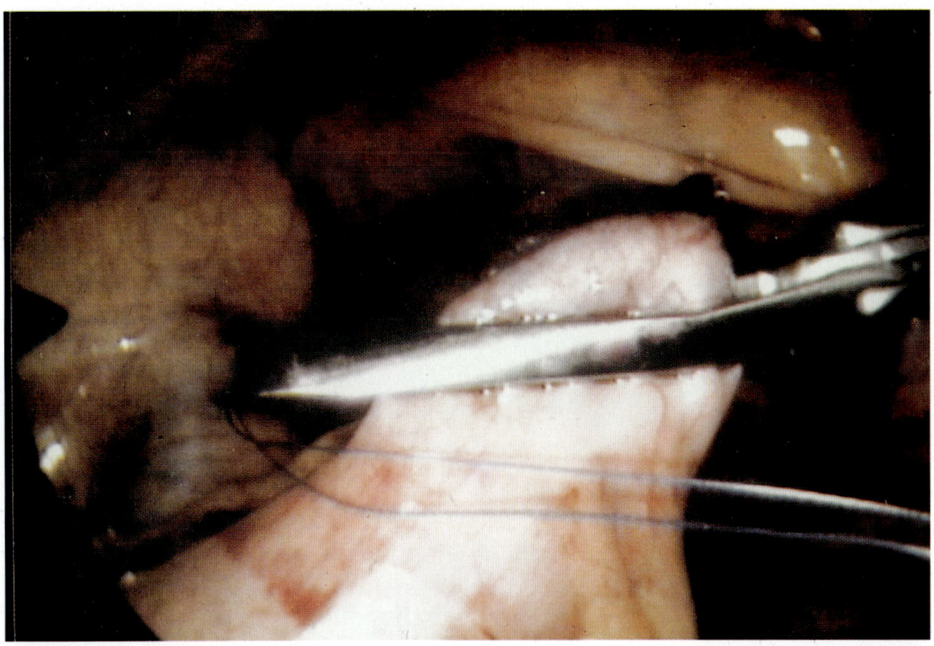

A

Fig. 19-6. (A) The needles are pulled toward the pursestring suture clamp and pulled through a trocar. *(Figure continues.)*

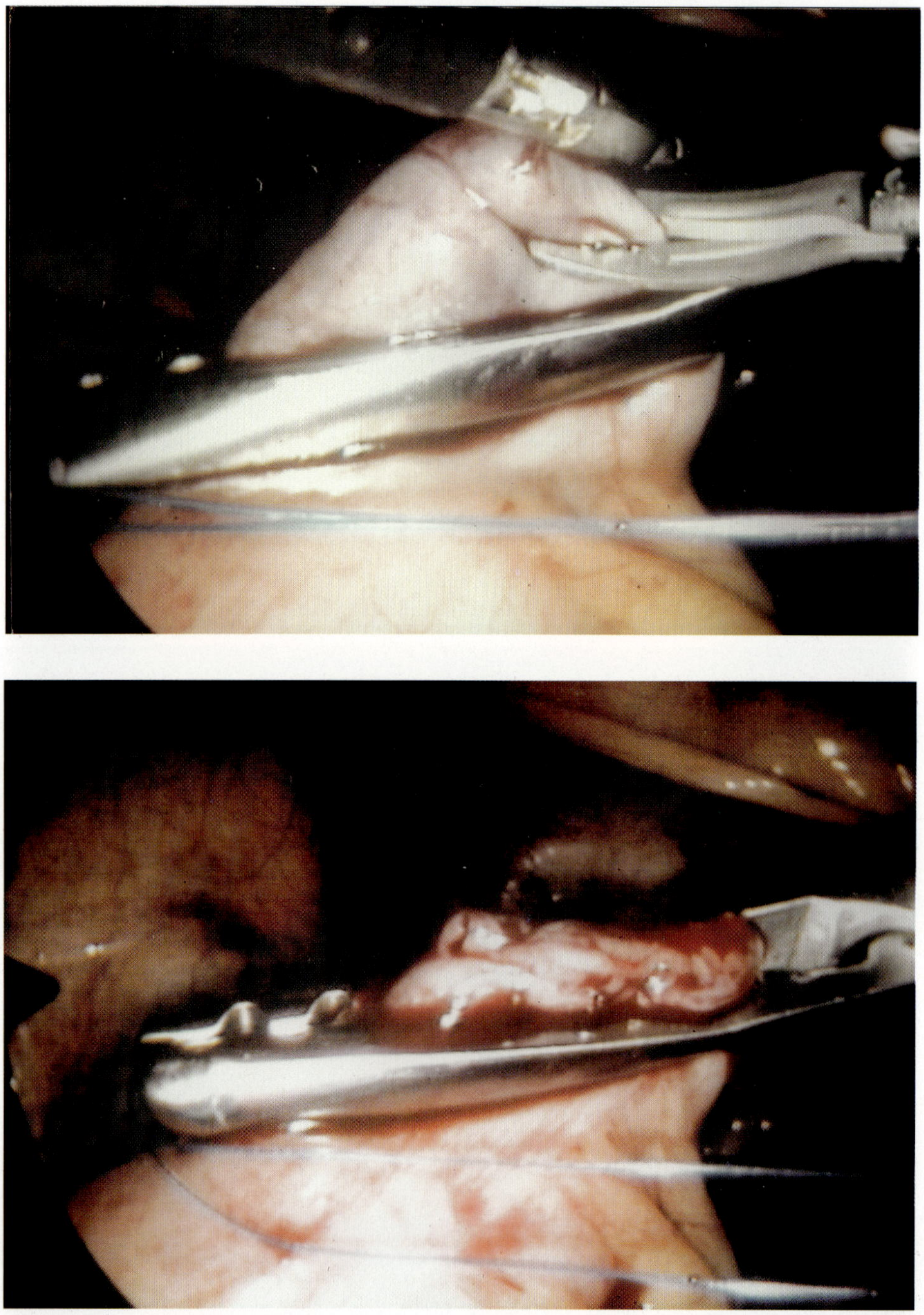

B

C

Fig. 19-6 *(Continued).* **(B)** The proximal bowel end that has been clamped in an antimesenteric direction can be opened. **(C)** Optical magnification represents an advantage in maintaining a correct tissue distance while creating a pursestring suture. *(Figure continues.)*

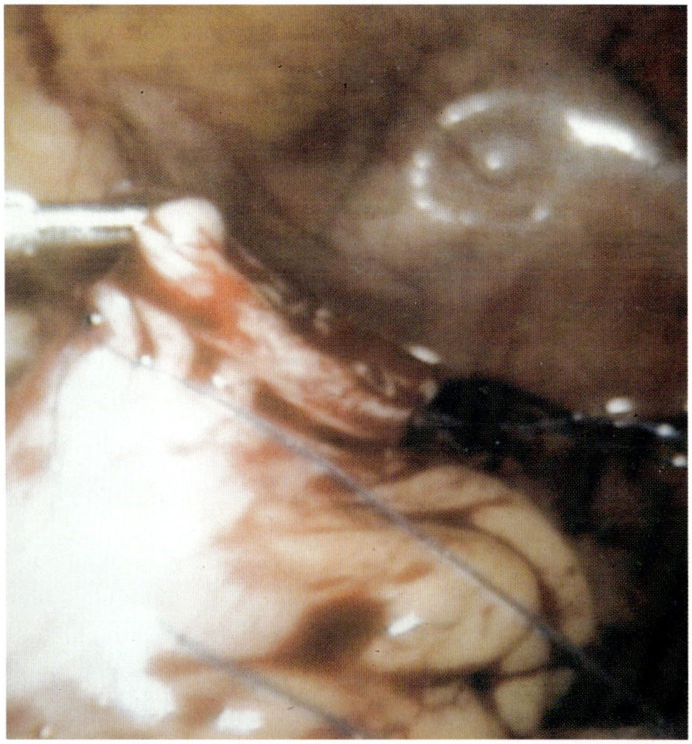

D

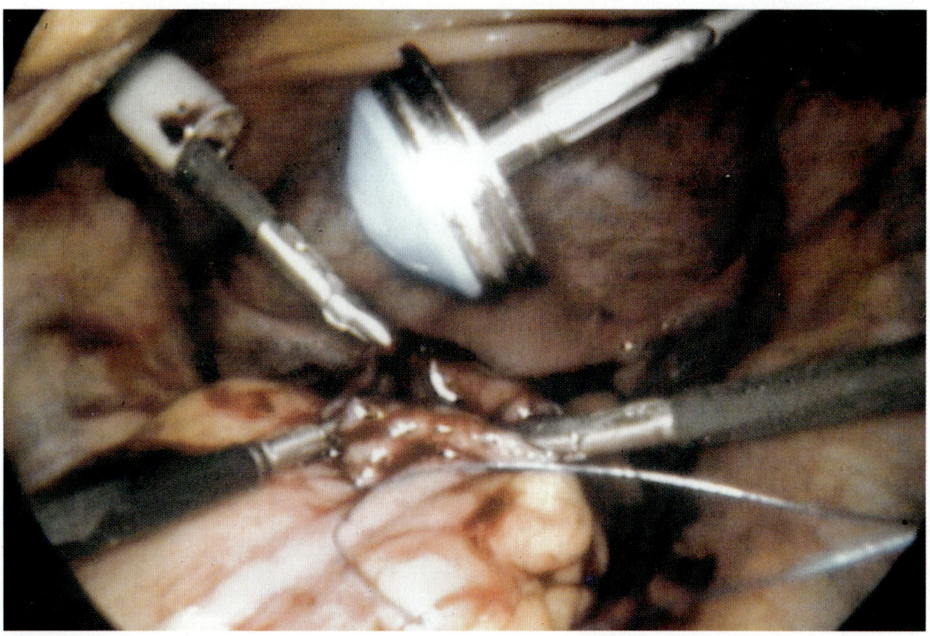

E

Fig. 19-6 *(Continued).* **(D)** After removal of the clamp, the bowel lumen can be opened with a grasping forceps. **(E)** The anvil of the gas-tight circular stapler is inserted into the abdomen over the 33-mm trocar and placed into the open lumen of the proximal bowel end.

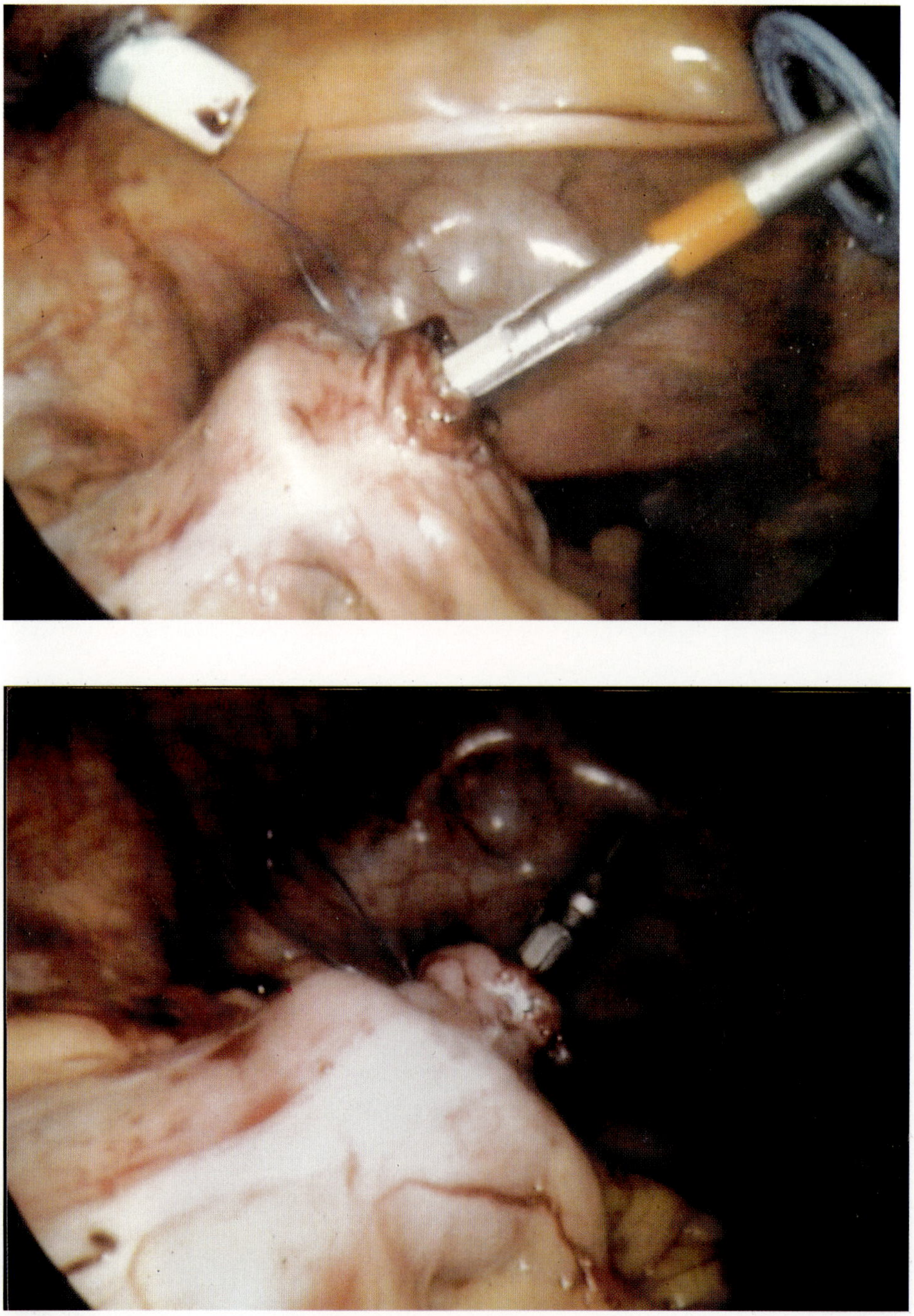

A

B

Fig. 19-7. (A) The knots on the pursestring suture are placed using normal surgical knots and a knot pusher. **(B)** The anvil can then be disconnected from the circular stapler with swabs on sticks. *(Figure continues.)*

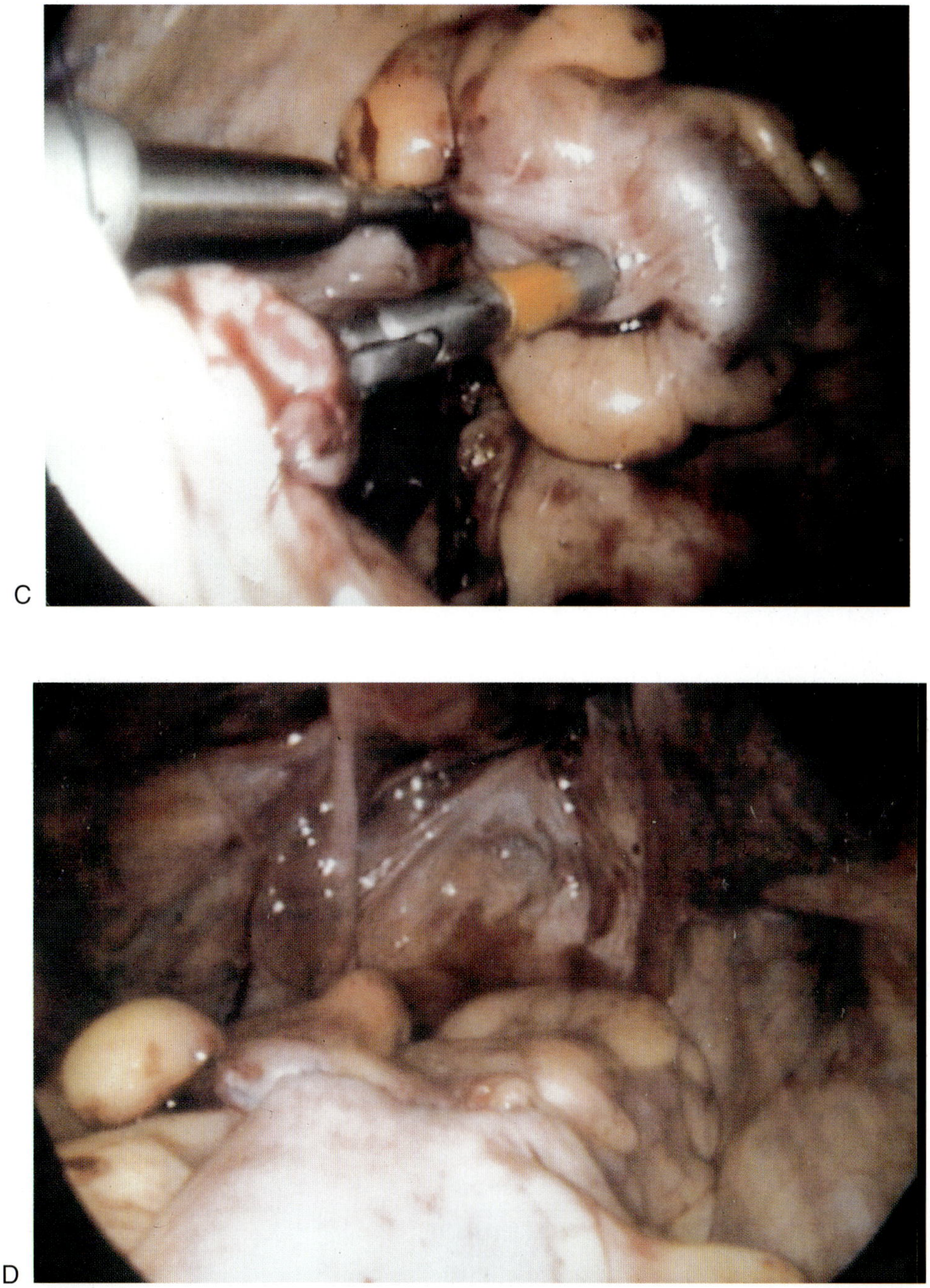

Fig. 19-7 *(Continued)*. **(C)** The circular stapler is inserted transanally, the central pin is pushed through the fat-free area of the rectal stump, and the instrument is reconnected. **(D)** Completion of the circular anastomosis. *(Figure continues.)*

E

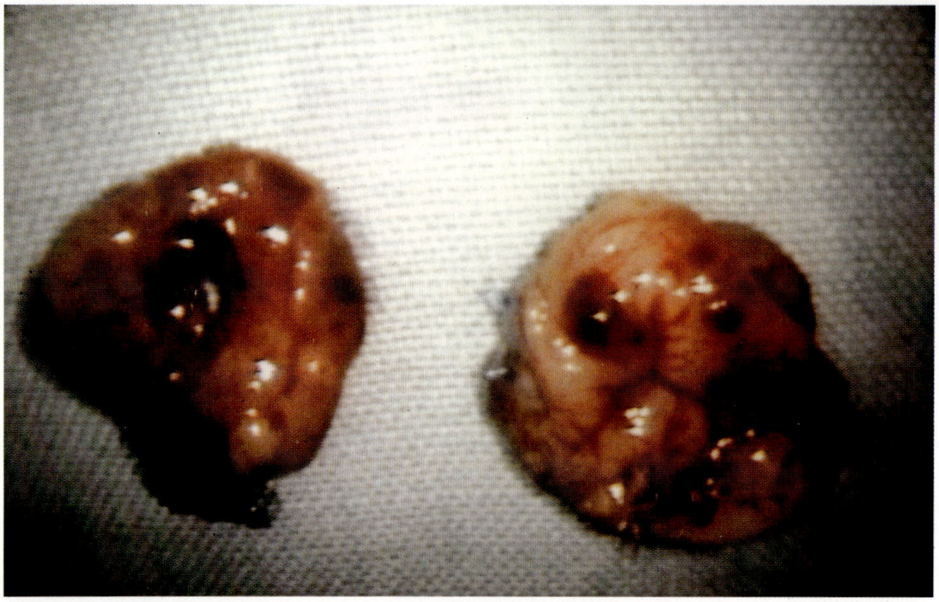

Fig. 19-7 *(Continued).* **(E)** Two complete and plump stapler doughnuts confirm a perfect anastomosis.

RESULTS

The results of our laparoscopic colorectal procedures are specified in Table 19-1. The operative time was 3 to 4 hours. The postoperative course was complication free, and we were able to discharge the patient after 8 days.

CONCLUSION

Based on our experimental studies and the technical prerequisites discussed, we introduced laparoscopic abdominoperineal rectal resection[4] and laparoscopic rectopexy into our clinical practice. Until now, specimen retrieval and safe anastomosing in colorectal surgery presented serious hindrances to a broader application. These problems led to the use of so-called assisted laparoscopic colorectal operations, especially in the United Kingdom and in the United States. The use of more or less large minilaparotomies for specimen retrieval and resection and the preparation of the proximal bowel end for anastomosing became popular in certain centers. We were dissatisfied with this idea, and for oncologic and surgical/technical reasons, we looked for a solution to achieve a completely intracorporeal resection and anastomosing technique.

The development of a laparoscopic triple-stapling anastomosis technique retrieval in an endopouch through a 33-mm trocar could not be clinically applied initially because the preparation of the proximal bowel wall and insertion of the anvil posed serious problems in patients with colon carcinoma and stenosing sigmoid diverticulitis.

The solution is the laparoscopic pursestring suture clamp that we have developed. The clamp permits preparation of the proximal bowel end for the anastomosis with insertion of the anvil in the same way as in conventional surgery. The simplicity of this technique permits the transference of conventional colorectal surgical techniques to laparoscopic surgery.

Nevertheless, the peculiarities of the laparoscopic technique must be introduced into the concrete resec-

Table 19-1. Results of Laparoscopic Colorectal Procedures

	No. of Procedure	Conversion	Complications
Laparoscopic rectopexy	15	—	—
Laparoscopic abdominoperineal excision of the rectum with high ligation of the inferior mesenteric artery	18	2 (11%) (severe adhesions, diverticulitis, and aneurysm of common iliac artery)	3 (16%) (sacral wound infection)
Laparoscopic oversewing of iatrogenic perforation	2	—	—
Laparoscopic sigmoid resection with pursestring suture clamp	10		
Laparoscopic-assisted colon resection	4	—	—

tion and anastomosis techniques. The simple creation of a proximal and distal pursestring suture in conventional surgery is less favorable because the proximal and distal bowel ends remain open for a long time. Also, the cancer-carrying colonic segment is not occluded. In addition, there is the problem of resection of the large bowel mesocolon. In this case, use of the linear cutter (not only in laparoscopic abdominoperineal proctectomy but also in sigmoid resection) has proved to be a rapid and safe procedure. The attempt to resect the mesocolon by identifying individual vessels is very time-consuming and can easily lead to bleeding.

We consider the junction of the colon and the mesocolon to be especially difficult to resect laparoscopically. The colon and the mesocolon can continuously be divided with the linear cutter. In addition to the oncologic and infectious problems, the technical difficulties can be solved using this technique. A feeling of safety, comparable to that achieved by conventional surgery, can be readily achieved with this operation. Preparation for anastomosis takes place only after successful, safe specimen retrieval. Thus, we are able to place a pursestring suture in the proximal bowel end in the antimesocolic region (i.e., avoiding the colonic wall/mesocolic junction), then introduce the anvil of the gas-tight circular stapler over the briefly opened bowel lumen and fixate it over the pursestring suture. Further steps in anastomosis correspond to the conventional procedures in double-stapling technique.

In addition to sigmoid resection, laparoscopic pursestring suture may well play a role in laparoscopic hemicolectomy, small bowel segment resection, and gastroenterostomy. The conventional linear stapler anastomosis techniques and the biofragmentable Valtrac rings may be recruited into the minimally invasive surgical repertoire. Other possible uses include laparoscopic management of iatrogenic colorectal perforations and placement of a laparoscopic pursestring suture in appendectomy.

REFERENCES

1. Jacobs M, Verdeja JC, Goldstein HS: Minimally invasive colon resection (laparoscopic colectomy). Surg Laparosc Endosc 1:144, 1991
2. Franklin ME, Jr, Ramos R, Rosenthal D et al: Laparoscopic colonic procedures. World J Surg 17:51, 1993
3. Kuramoto S, Ihara O, Sakai S et al: Intraoperative colonoscopy in the detection of nonpalpable colonic lesions—how to identify the affected bowel segment. Surg Endosc 2:76, 1988
4. Kockerling F, Gastinger I, Schneider B et al: Laparoscopic abdominoperineal excision of the rectum with high ligation of the inferior mesenteric artery in the management of rectal carcinoma. Endosc Surg 1:16, 1993

Editorial Comment I

Lars Påhlman

The technique described by Dr. Koeckerling and colleagues is interesting and probably offers some advantages in laparoscopic sigmoid resection. However, I fail to understand why the authors are concerned about doing a minilaparotomy. A minilaparotomy in the left lower quadrant is a quick procedure in our experience and does not prolong hospital stay substantially. Most patients recover well with little morbidity from the minilaparotomy.

By contrast, several problems can be identified with a total laparoscopic procedure. Although the pursestring suture technique described seems to be secure, it can be difficult to see whether the pursestring suture is tightened in a proper way around the central rod of the anvil. There is also a risk of spillage, however small, when the anvil is inserted in the open bowel.

An important factor is the tension in the anastomosis. It can be difficult to evaluate the length of the resected specimen if the operation is done purely as a laparoscopic procedure. I can see an advantage with a minilaparotomy. If the proximal bowel is taken out through a small laparotomy in the left lower quadrant, it is easier to evaluate the tension before the bowel is divided, taking appropriate measures to avoid tension in the anastomosis.

The authors' concern about specimen retrieval may not be valid if the specimen is taken out together with the proximal colon. Of course, a cell- and water-impermeable pouch can be used even for this purpose. The distal part of the proximal colon, including the specimen to be resected, can easily be placed in the pouch and taken out through the 33-mm trocar.

After resection of the cancer-containing colonic segment, the pursestring suture can be placed outside the abdomen. With this extracorporeal technique, the fecal spillage is avoided. Also, the pursestring suture can be placed under direct vision and tied tight around the central rod. In this fashion, the most important part of an anastomosis with a circular stapler (i.e., the pursestring suture) is created under direct vision. The descending colon is then inserted into the abdomen again, and the minilaparotomy is closed before the anastomosis is stapled.

Editorial Comment II

Steven D. Wexner

One of the major difficulties in laparoscopic surgery is that even after meticulous extensive dissection, resection, and anastomosis, the specimen still needs to be removed. This problem has led to most surgeons performing right hemicolectomies as assisted procedures. In these cases, the vessels are either divided intracorporeally or extracorporeally, but the bowel is extracorporeally divided and the anastomosis is extracorporeally performed. It is hardly justifiable based on presently available scientific data to spend the time necessary to perform complete intracorporeal vascular division, bowel division, and anastomosis creation. The possibility of intracorporeal contamination as well as the added time in most surgeons' hands make this option seem highly unattractive. Furthermore, as has been elegantly illustrated by Michelassi,[1] after such a herculean feat of technical wizardry, an incision in the abdomen is then generally made large enough through which to comfortably deliver not only the specimen but also the entire anastomosis and mesenteric defect. The time and expense necessary for such maneuvers is certainly questionable.

Certainly, left-sided procedures are separately classified, in that it is virtually impossible in all but the most emaciated patients to perform an assisted resection with extracorporeal vascular ligation in any oncologically meaningful fashion. Thus, left-sided resections have largely evolved into those that include intracorporeal vascular division and intracorporeal anastomosis with some form of specimen delivery. As Koeckerling and colleagues rightly note, transanal retrieval through an open rectal stump can lead to both technical and oncologic problems. It has been elegantly shown in the past that even the minimal transanal dilation such as that necessary to appropriately use a circular stapling device can lead to transient if not permanent impairment in internal anal sphincter function.[2] To date, none of the surgeons who routinely advocate the transanal specimen retrieval approach have provided any objective physiologic or even subjective functional data to support the advisability of this uncontrolled sphincter stretch.

To perform more elegant surgery, Koeckerling and colleagues have developed a modified triple-stapling technique using the laparoscopic pursestring suture. They beautifully outline numerous important points in their technical description. First, they always identify the left ureter. Second, they divide the inferior mesenteric artery at the level of the aorta and not, as many laparoscopic surgeons have shown, at the level of the sigmoidal vessels or even at the level of the superior rectal vessels at the sacral promontory. They also advocate the use of an impervious bag and a 33-mm trocar as double protection through which to remove the tumor. What the authors quite modestly did not mention is that they spent several *years* working in experimental facilities in the animal model developing their technique. Following that phase, they first operated only on benign disease. Dr. Koeckerling has mentioned this in numerous lectures, and the point is in contradistinction to what has been mentioned by other authors within this textbook. Clearly, the technical grace illustrated in this chapter shows the advantage of having developed an experimental routine in the animal model before embarking on these techniques in humans. This adage is particularly true when one considers that Dr. Koeckerling and co-workers are now performing attempted curative resections of malignancies in these patients. The issue of resection for malignancy is discussed in great detail throughout this textbook, and I will certainly not belabor it again at this juncture. However, several important points need to be made.

First, if one is operating for malignancy, one should first develop expertise in the animal model and expertise in resections of colorectal neoplasia in the open setting. Second, one must strictly adhere to oncologic principles, including adequate lymphovascular pedicle dissection and, when resecting rectal carcinomas, adequate lateral and distal margins. Dr. Koeckerling and coworkers limit their technique to sigmoid resections, and Stitz[3] from Australia also discourages the application of the laparoscope to low anterior resections based on presently available technology. Third, one should first embark on application of the laparoscope for treatment of benign pathology or palliation of malignancy. These resections should be done according to oncologic principles to gain expertise. However, if those principles are violated, the patient will not suffer. Fourth, and most important, when one eventually does fulfill the above four criteria and begins the performance of laparoscopic resection for attempted cure of malignancy, it should be done at the very least within the confines of an institutional review board/research protocol committee setting. Preferably, a prospective randomized trial should be undertaken. All patients must be told of the unproven nature of the technology, of the known incidence (at least 1.5 percent to as much as 21 percent) of port site recurrence, and of the need for diligent follow-up. Performance of such procedures must be made available for scrutiny not only by one's own colleagues in the institutional review board/research protocol committee and surgery department but also by the worldwide surgical community at large. Specifically, complications such as failure to locate a lesion during resection (see Ch. 22),[4–8] transecting a ureter, spilling tumor (P. Caushaj, personal communication, 1994), detecting port site implantation, or early local recurrence,[5,9–12] must be disseminated to the world at large, at the very least, in a letter to the editor in a peer-reviewed *Index Medicus*-listed reference journal, if not as a case report. It is only through diligent and academically critical examination of our collective results that an answer to the many questions existing today will be answered.

REFERENCES

1. Michelassi F: Laparoscopic ileocolonic resection with intracarporeal anastomosis for Cohn's ileitis. Video presentation at the American College of Surgeons 79th Annual Clinical Congress, San Francisco, October 1993
2. Horgan PC, O'Connell PR, Shinkain LA et al: Effect of anterior resection on anal sphincter function. Br J Surg 76:783, 1989
3. Stitz R: Laparoscopic colorectal surgery. Presented at the International Society of University Colon and Rectal Surgeons 15th Biennial Congress, Singapore, July 1994
4. Fingerhut A: Feasibility of laparoscopic colectomy. Presented at the 4th World Congress of Endoscopic Surgeons, Kyoto, Japan, June 1994
5. Gleeson NC, Nicosia SV, Mark JE et al: Abdominal wall metastases from ovarian cancer after laparoscopy. Am J Obstet Gynecol 169:522, 1993
6. Larach SW, Salomon MC, Williamson PR: Laparoscopic-assisted colectomy: experience during the learning curve. Coloproct 1:38, 1993
7. McDermott JP, Devereaux DA, Caushaj PJ: Pitfall of laparoscopic colectomy: an unrecognized synchronous cancer. Dis Colon Rectum 37:602, 1994
8. Monson RT, Darzi A, Declan-Carry P et al: Prospective evaluation of laparoscopic-assisted colectomy in an unselected group of patients. Lancet 340:831, 1992
9. Fusco MA, Paluzzi MW: Abdominal wall recurrence after laparoscopic-assisted colectomy for adenocarcinoma of the colon. Dis Colon Rectum 36:858, 1993
10. Guillou PJ, Darzi A, Monson JRT: Experience with laparoscopic colorectal surgery for malignant disease. Surg Oncol, suppl. 2:43, 1993
11. Nduka CC, Monson JRT, Menzies-Gow N, Darzi N: Abdominal wall metastases following laparoscopy. Br J Surg 1:648, 1994
12. Wexner SD, Cohen SM: Port site metastases after laparoscopic colorectal surgery for cure of malignancy. Br J Surg 82:295, 1995

20
Laparoscopic Right Colectomy

Rama M. Jager

Minimally invasive surgical resection, reconstruction, or repair of intra-abdominal disease is appealing because of the potential for reduction in postoperative incisional morbidity. The unprecedented metamorphosis of laparoscopic cholecystectomy, from an unknown and untested operative technique into the current standard of care,[1] has encouraged many abdominal surgeons to extend the minimally invasive surgical approach to the management of colorectal disease.[2,3] Multiple centers have conducted laparoscopic right colonic resection for both benign and malignant lesions.[4] Some propose that the laparoscopic approach to a colonic resection reduces postoperative morbidity and fosters rapid recovery, allowing the patient to return to work sooner.[5]

INDICATIONS

Indications for Laparoscopic Right Colonic Resection

- Benign colorectal disease
    - Colonoscopically nonresectable villous and villotubular adenomas
    - Lipomas
    - Inflammatory bowel disease
    - Ischemic colitis
    - Diverticulitis
    - Typhlitis
    - Post-traumatic stricture
    - Volvulus
- Malignant colorectal disease
    - Adenocarcinomas
    - Metastatic carcinomas
    - Carcinoid tumors
    - Smooth muscle tumors

Benign colonic lesions, such as colonoscopically nonresectable villous and villotubular adenomas, are the most common indications for the laparoscopic approach. Ileocecal Crohn's disease and right colonic primary adenocarcinomas are the other common indications.

Any right colonic lesion that is amenable to open resection can be approached by laparoscopic technique, although controversy exists regarding whether all colonic cancers can be curatively resected through the laparoscope. Minimal adenocarcinomas of the right colon, such as superficially invasive residual cancers at the site of colonoscopically resected polypectomy, can be removed laparoscopically. Also, right colonic cancers that have already metastasized to the liver and other distant organs are candidates for the laparoscopic resection because the extensive mesocolic and associated lymph nodal resection is not necessary to remove these advanced cancers.

Opinions differ, however, regarding the laparoscopic approach to invasive right colonic cancers that require curative resection. Some laparoscopic colorectal surgeons propose that laparoscopic right colonic resection is fully compatible with the current oncosurgical dogma, and that it is equivalent, if not superior, to the conventional open right hemicolectomy (see Ch. 2). Others point to port site cancer recurrence and technical difficulties in specimen removal without contamination of incision (see Ch. 26). They question the curative adequacy of the laparoscopic right colonic resection.

Also, those right colonic cancers invading adjacent organs such as the urinary bladder and uterine adnexa cannot be safely removed en bloc with the minimally invasive approach. Because the laparoscopic surgeon does not have the advantage of tactile sense, the resection of invaded adjacent organs with satisfactory margins requires the conventional open approach. By contrast, minimal invasion of the flank fascia and peritoneum by a right colonic cancer may be laparoscopically resectable en bloc. The feasibility of the more advanced laparoscopic resections depends on the experience of the laparoscopic surgeon.

General contraindications to any laparoscopic procedure—such as coagulopathy, portal venous hypertension associated with varicosities of the mesenteric veins, and extensive intraperitoneal adhesions from previous surgical procedures—also render the laparoscopic right colonic resection inappropriate. Previous abdominal operations and resultant adhesions may hinder safe laparoscopic access and dissection. When the patient has extensive intraperitoneal adhesions, the open approach to establishing a pneumoperitoneum and laparoscopic adhesiolysis may allow colonic resection. Crowding of the intraperitoneal space by a gravid uterus may also preclude the laparoscopic resection. Patients with severe cardiopulmonary insufficiency who cannot tolerate prolonged periods of pneumoperitoneum (see Ch. 7) may not be candidates for the laparoscopic approach. Note that laparoscopic colonic resection takes more time than its conventional counterpart, even for experienced laparoscopic surgeons.

PREOPERATIVE EVALUATION AND PREPARATION

A patient who cannot tolerate an open right colonic resection cannot tolerate a laparoscopic resection. Preoperative risk evaluation before the laparoscopic resection is similar to that done before the open resection. The patient's ability to undergo general anesthesia is decided, including cardiopulmonary and hepatorenal evaluations (see Ch. 3). The surgeon explains to the patient the rationale for the laparoscopic approach to colonic resection, the need for an abdominal incision for specimen removal, and possible conversion to a conventional open technique.

Mechanical and antibiotic bowel preparation, along with systemic preoperative antibiotics for the laparoscopic colon resection, is similar to the open technique. Gut lavage with polyethylene glycol (see Ch. 5) may at times produce fluid-filled small bowel loops that can interfere with laparoscopic dissection. Autologous preoperative blood donation is arranged only if the patient insists, because the risk of extensive blood loss during the right colonic resection is small.

PREOPERATIVE COLONOSCOPIC TATTOOING AND COLONIC IMAGING

Unless the right colonic lesion is large and involves the serosal surface, it may not be laparoscopically visible. Benign soft villous adenomas and small carcinomas require preoperative colonoscopic tattooing with sterile India ink or Indocyanine green[6,7] for laparoscopic identification. Colonoscopic tattooing can lead to pericolonic septic complications[8,9] such as pericolonic abscess, focal peritonitis, fat necrosis, and inflammatory pseudotumor formation. Thus, the tattooing should preferably be done as close to the day of colonic resection as possible. However, preoperative colonoscopy on the same day as laparoscopy should not be done for obvious reasons because of colonic dilation that may complicate peritoneal access. All four quadrants of the colonic wall near the lesion should be tattooed to ensure that the location of the lesion in the mesocolic or retroperitoneal side of the colon is laparoscopically visible.[10]

Intraoperative colonoscopy negates the need for tattooing and resultant infective complications. Also, the tattooing may not succeed in all instances. The laparoscopic surgeon should be prepared and the patient positioned for intraoperative colonoscopy even in patients who have had preoperative tattooing. Proper positioning of the patient to allow intraoperative colonoscopy avoids conversion of a laparoscopic operation to an open one. The abandonment of laparoscopic approach is not an uncommon occurrence when the preoperatively tattooed lesion is laparoscopically invisible because of inadequate or incomplete tattooing.

It is not necessary to do a colonic radiogram before an open colonic resection when the right colonic cancer is confirmed by colonoscopy. By contrast, a preoperative barium enema to localize the lesion in the right colon is often needed before a laparoscopic resection. Colonoscopic localization of right colonic lesions can be inaccurate unless the lesion is in the cecal cap or near the ileocecal valve. Preoperative colonic radiograms accurately locate colonic lesions even in patients who have had preoperative colonoscopy, avoiding the resection of a wrong colonic segment or inadequate length of the colon. Not uncommonly, what is described as a hepatic flexure carcinoma by the colonoscopist may prove to be a distal transverse colonic carcinoma, requiring left hemicolectomy instead of the originally scheduled right colonic resection.

PATIENT POSITIONING

The laparoscopic approach to right colonic resection differs from the open technique in some respects. Patient positioning is very important in laparoscopic surgery, more so than in the open resection. Thus, detailed discussion of the positional problems in laparoscopic surgery is in order.

Currently, three types of patient positions are common for the laparoscopic right colonic resection.

1. Supine position
2. Dorsolithotomy position
3. Left lateral position

These are usually combined with Trendelenburg's and reverse Trendelenburg's positions, depending on whether the dissection is done near the hepatic flexure of the colon or the ileocecum.

Proper positioning of the patient reduces operative frustration during laparoscopic dissection. The laparoscopic surgeon does not have the luxury of manually retracting the small intestinal loops by packing them away during laparoscopic right colonic mobilization. The presence of these interfering intestinal loops near the field of dissection intensifies the operative difficulty and promotes the risk of intestinal injury during mobilization, transection, and anastomosis. During the electrosurgical dissection with long, thinly insulated dissection scissors, electrical injury to the adjacent small intestinal loops from insulation failure, capacitive coupling, or direct coupling (see Ch. 9) can occur. Also, the site of injury may be laparoscopically invisible, and thus its recognition often may be delayed until the patient develops peritoneal septic complications.

Various laparoscopic retractors are currently available to allow endoscopic retraction. This technique, however, requires additional peritoneal cannulas to introduce the laparoscopic retractors. The risk of visceral injury from the retractors is small but not nonexistent. Also, laparoscopic retractors are less efficient than manual retractors.

Most laparoscopic surgeons operating on a supine patient use gravity to displace the small bowel loops by intraoperatively rotating the operating table. Unfortunately, the attainable safe rotation is limited because extreme rotation imperils the patient's stability on the table. The extreme degree of rotation may also contribute to neurovascular compression syndromes, especially if the surgeon uses mechanical barriers to prevent the patient from sliding off the table.

When the patient is in the dorsolithotomy position, the problem of compartment syndrome and other neurovascular complications should be considered.[11,12] Factors such as direct pressure on the posterior compartment of the calf, supracardiac leg elevation, prolonged operative time, pre-existent peripheral vascular disease, and intraoperative sequential compression devices all lead to anterior and posterior crural fascial compartment ischemia, producing myonecrosis. Reperfusion after taking the patient down from the lithotomy position produces capillary leak and tissue edema, increasing compartmental pressure with consequent neurovascular compromise. Proper precautions in dorsolithotomy positioning and perioperative monitoring of lower extremity perfusion status—either by pedal pulse oximetry or compartment pressure measurement, especially during prolonged operations—may reduce position-related neurovascular complications. Early detection and dermofasciotomy are the only ways to prevent permanent damage in the unfortunate event of compartment syndrome. Femoral neuropathy secondary to prolonged dorsolithotomy position has also been described.[13] By contrast, French laparoscopic surgeons use the dorsolithotomy position of the patient extensively with minimal positional complications. The dorsolithotomy position has the advantage of providing an extra standing space for the surgeon or the assistants and allows anal access for intraoperative colonoscopy.

Left lateral decubitus position has been proposed as the optimal position for laparoscopic right colonic resection.[14] Some positional complications from dorsolithotomy position are preventable by placing the patient in the left lateral decubitus position before draping. Also, gravity-aided displacement of small intestinal loops next to the operative field is maximized in the lateral decubitus position.

Neurovascular complications can also occur with the left lateral decubitus position. The surgeon and the anesthesiologist should take great care in putting the patient on the operating table in the left lateral decubitus position. The left arm is placed on a padded side arm board. The medial humeral epicondyle and the ulnar nerve are protected with foam rubber pads. A foam-rubber axillary pad protects the brachial plexus. The right arm rests over the patient's anterior chest wall, or an arm holder, and is taped securely to prevent intraoperative displacement (Fig. 20-1).

I have no experience in doing the laparoscopic right colonic resection with the patient in the dorsolithotomy position. My experience with patients who had a laparoscopic right colonic resection, with the patient in the left lateral decubitus position, is presented and compared with historical controls of the same operation done with the patient supine.

ANESTHETIC REQUIREMENTS

General, endotracheal, balanced anesthesia with excellent muscle relaxation is essential for a satisfactory laparoscopic resection. With inadequate muscle relaxation, it is difficult to raise and maintain the intraperitoneal pressure to an acceptable level. I notice that use of nitrous oxide as an inhalation anesthetic agent may lead to dilated small bowel loops, hindering laparoscopic dissection. Nitrous oxide inhalation may also increase intraperitoneal nitrous oxide concentration, thus enhancing the risk of an explosion from electrodissection. I request my anesthesiologist to avoid use of nitrous oxide during laparoscopic colon resection.

OPERATIVE TECHNIQUE

Well-planned arrangement of video equipment in the operating room reduces technical frustration and facilitates swift operation (Fig. 20-2). Two video monitors are positioned, one on either side of the operating

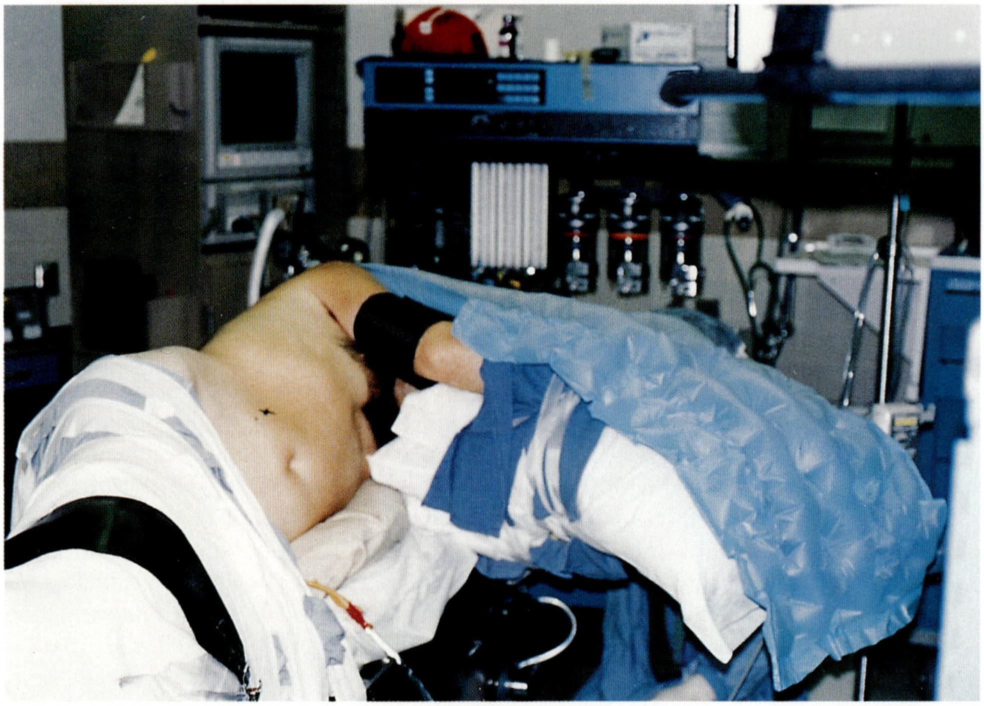

Fig. 20-1. Left lateral decubitus positioning of the patient with proper padding and arm placement.

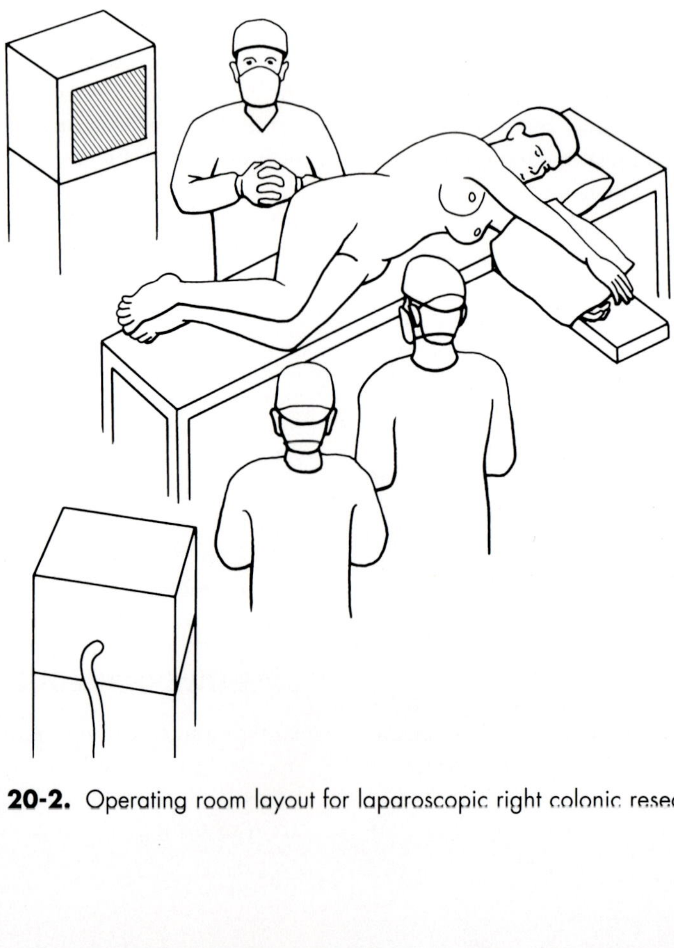

Fig. 20-2. Operating room layout for laparoscopic right colonic resection.

table. The room layout should allow their relocation cephalad or caudad, depending on the area of dissection. This option ensures a direct line of vision for the surgeon, evading the problem of paradoxical motion. The surgeon stands on the patient's right side and the assistant on the left side (Fig. 20-3).

A carbon dioxide pneumoperitoneum is produced through the inferior rim of the umbilicus with a Veress needle. Low or negative intraperitoneal pressure on insertion, a slow increase in the pressure with continued insufflation, and lowering of the pressure when the abdominal wall is lifted confirm the intraperitoneal location of the needle. Auscultation with an esophageal stethoscope during insufflation of carbon dioxide also confirms successful initiation of a pneumoperitoneum. This characteristic tympanic sound detects the pneumoperitoneum as soon as or sooner than did the other, standard methods such as the hanging drop technique.[15]

At times, the tip of the Veress needle may land anteriorly to the peritoneum and lead to extraperitoneal insufflation of carbon dioxide. Extraperitoneal insufflation is a common complication and can be difficult to rectify. Some surgeons use the extraperitoneal tissue space produced by carbon dioxide to place the Veress needle into the peritoneal cavity under direct vision.[16] Elevation of the peritoneum that obliterates extraperitoneal space confirms the successful establishment of a pneumoperitoneum.

When Veress needle insertion is not feasible, an open incision and placement of a blunt trocar establish the pneumoperitoneum. The open incision technique is especially useful in patients who have extensive intraperitoneal adhesions.

The intraperitoneal pressure is raised to 15 mm Hg before insertion of the primary peritoneal trocar. In elderly patients, cold carbon dioxide may contribute to hypothermia. Also, cold carbon dioxide fogs laparoscopes. Hypothermic stress from carbon dioxide pneumoperitoneum insufflation can be reduced by warming the insufflated carbon dioxide gas to 30°C.[17]

A 12-mm cannula for a 30-degree videolaparoscope is advanced into the peritoneal cavity. Additional peritoneal cannulas are placed under direct vision in the suprapubic midline and midway between umbilicus and xiphisternum in the midline. Once the additional ports are placed, carbon dioxide is insufflated through a different port than the port lodging the laparoscope to avoid fogging of the scopes. Preoperative Foley catheterization avoids undesirable trocar cystotomy. Nasogastric intubation and decompression allow safe dissection of the hepatic flexure. Five- or 10-mm cannulas, as required, are also placed in the right upper quadrant and right lower quadrant of the abdomen lateral to the rectus. When the patient is lying supine or in the dorsolithotomy position, the left lower or upper quadrant abdominal cannulas can be introduced as

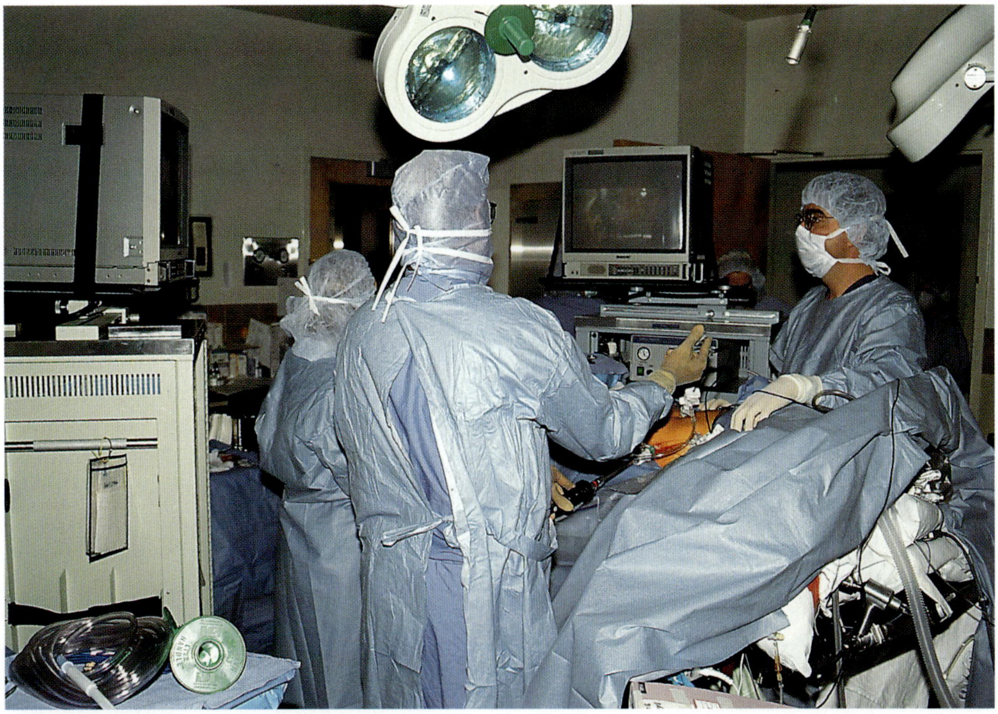

Fig. 20-3. Personnel and monitoring positioning for laparoscopic right colonic resection.

needed with ease. Cannulas to the left of the linea alba are awkward to place when the patient is lying in the left lateral decubitus position. These cannulas in the left side of the abdomen, however, are rarely indispensable for the laparoscopic right colonic resection.

Obesity in the patient is a challenge in laparoscopic colorectal surgery. Port placement in obese patients may require longer cannulas because standard laparoscopic ports may be too short for use in obese patients. When long cannulas are not available, an endotracheal tube as an overtube can overcome this problem.[18]

Magnetic resonance imaging (MRI) studies of the anterior abdominal wall suggest (and the experiences of most laparoscopists concur) that the technique of insertion of a Veress needle and peritoneal ports is different in obese patients compared with nonobese patients. The optimal location of the insertion point and the insertion angle of the Veress needle (and the primary port) vary depending on the patient's weight. In the nonobese patient, both the Veress needle and the port can be inserted at 45 degrees, at the inferior rim or the base of the umbilicus, with little risk of preperitoneal insertion. When the patient is obese, the angle of insertion can be 45 degrees, but the optimal insertion point is through the base of the umbilicus rather than the inferior rim. This position lessens chances of preperitoneal insertion. In very obese patients, both the Veress needle and the trocar have to be inserted through the base of the umbilicus at or near 90 degrees to avoid preperitoneal placement. As in patients with extensive intraperitoneal adhesions, an open laparoscopic technique may be necessary in obese patients.[19] Morbid obesity may be a relative contraindication to laparoscopic right colonic resection because of difficulty with peritoneal access and prolonged operative time in these patients.

Careful laparoscopic evaluation of the entire peritoneal cavity should be done before starting the laparoscopic dissection. Hepatic evaluation is optimally achieved with the 30-degree laparoscope. Rotation of the scope and axial movement enable inspection of all accessible hepatic surfaces. Laparoscopic ultrasound transducers also help to exclude hepatic metastases (see Ch. 10). The surgeon should inspect the ovaries to exclude metastatic disease.

When the patient is supine, small intestinal loops may hinder visualization and dissection of the ileocecal region and the hepatic flexure. Rotation of the patient and retraction by endoscopic retractors may help clear the operative field. Placement of lower quadrant cannulas in a patient placed in the dorsolithotomy position requires attention to reduce restriction of instrumental movement from the unyielding iliac crest and the right costal margin.

Not uncommonly, intra-abdominal adhesions from previous cholecystectomy or appendectomy pose problems with visualization or dissection of the right colon. Even additional port placement may require laparoscopic adhesiolysis. When a second cannula cannot be inserted because of adhesions, using a sidearm or therapeutic laparoscope through the primary port will help clear the anterior abdominal wall for additional port placement. Using bipolar coagulation forceps rather than monopolar electrosurgical scissors reduces the risk of visceral injury when the small intestinal loops adhere to the anterior abdominal wall.

When the patient is in the left lateral decubitus position, an excellent laparoscopic view of the terminal ileum, cecum, and the ascending colon is gained because small intestinal loops fall away from the ascending colon. The avascular plane of the right paracolic gutter and the hepatocolic ligament appear appealingly uncluttered. Dissection and mobilization of the right colon are accomplished by using the monopolar endoscopic electrodissecting scissors and endoscopic atraumatic Babcock forceps. An endoscopic Babcock forceps is inserted through a suprapubic midline port for colonic traction, and the electrosurgical scissors is inserted through the supraumbilical midline port. (This port selection may have to be reversed for the left-handed surgeon.)

Endoscopic Babcock forceps can traumatize the colonic wall with relative ease; thus, the traction should be done with great care. Five-millimeter cannulas placed in the right upper and lower quadrant of the abdomen will allow the use of atraumatic U-handle bowel graspers to tense the paracolic gutter and the hepatocolic ligament during the paracolic dissection. The vermiform appendix often is adherent to the posterior serosal peritoneum and requires mobilization. The right ureter is easily identified in normasthenic patients but requires retroperitoneal dissection in obese patients. The surgeon should reduce or avoid monopolar electrodissection near the right ureter to prevent ureteral thermal injuries and consequent postoperative ureteral strictures. Injury to the infundibulopelvic ligament can create problems with hemostasis during ileocecal mobilization.

Division of the hepatocolic ligament to free the hepatic flexure may require changing the camera to the supraumbilical port and the dissecting scissors to the right upper quadrant port. Similar shuffling of instruments and camera may also be necessary during the ileocecal dissection. The pulsating common and external iliac artery serves as a landmark during ileocecal mobilization. The gallbladder often adheres to the hepatic flexure and the proximal transverse mesocolon and should not be grasped. Gentle retraction with an atraumatic closed forceps and sharp dissection separate the gallbladder from the mesocolon. Dissection of the gastrocolic ligament can often be done through the avascular plane, although adipose omentum may lead to bloody dissection. The use of a bipolar electrocoagulator, not only to dissect and create windows in adipose planes but also for hemostasis, facilitates dissection of an adipose gastrocolic ligament. Vessels too large to coagulate can be ligated with endoscopic clip applicators and endoscopic ligators such as an endoloop. Tilting the patient into Trendelenburg's position eases the dissection of the ileocecal region, and reverse Trendelenburg's position eases the dissection of the hepatic flexure and hepatocolic ligament.

When the intraluminal colonic lesion is small or soft and thus laparoscopically invisible or nonpalpable, intraoperative colonoscopy (Fig. 20-4) can well be done by the surgeon or the assistant, changing only the perineal drapes after colonoscopy. This method obviously is feasible only when the patient is placed in the left lateral decubitus or dorsolithotomy position. The image from the videocolonoscope is projected on a third monitor placed to the left of the patient's feet or on top of the laparoscopic monitor on the patient's left side, avoiding the problem of too many monitors in a small room. The colonoscopic image can also be hooked to a separate input jack of the laparoscopic video monitors.

The air insufflated through the colonoscope rarely produces massive enough dilation of colon to hinder further colonic dissection. However, small bowel dilation from insufflation escaping cephalad through an incompetent ileocecal valve can render further continuation of laparoscopic dissection next to impossible. Occlusion of the distal ileum with an atraumatic bowel clamp before starting colonoscopy should be done. The other approach is to use carbon dioxide rather than air to insufflate the colon during colonoscopy. Any carbon dioxide escaping into the small intestine will be absorbed rapidly, thus avoiding problems with dilated small bowel loops.

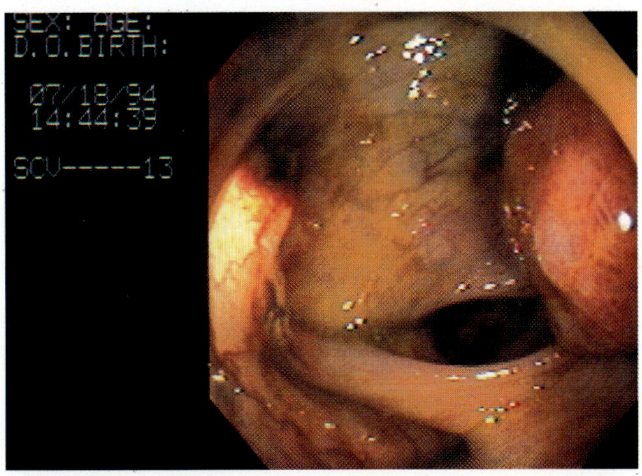

Fig. 20-4. Intraoperative colonoscopy showing the right colonic lesion and the transmitted light from the laparoscope.

Once the laparoscopically invisible intraluminal colonic lesion is identified by colonoscopy, the laparoscopist can place an endoscopic clip or use coagulation to mark the lesion on the colonic serosa and proceed with the operation. After mobilization of the right colon, the right colic vessels are dissected initially, coagulated with bipolar electrocoagulation forceps, transected, and then ligated with an endoclip applicator. When the patient is positioned in the left lateral decubitus position, dissection and ligation of the right colic vessels are preferably conducted before the right paracolic gutter dissection, thus avoiding the problem of any paracolic bleeding, obscuring the paraduodenal and right colic vascular dissection. The right half of the transverse colon, transverse mesocolon, and terminal ileum are transected with an endoscopic stapler. To remove the surgical specimen, a 4- to 5-cm muscle-splitting incision is made over the right lower quadrant or upper quadrant of the abdomen (Fig. 20-5). The ideal site for the incision is selected by bringing the ileal and transverse colonic ends toward the anterior abdominal wall. An attempt is made to include one of the cannula entrance sites in the abdominal incision made to deliver the specimen. Muscle-splitting incision is preferred to muscle-cutting incision. The wound edges are protected by gauze pads or a Vi-drape to prevent wound contamination by cancer cells or microbes during delivery of a specimen containing cancer. Even bulky right colonic resected specimens can be removed via small muscle-splitting incisions (Fig. 20-6).

In some patients, exteriorization of the mobilized colon through the muscle-splitting incision and further extracorporeal transection of the colon and mesocolon followed by the anastomosis may be appropriate rather than laborious and tedious intracorporeal dissection. For example, an adipose greater omentum or transverse mesocolon may prevent swift endoscopic colonic dissection and transection. The ligation of right colic vessels may not be endoscopically feasible because of large metastatic lymph nodes at the right colic artery's origin from the superior mesenteric artery. Also, intraoperative colonoscopy may not be possible, or the scope could not be advanced into the ascending colon for any number of reasons. After completion of the extracorporeal anastomosis, either by the hand-sewn or stapling technique, it is dropped into the peritoneal cavity, and the abdominal incision is repaired (Fig. 20-7).

Complete intraperitoneal ileotransverse colonic anastomosis is certainly feasible with existing endoscopic staplers. The potentially prohibitive number of cannulas and staplers needed to conduct totally intracorporeal anastomosis and the need for a small incision for specimen retrieval even after intraperitoneal anastomosis convince me to hand sew the ileocolic anastomosis.

Reports of port site hernias abound. Some German laparoscopists cite the absence of trocar site hernias in

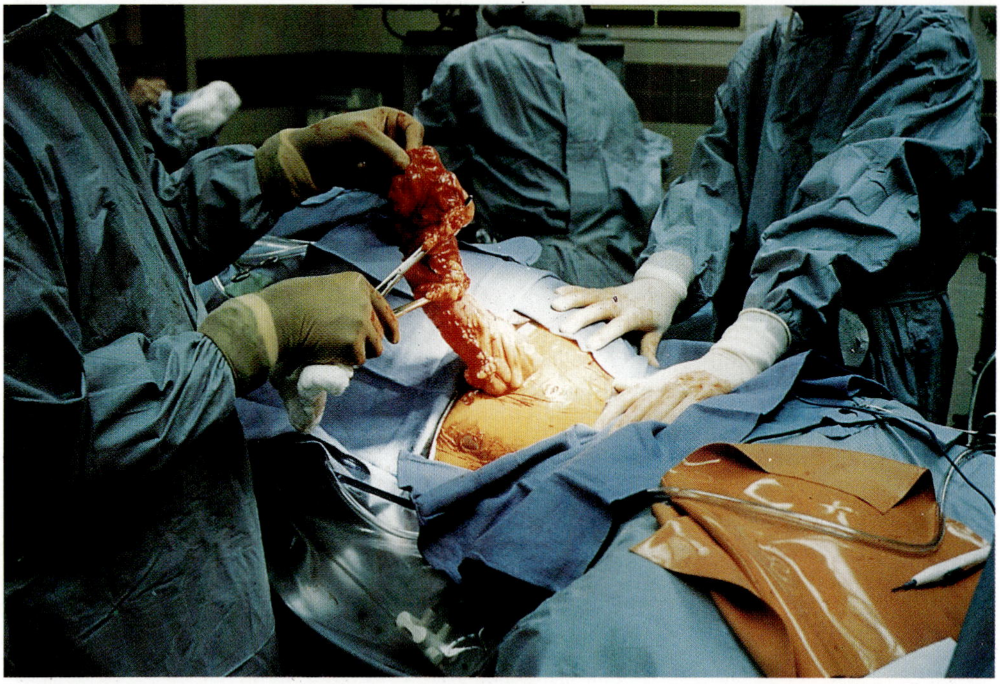

Fig. 20-5. Retrieval of a right colon with ileocolic Crohn's disease through a small incision.

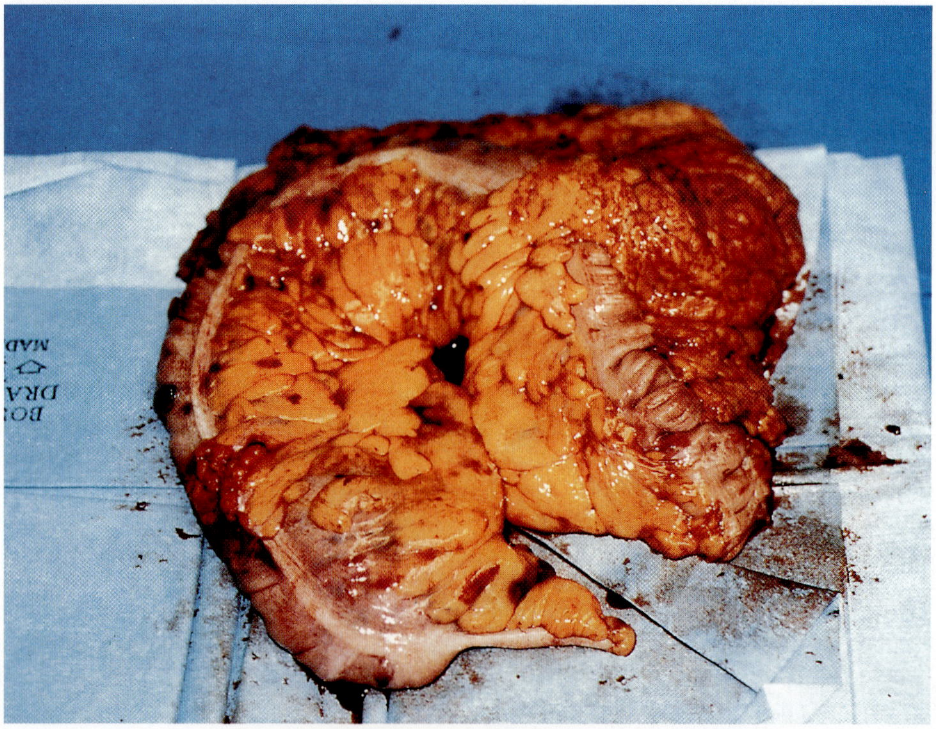

Fig. 20-6. A laparoscopically resected right colon with ascending colon cancer.

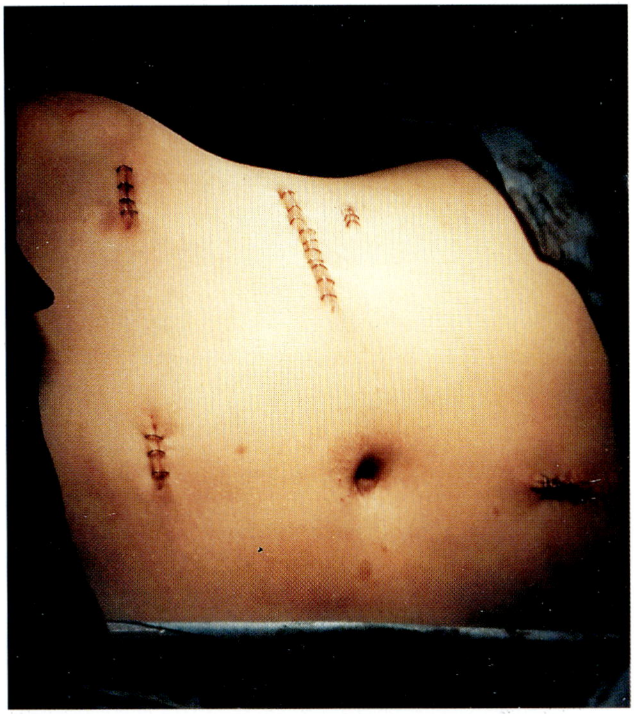

Fig. 20-7. Port sites and incision for specimen retrieval (patient positioned in left lateral decubitus position).

their vast experience with laparoscopy and suggest that the pyramidal trocar commonly used by North American laparoscopists may contribute more fascial damage and consequent herniation (G. Beuss, personal communication, 1993). Although the causal factors are unknown, incisional hernias frequently develop at the port entrance sites. Early incisional hernias seem to occur more commonly with 12-mm port entrance sites and in the midline. The frequency of incisional hernias at extraumbilical 12-mm trocar insertion sites can be as high as 3.1 percent.[20] Incisional hernias are also significantly more common if the fascia is left open, although hernias at 12-mm trocar sites occurred in some patients even after attempted closure of the fascial wound.[21] Omental evisceration[22] and Richter's hernia formation have also been described at the port entrance sites.[23]

The surgeon should repair the cannula entrance wounds before closure of the abdominal incision. All fascial defects are approximated by absorbable sutures. When practicable during closure, a malleable metal retractor is placed via right lower quadrant incision to protect small intestinal loops subjacent to the fascial wounds. Other fascial wounds at cannula sites distant from the incision made for specimen removal are repaired by inserting a Foley catheter through the port entrance site, inflating the balloon to displace the subjacent intestinal loops, and withdrawing the catheter after completion of fascial closure (Fig. 20-8).

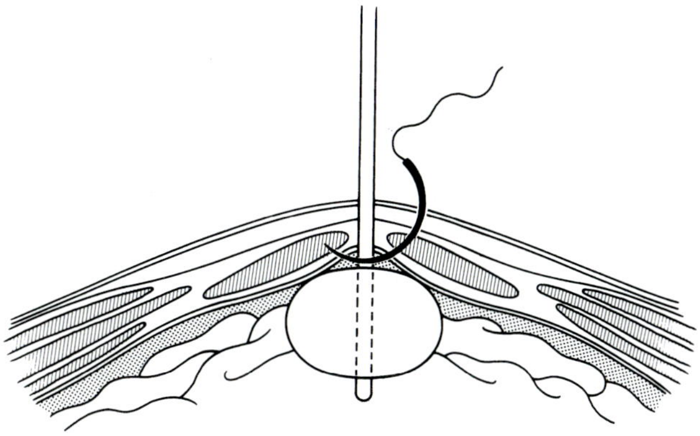

Fig. 20-8. Safe closure of fascial defect at port entrance sites using a Foley catheter balloon to displace subfascial small bowel loops.

All wounds are infiltrated with local anesthetic such as 0.25 percent bupivacaine solution with epinephrine before closure. In addition, intraperitoneal instillation of local anesthetic solution promotes postoperative analgesia without systemic toxicity.[24] Postoperatively, analgesia is provided by parenteral narcotics, replaced with oral narcotics as soon as the patient can take liquids. The patient is allowed to take liquids as soon as bowel sounds are present. The patient can be sent home on the fourth or fifth postoperative day when a liquid diet is tolerated (Fig. 20-9).

RESULTS

Data on 17 patients who had laparoscopic right colonic resection were collected and tabulated prospectively (Table 20-1). My experience with laparoscopic right

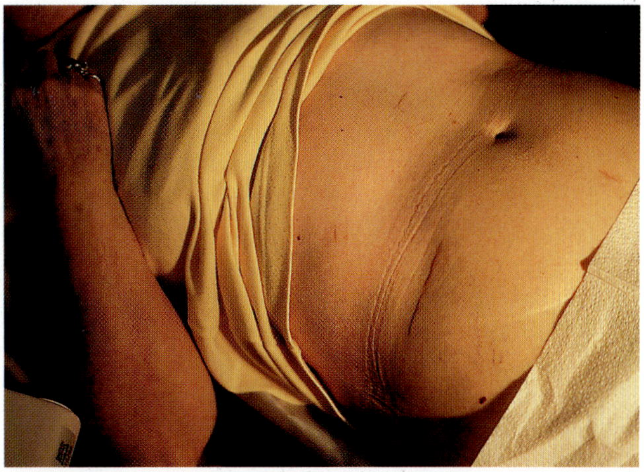

Fig. 20-9. A surgical scar from laparoscopic right colonic resection.

Table 20-1. Clinical Data on Laparoscopic Right Colonic Resections in 17 Patients

	Left Lateral Decubitus Position	Supine Position
Age distribution (mean and range in years)	55 (29–74)	66 (47–80)
Sex distribution (M/F)	2:3	9:3
Diagnosis		
Crohn's	1	1
Villous adenoma	3	5
Carcinoma	1	6
Total no.	5	12
Operative time (mean and range in minutes)	122 (67–155)	172 (109–245)
Duration of ileus (mean and range in days)	1.8 (1–2)	2.4 (1–4)
Hospital stay (mean and range in days)	5.4 (4–7)	8.6 (6–13)

colonic resection in 12 patients with the patient supine preceded my experience in 5 patients who had the operation in the left lateral decubitus position. The clinical course of those five patients is reported below.

1. A 29-year-old woman with an enlarging right lower quadrant mass underwent laparoscopic right colonic resection in the left lateral position. After mobilization of the colon, the colonic mass was brought out through a 4-cm incision, and the anastomosis was conducted extraperitoneally. The patient had normal bowel sounds on the second postoperative day and tolerated liquid diet well by the third postoperative day. She went home on the fourth postoperative day. The lesion proved to be chronic Crohn's disease with transmural inflammation and abscess formation with no neoplastic transformation.
2. An exophytic hepatic flexure colon carcinoma in a 74-year-old woman was resected by laparoscopic right colonic resection with the patient in the left lateral position. Colonic mobilization was conducted laparoscopically, and the ileum was transected with an endoscopic stapler. After the wound edges were protected with lap pads, the surgical specimen with the cancer was removed through a 4-cm incision. The transverse colon was transected extraperitoneally because of extremely adipose greater omentum, which hindered swift laparoscopic dissection. The anastomosis was done extraperitoneally. The patient had normal bowel sounds on the second postoperative day and went home on the fourth postoperative day when she could take a liquid diet.
3. A 60-year-old man had a 2-cm flat, sessile, wide-based villous cecal adenoma that could not be resected colonoscopically. The patient was placed in the left lateral position. The cecum and ascending colon were mobilized laparoscopically. Through a 4-cm muscle-splitting incision, the cecum and the ileum were delivered out of the peritoneal cavity. The polypoid lesion was present along the inferior lip of the ileocecal valve, and the excision of the cecal cap was done under direct vision to ensure that the villous adenoma was completely excised, still preserving most of the ileocecal valve. The neocecum was reconstructed extraperitoneally. Because of the need for excision of a portion of the inferior lip of the ileocecal valve, neocecal reconstruction was hand sewn. Postoperatively, the patient had normal bowel sounds on the second day, was able to tolerate liquid diet by the fourth day, and was sent home on the fifth day.
4. A 59-year-old woman had a 2-cm midascending colonic sessile, wide-based tubulovillous adenoma that could not be endoscopically resected. The patient was placed in the left lateral position. The ascending colon was mobilized laparoscopically, and the polyp-containing segment was identified with the aid of a transoperative colonoscopy. Through a 5-cm incision in the right lower quadrant of the abdomen, the segment of ascending colon was delivered out of the peritoneal cavity, resected, and an end-to-side anastomosis was done. The patient had normal bowel sounds on the first postoperative day, tolerated a liquid diet by the third postoperative day, and was discharged on the fifth postoperative day.
5. A 65-year-old woman with a large ascending colonic carcinoma underwent laparoscopic mobilization of the ascending colon in the left lateral decubitus position. During the paraduodenal dissection, large lymph glands were identified along the base of the right colic artery. A right upper quadrant muscle-splitting incision was made. The colonic resection and anastomosis were done extraperitoneally. The

patient had normal bowel sounds the second postoperative day and was discharged on the fifth postoperative day.

CONCLUSION

Laparoscopic right colonic resection both for benign and malignant disease is feasible. Improving instrumentation will increase the facility with which colonic mobilization and resection can be conducted. More so than in the conventional open colonic resections, proper positioning of the patient is of major significance in laparoscopic operations. The laparoscopic visualization, dissection, mobilization, and transection of the ileum and right hemicolon can at times be demanding because of overlying small bowel loops. When the table is rotated with the patient supine, these loops interfering with laparoscopic dissection can be displaced by gravity. The operative advantage from gravity-aided small intestinal displacement is disappointingly limited when the patient is lying supine. However, extreme rotation endangers the patient's stability on the operating table. The left lateral position, combined with Trendelenburg's and reverse Trendelenburg's position, promotes displacement of the small bowel loops more optimally than the supine position and lets the surgeon dissect and mobilize the right hemicolon and paraduodenal regions safely and swiftly.

Positioning of the patient can be done properly and securely before draping the patient. Proper padding of critical neurovascular areas (medial epicondyle and ulnar nerve, fibular neck and peroneal nerve, etc.) prevents positional complications. Padding of all critical areas can be done more proficiently if the patient is positioned before draping rather than relying on rotation transoperatively to obtain a virtual left lateral position.

I was concerned that establishing a pneumoperitoneum with the patient lying in the left lateral position might be difficult, because most laparoscopic surgeons are accustomed to working on the horizontal, flat anterior abdominal wall. However, a pneumoperitoneum can be produced quite well when the patient is lying in the left lateral position, either by the blind technique using a Veress needle, or by an open incision technique. Because the intestinal loops are displaced to the left side and the needle is introduced caudally and slightly to the patient's right side, intestinal and aortic injuries from the Veress needle or the peritoneal cannulas will be minimized. Making a muscle-splitting incision to deliver the right colon out of the peritoneal cavity can also be done without difficulty when the patient is in the left lateral position.

The advantage of colonic tethering to the abdominal wall in mesocolic dissection is appreciated by most laparoscopic colorectal surgeons. The mobile sigmoid colon is often tethered to the anterior abdominal wall during laparoscopic sigmoid colectomy. Similarly, the right colon is anatomically tethered to the right paracolic gutter, when the patient is lying in the left lateral position. In this position, the ileocolic and right colic vessels can be preferentially dissected and ligated before mobilizing the right colon off the paracolic gutter. This technique deters the freed ascending colon from falling over the paraduodenal region, hindering the dissection and ligation of the right colonic vessels at their origin. Reverse Trendelenburg's position and consequent hepatic descent while the patient is lying on the left side pose no problem in hepatic flexure dissection.

When the anastomosis is done extraperitoneally, the left lateral position also reduces the need for a longer incision. There is no need for medial retraction of interfering small intestinal loops with the patient in the left lateral position, as the surgeon often notices when the patient is supine. This enables delivering the mobilized right colonic segment through a small incision with little interference from the small intestinal loops.

One other advantage of the left lateral position is the availability of anal access. Transoperative colonoscopy can be conducted with no difficulty when the patient is placed in the left lateral decubitus position. By placing a third video monitor on the patient's left side or hooking the videocolonoscope to a different input jack on the laparoscopic monitor, the surgeon or the assistant can insert the videocolonoscope transanally to identify the nonpalpable intraluminal colonic lesion that is in question. While the colonoscopist identifies the lesion, the laparoscopic surgeon can grasp the colon with the endoscopic forceps and mark the site serosally with a metal clip, enabling removal of nonpalpable intraluminal lesions (see Ch. 12).

No position-related complications occurred in my experience with five patients who had right colonic resection in the left lateral position. Proper preoperative padding of the patient is imperative. As much as 15 minutes of operating room time may be consumed during the initial positioning. This time consumption is offset by the facility during right colonic mobilization and transection. Also, the increased safety—by protection from electrosurgical injury to the small intestinal loops near the area of dissection and avoidance of additional peritoneal cannulas for laparoscopic retractors—compensates for any lost time. Thus, the left lateral position improves the operative facility and efficiency with only minimal time loss from initial positioning.

The left lateral decubitus positioning of the patient during laparoscopic right colonic resection improves visualization and facilitates dissection and mobilization, along with transection of the right hemicolon. In addition, the left lateral decubitus position enables safe, swift, and satisfactory intraperitoneal or extraperitoneal anastomosis by maximizing gravity-aided displacement of interfering small bowel loops.

The laparoscopic right colonic resection in 12 patients (with the patients supine) reported preceded the experience in the last five patients who had the operation in the left lateral decubitus position. The sampling error, selection bias, and small sample size as well as the different disease distribution in the two groups render the noticed improvement insignificant. The learning curve may well explain the difference in operative times and hospital stay between the groups. The phenomenon of the learning curve can be appreciated by all surgeons from the time they begin conducting laparoscopic surgery. Training and practice improve any surgical skill, and laparoscopic colectomy is no exception.[25]

The issue of whether laparoscopic resection is compatible with current oncosurgical dogma is generating a healthy debate. The recent reports of port site recurrence[26,27] raise a serious concern in applying laparoscopic techniques to colorectal malignancies because of the possibility of tumor spillage and seeding. Whether the incidence of port site recurrences after laparoscopic cancer resection is more than that of incisional tumor implantation after conventional open cancer resection is unknown.

Minimal experimental data deal with port site recurrence. A murine model of peritoneal tumor implantation, using a bladder tumor, showed more tumor cells at the sites of peritoneal disruption. This phenomenon is partially prevented by intraperitoneal instillation of substances such as heparin that decrease cell adherence.[28] Whether the inevitable, intraoperative microscopic tumor seeding is more dangerous in laparoscopic operations than it is in conventional open operations is yet to be determined. It is hard to understand or explain the increase in tumor implants at the peritoneal access sites after laparoscopy compared with laparotomy. The degree of peritoneal disruption after open laparotomy is significantly more than any laparoscopic procedure, even with use of multiple trocars. The role of a carbon dioxide pneumoperitoneum, the major difference between open and laparoscopic procedures, in the pathogenesis of port site recurrence of cancer needs further investigation. If future experimental or clinical data suggest that the pneumoperitoneum promotes port site recurrence and compromises a curative cancer resection, the gasless approach to laparoscopic surgery using an abdominal wall lift may gain more attention.[29]

It can be argued that, at the current state of knowledge, colon cancers should not be resected laparoscopically until data from the randomized controlled trials are collected. Because most of the colon cancer recurrences develop within 2 years after the surgical resection,[30] the question of whether laparoscopic resection increases abdominal or intraperitoneal recurrences will be answered in the very near future by the proliferation or paucity of port site recurrences.[31]

Controlled trials are needed to compare laparoscopic resection versus conventional open resection. However, the problem of port site recurrence and other signs of inadequate cancer resection should become clear to the clinical surgeon long before the results of the trial become available. The systematic comparative clinical observation of current clinical experience and historical controls should yield information that is complementary to that gained from randomized clinical trials in finding the oncosurgical superiority or inadequacy of laparoscopic resection colon cancer.

The laparoscopic approach to right colonic resection is feasible and demonstrated to be safe in multiple centers. The applicability of the minimal access approach to colonic malignancy is currently being studied both by randomized controlled trials and retrospective clinical data collection. Attention to technical details such as proper preoperative preparation; positioning; localization of the lesion, either by preoperative tattooing or intraoperative colonoscopy; and adherence to established surgical principles are essential to gain the benefits from the laparoscopic resection of right colonic lesions.

REFERENCES

1. Soper NJ, Stockmann PT, Dunnegan DL et al: Laparoscopic cholecystectomy. The new "gold standard?" Arch Surg 127:917, 1992
2. Falk PM, Beart RW, Wexner SD: Laparoscopic colectomy: a critical appraisal. Dis Colon Rectum 36:28, 1992
3. Guillou PJ, Darzi A, Monson JR: Experience with laparoscopic colorectal surgery for malignant disease. Surg Oncol, suppl. 1:43, 1993
4. Monson JR, Darzi A, Carey PD et al: Prospective evaluation of laparoscopic-assisted colectomy in an unselected group of patients. Lancet 340:831, 1992
5. Jacobs M, Verdeja JC, Goldstein HS: Minimally invasive colon resection (laparoscopic colectomy). Surg Laparosc Endosc 1:144, 1991
6. Hammond DC, Lane FR, Mackeigan JM et al: Endoscopic tattooing of the colon: clinical experience. Am Surg 59:205, 1993
7. Lightdale CJ: India ink colonic tattoo: blots on the record. Gastrointest Endosc 37:99, 1991
8. Park SI, Genta RS, Romeo DP et al: Colonic abscess and focal peritonitis secondary to India ink tattooing of the colon. Gastrointest Endosc 37:68, 1991
9. Coman E, Brandt LJ, Brenner S et al: Fat necrosis and inflammatory pseudotumor due to endoscopic tattooing of the colon with India ink. Gastrointest Endosc 37:65, 1991
10. Hyman N, Waye JD: Endoscopic four quadrant tattoo for the identification of colonic lesions at surgery. Gastrointest Endosc 37:56, 1991
11. Schwartz LB, Stahl RS, DeCherney AH: Unilateral compartment syndrome after prolonged gynecologic surgery in the dorsolithotomy position. A case report. J Reprod Med 38:469, 1993
12. Mulhall JP, Drezner AD: Postoperative compartment syndrome and the lithotomy position: a report of three cases and analysis of potential risk factors. Conn Med 57:129, 1993
13. Hakim M, Katirji B: Femoral mononeuropathy induced by the lithotomy position: a report of five cases with a review of literature. Muscle Nerve 16:891, 1993

14. Jager RM: Laparoscopic right colonic resection in left lateral position. Surg Laparosc Endosc 4:321, 1994
15. Beckmann CR, Dadabhoy Z, Beckmann CA et al: Auscultation with an esophageal stethoscope. A new test for pneumoperitoneum. J Reprod Med 36:298, 1991
16. Kabukoba JJ, Skillern LH: Coping with extraperitoneal insufflation during laparoscopy: a new technique. Obstet Gynecol 80:144, 1992
17. Ott DE: Correction of laparoscopic insufflation hypothermia. J Laparoendosc Surg 1:183, 1991
18. Bradpiece H, Andrews SM, Rennie JA: A novel means of securing a laparoscopic port in the obese patient. Ann R Coll Surg Engl 75:252, 1993
19. Hurd WH, Bude RO, DeLancey JO et al: Abdominal wall characterization with magnetic resonance imaging and computed tomography, the effect of obesity on the laparoscopic approach. J Reprod Med 36:473, 1991
20. McMurrick PJ, Polglase AL: Early incisional hernia after use of the 12-mm port for laparoscopic surgery. Aust N Z J Surg 63:574, 1993
21. Kadar N, Reich H, Liu CY et al: Incisional hernias after major laparoscopic gynecologic procedures. Am J Obstet Gynecol 168:1493, 1993
22. Bloom DA, Ehrlich RM: Omental evisceration through small laparoscopy port sites. J Endourol 7:31, 1993
23. Wegener ME, Chung D, Crans C et al: Small bowel obstruction secondary to incarcerated Richter's hernia from laparoscopic hernia repair. J Laparoendosc Surg 3:173, 1993
24. Narchi P, Benhamou D, Fernandez H: Intraperitoneal local anesthetic for shoulder pain after day-case laparoscopy. Lancet 28:338, 1991
25. See WA, Fisher RJ, Winfield HN et al: Laparoscopic surgical training: effectiveness and impact on urological surgical practice patterns. J Urol 149:1054, 1993
26. Cavanagh D: Abdominal wall metastases from ovarian cancer after laparoscopy. Am J Obstet Gynecol 169:522, 1993
27. Patsner B, Damien M: Umbilical metastases from a stage I-B cervical cancer after laparoscopy: a case report. Fertil Steril 58:1248, 1992
28. Goldstein DS, Lu ML, Hattori T et al: Inhibition of peritoneal tumor-cell implantation: model for laparoscopic cancer surgery. J Endourol 7:237, 1993
29. Kitano S, Tomikawa M, Iso Y et al: A safe and simple method to maintain a clear field of vision during laparoscopic cholecystectomy. Surg Endosc 6:197, 1992
30. Galandiuk S, Wieand HS, Moertel CG et al: Patterns of recurrence after curative resection of carcinoma of the colon and rectum. Surg Gynecol Obstet 174:27, 1992
31. Ramos JM, Gupta S, Anthone GJ et al: Laparoscopic and colon cancer: is the site at risk? Arch Surg 129:897, 1994

Editorial Comment I

John A. Coller

INDICATIONS

The caveats relative to limitations of laparoscopy for right colon resection are certainly well taken. This is particularly true in regard to cancer. Port site recurrences appear to be a unique presentation of laparoscopic cancer resection, and they have not all been in the specimen extraction site. The possibility that the pneumoperitoneum environment may potentially alter cancer cell dissemination must be considered. The pneumoperitoneum could involve altered systemic dissemination as well as intra-abdominal aerosolization of viable cancer cells. By contrast, alteration of certain immune mediators may have an inhibitory effect on cancer dissemination when compared with standard surgical technique. These are areas of speculation and uncertainty and must temper any wholesale enthusiasm for laparoscopic colectomy for cancer.

Those of us who perform laparoscopic resection on selected patients with cancer must recognize that our selection criteria are both arbitrary and presumptive. Although it is difficult to see how patients with stage A cancer would be injured by a laparoscopic approach that follows cancer surgery principles, this teleological assumption must await an outcome proof. Likewise, just because the cancer presentation is metastatic and noncurative, it cannot be assumed that a palliative laparoscopic approach would not adversely alter survival as compared with traditional therapy. Prospective clinical trials to assess the efficacy of laparoscopic colon cancer resection are underway. For the time being, surgeons should strongly consider limiting their laparoscopic cancer resection efforts to within the framework of such trials.

Whether for cancer or benign disease, the selection of patients for laparoscopic colon resection should avoid those patients in whom the disease process or prior operative intervention has extensively disturbed or obliterated normal tissue planes of dissection.

POSITIONING

Dr. Jager has thoroughly described the left lateral decubitus position, which maximizes the use of gravity for small bowel displacement. I prefer to combine oblique body rotation with a modified Lloyd-Davies position using Allen stirrups. As with the left lateral decubitus position, this combined position requires a great deal of care in positioning to avoid pressure complications as described by Dr. Jager.

A 45-degree foam wedge is placed beneath the right flank. The arms are allowed to stay at the patient's sides. The foot of the table is dropped out of the way; both legs, with Venodyne compression boots, are placed in Allen stirrups. Both thighs must be positioned so that there is no hip flexion, and the flexed legs will be angled toward the floor. Any flexion of the thigh will interfere with instrument movement. The left buttock must be carefully positioned to ensure adequate cushioning to avoid injury to the sciatic nerve. The legs will be below the level of the table when it is level but will be even with the body when the table is in Trendelenburg's position.

Although positioning is sometimes tedious, the result offers certain advantages. Dependent displacement of the small bowel can be augmented by adding, as needed, up to 30 degrees of table rotation to the prepositioned 45 degrees. Having access to the perineum, between the Allen stirrups, provides an excellent vantage point for working up the right lateral gutter. This provides three operating positions (one between the legs and two on the left side) that have forward in-line views of the operating field. Furthermore, ready entry is available should intraoperative colonoscopy be indicated.

PRELIMINARY ASPECTS OF DISSECTION

At the onset of dissection, the field of dissection should be cleared of confusing anatomy. Dr. Jager has already mentioned the need to remove postappendectomy or cholecystectomy adhesions. Not infrequently, attachments are present between the distal ascending colon and the proximal transverse colon. These should be incised before dissection of the right colon itself, thus simplifying dissection of the right colon. Careful adhesiolysis simplifies dissection of the mesentery in the vicinity of the hepatic flexure. Likewise, if the omentum is dropped from the transverse and is adherent to the sigmoid or other lower abdominal structures, it should be liberated early on. These simple preliminary maneuvers will save considerable time and confusion.

Editorial Comment II

Steven D. Wexner

Dr. Jager provides a good background, including a rather comprehensive list of potential indications. Again, one must preface the entire chapter by stating that, at the present time, any pathology requiring resection is potentially addressable as a laparoscopic resection. The only point unanswered is whether curative resection of malignancy is acceptable. I will not reiterate at this juncture what I have stated at numerous other points in the text concerning the various issues relating to this question. I will, however, again state that at the time of writing this textbook, curative resection for carcinomas outside the confines of a prospectively randomized trial is inappropriate.

Dr. Jager discusses the time commitment to perform laparoscopic right hemicolectomy. Of my first 100 laparoscopic colorectal procedures, 47 included segmental resection such as right hemicolectomy. In the first 15 cases, the mean operative time was 3.5 hours, but in case numbers 31 to 47, the mean time was 2 hours. This almost 50-percent reduction in time was indeed significant ($P<0.05$) and allowed a final laparoscopic time not statistically significantly different from that entailed for open surgery. However, additional time is spent in setting up the instruments and removing them at the end of the case. These phases can add almost 1 hour to the procedure and are not reported by any author.

Dr. Jager raises many excellent points in this chapter. First, it is a fallacy to think that patients who are too sick for standard colectomy can safely undergo a laparoscopic procedure. He rightly notes that a patient who cannot tolerate an open procedure cannot and should not be subjected to a laparoscopic procedure. Second, Dr. Jager discusses the importance of tattooing small lesions or large polyps that have been completely removed. He also discussed intraoperative colonoscopy. I personally favor the latter technique, and from every patient scheduled for laparoscopic or laparoscopic-assisted surgery I also obtain consent for and schedule them for intraoperative colonoscopy. Dr. Jager's point of clamping the terminal ileum before colonoscopy is well made. I disagree with him relative to obtaining a preoperative barium enema. I believe that the expense is unnecessary, the procedure is inconvenient for the patient, and its usefulness is made redundant if intraoperative colonoscopy is always scheduled. Third, Dr. Jager discusses problems with the dorsolithotomy position. I perform virtually all open and laparoscopic colorectal procedures in the dorsolithotomy position. All patients have sequential compression stockings supplied before the induction of anesthesia; these stockings are worn until patients are fully ambulatory. Patients undergoing laparoscopic surgery also receive prophylactic subcutaneous heparin. Fourth, Dr. Jager makes an excellent point about paradoxical motion and the need for multiple video monitors. His technical treatise is superb. I have little to add other than to state that I use all 10-mm ports so that the camera and all of the instruments can be inserted through each and every port. To his discussion of right colonic mobilization, I add that I like to visualize both the ureter and the duodenum before any vessel transection.

Fifth, I fully agree with Dr. Jager that complete intraperitoneal anastomosis is, at the present time, not justifiable. I believe that such a maneuver represents a triumph of technology over common sense. He rightly notes that whereas one may spend an unreasonable amount of time and money performing complete intracorporeal vessel ligation, bowel transection, and anastomosis, one must then make an incision for specimen retrieval. The logic of such an approach defies me. I believe that completely intracorporeal right hemicolectomy represents more of an advantage to the surgeon's ego than to the patient's recovery. Perhaps at some point in the future, I will be proven wrong through a prospective randomized trial comparing laparoscopic-assisted and completely laparoscopic right hemicolectomy. However, at the present time, my cynical view is difficult to challenge. Fortunately, Dr. Jager thinks the same way. Sixth, he notes the problem of port site herniation. Several instruments are now commercially available to facilitate closure of 10-mm punctures. Finally, Dr. Jager discusses local anesthetic infiltration into the wounds. I suggest that such a maneuver might well be applied to the open setting and result in a similar decrease in postoperative pain and increase in rapidity of recovery. One of my former mentors, Dr. Charles O. Finne, of Minneapolis, has routinely employed such a maneuver during the last two decades. In general, residents passing through his tutelage dismissed the maneuver readily as dispensable. However, laparoscopy has taught us that reduction in pain can tremendously enhance recovery, and I believe that many more surgeons will now adopt Dr. Finne's technique.

I apologize to readers that I am unable to be more controversial regarding this chapter. However, I believe that debate about the scientific merits of the procedure are more important than arguments relative to technical trivia. Regardless of the specific technique employed for right hemicolectomy, the surgeon must at each step of the procedure question whether that particular maneuver is acceptable in an open setting. If the maneuver is not acceptable, then the surgeon should rethink the operating method and change tactics. If an alternative approach is found and is still not acceptable in the open setting, then a conversion to a laparotomy should be made. A conversion should never be considered a failure but should instead be regarded as sound judgment.

21

Laparoscopic Surgery for Intestinal Obstruction

Petachia Reissman and Steven D. Wexner

The indications for laparoscopic surgery have steadily diversified over the past few years, and a growing number of general surgical procedures are being performed using this technique.[1–6] Attracted by the many potential advantages of laparoscopic surgery compared to open surgery such as decreased postoperative pain, shorter ileus and hospitalization, faster return to normal activity, and better cosmesis, surgeons have been inclined to perform more procedures using the laparoscopic technique. As more experience is gained with simple procedures, larger and more complex procedures such as laparoscopic gastric, colorectal, pancreatic, and adrenal procedures can be successfully accomplished. Simultaneously, conditions initially considered as contraindications for laparoscopic surgery have been generally abandoned. Specifically, previous abdominal surgery and suspected intestinal adhesions were, until recently, considered a contraindication for laparoscopy because of the risk of bowel injury and limited visualization. Increased surgical experience, and improved surgical instrumentation, optics, and video monitoring equipment have all facilitated these advances.

Today, laparoscopic procedures are performed in patients who had previous abdominal surgery. In such cases, insufflation of the peritoneal cavity can be performed by an open technique of inserting a blunt-tip trocar under vision through a small fascial incision (Hasson's technique). Alternatively, the Veress needle could be placed distant to previous scars. Finally, newer ports include the optical capability to allow camera-guided placement without either a Veress needle or a Hasson cannula. Adhesions, which are often present, are sharply lysed to provide adequate exposure for the planned laparoscopic procedure. This led to the concept that laparoscopic adhesiolysis of intestinal adhesions that are due to previous abdominal surgery may be feasible even when the surgical indication is intestinal obstruction.

INDICATIONS

The most frequent cause of intestinal obstruction is adhesions caused by previous abdominal surgery.[7–9] Although a large variety of substances have been tried for prevention of adhesion formation, to date, there is still no effective preventive measure of this occurrence.[8–11] In most patients, intestinal adhesions are asymptomatic and well tolerated. However, symptoms that are due to variable degrees of intestinal obstruction may occur any time after the surgery. The spectrum of adhesion-related clinical symptoms ranges from transient recurrent abdominal pain and intestinal transient disturbances to frequent acute intestinal obstruction to peritonitis with perforated or gangrenous bowel.

In the absence of acute intestinal obstruction, the presence of intra-abdominal adhesions may be hard to confirm by imaging studies.[9,11] Radiographic contrast studies, abdominal computed tomography (CT), or magnetic resonance imaging (MRI) may be inconclusive. Therefore, clinical judgment and a high index of suspicion based on the past surgical history and symptomatology may be of utmost importance in the diagnosis and treatment of adhesion-related chronic recurrent abdominal pain.

Obviously, the aim of surgery for intestinal adhesions is relief of the obstruction, if possible, with prevention of recurrent obstruction. Therefore, the indications for laparoscopic adhesiolysis include patients who had previous abdominal surgery and present with transient recurrent episodes or an acute progressive onset of intestinal obstruction. The criteria for laparoscopic surgical treatment of an acute intestinal obstruction are similar to those for a laparotomy and include failure of conservative treatment with increasing pain, progressive dilation of bowel loops on repeated radiographs, leukocytosis, fever, and development of localized rebound tenderness with peritoneal signs. In chronic recurrent intestinal obstruction, additional findings may include weight loss, postprandial bloating, and alternating diarrhea and constipation.

PREOPERATIVE EVALUATION

When elective laparoscopic adhesiolysis is considered, careful preoperative evaluation of the patient is mandatory. First, if possible, clinical and radiographic documentation of previous transient episodes of obstruction may be helpful in establishing the diagnosis. Second, in addition to the routine preoperative evaluation, a thorough study of the gastrointestinal (GI) tract is required to exclude the GI disorders that may be responsible for the patient's symptoms. Therefore, lower GI contrast studies or colonoscopy followed by upper endoscopy and enteroclysis are indicated. Further studies may include CT scan or MRI of the abdomen and pelvic and abdominal ultrasound to exclude other causes of chronic recurrent abdominal symptoms. In an acute intestinal obstruction, the preoperative evaluation may be limited to plain abdominal radiographs and water-soluble contrast studies.

In some instances, even though preoperative evaluation is normal, laparoscopy may reveal unexpected pathology such as tumor, metastases, volvulus, internal hernia, intussusception, or an incarcerated groin or incisional hernia. Based on the findings, the procedure will either continue laparoscopically or be converted to laparotomy. Several conditions such as hernias, intussusception, or localized tumors may be successfully managed as a laparoscopic or laparoscopic-assisted procedure.

CONTRAINDICATIONS

The absolute contraindications for laparoscopic adhesiolysis in chronic, recurrent, or acute episodes are similar to those other laparoscopic procedures and include bleeding disorders and inability to tolerate general anesthesia. Relative contraindications include the following:

1. *Severe abdominal distension with massively dilated small bowel:* this condition may be associated with higher risk of bowel injury during the insufflation and dissection as well as limited exposure and visualization
2. *Peritoneal signs:* in cases of localized or diffuse peritonitis, perforated or gangrenous bowel may already be present; if compromised bowel is indeed found, it may increase the risk of septic complications following surgery; laparotomy with prompt resection and rapid completion of the procedure is desired
3. *The final relative contraindication, and perhaps the most important, relates to the surgeon's sound judgment concerning safety during the procedure:* in the presence of extremely dense adhesions and fused loops of bowel, the risk of enterotomy is increased. In such cases, laparotomy will ensure the patient's safe outcome.

Conversion to laparotomy must not be considered as a failure of laparoscopy. In fact, all the above conditions should lower the surgeon's tolerance for converting the procedure to open laparotomy.

SURGICAL TECHNIQUE

In preparation for laparoscopic adhesiolysis, the stomach and bladder are drained before the procedure. Additionally, in cases of previous pelvic surgery, radiation, prior pelvic sepsis, or multiple lower abdominal surgeries, ureteric stents are extremely useful for fast and safe intraoperative identification of the ureters. For cases in which preoperative evaluation was inconclusive about intraluminal obstruction, intraoperative colonoscopy or enteroscopy should be considered. Therefore, placement of the patient in a modified lithotomy position may be helpful. The operating room setup should include at least two video monitors to enable comfortable inspection for both the surgeon and assistants.

The initial creation of the pneumoperitoneum should be carefully planned and executed. When choosing the site for placement of the first trocar, previous incisions, including scars from previous laparoscopy should be avoided, if possible, because bowel or omentum may be adherent. After the site is chosen, an open technique is used to insert a blunt-tip Hasson trocar or a 10-mm port with video capability. For the Hasson technique, a 10-mm or larger skin incision is made followed by incision of the fascia and peritoneum under direct vision. If the site is away from the midline, careful muscle splitting is performed to avoid injury to the epigastric vessels. Once the peritoneal cavity is entered, either a pursestring suture or two stay sutures of the fascia are placed. The blunt-tip trocar or the 10-mm port are now introduced, and the fascial sutures are snugly secured. Therefore, even if a longer skin incision was made, no air leakage will occur. If the initial site is amid multiple adhesions, an effort should be made to close the fascia to prevent air leakage, and an alternate site is chosen. Alternatively, the Veress needle may be used when placed in an incision-free area. In such cases, after the needle is inserted, a 10-ml syringe is used for insufflation and evacuation followed by the drop test to confirm proper positioning. Once the proper intraperitoneal position is established, a low-flow (1 to 2 L/min) insufflation is started. A rapid increase in the intra-abdominal pressure may indicate improper positioning of the needle. If insufflation continues without difficulty, the tip of the needle may be swept in a circular motion to locate potential adhesions in its vicinity. When the tip of the needle contacts the adhesions, a sudden increase of pressure with a decrease or interruption of the carbon dioxide flow is noted. Hence, the needle can be held in the opposite direction until the desired pneumoperitoneum pressure is achieved, and the first trocar should be placed directed away from the suspected adhesions. A new technique allows video camera-directed placement of blunt-tipped optical ports.

After placement of the first trocar, the laparoscope is inserted, and careful inspection ensues. Most often, visibility is limited because of adhesions, and at least one other port should be inserted under direct vision before exploration is carried out. All ports should be 10/12 mm in size to provide flexibility in camera and instrument positioning. The second port is used for sharp lysis of adhesions to the abdominal wall, using a 10-mm scissors; cautery is used as needed for hemostasis. As the adhesions are lysed and more of the peritoneal cavity can be inspected, additional ports are placed for traction, exposure, and suction-irrigation. Repositioning of the camera and instruments in different ports is usually required when adhesions of omentum and bowel to the abdominal wall are divided. Once the abdominal wall is cleared of adhesions, careful inspection of the bowel is undertaken. This maneuver may be facilitated by positioning the operating table in different angles such as steep Trendelenburg's position, reverse Trendelenburg's position, and tilt to the sides. A thorough inspection of the small bowel should be performed by using two atraumatic Babcock clamps to examine the bowel in a retrograde fashion starting at the terminal ileum and moving proximally toward the ligament of Treitz. This maneuver is performed using a two-hand technique whereby one clamp grasps the antimesenteric portion of the small bowel and a 10- to 15-cm segment is inspected as the second clamp grasps the bowel at the end of the inspected segment. The first clamp is then released and placed close to the second one. This maneuver is repeated until inspection of the full length of the small bowel is completed. The camera, held by an assistant, should be placed in the same direction as the instruments for easier orientation. Because it is often difficult to assess which of the adhesions were responsible for the clinical symptoms, especially in elective cases, sound judgment should be used, and all suspected symptomatic adhesions should be lysed. If a loop of bowel needs to be resected, general principles of laparoscopic colorectal surgery should be applied. The anastomosis is best performed extracorporeally after the bowel is exteriorized through a small incision such as in a laparoscopic-assisted colectomy.

After completion of the lysis of adhesions and bowel inspection, irrigation of the peritoneal cavity is performed followed by careful inspection for hemostasis; after hemostasis is confirmed, the procedure is concluded. An attempt to close the fascia at all port sites should be made to avoid port site hernias, which may then lead to acute intestinal obstruction.

POSTOPERATIVE COURSE AND COMPLICATIONS

The specific complications of laparoscopic adhesiolysis are similar to those following laparoscopic colorectal procedures and therefore are not discussed in this chapter. Because of handling of the bowel, a prolonged ileus may be expected. Routine nasogastric decompression should be continued in the postoperative period in all cases of emergency surgery or should be based on the intraoperative findings.

EARLY RESULTS

Because the potential benefits of laparoscopic treatment of symptomatic intestinal adhesions have only recently been realized, a few series with short follow-up have been published. These series followed several anecdotal reports of successful laparoscopic adhesiolysis in patients who suffered from variable degrees of intestinal obstruction following abdominal surgery.[12–15] The first series of 42 patients (38 women and 4 men) operated on over a 5-year period was reported by Daniell.[16] All of these patients had undergone previous abdominal surgery and suffered variable degrees of recurrent intestinal obstruction. All the patients had undergone a minimum of two previous laparotomies (range, 2 to 17) for this reason. The initial operation included hysterectomy in 22 patients, ruptured appendix in 12, cholecystectomy in 4, perforated bowel due to blunt abdominal trauma in 2, and ruptured spleen in 2. The technique for establishing the pneumoperitoneum included both the standard Veress needle or the open technique. The lysis of adhesions was performed by a combined aquadissection and laser or electric cautery. Two operations were converted to laparotomy because of bowel injury and inadequate exposure. Five patients had a prolonged ileus, but 36 patients were discharged less than 48 hours after the procedure. During a mean follow-up of 4 months, 28 patients (67 percent) indicated a significant improvement of their symptoms, whereas 14 patients (33 percent) did not improve or were actually worse. Ten patients underwent subsequent laparotomy within 6 months after the laparoscopy because of persistence of symptoms. However, the outcome of these patients after the laparotomy was not reported.

In a later series, Franklin and colleagues[17] reported their experience with 23 patients (18 women and 5 men) who were operated on over a period of 2 years. All the patients had an acute intestinal obstruction that did not respond to conservative treatment. In all the patients, the authors determined the point of obstruction during the laparoscopy. Three procedures were converted to laparotomy because of severe adhesions, inability to completely examine the bowel, and suspected necrotic bowel. The cause of obstruction included an internal hernia in 5 patients (4 diaphragmatic and 1 through a defect in the broad ligament), adhesions from previous abdominal surgery in 10, abdominal wall or groin hernias in 6, gallstone ileus in 1, and obstructing splenic flexure carcinoma in 1. The other 20 patients were successfully treated using laparoscopy. Specifically, adhesiolysis, herniorrhaphy, repair of hernia, bowel resection, and repair of cholecystoduodenal fistula were successfully performed. The average operating time for the entire series was 1 hour and 15 minutes. The mean length of hospitalization was 2.5 days. Major morbidity in the series was noted in four patients and included abdominal sepsis, atelectasis with urinary sepsis, small bowel perforation, and gangrenous cholecystitis. Although the authors did not include the length of follow-up, they report good results in all the 20 patients who were treated laparoscopically (87 percent success).

In a series by Francois and colleagues,[18] the authors reported their experience with 52 patients (40 women and 12 men), who underwent laparoscopic adhesiolysis for acute intestinal obstruction (17 patients), or chronic recurrent abdominal pains with transient obstruction (35 patients). All the patients had a mean of 2.4 previous laparotomies. Three patients were converted to laparotomy because of bowel injury and severe adhesions. Perioperative morbidity was noted in seven patients (13 percent), and included bowel injury in five patients and postoperative intestinal obstruction in two patients. These two latter patients required repeat laparotomy during the postoperative course. The mean length of hospital stay was 3 days. The mean follow-up for this series was the longest one reported to date, 24 months. During this period, 32 patients were asymptomatic and 13 patients indicated an improvement. Five patients had no improvement of their symptoms. These results represent a clinical success of 90 percent.

The most recent and also the largest series reported to date was by Freys and colleagues.[19] This series included 58 consecutive patients (40 women and 18 men) who underwent laparoscopic adhesiolysis for recurrent intestinal obstruction or chronic recurrent abdominal pains that were due to adhesions. Six patients (10 percent) suffered major complications, which included enterotomies, omental hemorrhage, and peritonitis. The mean length of the procedure was 80 minutes, and the mean hospital stay was 5 days. Although the mean follow-up period is not reported, the range was up to 30 months after surgery. Complete remission of symptoms or improvement was noted in 45 percent and 35 percent of patients, respectively. Twenty percent of patients had persistent complaints. This represents an overall success rate of 80 percent.

SUMMARY

Intestinal adhesions caused by previous abdominal surgery are no longer considered a contraindication for laparoscopic surgery. Furthermore, because of cumulative experience and recent advances in techniques and instrumentation, such adhesions, which may frequently cause intestinal obstruction, may be successfully managed laparoscopically. Although laparoscopic adhesiolysis for intestinal obstruction is still relatively new, early reports are promising. Laparoscopy may also be an efficient diagnostic as well as therapeutic modality in cases of an undetermined cause of intestinal obstruction.

Thus, bearing in mind the many potential advantages of minimally invasive surgery, laparoscopic adhesiolysis may become a preferred alternative to laparotomy for selected cases of chronic recurrent or acute intestinal obstruction. However, larger series with longer follow-up are necessary before a final conclusion concerning the role of laparoscopy in the treatment of intestinal obstruction may be reached.

In any event, the laparoscopic option must not alter the indications for surgical intervention in intestinal obstruction. When surgical treatment is indicated, however, laparoscopy may be considered in properly selected patients. This procedure requires advanced laparoscopic skills and therefore should be performed only by a well-trained and experienced laparoscopic surgical team.

REFERENCES

1. MacFadyen BV, Wolfe BM, McKernan JB: Laparoscopic management of the acute abdomen, appendix, and small and large bowel. Surg Clin North Am 72:1169, 1992
2. Graves HA Jr, Ballinger JF, Anderson WJ: Appraisal of laparoscopic cholecystectomy. Ann Surg 213:655, 1991
3. Dubois F: Laparoscopic cholecystectomy: personal experience. Dig Surg 8:97, 1991
4. Cuschieri A: Laparoscopic cholecystectomy: indications, techniques and results, pros and cons. Dig Surg 8:104, 1991
5. Wexner SD, Johansen OB, Nogueras JJ, Jagelman DG: Laparoscopic total abdominal colectomy: a prospective assessment. Dis Colon Rectum 35:651, 1992

6. Wexner SD, Cohen SM, Johansen OB et al: Laparoscopic colorectal surgery: a prospective assessment and current perspective. Br J Surg 80:1602, 1993
7. Ellis H: The cause and prevention of intestinal adhesions. Br J Surg 69:241, 1982
8. Fabri PJ, Rosemurgy A: Reoperation for small bowel obstruction. Surg Clin North Am 71:131, 1991
9. Manyies D, Ellis H: Intestinal obstruction from adhesions: how big is the problem. Ann R Coll Surg Engl 72:60, 1990
10. Reissman P, Bloom A, Roisman I et al: Prevention of postlaparotomy adhesions using a foam composite. Res Surg 5:36, 1993
11. Siegel B, Golub RM, Loiacono LA et al: Technique of ultrasonic detection and mapping of abdominal wall adhesions. Surg Endosc 5:161, 1991
12. Kleinhaus S: Laparoscopic lysis of adhesions for postappendectomy pain. Gastrointest Endosc 5:304, 1984
13. Mouret P, Francois Y, Gelez C et al: L'adhesiolyse Coelioscopique. p. 52. Edition Malonie, Paris, 1991
14. Reissman P, Ligumsky M, Bloom A, Durst AL: Laparoscopic adhesiolysis: a treatment for recurrent intestinal obstruction due to adhesions. Min Inv Ther 3:103, 1994
15. Silva PD, Coghill TH: Laparoscopic treatment of recurrent small bowel obstruction. Wis Med J 90:169, 1991
16. Daniell JF: Laparoscopic enterolysis for chronic abdominal pain. J Gynecol Surg 5:61, 1989
17. Franklin ME Jr, Dorman JP, Pharand D: Laparoscopic surgery in acute small bowel obstruction. Surg Laparosc Endosc 4:289, 1994
18. Francois Y, Mouret P, Tomaglu K, Vignal J: Postoperative adhesive peritoneal disease. Surg Endosc 8:781, 1994
19. Freys SM, Fuchs KH, Heimbucher J, Thiede A: Laparoscopic adhesiolysis. Surg Endosc 8:1202, 1994

Editorial Comment

Rama M. Jager

The conventional approach to surgical treatment of acute small bowel obstruction often involves a vertical midline laparotomy. The rapid adoption of laparoscopic techniques by gastrointestinal surgeons led to the recent application of the minimally invasive approach to the management of acute intestinal obstruction. Drs. Reissman and Wexner discuss the technical aspects of laparoscopic treatment of acute intestinal obstruction and review the currently published experience with this new technique to the age-old, distressingly common problem of intestinal obstruction.

INDICATIONS AND TECHNIQUES

I agree with Drs. Reissman and Wexner that the indications for laparoscopic adhesiolysis are similar to that of open laparotomy for adhesiolysis. Any patient who cannot tolerate laparotomy cannot safely undergo laparoscopic adhesiolysis. The rate of conversion of laparoscopy to laparotomy in the treatment of peritoneal adhesive disease is high enough to support this dogma. By contrast, laparoscopic adhesiolysis has many contraindications. Establishing a pneumoperitoneum to facilitate laparoscopic inspection in a patient with diffuse peritonitis may not be appropriate. However, a mini-incision and laparoscopic examination of the peritoneal cavity using abdominal wall-lifting devices may be acceptable in a patient with signs of localized or generalized peritonitis. Also, if the review of previous operative reports detailing the degree of difficulty in laparotomy and adhesiolysis during the past operations indicate severe adhesions, it is likely that laparoscopic adhesiolysis may not be feasible.

The open technique to induce a pneumoperitoneum is preferred to the use of the Veress needle in this group of patients with intestinal obstruction to avoid visceral injury from the needle. I find it helpful to digitally explore the peritoneal cavity through the fascial incision and gently sweep away adhesions around the trocar entrance site before insertion of the trocar. Similar digital dissection, but under laparoscopic guidance, may also be helpful at the secondary trocar sites.[1]

INTESTINAL OBSTRUCTION FROM CAUSES OTHER THAN ADHESIONS

Intestinal obstruction from causes other than intra-abdominal adhesions is also amenable to laparoscopic treatment. Gallstone ileus is a rare cause of ileal obstruction. Diagnosis of the site of obstruction and retrieval of gallstone through a mini-incision to deliver the affected loop for enterolithotomy has been described.[2] Laparoscopic management of the choledochoduodenal fistula that led to gallstone ileus is also feasible,[3] although the experience and expertise of the laparoscopist dictate the choice of the operative technique.

Intestinal obstruction secondary to volvulus from Meckel's diverticulum[4] can be managed by laparoscopic approach. It is technically tempting to resect the Meckel's diverticulum at its base using an endoscopic stapler. However, this may lead to excessive narrowing of the ileal lumen by the metallic staple line. Enlarging the trocar entrance site to a 3-cm incision to deliver the affected ileal loop for extracorporeal resection and anastomosis may be more satisfactory. Shoop and Sackier[5] have described laparoscopic cecopexy for intestinal obstruction from cecal volvulus.

INTESTINAL OBSTRUCTION FROM PREVIOUS LAPAROSCOPIC PROCEDURES

Paradoxically, postlaparoscopic intestinal obstruction secondary to the trocar site herniation following laparoscopic procedures is also common.[6–10] Any fascial defect at a trocar site larger than 5 mm should be repaired with great care. Also, the trocar sheath should be opened to atmospheric air when it is being removed. This technique prevents development of a vacuum, which may pull an intestinal loop into the fascial incision, facilitating Richter's herniation.[11] All other trocar sites should be closed under direct vision with the aid of any of the commercially available port site closure devices. The camera is repositioned through the other ports to allow direct visualization of each site closure to reduce the possibility of subjacent bowel injury by the fascial sutures.

PREOPERATIVE AND INTRAOPERATIVE MEASURES TO AID LAPAROSCOPIC DIAGNOSIS

Laparoscopic technique suffers from the lack of tactile sense that is helpful for proper operative diagnosis. Berthelot and Dubois[12] have reported missing a left colonic cancer as a cause of intestinal obstruction in their published experience with laparoscopic management of intestinal obstruction. No preoperative imaging technique is equivalent to the intraoperative palpation of the viscera in diagnostic accuracy. However, proper and comprehensive preoperative diagnostic studies including ultrasonography, enteroclysis, contrast studies of the colon, colonoscopy, abdominal CT scanning, and/or MRI are helpful to diagnose the location and cause of intestinal obstruction.

I noticed that the intraoperative colonoscopy does not hamper laparoscopic visualization or dissection. The intraoperative enteroscopy as discussed by Drs. Reissman and Wexner, on the other hand, may lead to massive distension of small bowel loops. The dilated loops following enteroscopy render further laparoscopic dissection difficult if not impossible. Endoscopic insufflation of carbon dioxide instead of room air during the intraoperative endoscopic procedures is one option to facilitate rapid return of the distended bowel loops to preinsufflation status, thus enabling continuation of the laparoscopic dissection.

It is difficult to determine laparoscopically whether an incarcerated segment of bowel that is released from a hernial sac is viable and thus can be preserved. Intraoperative ultrasonographic Doppler and use of intravenous fluoroscein are suggested to evaluate the enteric ischemia and the vascular status of an incarcerated intestinal segment.[13] However, unless the segment of bowel completely returns to normal appearance after laparoscopic release from a hernial sac or volvulus, a minilaparotomy may be necessary for optimal evaluation and possible segmental resection followed by the anastomosis.

CONCLUSION

Like any other surgical technique, proper selection of patients is an important factor that decides the rate of success with the laparoscopic management of intestinal obstruction. Not all patients with intestinal obstruction are candidates for laparoscopic treatment. Even when the operation starts as a laparoscopy, needed conversion to a laparotomy is not a sign of technical failure but reflects surgical maturity.

REFERENCES

1. Tonietto G, Pintaldi S: Finger-assisted laparoscopic surgery. J Laparoendosc Surg 4:205, 1994
2. Montgomery A: Laparoscope-guided enterolithotomy for gallstone ileus. Surg Laparosc Endosc 4:310, 1993
3. Franklin ME Jr, Dorman JP, Schuessler WW: Laparoscopic treatment of gallstone ileus: a case report and review of the literature. J Laparoendosc Surg 4:265, 1994
4. Negro P, Catarci M, Zaraca F et al: Laparoscopic diverticulectomy for ileal volvulus on Meckel's diverticulum. G Chir 15:134, 1994
5. Shoop SA, Sackier JM: Laparoscopic cecopexy for cecal volvulus. Case report and a review of the literature. Surg Endosc 7:45, 1993
6. Burney TL, Jacobs SC, Naslund MJ: Small bowel obstruction following laparoscopic lymphadenectomy. J Urol 150:1515, 1993
7. Tsang S, Normand R, Karlin R: Small bowel obstruction: a morbid complication after laparoscopic herniorrhaphy. Am Surg 60:332, 1994
8. Spier LN, Lazzaro RS, Procaccino A, Geiss A: Entrapment of small bowel after laparoscopic herniorrhaphy. Surg Endosc 7:535, 1993
9. Kurtz BR, Daniell JF, Spaw AT: Incarcerated incisional hernia after laparoscopy. A case report. J Reprod Med 38:643, 1993
10. Wegener ME, Chung D, Crans C, Chung D: Small bowel obstruction secondary to incarcerated Richter's hernia from laparoscopic hernia repair. J Laparoendosc Surg 3:173, 1993
11. Kreutzer ER, Lerner SE, Kahan NZ, Melman A: Laparoscopic treatment of small bowel obstruction following laparoscopic lymphadenectomy. Urology 44:768, 1994
12. Berthelot G, Dubois F: Celioscopic treatment of acute obstructions of the small intestine. Immediate results in 25 patients. Ann Chir 47:497, 1993
13. Duh QY: Laparoscopic procedures for small bowel disease. Baillieres Clin Gastroenterol 7:833, 1993

22

Laparoscopic-Assisted Colonic Resection: The French Experience

Abe Fingerhut

Colonic resection is being accomplished more and more frequently under videolaparoscopic control. Because results are not concordant, controversy has risen.[1,2] Although some state that laparoscopic colonic resection presents the same advantages as laparoscopic cholecystectomy (e.g., shorter hospital stay, less postoperative pain and ileus, and quicker return to normal activity),[3] these theoretical advantages have not been borne out by all.[2,4] In this chapter, the initial experience of a prospective study of 224 unselected laparoscopic colonic resections performed by 39 members of four French associations for surgical research is reported. In addition, the results regarding the hypothetical advantages of laparoscopic surgical technique over traditional colorectal resections are presented.

PATIENTS AND METHODS

During an 18-month period (October 1991 until March 1993), 224 patients (110 women and 114 men), with a mean age of 62.3 ± 14.5 years (range, 18 to 84 years) from 22 centers were considered candidates for laparoscopic colonic resection. The indications included carcinoma in 92 patients; colonic diverticulosis in 71 (35 had recovered from a complication within 1 month before the laparoscopic resection); polyps (two instances of familial polyposis) in 42 (inability to remove the tumor endoscopically in 32 and/or invasion of the pedicle in 13); colectomy for appendicular carcinoid in 2, appendicular mucocele in 1, and malignant transformation of polyp in 4; recurrent volvulus in 4; and endometriosis, cure of rectocolic fistulae, and perforation during colonoscopy in 1 patient each.

RESULTS

Overall, 54 conversions (24.1 percent) were made. Thirty-three conversions took place before laparoscopic resection for the following reasons: dissection was deemed too hazardous or difficult (19 patients); accident occurred during trocar insertion (three instances of hemorrhage, one intestinal perforation); uncontrollable hemorrhage during dissection (6 patients); and inability to create a pneumoperitoneum (2 patients) or to find the tumor on exploration (polyps in both patients). Seventeen conversions took place during or after resection. The reasons were uncontrollable hemorrhage in 8 patients, failure to locate the tumor(s) or the specimen in 3, a mechanical device mishap in 3, and inability to perform anastomosis in 2. The reasons for conversion were undocumented in 3 patients. In 4 patients, the operator abandoned the laparoscopic technique because he had overrun the 4-hour time limit he had set for himself to accomplish the operation.

Overall, 164 resections were performed (73 percent of attempted resections).

Types of Resection[a]

Sigmoidectomy (77)
Left colectomy (28)
Right colectomy (24)
Cecal resection (11)
Anterior resection (4)
Transverse colectomy (4)
Polypectomy (6)

[a]Number in parentheses.

There were a total of 158 anastomoses, including 101 colorectal, 22 colocolonic, and 35 ileocolonic. Sixty-one anastomoses were intra-abdominal, and 92 were extra-abdominal. The specimen was extracted through various sites; the right lower quadrant was used most often.

Extraction of Specimen[a]

Per anus (6)
Trocar aperture (17)
Right lower quadrant incision (58)
Left lower quadrant incision (38)
Transverse incision
  Supraumbilical (16)
  Infraumbilical (8)
Suprapubic incision (9)
Pfannenstiel incision (18)

[a]Number in parentheses.

The mean duration of operation was 218 ± 82 minutes (range, 45 to 600 minutes). The mean interval before return of flatus was 3.2 ± 1.7 days (range, 6 hours to 10 days). Postoperative analgesia was administered for a mean of 1.6 days (range, 0 to 6 days).

Postoperatively, there were 16 anastomotic fistulas (9.5 percent) (four patients had radiologic fistulas only), eight of which required repeat surgery. Six patients died (three with fistulae; one myocardial infarction; the cause of death for others undocumented). The mean hospital stay was 9.2 ± 4.8 (2 to 31) days overall, whereas that for patients without complications was 7.7 ± 2.8 (2 to 13) days. Sixty-nine (45 percent) patients were discharged in fewer than 7 days, whereas 24 (16 percent) patients were discharged in more than 14 days. Postoperative complications are indicated below.

Postoperative Complications[a]

Pneumonia (5)
Wound problems
  Abscess (2)
  Hematoma (3)
Obstruction
  Bands (2)
  Unrecognized tumor (2)
  Ischemic stricture (1)

Continues

Cancer
  Seeding of cancer (3)
    Dukes' A (1)
    Dukes' B (2)
  Early recurrence (3)

[a]Number in parentheses.

The pathology reports showed that the number of lymph nodes removed per specimen was 5.7 ± 4.1 (0 to 28). In six specimens, no lymph nodes were found.

DISCUSSION

Although few true comparative trials have been conducted, laparoscopic surgery has been shown to reduce the insult of peritoneal access and to improve the quality of recovery after operation, notably after cholecystectomy.[3,5] The same benefits may be expected after laparoscopic colonic surgery.[6,7] Colonic resection, however, is technically more demanding. New problems have arisen as outlined elsewhere, including tissue handling,[4] increased morbidity, proper identification of tumor and extension,[8] difficulty of anastomosis, specimen retrieval,[4] peritoneal dissemination of disease at trocar sites,[9–13] and the learning of adequate techniques.[14]

It is known that adding a simple technique such as tubal ligation to diagnostic laparoscopy will double the morbidity.[15] There is no place for imperfect technique in laparoscopic surgery, which can increase the morbidity rate and the recurrence rate in carcinoma.[16,17] Adequate tissue resection is essential in colonic resection for malignancy.[18] Adequate treatment of cancer must not be compromised by minimal invasive surgery.[4,17,19] Several reports have emphasized mesenteric, nodal, and longitudinal resection of malignant colorectal disease being equivalent to those in open resection.[4,6,7,19] However, there have been few reports on the adequacy of circumferential margins of resection, which, if positive, are associated with a local recurrence rate as high as 87 percent in open surgery.[17] It is hoped that modern imaging such as magnetic resonance, transluminal ultrasound, and immunoscintigraphy will enable the surgeon to better detect locally invasive tumors and to determine the proper indications for laparoscopic versus conventional surgery.[19]

Carcinoma at the sites of cannula insertion after laparoscopy has been reported after cholecystectomy for unsuspected gallbladder carcinoma.[10–12] Of concern is the increasing number of local port site recurrences reported after resection for colonic carcinoma. Because only sporadic patients have been reported to date, it is difficult to estimate this risk in laparoscopic surgery correctly, which in open surgery has been estimated to be 0.7 percent (11 patients with recurrence associated with the laparotomy incision or drainage site in 1,603 patients).[20] Earlier in this century, Von Mikulicz of Bresaul[21] described colonic resection through an extracorporeal technique. Although the procedure was widely acclaimed to reduce perioperative mortality, it was heavily criticized and then abandoned because of an inordinately and unacceptably high rate of recurrence.[22] That recurrence can occur in port sites that are not used for the extraction of the specimen leads to speculation that direct dissemination or wound contamination is not the cause. Enveloping the specimen in a plastic bag for extraction does not suffice to prevent recurrence. Manipulation of tumor can cause viable malignant cells to exfoliate,[23,24] and these cells are known to implant and grow in healing colonic anastomosis. Tumor cell growth is known to be enhanced by tissue injury, and through the circulation, tumor cells can seed in injured tissues[25] or the laparotomy wound.[26] Incomplete excision of mesorectum is also claimed[17,27,28] to be a further source of tumor cells that may give rise to distant growth. Skipper et al[13] have determined experimentally that enhanced tumor cell proliferation is 1,000-fold in the healing tissues. Moreover, tumor cell dispersion into the port sites may in some way be facilitated by the pneumoperitoneum.[19]

The number of lymph nodes removed with specimens is important. First, the retrieval of lymph nodes in the mesocolon or at the origin of the inferior mesenteric vein in left colonic carcinoma[29] (although this will not influence outcome) can help determine the exact stage of disease, an element that is to decide the need for further adjuvant chemotherapy. The size of the primary tumor, its level of penetration into the bowel wall, and the histologic differentiation do not allow consistent prediction of the presence or absence of lymph node metastases.[18,30] Only a reliable count of resected lymph nodes is a valuable parameter for cancer prognosis.

Philips et al[7] reported an average yield of 14 lymph nodes (range, 8 to 22) in their 24 patients undergoing laparoscopic colectomy. This rate is higher than those published by Vara-Thorbeck et al[8] (mean, 8.5; range, 7 to 12) and in our series (reported here) but is far lower than the 34 (range, 0 to 88) found per specimen by Herrera and Villarreal[30] in open colorectal resections. It is fairly obvious that the rate of lymph node metastases increases proportionately to the number of lymph nodes examined.[30,31] The number of lymph nodes found in surgical specimens is known to differ according to variation in patients' anatomy, in individual surgical expertise and technique, and in the interest generated by pathologists to search for them.[30] In most centers, lymph nodes are obtained for pathology after recognition by sight and palpation. Because this method relies on the diligence and experience of the pathologist, it may be a source of potential problems in general hospitals that have pathologists of different levels of experience or interest, not to mention the time and cost constraints of large volume of specimens.

Missed tumors have not been reported often. In the series of 18 patients of Vara-Thorbeck et al,[8] however, one patient had to undergo a standard resection of a Dukes' B-2 cancer 10 cm from the anastomosis 9 months after the colonic resection. McDermott et al[32] reported another instance of unrecognized synchronous cancer revealed 2 weeks after the initial left colonic resection by obstruction. Synchronous cancer is reported in up to 5 percent of patients.[33] Colonoscopy has a false-negative rate of 3 to 8 percent.[33,34] Manual palpation is difficult or impossible in laparoscopic surgery (for the colonic tumor as well as for the hepatic metastases) as reported by these authors. Consequently, we conclude that a complete endoscopic or radiographic workup is necessary before engaging in laparoscopic resection. In the absence of such a workup, intraoperative colonoscopy should be done.

Bohm and Milsom[35] and Milsom et al[36] have stated that, contrary to other procedures in laparoscopic surgery, atraumatic handling of intraperitoneal organs, achievement of hemostasis, dissection of mesocolon with adequate lymphadenectomy, and high ligation of vessels are skills that cannot be learned in inanimate training models. Animal models along with proctoring are essential to training in colorectal surgery.[36]

The rate of anastomotic leakage (9.5 percent) in the series reported in this chapter may seem surprising, but anastomotic failure rates as high as 18 percent have been reported in laparoscopic surgery.[7] Infection increases the mortality and perioperative and late morbidity and is known to promote recurrence.[37] In multivariate analysis, our group (unpublished data) showed that intraoperative contamination was a predictive factor of anastomotic leakage. Anastomoses performed under videolaparoscopy are usually closed, the preparation is the same, but it is more difficult to occlude the intestinal lumen or protect the operative field from fecal contamination.

Other authors stated that return of postoperative bowel function and length of hospital stay are shorter in patients undergoing laparoscopic colonic resection as compared with conventional surgery.[7] This result was not confirmed by Wexner et al,[2] Milsom et al,[36] or this study. More recently, a prospective randomized trial has shown that early oral intake (less than 24 hours after surgery) was well tolerated after laparotomy and was therefore not limited to laparoscopy.[38] Moreover, the possibility of earlier discharge may well be annulled by life-threatening complications that may occur at home, making patient counseling and communication with home health services mandatory.[4]

The scope of laparoscopic or laparoscopic-assisted colorectal surgery for carcinoma varies with the location of the cancer. Right hemicolectomy is probably the easiest, but sigmoidectomy the most commonly performed procedure.[39] The main limiting factor is the size of the incision necessary for the extraction of the tumor. Anterior resection of the rectum poses the problem of adequate wide excision[4,27] and extraction of the tumor. The transanal route could be a factor in tumor spillage, breach of aseptic technique, and possible damage to the anal sphincter. In the left colonic rectal cancers, early division of the inferior mesenteric artery is facilitated by the mechanical stapling device.[19] Between the two ends of the large intestine, laparoscopic resection becomes more technically difficult and less valuable.[19] Although feasible, the extra time necessary to fully and safely mobilize the hepatic and splenic flexures is presently a limiting factor to widespread application of laparoscopic colonic resection.[19] By contrast, rectopexy and anterior resection for benign disease may be a highly desirable indication for laparoscopic or laparoscopic-assisted resection of colorectal disease. In diverticular disease, however, if resection of the rectosigmoid juncture is to be achieved, the colorectal anastomosis can only be performed intra-abdominally.

CONCLUSION

Laparoscopic resections and colonic anastomoses are feasible.[40] The safety, operative morbidity, facility with abdominal and intestinal exploration, and oncologic adequacy of resection are less than ideal in the population of patients we studied. Echoing Alexander et al,[9] we caution that laparoscopic surgery for rectal cancer is not recommended in all cancer patients and in all surgical centers. Some institutions have restricted their indications for laparoscopic colorectal resection to benign disease, malignant lesions requiring minimal or limited resections,[7] to patients with incurable disease, or those with contraindications to open surgical resection.[8] Improved laparoscopic skills in the general surgical community, instrumentation, and techniques of localization are necessary. Because uncontrolled trials performed to date do not seem to show any difference in the length of hospital stay or a decrease of postoperative pain as compared with standard techniques, and because operative morbidity seems high, controlled trials should help to determine whether laparoscopic colonic resection is of any real benefit to a patient with colorectal cancer.

ACKNOWLEDGMENTS

The following physicians were involved in the series reported in this chapter and in the writing of this chapter: Patrice Lointier, M.D., Bertrand Millat, M.D., Bruno Desrousseaux, M.D., Pierre Magdeleinat, M.D., Francois Desmaiziers, M.D., and Jean-Marie Hay, M.D. The following French Associations for Research in Surgery were also a part of the series reported here: Association de Recherche en Chirurgie, Association de Recherche Universitaire en Chirurgie, Association de Recherche en Chirurgie de I'Ile de France, and Association de Recherche en Chirurgie Viscérale du Languedoc.

REFERENCES

1. Franklin M: Is laparoscopic colon resection feasible?, abstracted. Minimal Invas Ther, suppl. 1:85, 1992
2. Wexner SD, Cohen SM, Johansen OB et al: Laparoscopic colorectal surgery: a prospective assessment and current perspective. Br J Surg 80:1602, 1993
3. Barkun JS, Barkun An, Sampalis JS et al: Randomized controlled trail of laparoscopic versus mini-cholecystectomy. Lancet 340:1116, 1992
4. Tate JJT, Kwok S, Dawson JW et al: Prospective comparison of laparoscopic and conventional anterior resection. Br J Surg 80:1396, 1993
5. Reddick EJ, Olsend DO: Laparoscopic laser cholecystectomy: a comparison with mini-laparotomy cholecystectomy. Surg Endosc 3:131, 1989
6. Monson JRT, Darzi A, Carey PDD et al: Prospective evaluation of laparoscopic-assisted colectomy in an unselected group of patients. Lancet 340:831, 1992
7. Phillips EH, Franklin M, Cartoll BJ et al: Laparoscopic colectomy. Ann Surg 216:703, 1992
8. Vara-Thorbeck C, Garcia-Caballero M, Salvi M et al: Indications and advantages of laparoscopy assisted colon resection for carcinoma in elderly patients. Surg Laparosc Endosc 4:110, 1994
9. Alexander RJT, Jacques BC, Mitchell KG: Laparoscopically-assisted colectomy and wound recurrence. Lancet 341:249, 1993
10. Fusco MA, Paluzzi MW: Abdominal wall recurrence after laparoscopic-assisted colectomy for adenocarcinoma of the colon. Dis Colon Rectum 36:858, 1993
11. Nduka CC, Monson JRT, Menzies-Gow N et al: Abdominal wall metastases following laparoscopy. Br J Surg 81:648, 1994
12. O'Rourke N, Price PM, Kelly S et al: Tumor inoculation during laparoscopy, letter. Lancet 342:368, 1993
13. Skipper D, Jeffrey MJ, Cooper AJ et al: Enhanced growth of tumor cells in healing colonic anastomoses and laparotomy wounds. Int J Colorectal Dis 4:172, 1989
14. Pappas TN: Laparoscopic colectomy: the innovation continues. Ann Surg 216:701, 1992
15. Chamberlain G, Brown J: Report of the Working Party of the Confidential Inquiry into Gynecological Laparoscopy. Royal College of Obstetricians and Gynecologists, London, 1978
16. Fielding LP, Stewart-Brown S, Dudly HAF: Surgeon-related variables and the clinical trial. Lancet 2:778, 1986
17. Quirke P, Durdey P, Dixon MF et al: Local recurrence of rectal adenocarcinoma due to inadequate surgical resection. Lancet 2:996, 1986
18. Michiels C, Boutron MC, Chatelain N et al: Facteurs pronostiques des adenocarcinomes colorectaux de stade B de Dukes'. Etude d'une serie de population. Gastroenterol Clin Biol 18:456, 1994

19. Gillou PJ: Laparoscopic surgery for diseases of the colon and rectum quo vadis? Surg Endosc 8:669, 1994
20. Hughes ES, McDermott FT, Polgase AI et al: Tumor recurrence in the abdominal wall scar tissue after large bowel cancer bowel surgery. Dis Colon Rectum 26:571, 1982
21. Von Mikluicz J: Small contributions to the surgery of the intestinal tract. Boston Med Surg J 148:608, 1903
22. Sistrunk WE: Mikulicz operation for resection of the colon. Its advantages and dangers? Ann Surg 88:597, 1928
23. Fermor B, Umpleby HC, Lever JV et al: Proliferative and metastatic potential of exfoliated colorectal carcinoma cells. Br J Surg 71:659, 1984
24. Umpleby HC, Fermor B, Symes MO et al: Viability of exfoliated colorectal carcinoma cells. Br J Surg 71:659, 1984
25. Alexander JW, Altemeier WA: Susceptibility of injured tissues to hematogenous metastases; an experimental study. Ann Surg 85:933, 1964
26. Murphy P, Alexander P, Senior PV et al: Mechanisms of organ selective tumor growth by bloodborne cancer cells. Br J Cancer 57:19, 1988
27. Heald RJ, Husband EM, Ryall RDHH: The mesorectum in rectal cancer surgery: the clue to pelvic recurrence? Br J Surg 69:613, 1988
28. MacFarlane JK, Ryall RDH, Heald RJ: Mesorectal excision for rectal cancer. Lancet 341:457, 1992
29. Rouffet F, Hay JM, Vacher B et al: Curative resection for left colonic carcinoma: hemicolectomy versus segmental colectomy. A prospective, controlled, multicenter trial. French Association for Surgical Research. Dis Colon Rectum 37:651, 1994
30. Herrera L, Villarreal JR: Incidence of metastases from rectal adenocarcinoma in small lymph nodes detected by a clearing technique. Dis Colon Rectum 35:783, 1992
31. Cawthorn SJ, Gibbs NM, Marks CG: Clearance technique for the detection of lymph nodes in colorectal cancer. Br J Surg 73:58, 1986
32. McDermott JP, Devereaux DA, Caushaj PF: Pitfall of laparoscopic colectomy. An unrecognized synchronous cancer. Dis Colon Rectum 37:602, 1994
33. Byrd RL, Boggs HW, Stragle GW et al: Reliability of colonoscopy. Dis Colon Rectum 32:1023, 1989
34. Abrams JS: A hard look at colonoscopy. Am J Surg 133:111, 1977
35. Bohm B, Milsom JW: Animal models as education tools in laparoscopic colorectal surgery. Surg Endosc 8:707, 1994
36. Milsom JW, Lavery IC, Church JM et al: Use of laparoscopic techniques in colorectal surgery. Preliminary study. Dis Colon Rectum 37:215, 1994
37. Sauven P, Playforth MJ, Evans M et al: Early infective complications and late recurrent cancer in stapled colonic anastomoses. Dis Colon Rectum 32:33, 1989
38. Binderow SR, Cohen SM, Wexner SD: Must early postoperative oral intake be limited to laparoscopy? Dis Colon Rectum 37:584, 1994
39. Lirici MM, Beuss G, Melzer A et al: New technique for sigmoid colectomy. Br J Surg 80:1606, 1993
40. O'Rourke NA, Heald RJ: Laparoscopic surgery for colorectal cancer. Br J Surg 80:1229, 1993

Editorial Comment

Steven D. Wexner

Throughout this book, numerous contributors have offered their expertise and shared their experience. The common thread throughout virtually the remainder of this textbook is that the authors cite their own individual experiences or the experiences accumulated within their individual departments. Many of these individuals, therefore, tend to offer a rather glowing endorsement of the technique. It must be remembered, however, that a steep learning curve needs to be surmounted before the appreciation of such good results. The problem with the learning curve is that it cannot be inherited or shared; it must be individually conquered.

Dr. Fingerhut provides insight into the type of problems that can arise when the "average" surgeon initially performs laparoscopic colorectal surgery. Again, it is tempting to try to extrapolate complication and success rates from surgeons who perform several hundred colorectal procedures per year and can, therefore, even with selective application, easily perform several laparoscopic resections per week. In this chapter, 39 surgeons from 22 centers contributed 224 patients over an 18-month period. Thus, the average contribution per surgeon was approximately six laparoscopic cases over an 18-month period, or one case per 3 months. In other words, this chapter represents reality rather than academic hyperbole. In a recent survey, an estimate was made that given 165,000 new cases of colorectal carcinoma per year and 25,000 practicing surgeons, the average general surgeon performs less than seven colorectal resections for cancer per year. Furthermore, most practicing general surgeons perform very few resections for inflammatory bowel disease and may perform a few resections for diverticular disease, trauma, volvulus, or other miscellaneous indications. However, the numbers are artificially inflated because one must realize that the surgeons certified by the American Board of Colon and Rectal Surgery perform a large share of this surgery. The presence of surgical oncologists further imbalances the equation. This editorial is not meant to be a mathematical treatise but does intend to establish a point. Specifically, if a surgeon is to perform between 6 and 12 colorectal resections per year (ranging from 1 per month to 1 every other month), the learning curve for laparoscopy will take a long time to surmount. A recent survey[1] indicated that even among enthusiastic colorectal laparoscopic surgeons, the penetrance of laparoscopy within the individual practices ranged from only 10 to 20 percent. Thus, the average general surgeon may realistically perform one to two laparoscopic colorectal resections per year. Therefore, the average of four laparoscopic resections per year being contributed in this French study shows a certain degree of enthusiasm and dedication.

Despite this enthusiasm and dedication, the learning curve still reared its typical appearance. The 24-percent conversion rate in no way represents failure. However, the reasons for conversion are certainly somewhat disturbing, in that they include dissection "deemed too hazardous or too difficult," hemorrhage or intestinal perforation during trocar insertion, uncontrolled hemorrhage during dissection, inability to locate the lesion, or excessive time spent performing the procedure. All of these complications are potentially avoidable with time. Thus, although conversion itself is not considered a failure, 21 of 54 conversions in this study were because of complications such as hemorrhage or intestinal perforation. The best indication for conversion was actually that some surgeons thought that they were spending too long a time operating. I personally endorse the view that if the entire procedure cannot be completed within a maximum of 3 to 4 hours or if a single phase of the procedure cannot be satisfactorily completed within 30 to 60 minutes, then the procedure should be converted. Again, to review my definition of conversion, a laparoscopic procedure is one in which all vascular control, bowel division, and anastomotic creation is performed intracorporeally with the pneumoperitoneum under visual guidance through a variety of ports. A laparoscopic-assisted procedure is one in which any one or more of the steps (vascular control, bowel division, anastomotic creation, specimen retrieval, mesenteric defect repair) is performed through any sized incision rather than a port. A converted procedure is one in which an incision was either unplanned, or made either sooner than planned or larger than planned.

The French study shows the typical findings of the average laparoscopic neophyte. The mean duration of operation was 3.5 hours, and the upper limit of time spent was 10 hours. Clearly, after experience has been gained, such lengths of time will be greatly reduced. A major problem of the study was that an anastomotic leak rate of 9.5 percent was found, resulting in three deaths. Similar to the study by Phillips et al,[2] in which the incidence of incomplete donuts during laparoscopic coloproctostomy was 18 percent, one must worry about the anastomosis. The major difference herein may be that Phillips and his group were sufficiently experienced to recognize and repair these defects without adverse sequelae, whereas, the average surgeon either did not recognize or could not adequately fix the defect.

As has been shown throughout this textbook, the mean hospital stay was 9.2 days, ranging up to 31 days. Even in the absence of complications, the mean stay was still 7.7 days. One recent study has reviewed all published series of laparoscopic colorectal resections and found that these 808 patients had a mean hospital stay of 7.1 days.[3] Therefore, Fingerhut and colleagues have achieved the world mean in length of stay for this procedure.

Dr. Fingerhut quite aptly addresses some of the problems of lymph node harvest. In six specimens resected for cancer, no lymph nodes were found. Clearly, the mean of 5.7 nodes per specimen was far below an appropriate number. As Cohen and colleagues have shown,[4] the number of nodes identified is greatly contingent on the technique of mesenteric analysis and the enthusiasm of the pathologist. Once again, a recent compilation of laparoscopic series has revealed that the mean number of nodes in the various published series is approximately 10 or approximately one-half of the minimally acceptable number.[5] In fact, even though my series includes the largest mean number of laparoscopically retrieved nodes (18),[6] that number still falls 10 percent short of the ideal mean harvest. Fingerhut has quite clearly emphasized the need to harvest more nodes to prognosticate and to allow assignment to various adjuvant therapies.

Fingerhut is one of only a few individuals who have estimated a national incidence for port site recurrence after curative laparoscopic resection of colorectal neoplasia. Ngoi in Singapore[7] has estimated an incidence of 4.5 percent, very close to the 3.2 percent incidence noted herein by Fingerhut, and Berends et al[8] estimated a 21-percent incidence. Several hypotheses are offered, but at the moment, there is no good answer as to why this problem occurs. I wholly support the admonition by Fingerhut. Specifically, appropriately trained surgeons can quite reasonably offer and perform laparoscopic resections for benign disease in appropriately selected patients. Similarly, these same surgeons can most definitely offer some benefit when performing laparoscopic resection for palliation of malignancy. However, no surgeon at the present time should perform laparoscopic colorectal surgery for cure of cancer outside the confines of a prospectively randomized trial. The honest discussion of port site recurrence within this chapter shows us that even after attempted curative resection of Dukes' A or Dukes' B lesions, this inexplicable phenomenon can occur. Thus, regardless of the magnitude of the technical or cosmetic triumph, the patient who has a port site implantation within 18 months of attempted curative resection of a Dukes' A lesion has been ill served by laparoscopy.

REFERENCES

1. Wexner SD (panelist): Laparoscopic considerations in colon and rectal surgery (expert exchange). p. 245. In Beart R (moderator): Perspectives in Colon and Rectal Surgery. Vol. 7. Quality Medical Publishing, St. Louis, MO, 1994
2. Phillips EH, Franklin M, Carroll BJ et al: Laparoscopic colectomy. Ann Surg 216:703, 1992
3. Reissman P, Cohen SM, Weiss EG et al: Laparoscopic colorectal surgery: ascending the learning curve. World J Surg (in press)
4. Cohen SM, Wexner SD, Schmitt SL et al: Does xylene mesenteric fat clearance improve lymph node harvest after colon resection. Eur J Surg 160:693, 1994
5. Teoh TA, Wexner SD: Laparoscopic surgery in colorectal cancer. In Williams N (ed): Colorectal Cancer. Churchill Livingstone, London (in press)
6. Wexner SD, Cohen SM et al: Laparoscopic colorectal surgery: a prospective assessment and current perspective. Br J Surg 80:1602, 1993
7. Ngoi SS: Laparoscopic colorectal surgery. Presented at the International Society of University Colon and Rectal Surgeons 15th Biennial Congress, Singapore, July 1994
8. Berends FJ, Kazemjer G, Bonjer HJ, Lange JF: Subcutaneous metastases after laparoscopic colectomy (letter). Lancet 344:58, 1994

23 Developing Laparoscopic Expertise

Eric G. Weiss and Steven D. Wexner

Laparoscopic surgery has changed the practice of surgery. Although not a new technique, its application to general surgery and, specifically, colorectal surgery is a relatively new addition. Since the introduction of laparoscopic cholecystectomy,[1] the laparoscopic revolution has taken place. Along with this progress come many questions, concerns, and issues regarding proper credentialing and training. These areas are discussed in this chapter.

Historically, a new technique or instrument is introduced to the surgical community in one of several forms. A surgeon or group of surgeons who treat a particular disorder in a new or innovative way publish their results in a peer-reviewed journal after presentation at a major meeting of a national or an international society. Once efficacy has been scientifically proven, other surgeons may begin applying that technique to their own patients. Depending on the complexity, the individual confidence, and skills, no further training may be necessary to perform the new operation. Conversely, if the technique is significantly different or new, a course or preceptorship may be necessary to obtain adequate training.

Similarly, new instrumentation may be introduced in meetings or in publications but more commonly is detailed by representatives of the companies manufacturing the instruments. The representatives often show the product to surgeons, hoping that they will try the instrument in the operating room. Often, the company will have a well-known, well-respected spokesperson in a given field endorsing the use of the product. Similarly, if special training is necessary, it is often provided by the company manufacturing or marketing the product. The endorsing physician may provide training to other physicians during courses or personal training sessions. Finally, exposure in the lay press introduces both the public and physicians to new techniques and instruments with which to treat diseases.

Seldom, if ever, have all these forces converged on a new method of surgery. Through a combination of potential benefits to patients (through reduced pain and morbidity) and to technology shareholders (through increased sales and profits), the field of laparoscopic surgery rapidly burgeoned. As soon as a few anecdotal reports suggested these benefits, surgeons, patients, biomedical engineers, medical writers, Wall Street pundits, and others began extrapolating the applications. The initial limits were imposed not by the technology or the technicians (surgeons), but by the imagination. However, somewhere within this Gordian nexus of competing factors lie a number of questions relating to the requisite qualifications to perform the procedures.

The training of surgeons has evolved from that of unorganized preceptorships to that of organized residency programs designed to incorporate all facets necessary in any given field to allow adequate training. Residents are given increasing responsibility in the operating room, with varying amounts of supervision, depending on both their own abilities and the difficulty of the given case. Techniques are read in textbooks or observed on videos, then assisted in the operating room, and eventually performed by the resident. This process, with some modifications, should continue as the model for laparoscopic surgery.

Several issues need to be explored to develop expertise in laparoscopic colorectal surgery. First and foremost, a surgeon should be a qualified surgeon. In laparoscopic colorectal surgery, advanced training in colorectal surgery beyond that of general surgery is required. However, this special training and subspecialization are not available in every country. In the United States and Canada, subspecialization means fellowship training in 1 of 30 approved colorectal residency programs. In other parts of the world, subspecialty training varies. Before embarking on laparoscopic colorectal surgery, the surgeon should be comfortable with all facets of diagnosis and treatment of colorectal pathology in the traditional manner.[2–5]

Next the surgeon must obtain basic laparoscopic skills. For those surgeons currently in training, this goal has been incorporated into the surgical residency curriculum.[6,7] However, for the majority of surgeons who have already completed residency training, attendance at a course to obtain this advanced training is required. The nature, duration, faculty, and cost of these courses vary. When laparoscopic surgery was first introduced, weekend courses were used to train prospective surgeons in the basic techniques of laparoscopic surgery and the specifics of laparoscopic cholecystectomy.[8–10] Most courses involved a didactic session where theory, instrumentation, operation room setup, and technique were discussed. Then "dry labs" using models, inanimate trainers,[11] and other teaching devices were used to acquaint surgeons with the procedures, skills, and instrumentation. Last was the performance of the procedure in "wet labs" using live animal models. Many of these models were not ideal, because the anatomy was significantly simplified in the animal model as compared with a human. Nevertheless, on completion of these courses, many surgeons immediately performed laparoscopic surgery on their patients.[12] See et al,[13] in a survey of 297 urologists, compared complication rates among those who completed laparoscopic training courses. They assessed complications from laparoscopic urological procedures at both 3 and 12-month intervals with respect to (1) any additional laparoscopic training, (2) additional training course with a designated laparoscopic assistant, and (3) the type of assistant used during laparoscopic procedures. At the 3-month interval, those urologists who had no further training beyond their initial training course were almost 3.5 times more likely to have a complication compared with those who sought additional training. Similarly, at the 12-month interval, those surgeons who attended the course alone, were in solo practice, or used a variable assistant, were at least 4.5 times more likely to have a complication. Finally, the likelihood of complications was inversely related to the number of operations performed. There is no reason to think that a similar process does not occur within other fields of surgery. Therefore, laparoscopic courses do not provide sufficient training to perform advanced laparoscopic surgery. Furthermore, the skills requisite to perform simple laparoscopic procedures such as a cholecystectomy, appendectomy, and herniorrhaphy are neither translatable nor requisite to the performance of laparoscopic colectomy.

Laparoscopic colorectal surgery is different from most other laparoscopic procedures in five ways.[14] First, most laparoscopic procedures are single-quadrant procedures. Herniorrhaphy, cholecystectomy, and fundoplication are all performed in a single, localized region of the abdomen. Once the trocars are placed, the monitors arranged, and the camera placed to view the respective organ or region, little to no movement is necessary to proceed with the operation. Instrumentation may need to be exchanged, but the monitors, ports, camera, and personnel do not need to move. Conversely, in laparoscopic colorectal surgery, multiple rearrangements of all of the above components frequently occur.

Second, either small single vessels or no vascular structures need to be ligated in most other laparoscopic procedures. In most instances, a small or single vessel needing ligation can be accomplished with hemostatic clips or, at most, a pretied vessel ligature. However, the broad-based mesentery of the colon will not allow such simple control of most vessels. Usually multiple large vessels, often embedded in a thickened mesocolon will be present and will require ligation. Ligation may be accomplished more rapidly with a vascular stapler, but at a significantly increased cost. The alternative is a time-consuming, tedious dissection with multiple applications of clips or loops to ligate the mesocolic arcade.

Third, in most other laparoscopic procedures, there is either a small specimen or no specimen. Thus, specimen retrieval is through a standard 10- to 12-mm port, as in the case of appendectomy, or a slight enlargement of a trocar site, as in the case of cholecystectomy. In colorectal surgery, an incision of varying size or enlargement of a trocar site to a less conventional size such as 18 mm or larger may be required.

Fourth, once the defect is repaired or the organ is removed in most other laparoscopic procedures, the procedure is essentially complete. However, in laparoscopic colorectal surgery, an anastomosis usually needs to be performed. The skills to perform a laparoscopic, tension-free, well-vascularized and circumferentially intact anastomosis are far different from those used to extirpate a small end organ.

Finally, although laparoscopy has been applied to malignant diseases in other organ systems, most laparoscopically treated pathology of other organs is benign. Recurrences of reflux or an inguinal hernia or a common duct injury, although bothersome, are of a far different magnitude than is an early recurrence of a port site recurrence after a theoretically curvation resection of a Dukes' A or B colorectal carcinoma.[15–23] Thus, advanced colorectal procedures require further training beyond the basic laparoscopic training courses. The differences in techniques, instrumentation, and potential complications of any of these procedures mandates further training. Initial training entails attendance at a colorectal course.

Further practice of techniques beyond training courses is extremely valuable. Continued use of inanimate trainers, cadaver or animal models, and simulators in the future may prove invaluable in allowing surgeons to obtain greater expertise in laparoscopy. Preceptorships and subsequent observation by proctors should form the next phases of training.[26–28] Several studies have shown a steep learning curve in laparoscopic surgery.[27,28] Complications are relative to the number of cases performed and the type of procedure performed. This curve may be flattened by continued training and practice as mentioned above.

Once the surgeon has obtained this basic or advanced training, further issues regarding privileging and credentialing are left up to the individual institutions. Several authors[26,29] have written about the numbers of cases that should be assisted, proctored, and then independently performed before granting of privileges to perform a given procedure. However, a lack of uniformity among hospitals has led New York state to mandate certain instructions to physicians before allowing them to perform laparoscopic surgery.[12] Thus, a well-trained professor of surgery is viewed in the same context as a nonboard-certified recent graduate. It is hoped that cautious, conservative development of laparoscopic colorectal surgery will obviate the recurrence of such a problem.

A concept not previously addressed is that of a laparoscopic team. More so in laparoscopic surgery than in traditional surgery, a surgeon depends on others in the team for assistance. The camera person acts as the eyes for all the members of the team; thus, the assistant must understand and be as accomplished a laparoscopist as the surgeon. This fact is particularly relevant in more advanced procedures in which exposure and retraction are more important and difficult than the actual dissection or mobilization. Operating with the same person has been shown to decrease the number of complications.[13] Also, communication is awkward in laparoscopic surgery. It is difficult to show others where to grasp, where to coagulate, and where to cut. This problem is due to several factors: a tunnel field of vision, the inability to point because both hands are often simultaneously used for holding instruments, and that several monitors are used, not allowing simple pointing to be perceived by all personnel. Verbal communication and slow, deliberate movement of intra-abdominal instrumentation are necessary.

To date, policy statements have been issued by the American College of Surgeons, the American Society of Colon and Rectal Surgeons, and the Society of Gastrointestinal and Endoscopic Surgeons regarding laparoscopic surgery.[2,30–33] The common denominator among all these statements is that they fail to list specific guidelines and are merely philosophic dicta.

Recommended Steps for Becoming an Accomplished Laparoscopic Colorectal Surgeon

These recommendations can be extrapolated to any laparoscopic procedure.

1. For any laparoscopic procedure, one must have privileges in the traditional open procedure
2. Training in basic laparoscopic technique must be obtained before performing the more complex therapeutic laparoscopic procedures on patients
   A. Residents will obtain such training in surgical residency programs
   B. Others will need to obtain outside training in laparoscopic courses
3. Advanced laparoscopic training similarly must be obtained
4. Further training beyond courses—including continued practice in "dry labs," animal models, cadaver models, and simulators—should be encouraged
5. Institutional policies should be devised in an attempt to ensure proper training and proctoring, including a period of preceptoring. The exact number of cases assisted, preceptored, and performed before independent privileges is up to the individual institutions. It is hoped that national and international guidelines will become available to help in these matters
6. Training and performance of complex laparoscopic procedures should involve a dedicated laparoscopic team
7. Participation in organized studies to evaluate the effectiveness and complications of laparoscopic surgery will improve the participant's laparoscopic skills

Laparoscopic surgery is still in its infancy, and long-term follow-up data are lacking for most laparoscopic procedures, especially newer techniques such as laparoscopic colorectal surgery. All surgeons who perform laparoscopic surgery should keep records tracking their patients' regarding long-term outcome. Most notable in the cases performed for cancer are long-term survival, recurrences, and any specific complications that are due to laparoscopy such as port site recurrence. If trends inconsistent with similar stage patients done in a traditional manner occur, it should be that surgeon's responsibility to inform other surgeons of these potential shortcomings. This information can be in the form of a letter to the editor or correspondence and does not necessarily need to be a well-planned paper. Participation in multi-institutional trials may give answers to potential problems with regard to laparoscopy sooner than awaiting the filtering data of case presentations. All surgeons should be encouraged to participate in these trials and to submit their data so that collective results can be obtained.

Because the long-term results of laparoscopic resection for carcinoma are not known, and there is no consensus regarding the benefits of laparoscopy in colorectal surgery, surgeons must be honest with their patients. The published series on laparoscopic colorectal surgery to date are not consistent. They vary with regard to length of stay, complications, degree of pain, return to activity, and other criteria. Only cosmesis is a universally accepted benefit at the present time. Patients must be told that there may be no benefits other than cosmesis and that potential problems not found with traditional surgery may occur. Patients should give informed consent. By following the above steps (including data collection and review), one can become an accomplished laparoscopic colorectal surgeon.

REFERENCES

1. Perissat J, Collet D, Belliard R: Gallstones, laparoscopic treatment, cholecystectomy, cholecystectomy and lithotripsy: our own technique. Surg Endosc 4:1, 1990
2. Statement on laparoscopic and thoracoscopic procedures. Bull Am Coll Surg 78:48, 1993
3. Cuschieri A, Berci G, McSherry CK: Laparoscopic cholecystectomy. Am J Surg 159:273, 1990
4. Cuschieri A: The dust has settled—let's sweep it clean: training in minimal access surgery, editorial. J R Coll Surg Edinb 37:213, 1992
5. Cuschieri A: The laparoscopic revolution—walk carefully before we run, editorial. J R Coll Surg Edinb 34:295, 1989
6. Bailey RW, Imbembo AL, Zucker KA: Establishment of laparoscopic cholecystectomy training program. Am Surg 57:231, 1991
7. Laws HI: Credentialing residents for laparoscopic surgery: a matter of opinion. Curr Surg 684, 1991
8. Dent TL: Training, credentialing, and evaluation in laparoscopic surgery. Surg Clin North Am 72:1003, 1992
9. Greene FL: Training, credentialing, and privileging for minimally invasive surgery. Probl Gen Surg 8:502, 1991
10. Gillou PJ: Laparoscopic surgery for diseases of the colon and rectum-quo vadis? Surg Endosc 8:669, 1994
11. Sackier JM, Berci G, Paz-Partlow M: A new training device for laparoscopic cholecystectomy; technical note. Surg Endosc 593:158, 1991
12. Altman LK: Surgical injuries lead to new rule. New York Times, June 14, 1992
13. See WA, Cooper CS, Fisher RJ: Predictors of laparoscopic complications after formal training in laparoscopic surgery. JAMA 270:2689, 1993
14. Cohen S, Wexner SD: Laparoscopic colectomy and appendectomy. In Condon R (ed): Shackelford's Surgery of the Alimentary Tract. 4th Ed. WB Saunders, Philadelphia (in press)
15. Alexander RJ, Jaques BC: Laparoscopically-assisted colectomy and wound recurrence, letter. Lancet 341:249, 1993
16. O'Rourke N, Price PM, Kelly S et al: Tumor inoculation during laparoscopy, letter. Lancet 342:368, 1993
17. O'Rourke NA, Heald RJ: Laparoscopic surgery for colorectal cancer. Br J Surg 80:1229, 1993
18. Fusco MA, Paluzzi MW: Abdominal wall recurrence after laparoscopic-assisted colectomy for adenocarcinoma of the colon. Report of a case. Dis Colon Rectum 36:858, 1993
19. Gillou PJ, Darzi A, Monson RT: Experience with laparoscopic colorectal surgery for malignant disease. Surg Oncol, suppl. 1:3, 1993
20. Ngoi SS, Kum CK, Goh PMY et al: Laparoscopic colon resection: the Singapore experience. Poster presentation (P56) at the Tripartite Colorectal meeting. Sydney, Australia, October 1993
21. Fingerhut A: Laparoscopic colorectal surgery. Presented at the World Congress of Endoscopic Surgery, Kyoto, Japan, June 1994
22. Nduka CC, Monson JRT, Menzies-Gow N et al: Abdominal wall metastasis following laparoscopy. Br J Surg 86:648, 1994
23. Wade TP, Comitalo JB, Andrus Ch et al: Laparoscopic cancer surgery. Surg Endosc 8:698, 1994
24. Asbun HC, Reddick EJ: Credentialing in laparoscopic surgery: a survey of physicians. J Laparoendosc Surg 2:27, 1992
25. Cuschieri A, Bailey JM, Jago R: Report of working party to council of the state. R Coll Surg Edinb, July 1993
26. Proctoring and hospital endoscopy privileges, letter. Gastrointest Endosc 37:667, 1991
27. Larach SW, Solomon MC, Williamson PR et al: Laparoscopic-assisted colectomy: experience during the learning curve. Coloproctology 15:38, 1993
28. Reiver D, Kmiot WA, Cohen SM et al: A prospective comparison of laparoscopic and open procedures in colorectal surgery, abstracted. Dis Colon Rectum 37:P22, 1994
29. Dent TL: Training, credentialing, and granting of clinical privileges for laparoscopic general surgery. Am J Surg 161:339, 1991
30. American Society of Colon and Rectal Surgeons: Approved statement of laparoscopic colectomy. Dis Colon Rectum 37:638, 1994
31. Society of American Gastrointestinal Surgeons: Position Statement. Society of American Gastrointestinal Surgeons, 1992
32. Society of American Gastrointestinal Surgeons: Guidelines for Granting Privileges for Laparoscopic General Surgery. SAGES publication No. 0014. Society of American Gastrointestinal Surgeons, 1992
33. European Association of Endoscopic Surgeons: Training and assessment of competence. Surg Endosc 8:721, 1994

Editorial Comment

Rama M. Jager

Drs. Weiss and Wexner address an important issue: How does a novice laparoscopic surgeon develop expertise in laparoscopic colorectal surgery? Unless the surgeon has just completed the formal residency training in an institution with surgical teaching staff experienced in laparoscopic colorectal surgery, every practicing abdominal surgeon faces the problem of acquiring the new skills in the new and rapidly expanding field of laparoscopic surgery. Surgeons have to master the hand-eye coordination while watching a two-dimensional video view, obtain perfect and a more meticulous hemostasis to avoid degradation of the video image, and conquer the problem of safe extrication of resected colon through a minuscule incision.[1]

No surgeon in active practice or teaching can escape the need to learn laparoscopic surgery. Many surgical procedures that were routinely done by open laparotomy until recently may be done by the laparoscopic approach in the very near future. Laparoscopic colorectal surgery brings up different problems related with surgical training because of its adolescence. Even a surgeon who is extremely talented and skilled in open colorectal surgery may painfully face the video demonstration of hand-eye incoordination to the entire operating room in a magnified view, when attempting a laparoscopic procedure. The simple act of suture ligating a blood vessel may involve multiple false steps and unwanted frustration.

Laparoscopic training should begin with inanimate models and animal laboratory training. It should be applied progressively on patients working in conjunction with a trained surgeon.[2] Preceptorship and proctoring are becoming more common. Also, the traditional apprenticeship system—either through a formal residency, a fellowship, or a mini-residency—still remains an important facet of surgical training.[3]

LEARNING CURVE

As with any other motor skill, laparoscopic colorectal surgery imposes the penalty of a learning curve on the surgical student.[4] All surgeons face failure, high rate of conversion to open technique, and myriad complications during their initial attempts at laparoscopic colorectal surgery. The rate of complications associated with the anticipated clinical learning curve can be decreased by additional education following an initial didactic and animal laboratory course in laparoscopy. An ongoing clinical association with more experienced surgeons performing similar procedures, either through preceptorship or proctoring, can reduce the severity and frequency of complications.[5] Most of the published studies on the impact of learning curve on laparoscopic surgical skills deal with urologic laparoscopy. One of the studies involved laparotomy following the initial laparoscopic pelvic lymphadenectomy in 30 patients with prostatic cancer.[6] The study was designed to determine the adequacy of lymph nodal harvest by the laparoscopic approach. The amount of remaining lymph nodes after laparoscopic lymphadenectomy progressively decreased with time, especially after the first 20 patients. A similar learning curve may be true with laparoscopic colorectal surgery. Increasing experience, however, does not make one immune from complications,[7] and continued careful attention and steps to avoid known complications is essential.

LAPAROSCOPIC SUTURING AND ULTRASOUND

Although increasingly sophisticated instruments such as laparoscopic staplers make laparoscopic repair and reconstruction safe and swift, laparoscopic suturing is still a necessary component of every laparoscopic surgeon. The suturing skills such as needle loading, driving, and knot tying[8] require extensive practice. The laparoscopic surgeon should also master the skills in using laparoscopic ultrasound, an increasingly useful tool in the localization and examination of hepatic and retroperitoneal focal lesions.[9]

TRAINING MODELS

Various inanimate models and use of graded exercises are available in learning laparoscopic skills.[10,11] The novice laparoscopic surgeon should practice on the bench to learn hand-eye coordination and orientation, watching a two-dimensional video image in a closed inanimate trainer. The surgeon should learn handling the instruments and practice the different steps of the procedure such as ligation of mesocolic vessels, colonic transection and stapling, and placement of the resected specimen in an impermeable bag. The use of explanted organs positioned in the models may be helpful in these exercises. Pulsatile perfused organs placed in an inanimate model also serve as training devices providing optimum simulation of intraoperative status.[12]

Laparoscopic surgical procedures in an animal laboratory are helpful, although the differences of animal colorectal anatomy from the human anatomy diminish the learning benefits. Henkel et al,[13] from Germany, suggested the use of a "laptent" to cover the operative site after laparotomy and completion of the operation with laparoscopic instruments under continuous video monitoring to train surgeons in laparoscopic surgery. This may not be pragmatic, feasible, or acceptable in many health-care centers. With increasing sophistication of video-simulation systems, virtual reality surgical simulators may become effective in laparoscopic surgical training and more acceptable than the extant inanimate models.

As Drs. Weiss and Wexner point out, the skills required for laparoscopic colorectal surgery are more sophisticated than those needed for laparoscopic cholecystectomy. Although helpful, no amount of didactic instruction, inanimate model training, and animal laboratory experience will train one to become a skilled laparoscopic colorectal surgeon. In the absence of formal residency programs in advanced laparoscopic procedures, working with a more experienced laparoscopic colorectal surgeon may be the most effective learning tool. As reported in the cited studies dealing with the laparoscopic learning curve, one's laparoscopic surgical skills evolve and mature with increasing experience.

REFERENCES

1. Monson JR: Advanced techniques in abdominal surgery. BMJ 307:1346, 1993
2. Bedat B, Hugonnet C, Merlini M: Laparoscopy: obstacle or revolution in the development of surgery? Helv Chir Acta 60:783, 1994
3. Jakimowicz JJ: The European Association for Endoscopic Surgery recommendations for training in laparoscopic surgery. Ann Chir Gynaecol 83:137, 1994
4. Meinke AK, Kossuth T: What is the learning curve for laparoscopic appendectomy? Surg Endosc 8:371, 1994
5. See WA, Cooper CS, Fisher RJ: Predictors of laparoscopic complications after formal training in laparoscopic surgery. JAMA 270:2689, 1993
6. Guazzoni G, Montorsi F, Bergamaschi F, Bellinzoni P et al: Open surgical revision of laparoscopic pelvic lymphadenectomy for staging of prostate cancer: the impact of laparoscopic learning curve. J Urol 151:930, 1994
7. Wexler MJ, Hinhey EJ, Sampalis J, Barkun J: Canadian laparoscopic surgery survey. Can J Surg 36:217, 1993
8. Hunter J, Berci G, Sackier J, Cuschieri A: Analysis of surgical movements during suturing in laparoscopy. Endosc Surg Allied Tech 2:55, 1994
9. Velez PM, Robertson DW: A method for training surgeons in laparoscopic ultrasound. Endosc Surg Allied Technol 2:155, 1994
10. Shapiro SJ, Gordon LA, Daykhovsky L, Senter N: The laparoscopic hernia trainer. The role of a life-like trainer in laparoendoscopic education. Endosc Surg Allied Tech 2:66, 1994
11. Steele RJ, Hosking SW, Chung SC: Graded exercises for basic training in laparoscopic surgery. J R Coll Surg Edinb 39:112, 1994
12. Szinicz G, Beller S, Bodner W, Zerz A et al: Simulated operations by pulsatile organ-perfusion in minimally invasive surgery. Surg Laparosc Endosc 3:315, 1993
13. Henkel TO, Potempa DM, Rassweiler J et al: Lap simulator, animal studies, and the laptent. Bridging the gap between open and laparoscopic surgery. Surg Endosc 7:539, 1993

24

Laparoscopic Complications

David E. Beck and Frank G. Opelka

Laparoscopy, like any invasive procedure, has associated complications. The rapid adoption of this technology by general surgery and surgical subspecialties (e.g., colorectal surgery) and expansion to new procedures has produced a unique situation. Surgeons adopted this new technology without the benefit of traditional training such as residency and fellowships. An interim lack of organized progressive experience in colorectal laparoscopic surgery and the challenges of advanced procedures have contributed to complications. Complications are inversely related to the operating surgeon's experience. Multiple authors have documented a higher complication rate during a surgeon's early laparoscopic experience.[1–3] Laparoscopic colon and rectal surgical procedures are more difficult than other advanced laparoscopic procedures. Colorectal procedures require extensive mobilization of a large hollow organ with ligation of numerous large blood vessels. Laparoscopic intestinal surgery involves the extraction of a large specimen and restoration of bowel continuity.[2] Complications of laparoscopic procedures can be divided into those related to trocars, the pneumoperitoneum, and the procedure itself.

TROCAR-RELATED COMPLICATIONS

Although relatively safe, the placement and use of trocars and pneumoperitoneum needles (e.g., Veress needles) have been associated with complications. During trocar and needle insertion, every organ and structure in the abdomen has the potential for injury. A trocar injury to the bladder usually manifests itself by pneumaturia, hematuria, and occasionally by ballooning of the urinary drainage bag.[2] Injury to solid organs and major vascular structures is usually accompanied by hemorrhage. Multiple reports and presentations have documented these injuries, but their incidence is low. Mintz[4] reported an incidence of 0.05 percent in a survey of over 99,000 procedures. Several extensive reviews of diagnostic laparoscopic procedures identified a morbidity of 0.15 to 0.6 percent and a mortality of 0.04 to 0.13 percent.[5]

The use of a Veress needle to establish a pneumoperitoneum has the potential to injure organs, blood vessels, or bowel. The small diameter of this needle and its spring-loaded cover limit complications. Knowledge of vascular anatomy (e.g., the location of the epigastric arteries) is helpful in avoiding abdominal wall vascular injuries. Such methods as aspiration after needle placement, the saline drop test, and pressure monitoring during gas insufflation also help minimize complications. Improper placement of a Veress needle leads to insufflation in the preperitoneal space or possible intestinal insufflation. One study found that 1.5 percent of patients studied with perioperative abdominal films had documentation of air insufflation of an intestinal loop that was due to use of a Veress needle.[6]

To eliminate the potential complications from use of a Veress needle and the initial trocar insertion, some surgeons avoid the use of an insufflation needle; instead, they insert the first trocar with an open or Hasson's technique.[7] The open technique, however, has associated complications, such as avulsion of adhesions. Comparison of complications using an open versus a closed technique have shown fewer complications with the open method, but the difference has been small.[8]

The major risk with trocars is related to the initial trocar insertion. Because this is a blind procedure, organs adhered to the abdominal wall may be inadvertently injured. Other trocars, inserted under direct vision from the laparoscopic camera, placed through the initial trocar, have a lower potential for injury. Most trocar injuries result from technical problems, such as an inadequate skin incision (which causes increased insertion force), extraperitoneal location of the trocar (usually from failure to penetrate a loose peritoneal layer), excessive depth of insertion (usually from excessive force), and faulty instruments.[9] An adequate pneumoperitoneum moves the abdominal wall away from the intraperitoneal organs and lessens the chances of organ injury.

Trocar site hernias are rare, and their occurrence is related to the location and size of the trocar (or cannula) wound. Hernias are more frequent if the cannulas are placed through the linea alba rather than placed through the rectus muscle. The reported incidence when using small cannulas is one in 5,000 to 10,000 cases.[10] The instruments used in laparoscopic colorectal procedures require larger cannulas (10 to 33 mm). As larger trocars become more common and the use of laparoscopic surgery expands, the previous hernia incidence will increase. To minimize the occurrence of hernia, the fascia on all trocar wounds 10 mm or larger requires closure.[11]

Wound infection of trocar sites has been rare. Most infections have been associated with intra-abdominal contamination (e.g., ruptured appendicitis) or with specimen removal (e.g., appendicitis or cholecystitis). These small, deep wounds—if not appropriately managed—have the potential to progress to necrotizing fasciitis, a potentially lethal but uncommon problem. Because many laparoscopic patients are discharged from the hospital in the early postoperative period, it is important to instruct patients on the signs and symptoms of wound infections. Development of wound erythemia, drainage, or increasing pain should prompt the patient to seek medical attention. Any suspected wound infection requires exploration (opening), debridement, and drainage of any fluid collection.

PNEUMOPERITONEUM-RELATED COMPLICATIONS

A carbon dioxide pneumoperitoneum results in several physiologic changes, including alterations in acid base, pulmonary mechanics, and cardiopulmonary physiology.[2] Transperitoneal absorption of carbon dioxide results in elevation of arterial partial pressure of carbon dioxide, and all patients should have continuous monitoring of end-tidal carbon dioxide. While most patients can be managed by an increased ventilation rate, patients with cardiovascular diseases may develop hypercarbia and acidemia. Treatment of severe hypercarbia and acidosis requires prompt evacuation of the intraperitoneal carbon dioxide and mechanical hyperventilation.[12–14]

Hemodynamic and pulmonary complications that are due to increased intra-abdominal pressure have also been described.[15,16] The magnitude of these alterations is related to the amount of intra-abdominal pressure, baseline hemodynamic function, and the patient's volume status. It is recommended that the intra-abdominal pressure remain lower than 15 mm Hg to minimize these effects. The increased intra-abdominal pressure used in laparoscopy also raises the diaphragm and decreases pulmonary compliance. This effect can be compensated for by increasing the ventilator's inflation pressure.[15–17] Severe bradycardia can occur during the intraperitoneal insufflation of carbon dioxide, as the peritoneal distension increases vagal tone. Careful monitoring will identify these changes, and appropriate measures can be instituted.

Subcutaneous emphysema results from failure of an insufflating Veress needle to reach the peritoneal cavity or from carbon dioxide being forced into the abdominal wall during accidental withdrawal of trocars and their subsequent replacement. Minimal subcutaneous emphysema will resolve spontaneously. The presence of significant subcutaneous gas may lead to a pneumothorax or a pneumomediastinum, which requires prompt diagnosis and treatment. A large amount of sequestrated carbon dioxide can also overwhelm the endogenous clearance mechanisms and lead to hypercarbia and acidosis.[18]

The high flow and volume of gas used to obtain and maintain the pneumoperitoneum can cause problems. The temperature of carbon dioxide used to inflate the abdomen is generally 16° to 17°C when it contacts the peritoneum.[2] Prolonged exposure (more than 3 to 4 hours) to unheated gas leads to hypothermia. A core temperature below 32°C is associated with serious complications such as hypotension, cardiac arrhythmias, and clotting disorders. Hypothermia is minimized by the use of air or water warming blankets, warming intravenous fluids, irrigating fluids, anesthesia gases, and limitation of laparoscopic operating time. An extremely rare and potentially lethal complication is a gas embolus. Direct injection of carbon dioxide into a blood vessel results in the characteristic "mill wheel" murmur, which prompts initial treatment (100 percent oxygen, movement of the patient to left lateral and head-down position, and attempted aspiration of gas from the ventricle).[19]

PROCEDURE-RELATED COMPLICATIONS

Complications related to the procedure can be divided into those that occur early (during the procedure) and those that occur late (postoperative). A summary of the larger published laparoscopic bowel surgery series[20–23] is presented in Table 24-1. Intraoperative complications have ranged from 14 to 17 percent, whereas postoperative complications have varied from 8 to 33 percent. Early complications include conversion to an open procedure, organ injury, and hemorrhage.

Table 24-1. Reported Complications After Laparoscopic Colorectal Procedures

Author	Year	No. of Patients	Intraoperative Complications (%)	Postoperative Complications (%)
Phillips et al[20]	1992	51	16	8
Monson et al[21]	1992	40	16	18
Falk et al[22]	1993	66	17	33
Wexner[23]	1993	74	14	20

Conversion to an open procedure is not a complication but instead an indicator of good surgical judgment. The reasons for converting to an open procedure include unclear anatomy, excessive operating time, intraoperative complications (e.g., hemorrhage or organ injury), or inability to complete the procedure (usually as a result of adhesions, abscesses, etc.). The reported rates of conversion have varied from 8 to 50 percent. The large range reflects differences in patient selection, the surgeon's experience, and definitions of what constitutes conversion. Most studies have documented that patients who have their operations converted have more frequent complications, higher costs, and longer postoperative hospital stays.

Injury to organs can occur from trocars (as described in the previous section) or from energy from use of lasers (light amplification by stimulated emission of radiation), electrocautery, or trauma from instruments. Carbon dioxide lasers are commonly used in gynecologic procedures to vaporize endometriomas. However, carbon dioxide lasers have little to add to laparoscopic colon and rectal procedures. Laparoscopy results in loss of the surgeon's tactile ability, which is accentuated by the use of a noncontact laser. Use of a laser adds operative time and expense to the procedure, requires additional protective equipment, and offers no proven benefit in the majority of colorectal procedures.[24] In addition, several of the lethal complications resulting from laparoscopic procedures occurred after laser injuries to the portal vein and vena cava. Therefore, the laser is rarely used in laparoscopic colorectal procedures. Most colorectal laparoscopic surgeons use scissors or electrocautery.

The electrosurgical instruments used in laparoscopy are associated with a significant portion of laparoscopic complications. Injuries that occur as a result of energy transfer outside the visual field often go unrecognized. Injuries can also be due to defective insulation on the active electrode, capacity coupling, or direct coupling between the active electrode and metal instruments or electrode and the laparoscope itself.[2,25] An unrecognized thermal bowel injury may progress to a transmural perforation and present hours to days after the injury. Patients with this type of injury usually present with an ileus, signs of peritoneal irritation, fever, and leukocytosis.[2] These types of injuries are minimized by ensuring that the active electrodes come in contact with only the intended tissue. A bowel electrocautery injury is managed by imbrication of small injuries and resection and closure of more extensive burns. It is often best to manage these significant injuries with the abdomen open. Capacitance coupling is prevented by the use of metal cannulas that disperse the current through the abdominal wall or by modern plastic cannulas, which do not store current.

Minor bleeding can be controlled laparoscopically by occluding the bleeder with a laparoscopic clamp followed by ligaclip placement or endoloop ligation. Electrocautery is useful for small vessels only. Major hemorrhage is appropriately managed by expeditiously opening the abdomen. Ureteral injury is the most common urologic complication occurring during laparoscopic surgery.[26] Knowledge of pelvic anatomy as seen laparoscopically and good operative technique are essential to avoid ureteral injury. Exposing and visualizing the ureter at all times during the procedure minimizes its potential for injury. Electrocoagulation in the vicinity of the ureter should be avoided to prevent thermal injury. A preoperative computed tomography (CT) scan or intravenous pyelogram is used by some surgeons to confirm the location of the ureter and identify medial deviation associated with inflammatory or neoplastic conditions.[27] Stenting the ureters with standard or fiberoptic ureteral catheters or use of a laparoscopic Doppler probe may be helpful in difficult cases.[2] An injured ureter identified during laparoscopy has been repaired laparoscopically. The technique involves mobilizing the ureter, placing stents in an antegrade or retrograde manner, and suturing the injury with 4-0 chromic catgut.[2] More extensive repairs—such as a ureteroureterostomy or a ureterocystostomy—are best accomplished after a laparotomy. Unrecognized urinary injuries usually result in fever, abdominal and flank pain, leukocytosis, and peritoneal signs. An aggressive evaluation will identify the cause of the problem, and the patient is best managed in a multispecialty approach.

Inability to locate intraluminal lesions such as polyps or small tumors remains a problem with laparoscopy. Several reports have documented missing the intended lesion after a colectomy. Ideas to improve intraoperative identification of the target lesion include preoperatively tattooing the colon near the lesion, preoperative radiologic verification of lesion location, and intraoperative colonoscopy[2] (see also Ch. 12).

Because laparoscopic procedures are relatively lengthy, it is imperative that the patients be positioned correctly. Adequate padding of extremities and pressure areas is necessary to prevent pressure injuries. Special attention to the elbows and knees is important to prevent injury to the ulnar and peroneal nerves. Sequential compression stockings minimize the venous pooling in the lower extremities that is associated with operative procedures and the use of a pneumoperitoneum. The operating table is frequently moved and repositioned to assist the surgeon in intra-abdominal retraction and exposure during laparoscopy. To prevent the patient from slipping while in extreme positions, the patient must be securely attached to the operating table by the use of a beanbag or adhesive tape.

Late complications of laparoscopic colorectal surgery result from an anastomotic leak or contamination. All elective patients should receive a full mechanical and antibiotic bowel preparation.[28] Patients receiving left colon operations also undergo a rectal irrigation after induction of anesthesia. Some surgeons have used intraoperative colonoscopy to confirm a clean and decompressed colon before resection[29] (see also Ch. 12). Multiple technical maneuvers used to minimize contamination include wound protectors, specimen bags, and bowel occlusion devices or clamps. Current techniques of performing an intracorporeal anastomosis have a higher potential for contamination. The experience to date has demonstrated equivalent leak rates after comparable open and laparoscopic procedures.

Of special concern is the potential for metastatic tumor recurrence or dissemination to trocar sites. The reports currently available are anecdotal; prospective controlled trials have not been completed.[30–33] Factors to consider include the presence of ascites in some of the case reports. Experience from the gynecology literature documents the problem of tumor implantation in patients with carcinoma of the ovary associated with ascites. Some reports have involved patients with late-stage disseminated tumors; however, others occurring after small potentially curable colon cancers suggest violation of well-accepted cancer principles or risks related to the laparoscopic technique or pneumoperitoneum.[30–33] Until the results of prospective trials are available, some authors have recommended irrigation of trocar sites with sterile water,[2] while others have refrained from using laparoscopic techniques in potentially curative cancer patients outside of Institutional Review Board-approved protocols.

With any developmental technology and new procedures, complications will occur. Appropriate training and experience, as well as careful and objective review of results, should minimize morbidity to laparoscopic colorectal patients.

REFERENCES

1. See WA, Cooper CS, Fisher RJ: Predictors of laparoscopic complications after formal training in laparoscopic surgery. JAMA 270:2689, 1993
2. Ramos R: Complications in laparoscopic colon surgery: prevention and management. Semin Colon Rectal Surg 5:239, 1994
3. Deziel DJ, Millikan KW, Economou SG et al: Complications of laparoscopic cholecystectomy: a national survey of 4,292 hospitals and an analysis of 77,604 cases. Am J Surg 165:9, 1993
4. Mintz M: Risks and prophylaxis in laparoscopy: a survey of 100,000 cases. J Reprod Med 18:269, 1977
5. Lightdale CJ: Indications, contraindications, and complications of laparoscopy. p. 1039. In Sivak M (ed): Gastroenterologic Endoscopy. WB Saunders, Philadelphia, 1987
6. Reich H: Laparoscopic bowel injury. Surg Laparosc Endosc 2:74, 1992
7. Hasson HM: Window for open laparoscopy. Am J Obstet Gynecol 137:869, 1980
8. Hasson HM: Open laparoscopy vs closed laparoscopy. A comparison of complication rates. Adv Planned Parenthood 13:41, 1978
9. Borten M: Complications of trocar insertion. p. 286. In Friedman EA (ed): Laparoscopic Complications. Prevention and Management. BC Decker, Philadelphia, 1986
10. Kadar N, Reich H, Liu CY et al: Incisional hernias after major laparoscopic gynecologic procedures. Am J Obstet Gynecol 168:1493, 1993
11. McMurrick PJ, Polglase AL: Early incisional hernia after use of the 12-mm port for laparoscopic surgery. Aust NZ J Surg 63:574, 1993
12. Hall D, Goldstein A, Tynan E et al: Profound hypercarbia late in the course of laparoscopic cholecystectomy: detection by continuous capnometry. Anesthesiology 79:173, 1993
13. Hodgson C, McClelland RM, Newton JR et al: Some effects of the peritoneal insufflation of carbon dioxide at laparoscopy. Anesthesiology 25:382, 1970
14. Fitzgerald SD, Andrus CH, Baudendistel LJ et al: Hypercarbia during carbon dioxide pneumoperitoneum. Am J Surg 163:186, 1992
15. Safran DB, Orlando R: Physiological effects of pneumoperitoneum. Am J Surg 167:281, 1994
16. Wittgen CM, Andrus CH, Fitzgerald SD et al: Analysis of hemodynamic and ventilatory effects of laparoscopic cholecystectomy. Arch Surg 126:997, 1991
17. Nord HJ: Complications of laparoscopy. Endoscopy 24:693, 1992
18. Kent RB III: Subcutaneous emphysema and hypercarbia following laparoscopic cholecystectomy. Arch Surg 126:1154, 1991
19. Au-Yeung P: Gas embolism during attempted laparoscopic vagotomy. Anesthesiology 47:817, 1992
20. Phillips EH, Franklin M, Carroll BJ et al: Laparoscopic colectomy. Ann Surg 216:703, 1992

21. Monson JR, Darzi A, Carey PD et al: Prospective evaluation of laparoscopic-assisted colectomy in an unselected group of patients. Lancet 340:831, 1992
22. Falk PM, Beart RW, Wexner SD et al: Laparoscopic colectomy: a critical appraisal. Dis Colon Rectum 36:28, 1993
23. Wexner SD: Laparoscopic colectomy. p. 2434. In Keighley MEB, Williams NS (eds): Surgery of the Anus, Rectum and Colon. WB Saunders, London, 1993
24. Hunter JG: Laser or electrocautery for laparoscopic cholecystectomy? Am J Surg 161:345, 1991
25. Voyles CR, Tucker RD: Education and engineering solutions for potential problems with laparoscopic monopolar electrosurgery. Am J Surg 164:57, 1992
26. Evans RM, Hulbert JC, Reddy PK: Complications of laparoscopy. Semin Urol 10:164, 1992
27. Grainger DA, Soderstrom RM, Schiff SF et al: Ureteral injuries at laparoscopy: insights into diagnosis, management, and prevention. Obstet Gynecol 75:839, 1990
28. Beck DE: Mechanical bowel preparation. Perspect Colon Rectal Surg 7:97, 1994
29. Franklin M Jr, Ramos R, Rosenthal D et al: Laparoscopic colonic procedures. World Surg 17:51, 1993
30. Fusco MA, Paluzzi MW: Abdominal wall recurrence after laparoscopic assisted colectomy for adenocarcinoma of the colon. Dis Colon Rectum 36:858, 1993
31. Fermor B, Umpleby HC, Lever JV et al: Proliferative and metastatic potential of exfoliated colorectal cancer cells. J Natl Cancer Inst 76:347, 1986
32. Walsh DC, Wattchow DA, Wilson TG: Subcutaneous metastases after laparoscopic resection of malignancy. Aust N Z J Surg 63:563, 1993
33. Wexner SD, Cohen SM, Johansen OB et al: Laparoscopic colorectal surgery: a prospective assessment and current perspective. Br J Surg 80:1602, 1993

Editorial Comment I

Lars Påhlman

One complication not addressed in this chapter is the lack of adequate exposure and difficulty with satisfactory exploration of the abdomen. Because the surgeon cannot manually palpate, it can be difficult to exclude even large lymph nodes in the mesocolon along the aorta and the hepatoduodenal ligament. Although technologic advances such as Doppler and ultrasound probes may facilitate the laparoscopic exploration, none can replace manual palpation by the surgeon. In my own experience, I have found small bowel carcinoma in the proximal jejunum in one patient and gastric carcinoma in another patient by manual palpation, which I did not identify on laparoscopy. Both of these patients were in the early stages of our laparoscopic experience, and their operations were converted to an open technique because of technical difficulties. Those two episodes are anecdotal and rather rare but indicate that laparoscopic exploration of the abdomen is not perfect.

I totally agree that both the Veress needle and Hasson's technique have their own complications. In our practice, we always establish a pneumoperitoneum with a Veress needle if the patient has not been operated on before. If a midline incision has been performed earlier, we use the Hasson technique. It is also important to note that the risk of trocar site hernias increases with the use of larger trocars.

Patients undergoing colorectal surgery often are placed in a very steep Trendelenburg's position. The increased abdominal pressure from intraperitoneal carbon dioxide combined with the position of the patient can precipitate pulmonary edema during surgery. It is important that the anesthesiologists are aware of such a complication, which can be prevented by increasing the ventilator's inflation pressure in most patients.

It is also important, as Drs. Beck and Opelka state, that the extremities are adequately padded to prevent pressure injuries. Padding is of special interest when patients are placed in the lithotomy position. In placing the patient in the lithotomy position, combined with the head down to facilitate pelvic access, care must be taken to avoid crural compartment syndrome.

Drs. Beck and Opelka state that a conversion to an open procedure is not necessarily a complication. One must accept rather high rates of conversion, especially during the learning curve. If the conversion rate is too low and the operating time too long, the surgeon must consider whether the laparoscopic procedure is justified. I also want to stress that in all patients for whom the operation does not proceed smoothly, it is advisable to convert the procedure to an open technique.

We have had some bowel injuries with Babcock clamps and other types of grasping clamps. The injuries can be of two types. One is direct perforation of the bowel. Those perforations can be rather difficult to see, especially because the clamp is often opened outside the visual field, making it difficult to always see what is happening when a clamp is opened. Another situation is when appendix epiploica or the omentum has been caught by the clamp and not released before the clamp is taken out through a port. The handling of the instruments must be gentle when they are taken out to avoid an entrapment injury.

It is preferable to have a barium enema indicating exactly where the lesion is. If the surgeon relies only on preoperative colonoscopy, it is difficult to know exactly where the endoscopist has found the lesion. For example, 70 cm from the anal verge can be in the top of the sigmoid colon, but it can also be at the splenic flexure. Once the lesion has been identified, the bowel can easily be resected and the specimen retrieved.

An important aspect is the creation of the anastomosis. If the anastomosis is done via minilaparotomy, routine surgical procedures are used. On the other hand, if the anastomosis is totally laparoscopic—for instance, stapled anastomosis to the rectum—it is mandatory to test the anastomosis intraoperatively with air or dye to prevent an anastomotic dehiscence. If a leakage is found during this test, the defect can be identified and repaired laparoscopically or by an open procedure.

A very odd complication and one difficult to explain is port site metastases. If ascites or peritoneal carcinosis is present, such a complication can easily be understood. However, port site metastases have been reported in patients with Dukes' A colon cancer, which is rather difficult to explain. This can be from unsatisfactory handling with instruments with direct contact to the tumor. If cancer cells are free in the abdomen because of inadequate operative technique, an aerosol of malignant cells can be created by the carbon dioxide insufflation, which may spread the tumor cells to port sites.

Editorial Comment II

Steven D. Wexner

Drs. Beck and Opelka very nicely outline the complications of laparoscopic colorectal surgery. Once again, a few large series are available from which to glean data. However, it appears that intraoperative complication rates vary from 14 to 17 percent and that postoperative complications in general occur in between 18 to 33 percent of patients.[1–12] Unfortunately, most series to date have been small retrospective or prospective series, and obviously no prospective randomized trials exist. Many of the series to date have been presented and not published. Nonetheless, when comparing the myriad of smaller published and presented series to the four cited within this chapter, complication rates tend to, in general, remain within the ranges outlined by Drs. Beck and Opelka. Also alluded to by the authors is that the intraoperative complication rates and, quite possibly, the postoperative complication rates appear to decrease with increasing experience. Again, one must question whether the increasing experience represents only improved ability to perform the procedure and not also improved ability at patient selection. Selection criteria include the disease process as well as the patient's body habitus, prior operations, and ability to tolerate anesthesia. Other selection factors obviously include not only the surgeon's prowess but the availability of a dedicated team to perform the procedure. It is unwise, especially for the neophyte, to commence a laparoscopic colectomy late in the afternoon with assistants other than those individuals with whom the surgeon has trained. Ideally, the surgeon should train with one other surgeon and one or two nurses, who will then function as a team for all procedures. It is critical, in order to limit complications, that all members of the team be familiar with not only all phases of the operation but also with all of the instrumentation. Clearly, problems can occur with the technical components of the operation such as the electrocautery scissors or the stapling devices. However, complications limiting performance of the technique and increasing the morbidity of the procedure can be related to items as seemingly remote as the video monitor. Imperfect lighting with either too dark a field or with static on the screen can impair visibility and increase the risk for morbidity. Accordingly, the members of the team must be familiar not only with the surgical tools but also with the various electronic and video components, including the monitor, VCR, matrix printer, camera, suction irrigation device, electrocautery, and laser, if used. Relative to this latter aspect, I agree fully with Drs. Beck and Opelka that the laser adds an expensive instrument to an already expensive procedure and brings a large bulky component into an already crowded operating room. It adds setup time and added training. In addition, there are no known advantages to using a laser during any phase of a laparoscopic or even an open colorectal operation.

Certain points raised by Drs. Beck and Opelka need to be reinforced. Injuries can occur from both the Veress needle and Hasson's technique. To date, there is no uniform agreement on which method should be routinely employed. Basically, both techniques are acceptable, and each has its proponents. Regardless of the method of insertion of the first cannula, the additional cannulas are, in general, a minimum of 10 mm in diameter. Although a few surgeons who routinely perform laparoscopic colorectal surgery advocate the use of some 5-mm ports, the majority of such surgeons do not. The reason for the use of larger trocars is because the majority of instruments useful for colorectal surgery such as the range of clamps, smaller stapling instruments, scissors, and retractors fit through ports ranging in size from 10 to 12 mm. Some of the larger stapling instruments require 18- to 33-mm ports, which also prove useful for specimen delivery. Once again, unlike gallbladder or appendix surgery, port location needs to be varied and, in my experience, is best undertaken as a fluid motion. I never begin an operation by placement of all of the ports. I will always place the camera port for initial exploration and then add between one and three additional ports during the dissection. In general, two ports are useful for grasping and another is needed for dissection. For procedures as extensive as laparoscopic total abdominal colectomy, a total of five ports rather than four is necessary. However, because of tremendous variations in internal anatomy and body habitus, port placement can be quite varied. Again, when fixing inguinal or paraesophageal hernias or when removing gallbladders or appendices, the operations can always be performed in single quadrants through preset "cookbook" port site configurations. When performing colorectal procedures, such a template approach is seldom useful. Moreover, the actual number of ports necessary will also vary contingent on the factors outlined above.

Epigastric vascular injury during port placement has certainly been reported and continues to be a problem. The problem is particularly pronounced in obese patients in whom the epigastric vessels cannot be well illuminated. I have personally adopted the use of port sites *lateral* to the rectus muscles. First, epigastric vascular injury is avoided. Second, the ergonometrics are superior for dissecting the lateral reflection of Toldt and for isolating the ureter and other retroperitoneal structures during colonic mobilization. Third, this port placement helps maximize distance among ports, thereby decreasing intracorporeal interference among the instruments. The use of larger ports has obviously led to an increase in port site herniations as noted by the authors (see Ch. 22[13]). To help prevent this complication, port sites of 10 mm or larger may need to be closed. The problem, especially in obese patients, is that one needs to enlarge the skin incision merely to access the fascia to close it after the procedure. Unfortunately, such an approach obviates the only provable advantage of laparoscopic colorectal surgery: cosmesis. It is hardly justifiable to spend numerous hours painstakingly performing a laparoscopic or laparoscopic-assisted procedure at the end of which all of the incisions are enlarged to close the ports. To rectify this problem, several commercially available devices may facilitate closure of port sites. Drs. Beck and Opelka discuss conversion as an indicator of good surgical judgment. Once again, I applaud this logic. Conversion should never be considered a complication and is in no way synonymous with failure. During laparoscopic procedures, success should be mitigated by the ultimate best long-term outcome for the patient, not by the ultimate gratification to the surgeon's ego. As an example, assume the hypothetical patient who undergoes a completely laparoscopic colectomy. This hypothetical patient leaves the hospital the day of surgery, returning to work that evening and taking only acetaminophen for pain. This patient has no ileus, a minimal cosmetic insult, and no discernible disability. At the outset, the patient may sound like an overwhelming success. However, one must query additional details. For instance, did the procedure require a prolonged anesthetic and therefore cost an inordinate sum of money (6- to 9-hour cases, particularly early during the learning curve, are legion). Second, and most important, what was the long-term outcome? Assume that this same patient underwent an attempted curative resection for a Dukes' A or B colonic adenocarcinoma and returns with port site implantation soon after surgery or succumbs to metastatic disease at an early date. Surely, this same success represents a triumph of technology over common sense. While the surgeon may have gone home to celebrate the technical triumphs and wizardry on the evening of surgery, it is doubtful that the patient experienced similar elation on diagnosis of early recurrent metastatic disease.

Unfortunately, many of the surgeons who extol the virtues of laparoscopic colorectal surgery do so based on subgroup analysis.[2,9,11] All too often, reports discuss all of the cases but then somehow analyze the patients without complications separately from the patients who sustain complications or analyze the patients who successfully completed laparoscopically versus those who required conversion. Because neither of these subdivisions can be preoperatively made, it is inappropriate to perform such analyses. When perusing the oncologic literature, a similar subgroup analysis would lead to reporting a 100-percent cure rate in patients whose cancers did not recur versus a 100-percent mortality in patients whose cancers did recur; such logic is obviously fallacious. Nonetheless, some laparoscopic advocates, in the absence of solid scientific data to support their own personal biases, rely on inappropriate statistical manipulation and prosaic verbiage to attempt to convince the skeptical reader of their viewpoint.

Six complications discussed by Drs. Beck and Opelka warrant special discussion. First, they cite the case of a ureteric injury that was laparoscopically repaired. Although such a technical triumph may indeed be possible, I personally advocate only one course of action for the "average" laparoscopic surgeon who has been fortunate enough to intraoperatively recognize ureteric injury. That surgeon should immediately convert to a laparotomy. At the present time, the standard of care in the community is such that laparoscopic repair of ureteric injury is, in my view, indefensible if it is unsuccessful. Throughout history, surgeons have never been faulted for assuming the conservative tact. Laparoscopy is certainly no different.

Second, the use of stents was mentioned. Some laparoscopic enthusiasts have made statements to the effect that "attempts should be made to visualize the ureter."[9] I strongly disagree with this statement. The ureter *must* be visualized before any vascular ligation during a laparoscopic procedure. Although such visualization may be difficult (Monson et al[4] and Guillou et al[14] found the ureter in less than half of the cases in which they tried to find it), if the ureter cannot be visualized before vascular division, the procedure should be converted to a laparotomy. Again, the conservative approach will never be punished. Some surgeons have advocated the routine use of ureteric stents including even illuminated stents to facilitate the laparoscopic procedure. It is unethical and unjustifiable to routinely add such an expensive, invasive, and time-consuming procedure merely to gratify one's ego by facilitating the performance of a laparoscopic colectomy. Certainly, in selected cases, stents are advisable as they may well be in the standard open setting. However, routine stent use is mentioned only to be condemned.

The third issue is that anastomotic leaks may occur. While Drs. Beck and Opelka mention that to date equivalent leak rates have occurred, it is impressive to review the series of Philips et al,[15] in which 18 percent of patients in whom the anastomosis was formed with a circular stapling device had donuts that were incomplete. This problem represents an 18-fold increase in the accepted rate of incomplete donuts during an open procedure.[16] Although the authors might argue that no adverse clinical sequelae ensued, incomplete donuts do require being addressed by anastomotic reinforcement. Certainly, small isolated anterior defects may be suture reinforced or addressed by other means such as use of a hernia stapler.[17,18] However, larger posterior defects, especially those that occur within the mid or distal rectum, may be difficult or impossible to reinforce in the laparoscopic setting. Furthermore, once again, the conservative approach will never be punished. Any surgeon who converts to laparotomy after noting incomplete donuts will never be thought cavalier about this new technology. Conversely, surgeons who have performed only a few laparoscopic colectomies and whose patient undergoes laparoscopic repair of an anastomotic defect and subsequently develops a fistula or abscess may well be queried as to the soundness of their judgment in not having converted to a laparotomy. The laparoscopic enthusiasts might argue that the 18-percent incidence of incomplete donuts is unduly high and is a reflection of early experience; that intracorporeal reinforcement is in most cases necessary, obviating the need for conversion; and that no adverse clinical sequelae ensue in the vast majority of cases. Conversely, however, one might argue that many surgeons would have converted to laparotomy on those patients. Certainly, after a 4- to 6-hour laparoscopic anterior resection, one might be tempted to intracorporeally repair such a defect. However, one must remember that it is not an insult to one's ego to convert. It is, however, certainly quite frustrating after having invested so much time and effort to need to make an incision to finish a portion of the operation that probably would not have occurred had the entire operation been done as a laparotomy.

The fourth issue that requires special mention is deep venous thrombosis (DVT). Drs. Beck and Opelka discuss the use of sequential compression stockings. The problem of DVT has been addressed by Guillou et al,[14] who have actually noted an increase rather than a decrease in the incidence of this complication when comparing laparoscopic to traditional open surgery. They noted an increase in the incidence of not only DVT but also fatal pulmonary embolism. Thus, the advice of Drs. Beck and Opelka to use sequential compression stockings is wise. Many surgeons might also add the routine use of minidose subcutaneous heparin.

The fifth important complication that requires special mention is removal of the wrong segment of colon. Several permutations of this unfortunate occurrence have been reported. Monson et al[4] and O'Donovan and Larach[6] were the first two groups to publicly admit to having spent numerous hours toiling during a laparoscopic operation only to be rewarded by opening the specimen and finding that the lesion was, in fact, not in the resected piece of bowel. Despite psychological and physical fatigue and undoubtedly a sense of defeat on opening the specimen, these authors bravely but appropriately converted to laparotomy to resect the correct specimen. Once again, such complications are virtually unreported after standard laparotomy. Cohen and Wexner,[19] in a survey of the members of the American Society of Colon and Rectal Surgeons, identified 18 more cases in which the wrong segment of bowel was removed. The difference between the two procedures is obviously that tactile sensation is lost during the laparoscopic procedure. More recently, McDermott et al[20] and Fingerhut (see Ch. 22)[13] have independently reported several cases in which a postoperative bowel obstruction was due to an unrecognized synchronous proximal lesion. Drs. Beck and Opelka have discussed several methods of obviating this complication, including preoperative tattooing, routinely obtaining preoperative barium enemas in addition to colonoscopy, and routine use of intraoperative colonoscopy. Again, in the survey by Cohen and Wexner,[19] many surgeons have routinely added one or more of these measures to their practice to facilitate laparoscopic colectomy. My personal view is that the laparoscopic procedure is already expensive, long, and invasive enough without adding additional procedures. If a surgeon routinely requires those techniques to facilitate the laparoscopic procedure, then the procedure should instead be done as a laparotomy.

The last issue is the most controversial and the most important. At least 33 cases have been either presented at major national and international meetings or published describing port site recurrences.[21–25] These recurrences have been noted after curative resection of Dukes' A, B, and C lesions. They have occurred in ports through which the specimen has been withdrawn as well as through remote dissection ports. They have been noted in series in which only a few patients have undergone surgery and in large series. They have been seen when the specimen has been withdrawn directly through the skin and when the specimen has been withdrawn through the trocar or within a specimen protective bag. In general, these port site recurrences have occurred between 10 and 26 weeks after the attempted curative surgery. To date, only six series have quantified specific incidences, which have ranged from 1.5 percent to 21 percent, with a mean of 6.5 percent.

REFERENCES

1. Cohen SM, Nogueras JJ, Wexner SD: Laparoscopic colorectal surgery: ascending the learning curve. World J Surg (in press)
2. Hoffman GC, Baker JW, Fitchett CW, Vansant JH: Laparoscopic-assisted colectomy: initial experience. Ann Surg 219:732, 1994
3. Milsom JW, Lavery IC, Bohm B, Fazio VW: Laparoscopic-assisted ileocolectomy in Crohn's disease. Surg Laparosc Endosc 3:77, 1993
4. Monson JRT, Darzi A, Carey PD, Guillou J: Prospective evaluation of laparoscopic-assisted colectomy in an unselected group of patients. Lancet 340:831, 1992
5. Musser DJ, Boorse RC, Madera F, Reed JF III: Laparoscopic colectomy: at what cost? Surg Laparosc Endosc 4:1, 1994
6. O'Donovan SC, Larach SW: Postoperative herniation of small bowel through a laparoscopy port site. Coloproctology 16:98, 1994
7. Peters WR, Bartels TL: Minimally invasive colectomy: are these potential benefits realized? Dis Colon Rectum 36:751, 1993
8. Scoggin SD, Frazee RC, Snyder SK et al: Laparoscopic-assisted bowel surgery. Dis Colon Rectum 36:747, 1993
9. Senagore AJ, Luchtefeld MA, Macheigan JM et al: Open colectomy versus laparoscopic colectomy: are there differences? Am J Surg 59:549, 1993
10. Tate JJ, Kwok S et al: Prospective comparison of laparoscopic and conventional anterior resection. Br J Surg 80:1396, 1993
11. Vara-Thorbeck C, Garcia-Caballero M, Salvi M et al: Indications and advantages of laparoscopic-assisted colon resection for cancer. Surg Laparosc Endosc 4:110, 1994
12. Wexner SD, Cohen SM, Johansen OB et al: Laparoscopic colorectal surgery: a prospective assessment and current perspective. Br J Surg 80:1602, 1993
13. Fingerhut A: Feasibility of laparoscopic colectomy. Presented at the 4th World Congress of Endoscopic Surgeons, Kyoto, Japan, June 1994
14. Guillou PJ, Darzi A, Monson JRT: Experience with laparoscopic colorectal surgery for malignant disease. Surg Oncol, suppl. 2:43, 1993
15. Phillips EH, Franklin M, Carroll BJ et al: Laparoscopic colectomy. Ann Surg 216:703, 1992
16. Beck DE, Wexner SD: Fundamentals of Anorectal Surgery. McGraw-Hill, New York, 1992
17. Cohen SM, Clem MS, Wexner SD, Jagelman DG: An initial comparative study of two techniques of laparoscopic colonic anastomosis and mesentery defect closure. Surg Endosc 8:130, 1994
18. Reissman P, Wexner SD, Nogueras JJ, Jagelman DG: Complications in laparoscopic colorectal surgery. Surg Endosc 8:562, 1994
19. Cohen SM, Wexner SD: Laparoscopic colorectal surgery: are we being honest with our patients? Dis Colon Rectum (in press)
20. McDermott JP, Devereaux DA, Caushaj PF: Pitfall of laparoscopic colectomy: an unrecognized synchronous cancer. Dis Colon Rectum 37:602, 1994
21. Ngoi SS, Kum CK, Goh PMY et al: Laparoscopic colon resection: the Singapore experience. Poster presentation at the Tripartite Colorectal Surgery Meeting, Sydney, Australia, October, 1993
22. Alexander RJT, Jaques BC, Mitchell KG: Laparoscopic-assisted colectomy and wound recurrence, letter. Lancet 341:249, 1993
23. Fusco MA, Paluzzi MW: Abdominal wall recurrence after laparoscopic-assisted colectomy for adenocarcinoma of the colon. Dis Colon Rectum 36:858, 1993
24. Nduka CC, Monson JRT, Menzies-Gow N, Darzi A: Abdominal wall metastases following laparoscopy. Br J Surg 81:648, 1994
25. Wexner SD, Cohen SM: Port site metastases after laparoscopic colorectal surgery for cure of malignancy. Br J Surg 82:295, 1995

25

Immune Function After Laparoscopy and Laparotomy

Richard L. Whelan, Marc Bessler, and Michael R. Treat

Laparoscopic colectomy has been touted as being less stressful than a standard open colectomy. The parameters most often used for comparison include (1) length of hospital stay, (2) time to resumption of diet, (3) time to first flatus or bowel movement, and (4) the amount of pain medication consumed. Almost all would agree that a more rigorous and scientific comparison of open and laparoscopic bowel techniques is necessary to determine the specific physiologic and immunologic differences of the two methods. Until recently, little had been done to elucidate these differences in a well-controlled setting. A series of recent animal experiments carried out at Columbia University, as well as several other studies, suggest that cell-mediated immune function is better preserved after laparoscopy than after open surgery. The implications of such a difference may be far reaching. Improved postoperative immune function may translate into lower rates of post-procedure infection and, more important, lower recurrence rates or improved 5-year survival following resection of colon tumors. This chapter briefly reviews what is known about immune function after open surgery and presents the results of the recent animal studies mentioned above.

IMMUNE FUNCTION AFTER SURGERY

Almost all studies looking into postoperative immunosuppression have dealt with cell-mediated immune functions. Cell-mediated functions are thought to defend against infection and possibly to limit the spread of tumor cells.[1–6] It has been well documented that cell-mediated immunity is suppressed after major open surgical procedures. The degree of suppression roughly correlates with the magnitude of the surgical procedure. Decreased immune function is thought to last about 6 to 9 days after surgery in humans.[7] Impairment of the following cell-mediated functions have been found to occur: (1) lymphocyte and neutrophil chemotaxis, (2) natural killer T-cell activity, (3) lymphocyte and macrophage interactions, and (4) delayed type hypersensitivity (DTH) responses.[1,8–11] DTH testing is relatively inexpensive and easily performed in the clinical setting. It has been frequently used as a measure of cell-mediated immune function.

What is known about immune function after laparoscopy? Little research has been done in this area, thus far. Horgan et al[12] compared lymphocyte proliferation rates of mice undergoing either laparoscopy, laparotomy, or anesthesia alone. They found that the laparotomy group demonstrated significantly lower proliferation rates than did the control group. Similarly, proliferation rates in the open group were markedly lower than controls after stimulation of the lymphocytes with a mitogen. No significant differences were found between the laparoscopy group and controls. This study supports the concept that less immunosuppression occurs following laparoscopy.

Is cell-mediated immune function important postoperatively? Preoperative patients found to be anergic have a significantly higher incidence of sepsis and a higher mortality than normal DTH responders.[5] One study of 727 patients found a postoperative sepsis rate of 7.5 percent and a mortality rate of 4.6 percent in normal DTH responders, whereas anergic and relatively anergic patients had a 30-percent sepsis rate and a 23-percent mortality.[6]

Do anergic cancer patients fare worse than those with normal DTH responses? Interestingly, a surprisingly low percentage of cancer patients are found to be normal DTH responders (39 percent) when compared with controls without tumors (90 percent).[13] The reason for this is unclear. Nonetheless, there is a significantly higher incidence of normal responders in the population of patients with resectable tumors (55 percent) when compared with the inoperable group (20 percent). Even more striking is the correlation of resectability with the ability of a patient to normally respond to a 2 to 4-dinitrochlorobenzene (DNCB) challenge after initial sensitization. Ninety-five percent of such patients had resectable lesions. By contrast, 93 percent of DNCB nonresponders were found to have inoperable tumors. Furthermore, 90 percent of the few nonresponders who were found to have resectable tumors developed recurrences or metastases within 6 months.[13]

To summarize, cancer patients with intact cell-mediated immune function fare better than those with diminished function. Major open surgery causes temporary immunosuppression. If it were possible to eliminate or decrease the immunosuppression that occurs after major surgery, the perioperative morbidity and mortality might be favorably altered. Are laparoscopic procedures associated with the same degree of immunosuppression as open procedures? Little is known about the effects of laparoscopy on immune function. It is for these reasons that a series of animal studies comparing laparoscopy and open surgery were undertaken.

DTH EXPERIMENTS

A normal DTH response to antigen challenge requires that the subject has been previously sensitized to the antigen. The antigen is injected intradermally, and the size of the resulting wheal is measured at 24 and 48 hours. The normal DTH response has both a cognitive and an effector limb. The former consists of antigen presentation to a clonally specific T cell (CD4+ cell) by a macrophage or other antigen-presenting cell. The antigenic presentation is followed by the elaboration and secretion of cytokines by the stimulated T cell, which then attract and activate effector cells—including macrophages, lymphocytes, and endothelial cells. These latter cells are responsible for the characteristic induration and inflammation seen at the site of injection with a positive test result. In the clinical setting, the patient is challenged with a panel of five to seven common antigens without prior sensitization. Patients are considered to have normal function as long as they respond to at least two of the antigens. Patients with a single response are considered to be relatively anergic, whereas those without any response are labeled *anergic*. In the laboratory, animals are most often challenged with one or two antigens to which they have been sensitized earlier.

The first large animal study concerning laparoscopic-assisted colon resection (LACR) at our institution was completed in 1993. The purpose of the study was to compare the physiologic responses of the animals to open and laparoscopic-assisted colectomy. A total of 22 domestic pigs were studied; 11 underwent open resection, and 11 had LACR. The equivalent of a sigmoid resection was carried out, and a stapled circular end-to-end anastomosis (EEA) was performed in each animal. The open surgery was carried out through a 20-cm lower midline incision. Five 12-mm ports were used for the LACR. One port incision was extended to a 3-cm length to allow for removal of the specimen and placement of the EEA anvil and pursestring. Extensive hemodynamic measurements, blood testing, and DTH testing were carried out.[14,15] Only the DTH results are discussed here.[16]

Immediately following the colectomy, all pigs were challenged with an intradermal injection of Sow Bac-E, an antigen preparation of common pathogens with which the pigs had been immunized as piglets. Then, 48 and 72 hours after the procedure, the two largest diameters of the indurated wheal were determined for each animal, and the average of the two was reported as the DTH response.

Surprisingly, the laparoscopic group was found to have significantly larger wheals than the open surgery group at 48 and 72 hours[16] (Fig. 25-1). These results suggested that cell-mediated immune function, as measured by DTH, may be better preserved following laparoscopic bowel surgery than with standard open techniques. Although these results were exciting, we realized that there were several shortcomings to this study in regard to the DTH testing. A preoperative DTH test, which would have established a baseline response for the animals, was not carried out. Furthermore, no control animals were exposed only to the anesthesia. Finally, repeat postoperative challenges were not performed. Such testing would allow determination of the duration of the differences in DTH response between the groups. These results led to the following rat DTH experiment.

This second study compared DTH responses in rats who underwent either an open laparotomy, abdominal insufflation, or anesthesia alone.[17] This study compared the methods of exposure alone and did not involve a bowel resection or other intra-abdominal procedure. Keyhole limpet hemocyanin (KLH) and phytohemagglutinin (PHA) were used to test the DTH response. A positive response to intradermal KLH challenge is a classic example of cell-mediated immunity that requires proper functioning of both the cognitive and effector limbs to elicit the response. By contrast, PHA tests only the effector arm of the DTH response. PHA is a nonspecific stimulator of CD4+ T cells, and a positive response does not require antigen recognition by the T cell. Both KLH and PHA were included in this study in

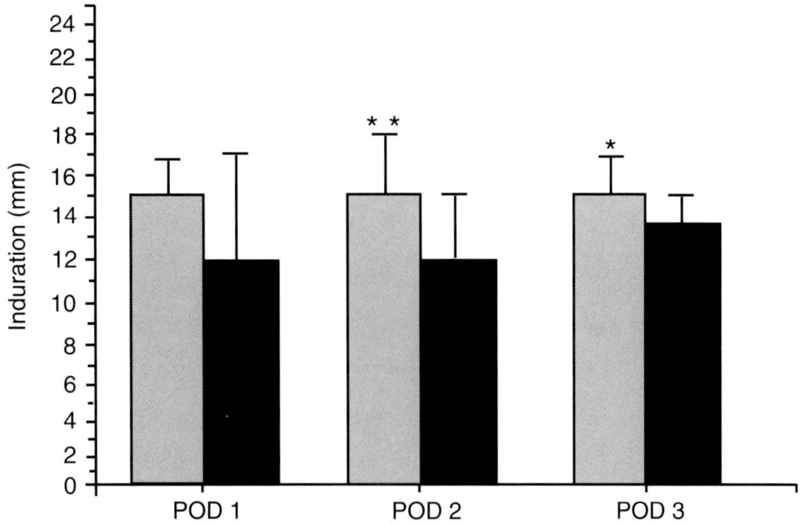

Fig. 25-1. Delayed type hypersensitivity. Shaded bars, laparoscopic group; solid bars, open surgery group; **, $P < 0.027$; *, $P < 0.05$.

an effort to examine both the cognitive and effector phases of the DTH response.

A total of 132 Sprague-Dawley rats, 44 in each of the three study groups, were included in the experiment. All animals were sensitized to KLH 2 weeks before the procedure. Ten days following the sensitization, the baseline DTH response to KLH and PHA challenge was then determined. On day 14, the animals were anesthetized and divided into three groups which underwent one of the following: group 1, laparotomy (midline incision, xiphoid to pubis); group 2, carbon dioxide pneumoperitoneum (6 to 8 mm Hg via 18-gauge angiocatheter); and group 3, anesthesia alone. All procedures were 30 minutes long. Immediately following, KLH and PHA were intradermally injected into each animal at separate sites. A third challenge of both KLH and PHA was administered on the third postoperative day. Responses to all challenges were measured 24 and 48 hours after injection.

Preoperatively, as expected, there were no significant differences in the mean DTH responses of the three groups to KLH. However, the laparotomy group demonstrated significantly smaller DTH responses than the other two groups after the first postoperative KLH chal-

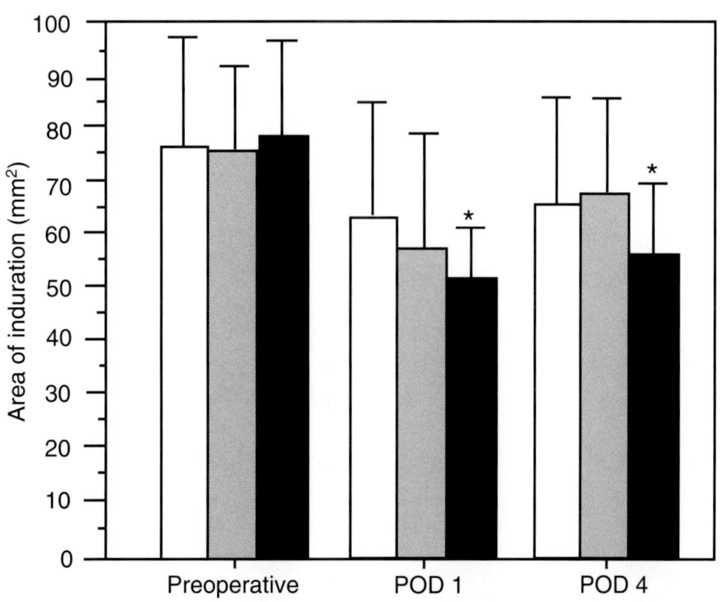

Fig. 25-2. Delayed type hypersensitivity response to keyhole limpet hemocyanin at 24 hours. Open bars, control group; shaded bars, insufflation group; solid bars, laparotomy group; *, $P < 0.005$ versus insufflation and control group.

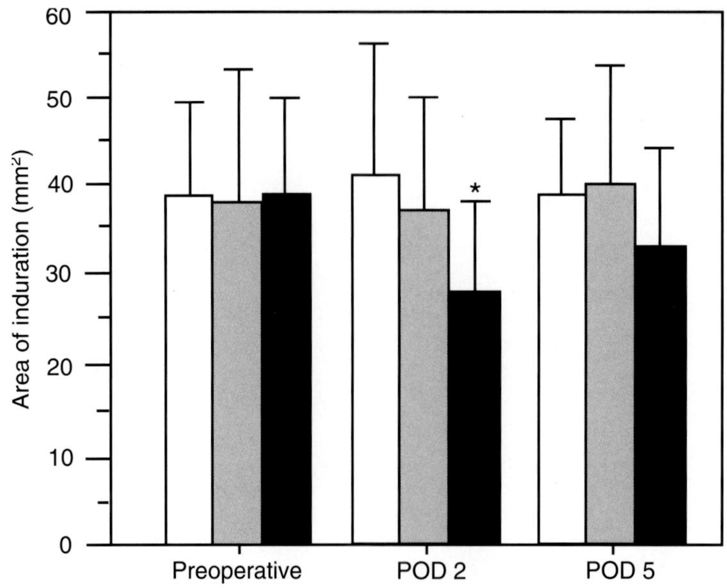

Fig. 25-3. Delayed type hypersensitivity response to keyhole limpet hemocyanin at 48 hours. Open bars, control group; shaded bars, insufflation group; solid bars, laparotomy group; *, *P* <0.001 versus insufflation and control group.

lenge at both 24 and 48 hours (Figs. 25-2 and 25-3). Similar results were noted after the postoperative day 3 KLH challenge at 24 hours. At 48 hours, no significant differences were found. No significant differences were found between the insufflation and anesthesia control groups at any of the time points.

PHA testing before the procedure revealed similar DTH responses in each of the three groups. The post-procedure challenges demonstrated significantly smaller responses in the laparotomy group at all four time points (Figs. 25-4 and 25-5). Again, no significant differences were found between the responses of the anesthesia and insufflation groups.[17]

These results suggest that the effector arm of the DTH response is the likely site of the alteration in immune response after laparotomy because similar changes in DTH response were noted after both KLH and PHA challenges. If the recognition portion of the response was the

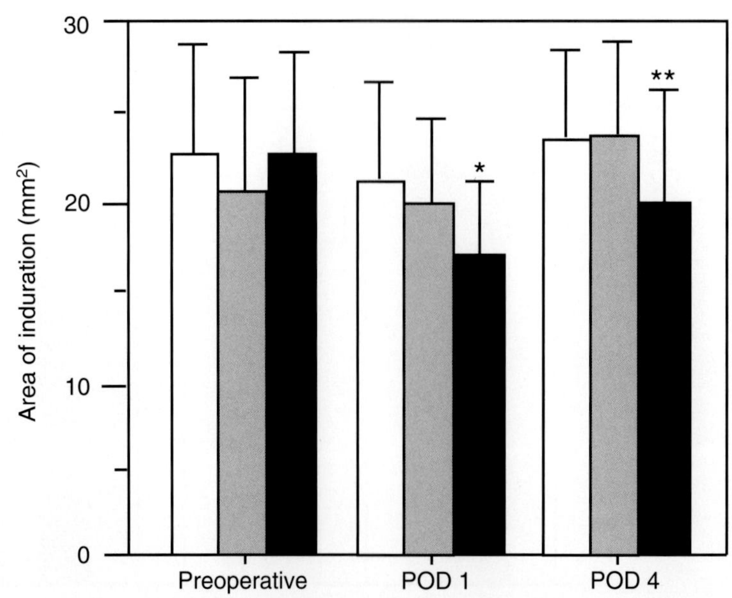

Fig. 25-4. Delayed type hypersensitivity response to phytohemagglutinin at 24 hours. Open bars, control group; shaded bars, insufflation group; solid bars, laparotomy group; *, *P* <0.005 versus insufflation and control group; **, *P* <0.01 versus insufflation and control group.

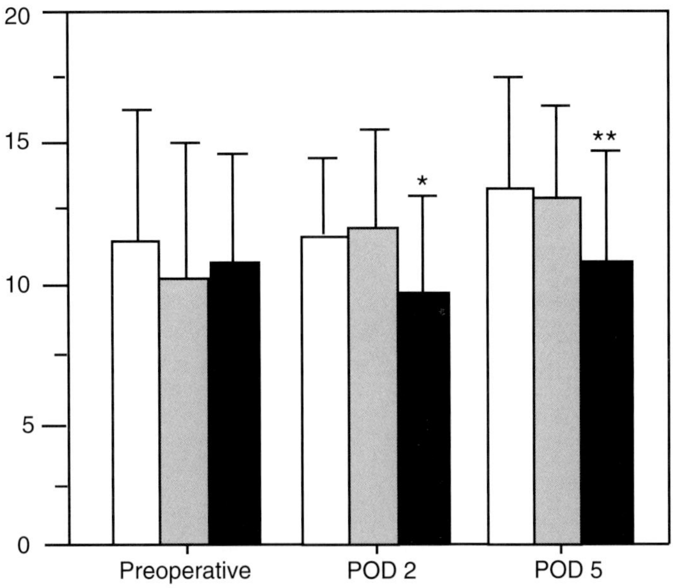

Fig. 25-5. Delayed type hypersensitivity response to phytohemagglutinin at 48 hours. Open bars, control group; shaded bars, insufflation group; solid bars, laparotomy group; *, $P < 0.07$ versus insufflation group and $P < 0.04$ versus control group; **, $P < 0.01$ versus insufflation and control group.

site, then the postprocedure PHA testing should have yielded similar results in all three groups.

These results lend further support to the hypothesis that significant cell-mediated immunosuppression occurs following laparotomy. Insufflation alone does not result in such changes. Would tumor growth rates or implantation rates be altered during the period of postoperative immunosuppression? The next series of studies addressed this important question.

TUMOR STUDIES

Several investigators have demonstrated that tumor growth in rats and mice is accelerated following laparotomy as opposed to anesthesia controls.[18–20] These increased growth rates are thought to be the result of the immunosuppression associated with open surgery. To determine whether the immunologic benefits seen with insufflation would include preservation of normal tumor growth rates, three additional animal studies were carried out. Tumor cells derived from the MC-2 mouse mammary carcinoma (MMC) cell lines were used for these experiments.[21] Tumor nodules that could easily be assessed were established by intradermally injecting the mice with tumor cells. Characteristically, once established, these MMC nodules will increase in size for about 12 days and then will begin to spontaneously regress. MMC tumor regression is thought to be immune mediated.[21]

The purpose of the first experiment was to determine if the growth and regression rates of established tumors was effected by either insufflation or laparotomy.[22] In this study, tumors were established preoperatively by injecting 35 mice with 1×10^{-6} MMC cells intradermally. After 7 days, the mice were examined. Only those with palpable tumor nodules were used for the study. A total of 33 mice were divided into three groups of 11 which underwent either insufflation, laparotomy, or anesthesia alone for 30 minutes. The mice were followed for 12 days postprocedure. Tumor volumes were assessed on postoperative days 3, 6, 10, and 12. Tumor volumes were calculated from length, width, and girth measurements taken with calipers by a blinded observer. The percentage of change in tumor volume from the volume noted at the time of procedure was calculated for all groups and compared (Fig. 25-6). Whereas the control and insufflation groups demonstrated the expected slow regression of tumor volumes, the laparotomy group tumors continued to grow. The changes in tumor volume at all points of measurement were greatest in the laparotomy group. Significant differences were found between the laparotomy group and both the insufflation and anesthesia control groups on postprocedure days 6 and 12. No significant differences were found between the insufflation and control groups at any point. Therefore, normal tumor growth rates were preserved with insufflation but not with laparotomy.

The purpose of the second experiment was to determine if the growth rates of tumor cells implanted at the time of surgery would differ when the two different exposure techniques were compared. A high dose of tumor cells, which results in tumor growth in practically all animals (1×10^{-6} MMC cells), was injected at the time of the procedure. A total of 46 mice were included in the study. These mice were divided into three groups, which under-

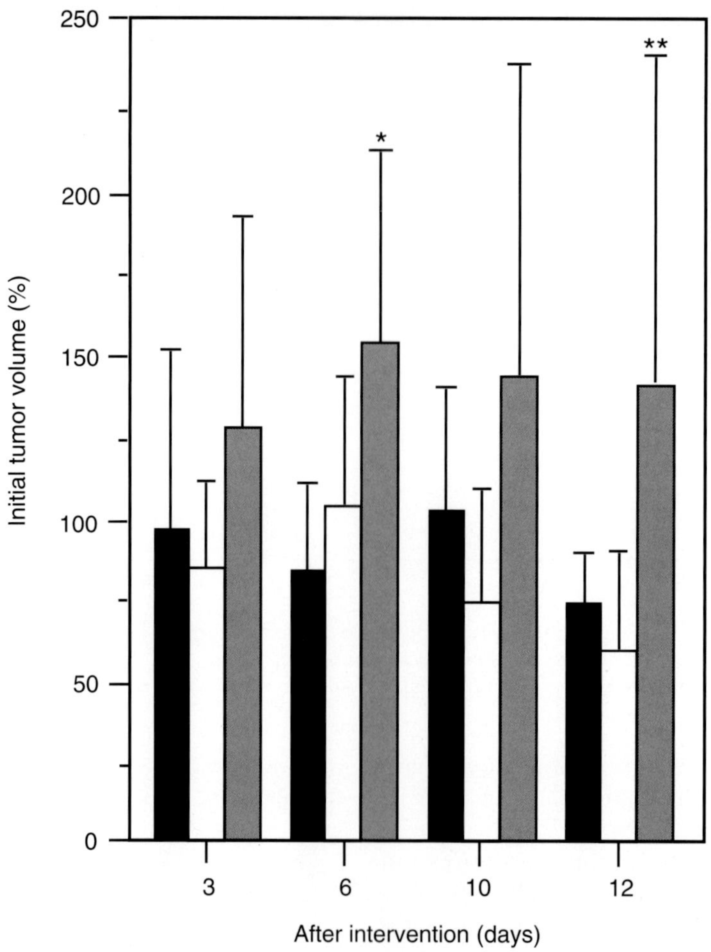

Fig. 25-6. Percentage of initial tumor volume. Open bars, insufflation group; shaded bars, laparotomy group; solid bars, anesthesia group. *, *P* <0.05 versus insufflation and anesthesia groups; **, *P* <0.05 versus insufflation and anesthesia groups.

went either laparotomy (n = 17), insufflation (n = 17), or anesthesia alone (n = 12) for 30 minutes. Twelve days after the procedure, the mice were killed, and the tumors were excised and weighed (Fig. 25-7). The laparotomy group's tumors were significantly larger than both the insufflation and control group's (control, 28 ± 13 mg; insufflation, 48 ± 32 mg; laparotomy, 87 ± 46 mg). Almost a threefold difference was found in the average size of the lesions when the laparotomy and control groups were compared (*P* <0.01 by analysis of variance [ANOVA]) and an 80-percent difference between the open and insufflation groups (*P* <0.01 by ANOVA).[22] Although significantly smaller than the open group's tumors, the insufflation group's lesions were larger than the anesthesia-alone lesions.

The purpose of the third experiment was to determine whether the rate of tumor establishment from cells implanted at the time of surgery following insufflation or laparotomy differed. In this experiment, a lower, threshold dose of cells was given (approximately 4×10^{-3}). In controls at this dose level, a minority of mice develop tumors. At the time of the procedure, 59 female mice were given intradermal injections of 4×10^{-3} tumor cells. Then 20 mice underwent laparotomy, 19 insufflation, and 20 anesthesia alone. The procedures were 30 minutes long. The mice were then followed for 30 days. A blinded observer on postprocedure days 14 and 30 palpated the mice and noted the presence or absence of tumor nodules. Two weeks after the procedure, tumors had grown in 15 of 20 of the laparotomy group, 7 of 19 of the insufflation group, and 1 of 20 of the control mice (Fig. 25-8). At 30 days, the results were identical, except that 5 of 20 of the control group had developed tumors. At both points of measurement, significantly more tumors developed in the laparotomy group than in either the insufflation or anesthesia control groups. On day 14, but not on day 30, a significant difference was found between the insufflation and control groups.[22] Therefore, tumors were more easily established after laparotomy than after insufflation.

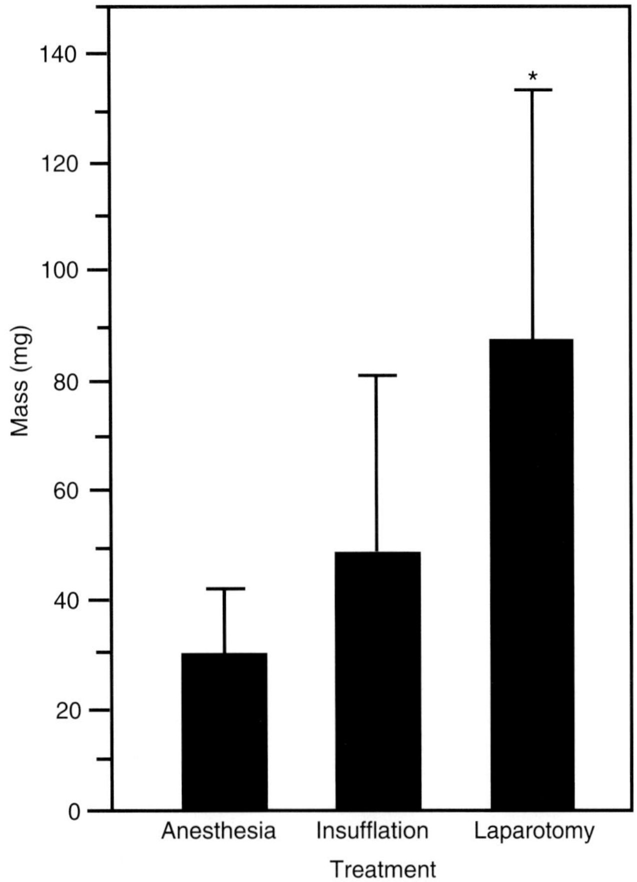

Fig. 25-7. Tumor mass: anesthesia (control), insufflation, and laparotomy treatment groups. *, P <0.01 versus insufflation group and P <0.01 versus insufflation and anesthesia groups.

SUMMARY

Significant suppression of cell-mediated immune function occurs after major open surgery. Smaller postoperative DTH responses (in humans and animals) and increased tumor growth rates (in animals) exemplify this immunosuppression. After laparoscopic colon resection in pigs, DTH responses are significantly larger than after open resection. Furthermore, DTH responses in mice were also found to be significantly larger after insufflation than after laparotomy. These results suggest that less cell-mediated immunosuppression occurs after laparoscopic procedures than after comparable open surgery.

The results of the mice tumor studies support the hypothesis that after laparotomy, it is easier for tumor cells to grow or implant. Similar but significantly less marked changes in tumor growth and implantation rates are seen after insufflation. Therefore, there appears to be a significant advantage to insufflation over laparotomy in regard to limiting tumor growth rates. It is not clear from these studies what is responsible for these changes in tumor growth and establishment, although it seems likely that suppression of the immune system is involved.

These studies have a number of important shortcomings. It will be important to determine whether the observed differences in growth rates are seen when other types of tumors are used. Differences observed with MMC may not be seen with other tumor types. Furthermore, will the differences in growth rates be preserved when an actual procedure is carried out in addition to the insufflation? Surely, a bowel resection is more stressful and traumatic than insufflation alone. Will humans demonstrate similar alterations in tumor growth rates? Finally, will such temporary differences in tumor growth and implantation rates be of sufficient magnitude to result in lower local recurrence rates and improved 5-year survival rates?

Clearly, this is an exciting area of research that deserves further study. It is crucial that we continue to search for the physiologic and immunologic differences between laparoscopic and open procedures. In the end, it will be the elucidation and documentation of such differences that will justify the continued use of and growth of laparoscopic bowel techniques.

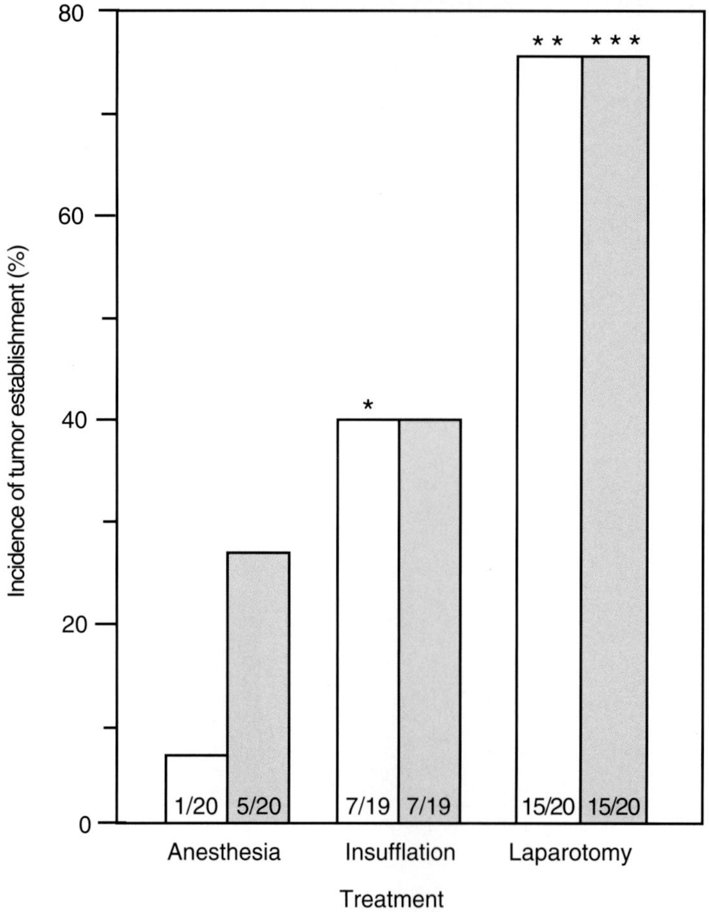

Fig. 25-8. Percentage of incidence of tumor establishment: anesthesia (control), insufflation, and laparotomy treatment groups. Open bars, day 14; solid bars, day 30. *, P <0.04 versus anesthesia group; **, P <0.04 versus insufflation group; and P <0.001 versus anesthesia group; ***, P <0.04 versus insufflation group and P <0.01versus anesthesia group.

REFERENCES

1. Nielsen HG, Pedersen BK, Moesgaard F: Effect of ranitidine on postoperative suppression of natural killer cell activity and delayed hypersensitivity. Acta Chir Scand 155:377, 1989
2. Young JD, Cohn ZA: How killer cells kill. Sci Am 258:28, 1988
3. Feldman M, Eisenbach L: What makes a tumor cell metastatic? Sci Am 259:40, 1988
4. Cook JL: Natural killer cell activity associated with human neoplasms. Sci Am 258:1324, 1988
5. Pietsch JB, Meakins JL, MacLean LD: The delayed hypersensitivity response: application in clinical surgery. Surgery 82:349, 1977
6. Christou NV, Meakins JL, MacLean LD: The predictive role of delayed hypersensitivity in preoperative patients. Surg Obstet Gynecol 152:297, 1981
7. Hammer JH, Nielsen HJ, Moesgaard F et al: Duration of postoperative immunosuppression assessed by repeated delayed type hypersensitivity skin tests. Eur Surg Res 24:133, 1992
8. Christou NV, Superina R, Broadhead M et al: Postoperative depression of host resistance: determinants and effect of peripheral protein-sparing therapy. Surgery 92:786, 1982
9. Lennard TWJ, Shenton BK, Borzotta A et al: The influence of surgical operations on components of the human immune system. Br J Surg 72:771, 1985
10. Nielsen JH, Moesgaard F, Kehlet H: Ranitidine for prevention of postoperative suppression of delayed hypersensitivity. Am J Surg 157:291, 1989
11. Hjortso NC, Kehlet H: Influence of surgery, age and serum albumin on delayed hypersensitivity. Acta Chir Scand 152:175, 1986
12. Horgan PG, Fitzpatrick M, Couse NF et al: Laparoscopy is less immunotraumatic than laparotomy. Min Invasive Ther 1:241, 1992
13. Eilber FR, Morton DL: Impaired immunologic reactivity and recurrence following cancer surgery. Cancer 25:362, 1970
14. Bessler M, Treat MR, Whelan RL et al: Controlled trial of laparoscopic versus open colon resection. Presented at the meeting of the Society of Minimally Invasive Surgery, Orlando, FL, November 1993. Surg Endosc (submitted)
15. Bessler M, Halverson A, Whelan RL: Stress response to laparoscopic colon resection. Presented at the meeting of the Society of Minimally Invasive Surgery, Orlando, FL, November 1993. Arch Surg (submitted)

16. Bessler M, Whelan RL, Halverson A et al: Is immune function better preserved after laparoscopic versus open colon resection? Surg Endosc 8:881, 1994
17. Trokel MJ, Bessler M, Treat MR et al: Preservation of immune response after laparoscopy. Surg Endosc 8:1385, 1994
18. Eggermont AM, Steller EP, Marquet RL et al: Local regional promotion of tumor growth after abdominal surgery is dominant over immunotherapy with interleuken-2 and lymphokine activated killer cells. Cancer Detect Prev 12:421, 1988
19. Goshima H, Saji S, Furata T et al: Experimental study on preventive effects of lung metastases using LAK cells induced from various lymphocytes—special references to enhancement of lung metastasis after laparotomy stress. J Jpn Surg Soc 20:1245, 1989
20. Ratajczak HV, Lange RW, Sothern RB et al: Surgical influence of murine immunity and tumor growth: relationship of body temperature and hormones with splenocytes. Proc Soc Exp Biol Med 199:432, 1992
21. Vaage J, Pepin K: Morphological observations during developing concomitant immunity against a C3H/HE mammary tumor. Cancer Res 45:659, 1985
22. Allendorf JDF, Bessler M, Kaytone ML et al: Incrased tumor establishment and growth after laparotomy vs. laparoscopy in a murine model. Arch Surg 130:649, 1995

Editorial Comment I

Heidi Nelson

Drs. Whelan, Bessler, and Treat provide not only a review of the effects of surgery on immune function and tumor growth but, more important, data suggesting an immunologic and tumor advantage for minimally invasive techniques. The possibility that laparoscopic surgery could offer such advantages in addition to patient-related benefits is encouraging and stresses the need for further investigations. To critically examine whether the immunologic and antitumor advantages—as described for laparoscopic surgery in animal models—are causally related and will likely translate into clinical advantages requires an appraisal of what is known about the effects of surgery on immune function and the relevance to tumor growth.

Substantial work has previously demonstrated (1) that cellular effector arms of the immune system can be used as antitumor therapy,[1] (2) that measures of cellular immune function are adversely affected after surgery,[2,3] and (3) that surgery provides growth advantage for tumors in some animal models.[4] It is attractive to assume that these findings describe a causal relationship between surgery, cellular immune dysfunction, and tumor growth. This is not necessarily so. Consider the study demonstrating that anergic cancer patients have less favorable surgical and cancer outcomes. Even though this study was important in illustrating the value of anergy as a marker of poor results, it did not prove that an abnormal delayed type hypersensitivity was the cause of poor outcome. Further, the premise that improving simple measures of cellular immune dysfunction after surgery will improve oncologic outcome must be challenged. Results from an interferon-γ clinical adjuvant trial illustrate this point. Even though interferon-γ enhanced the expression of HLA-Dr and Fc receptors on monocytes, disease-free survival was inferior in patients treated with interferon-γ when compared with controls.[5] The concept that cellular immune dysfunction and cancer outcome are causally related, although intuitively appealing, ignores the complexities of host-tumor interactions.

Uncontrolled tumor growth always signifies some measure of cellular immune dysfunction, yet the difficulty lies in understanding the complexities of host- and tumor-related mechanisms for uncontrolled tumor growth. It is known that tumors escape from normal immune-mediated destruction by such mechanisms as failure to provide a suitable target, through antigenic modulation and masking, or by secretion of immunosuppressive factors such as cytokines. In other cases, tumor growth may be favored by the hormonal environment, because many tumors are known to be sensitive to influences of hormones and growth factors.[6–8] Host-related hormonal, rather than immune factors, may allow the tumor burden to grow beyond that which can be reasonably eradicated by normal immune defenses, creating an irreversible tumor-favored condition. Because endocrine responses to injury and surgery are well established, it must be considered that these changes may be influential in tumor growth responses to surgery, especially for hormonally sensitive tumors. It is likely that many of the same factors that support growth and repair at sites of wounding also support tumor growth. To discover the intricate details of the relationship between surgical trauma, immunosuppression, and tumor growth is the challenge of the future.

Dr. Whelan and colleagues have initiated an important line of research, examining the impact of new minimally invasive techniques on immune function and cancer outcome. In these preliminary studies, the laparoscopic approach appears to provide an environment that is less stimulating for tumor growth. This is an important and intriguing observation. Follow-up studies with a model where a full pneumoperitoneum is established and a laparoscopic-assisted resection is performed will be crucial to substantiating these potential benefits. Future studies may also help to determine whether differences in tumor growth observed in the insufflation and laparotomy groups are related to differential delayed type hypersensitivity responses. Finally, because many factors may be essential to the clinical question of whether laparoscopic-assisted colectomy offers the same oncologic outcome as open colectomy, these issues must be addressed in clinical trials.

REFERENCES

1. Rosenberg SA, Lotze MT, Muul LM et al: A progress report on the treatment of 157 patients with advanced cancer using lymphokine-activated killer cells and interleukin-2 or high-dose interleukin-2 alone. N Engl J Med 316:889, 1987

2. Christou NV, Superina R, Broadhead M et al: Postoperative depression of host resistance: determinants and effect of peripheral protein-sparing therapy. Surgery 92:786, 1982
3. Lennard TWJ, Shenton BK, Borzotta A et al: The influence of surgical operations on components of the human immune system. Br J Surg 72:771, 1985
4. Weese JL, Ottery FD, Emoto SE: Do operations facilitate tumor growth? An experimental model in rats. Surgery 100:273, 1986
5. Wissenfeld M, Wieand HS, Gonchoroff NJ et al: Interferon-gamma as postoperative surgical adjuvant therapy for colon cancer: significant immune stimulation without evidence of therapeutic benefit, abstracted. Proc ASCO 11:167, 1992
6. Nelson H, Miller SH, Buck D et al: Effectiveness of prophylactic mastectomy in the prevention of breast tumors in C_3H mice. Plast Reconstr Surg 83:662, 1989
7. Sizeland AM, Burgess AW: The proliferative and morphologic responses of a colon carcinoma cell line (LIM 1215) require the production of two autocrine factors. Mol Cell Biol 11:4005, 1991
8. Watkins L, Levine AE: Differential role of transforming growth factor-α in two human colon carcinoma cell lines. Int J Cancer 47:455, 1991

Editorial Comment II

Rama M. Jager

Generalized temporary postoperative immunosuppression is a well-recognized component of a body's response to injury, including surgical injury.[1] This postoperative response involves the neuroendocrine axis, the T/B immune limbs, and the inflammatory effector apparatus along with complex intersystem interactions. The magnitude of surgical injury influences the magnitude of the body's response and postoperative morbidity.[2] Whether the postoperative immunosuppression has any teleologic beneficial effects is yet to be proven. Even if such benefits exist, immunosuppression from major abdominal surgical procedures may, in fact, promote unwanted postoperative septic complications.[3] The goal of laparoscopic surgery is to reduce the magnitude of operative injury and the postoperative morbidity. Careful study of immunosuppression from laparoscopic surgery, its quantification, and comparison with immunosuppression produced by laparotomy will help to decide whether laparoscopic surgery is truly less morbid and less invasive compared to the standard open abdominal surgery.

The immunosuppressive effect of laparoscopic surgery can be from anesthesia, pneumoperitoneum, surgical mini-incision, visceral dissection, or mobilization and anastomosis. Which of these various components of the laparoscopic surgical injury leads most to postoperative immunosuppression? Laparoscopic surgical injury differs from the injury following laparotomy in some respects. The differences include the duration of anesthesia, the need for a pneumoperitoneum, and the size of the abdominal incision. By contrast, both surgical approaches involve similar degrees of visceral dissection, mobilization, and anastomosis. It is possible that the differences in dermomyofascial injury, rather than the similarity of visceral injury, contribute most to any reduction in the degree of immunosuppression following laparoscopic surgery. Alterations of immune function to the body's detriment do occur from extensive surgical injury.[3] The advantages of reducing the degree of postoperative immunosuppression are obvious. The role of immune defenses against infections is well understood. The significance of immune defense against cancer induction is generally accepted. The effect of immunosuppression on the tumor growth in a tumor-bearing host with existing tumor-specific immune response depends on the degree and type of immunologic modulation. The aim of any surgical treatment is to accomplish the desired therapeutic goal with little undesirable alteration of the body's systems, including immune function. Does laparoscopic surgery achieve the therapeutic goal with less effect on the immune system compared to open laparotomy?

Data from Dr. Whelan's group suggest that laparoscopic surgery may be less immunosuppressive. Their data corroborate other experimental evidence showing attenuation of metabolic and cytokine responses following laparoscopic surgery compared with those changes that occur after standard open abdominal operations.[4,5] Whether reduction in postoperative immunosuppression is oncologically advantageous needs further verification. The experimental model of mouse mammary carcinoma in Dr. Whelan's studies evaluates the immunologic rejection of an allogeneic tumor transplant rather than tumor induction. The immunologic response of the host to allogeneic histocompatibility antigens is more powerful than is the response to less immunogenic tumor-associated antigens. The effect of postlaparoscopic immunosuppression on syngeneic tumor transplants and induction of autochthonous tumors may yield more definitive information on the advantages of laparoscopic surgery in patients with cancer. The role of the body's immune response to tumor-specific and tumor-associated antigens is complex. The immune response to tumor-associated antigens is not curative, as is evident by the coexistence of tumor-specific antibodies and T cells in cancer patients and continued cancer growth. Also, immunosuppression by carcinostatic chemotherapeutic agents and radiation therapy coexists with successful tumor eradication. Whether surgical injury-induced immunomodulation of tumor-associated immune response is beneficial or detrimental to the host is a fertile field of study.

Detailed analysis of the influence of laparoscopic surgery on immune response in general and various components of tumor-associated immunity is essential to understanding the advantages and disadvantages of laparoscopic surgery for colorectal cancer. Future experimental studies dealing with the effect of each component of laparoscopic surgical injury on various immune functions and on tumor growth in autoch-thonous tumor systems are in order. The data reviewed in this chapter are a good starting point. In these days of capricious and decreasing funding from the National Institutes of Health, health care reform, and the difficulty in justifying even the most crucial medical research, Dr. Whelan and associates deserve commendation for initiating studies analyzing the immune responses to laparoscopic surgery.

REFERENCES

1. Faist E et al: Depression of cellular immunity after major injury. Arch Surg 121:1000, 1986
2. Cruikshank AM et al: Response of serum interleukin-6 in patients undergoing surgery of varying severity. Clin Sci 79:161, 1990
3. Duignan JP et al: The association of impaired neutrophil chemotaxis with postoperative surgical sepsis. Br J Surg 73:238, 1986
4. Joris J, Cigarini I, Legrand M et al: Metabolic and respiratory changes after cholecystectomy performed via laparotomy or laparoscopy. Br J Anesth 69:341, 1992
5. Mealy K Gallagher H, Barry M, et al: Physiological and metabolic responses to open and laparoscopic cholecystectomy. Br J Surg 79:1061, 1992

26

Justifiability of Laparoscopic Colorectal Surgery

Stephen M. Cohen and Steven D. Wexner

The use of the laparoscope in the field of colorectal surgery is still in its early stages of development in terms of the ease, efficacy, and safety of colonic mobilization, resection, and anastomosis. Not only should the laparoscope be regarded as a new technique, but its role in the staging and treatment of one of the more common colorectal conditions, malignancy, has yet to be defined. In 1991 the American Society of Colon and Rectal Surgery stated that laparoscopic colon and rectal surgery should be undertaken only in a setting in which meaningful prospective data retrieval will occur.[1] Because of this statement, centers across the country have begun to assess prospectively the safety and efficacy of laparoscopic colon and rectal surgery by establishing registries to collect the data and establish its role.[2,3] Subsequently, the Society of American Gastrointestinal Endoscopic Surgeons proposed specific training and credentialing guidelines. The data being collected relate to the procedure's safety, as well as to the length of postoperative ileus, duration of hospital stay, and length of disability. Even though preliminary results have been encouraging, no prospective randomized trials or other statistically valid data prove the superiority or even the equivalence of laparoscopic colectomy as compared to standard laparotomy. This fact is especially germane when the diagnosis is colon or rectal carcinoma.

Laparoscopic colorectal surgery is notably different from all of the other procedures being performed to date. In point of fact, all of the other attempted procedures have several common denominators. First, all of these other procedures are performed in a relatively fixed intra-abdominal location. From a strictly practical point of view, this is fundamental, because there is virtually no need for intraoperative repositioning of instruments, ports, monitors, and personnel. The lesion is always in the anticipated position. Second, the other operations include either no vascular division (herniorrhaphy or fundoplication) or limited vascular division (cholecystectomy or appendectomy). Thus, vascular control can be rapidly and inexpensively undertaken. Conversely, the colonic mesentery includes numerous large vessels. Thus, vascular control requires considerably more time and, quite often, considerably more cost than do the other procedures. Third, in none of these procedures is an anastomosis fashioned. The dissection, mobilization, specimen retrieval, and laparoscopic suturing require certain skills and special instrumentation. However, the more advanced skills and equipment necessary for a tension-free, well-vascularized anastomosis differ markedly. Moreover, although the failure of sutures or staples after laparoscopic hernia or fundoplication may or may not result in recurrence, the failure may not lead to catastrophic complications. By contrast, the failure of a bowel anastomosis is a potentially lethal complication associated with significant increases in morbidity, length of hospitalization, cost, and survival. Fourth, the other procedures require either the removal of a small organ or no retrieval at all. Removal of a properly resected segment of colon with its attached mesentery requires either an incision or an extremely large port. Finally, none of the other currently performed laparoscopic procedures are undertaken to cure a malignancy. There is a marked difference in clinical sequelae between an asymptomatic hernia recurrence and a pelvic recurrence from a rectal carcinoma. Moreover, if such recurrences are asymptomatic and appropriate prospective randomized trials are not used, true rates of cancer recurrence after laparoscopic resection will be erroneously low in the absence of diligent routine long-term postoperative assessment.

To date, no prospective randomized trials have been published that demonstrate either the superiority or even the equivalence of laparoscopic colectomy. These data will only become available if qualified surgeons learn, develop, and apply these new techniques in a responsible and scientific manner. Currently, the steep part of the learning curve is still being ascended. As our skills develop in conjunction with the development of improved instrumentation, results also should improve. Thereafter, equivalent skills can be compared. It is inappropriate to compare the results of standard colectomy in the hands of a skilled specialist with the results from a laparoscopic novice.

CONTROVERSIES

One of the basic questions of paramount importance is the appropriateness of this technology for the treatment of colorectal carcinoma. The current standard of care for the treatment of colorectal carcinoma is an abundant excision of lymph-node bearing tissue, high ligation of the vessels, and adequate resection of the colon proximal and distal margins from the pathology. Because the counting of lymph nodes is relatively reproducible, this feature has seemingly become the sole fact on which laparoscopic enthusiasts have based their claims of success. However, reality is such that the number of lymph nodes harvested in a particular specimen depends on both the surgeon and the pathologist.

The institutional variability of the lymph nodes identified is great.[4] In the multicenter study conducted by Falk et al,[2] 66 patients who underwent laparoscopic or laparoscopic-assisted colon resections were analyzed. The authors demonstrated that, in both sigmoid and right hemicolectomy specimens resected for carcinoma, no statistically significant difference was found among laparoscopic, converted, or historical control patients. Similarly, Jacobs et al[5] compared the number of lymph nodes harvested by laparoscopic right hemicolectomy or rectosigmoid resections with traditional open surgery. The average number detected when a laparoscopic resection took place was actually more than with standard right colectomies (17 versus 14, $P =$ NS); but the reverse was true with rectosigmoid resections (6 versus 10). Dodson and co-workers[6] reported on their experience with three laparoscopic-assisted abdominoperineal resections. Again, comparable node samples were demonstrated between their laparoscopic-assisted cases and traditional controls (4.2 versus 7.2, respectively). One could argue that neither 7.2 nor 4.2 resected lymph nodes are adequate for a curative procedure. When we evaluated our own data,[7] 13 laparoscopic-assisted resections were performed for carcinoma. A mean of 19 (range, 3 to 84) lymph nodes were harvested. Two patients had Dukes' C lesions, but the majority were Dukes' A or B lesions.

These reviews clearly emphasize that, in most cases, the pathologist has control over the number of lymph nodes found in any given specimen. The impact of the pathologist on the number of evaluated lymph nodes cannot be overlooked. There is no incentive for the pathologist to find more lymph nodes. Because no study to date has clearly demonstrated an increased 5-year survival rate with the excision of more metastatic lymph nodes, location rather than the absolute number of harvested lymph nodes may be more important. Specifically, a recent study identified a 32-percent incidence in skip metastasis; patients with distant node metastases along the major vessels had no local node involvement.[8] Another problem is the growing enthusiasm to prove the merits of laparoscopic colectomy for cancer. There may be more enthusiasm among pathologists to help their surgical friends search more diligently when reviewing laparoscopic specimens. Thus, one must be especially critical of reports emanating from laparoscopic enthusiasts who justify oncologic radicality strictly based on the number of lymph nodes.

Another potential problem that has recently been recognized is one of local wound recurrence of tumor cells in port sites of patients who have undergone laparoscopic or laparoscopic-assisted colectomies for cancer. Popularized earlier this century, the Paul Mikulicz operation had an unacceptably high incidence of local wound recurrence.[9] Fusco and Paluzz[10] recently reported a trocar site abdominal wall recurrence 10 months after a laparoscopic-assisted right hemicolectomy. The patient was thought to have an early cancer based on preoperative workup; however, the final pathology revealed a T3N1M0 lesion, with 4 of 11 resected lymph nodes positive for metastatic carcinoma. Similarly, Alexander and co-workers[11] reported a 67-year-old woman who also presented with a port site recurrence 3 months after a laparoscopic-assisted right hemicolectomy for a Dukes' C adenocarcinoma. O'Rourke et al[12] reported two simultaneous port site recurrences in an 82-year-old woman who underwent a curative laparoscopic right hemicolectomy for a Dukes' B carcinoma; these recurrences unfortunately occurred 10 weeks after the operation. Numerous other port site recurrences have been noted.[13,14]

Other problems with resection of carcinoma exist, especially when the lesion is in the rectum. Tate and co-workers[15] compared 11 patients who underwent laparoscopic anterior resection with 14 patients who underwent laparotomy. Despite the mean tumor height of 20 cm in the former group as compared to 15 cm in the latter group, the distal resection margin was as small as 5 cm in the laparoscopic group. More recently, Darzi and collegues[16] compared 12 patients who underwent laparoscopic abdominoperineal excision to 15 patients in whom the excision was accomplished by laparotomy. Although the length of the procedure in the former group was almost doubled (195 versus 104 minutes, respectively), the mean radical margin was reduced by approximately 50 percent, from 9 mm in the open group to 5 mm in the laparoscopic group.

Only properly constructed, prospective, randomized trials will be able to truly elucidate whether laparoscopic colon and rectal surgery is suitable for patients with carcinoma.

Another area in which benefit is unproven is cost. In the 66 patients assessed by Falk and co-workers,[2] the laparoscopic procedures were statistically significantly more costly than were their open counterparts ($P<0.05$), although the mean postoperative stay for laparoscopically completed sigmoid or right hemicolectomy was significantly less than that after standard sigmoid or right hemicolectomy ($P<0.02$). Therefore, the total hospital cost was identical for both procedures. Moreover, none of the procedures included the use of intracorporeal staplers, which are very costly. Had staplers been used, the cost assessment would have favored the open procedures. More recently, Kmiot and co-workers[15] prospectively compared the effect of laparoscopic-assisted colectomy (n = 40) and open procedures (n = 40) with respect to the length of hospitalization, cost, and morbidity.[17] The two groups were matched for age, sex, diagnosis, and operation. No significant differences were found in operating time, duration of ileus, length of hospitalization or total cost. A trend toward decreased morbidity was noted in the laparoscopic-assisted group. This is the first such study to clearly demonstrate that there may not be a large difference between laparoscopic-assisted colectomies and open operations. Furthermore, three other recent reports compared their laparoscopic-assisted colectomies with standard open operations.[18–20] They both concluded that, despite the higher cost of operating room time and equipment, the total cost of laparoscopic-assisted colectomy was not statistically different from that noted during open resections. They claimed that the cost savings are due to a shortened hospital stay.

One of the most controversial topics is the length of hospitalization. Whereas several laparoscopic enthusiasts have claimed shorter lengths of stay for their laparoscopic patients, a critical look at their data often reveals two sets of criteria.[21] Patients in whom a standard open operation was performed were discharged from the hospital only after both tolerating a regular diet and moving their bowels. Laparoscopic patients, however, were discharged taking only clear fluids before they had moved their bowels. The disparity in results can certainly be accounted for strictly by application of two dramatically different sets of criteria to the two patient populations. Others, however, have demonstrated no difference in the length of ileus or hospitalization after laparoscopic or laparoscopic-assisted colectomy when both groups are managed in a similar manner.[22–25] Furthermore, Binderow and co-workers[26] and Reissman and collegues[27] have successfully challenged the notion that early oral intake is a unique postoperative feature to laparoscopy. In prospective randomized trials, they demonstrated earlier discharge in standard open colectomies when patients were allowed to eat immediately after their operation.

Another area of controversy is the question of intraoperative blood loss. Senagore et al[18] suggested that, when compared with open colectomies, laparoscopies yielded a subjectively significant decrease in intraoperative blood loss (157 ml ± 19 ml in open surgeries versus 687 ml ± 54 ml in laparoscopies). Peters and Bartels,[28] however, measured both preoperative and 24-hour postoperative hemoglobin levels as an indirect indicator of operative blood loss. Objectively, they demonstrated a trend toward a greater fall in hemoglobin in the laparoscopic group.

In order to demonstrate lower cost and shorter hospitalization, some surgeons have reverted to the long ago condemned technique of colotomy and polypectomy.[29] Lauroy and collegues[30] have reminded us of why we abandoned this inadequate technique. They reported on a performance of a colotomy and polypectomy in which a Dukes' A carcinoma was unexpectedly discovered. Nine months later the patient experienced isolated local recurrence at the port site, although not at the extraction site. Thus, the technical triumph of the procedure was rapidly replaced by the defeat at having converted a Dukes' A lesion into a Dukes' D lesion. In a similar mode, Jacobi and associates[31] have reported preferential tumor implantation at port sites but not at the laparotomy incision. Fleshman and Fry[32] have elegantly demonstrated that tumor cells preferentially select port sites for implantation under the influence of pneumoperitoneum.

Many unanswered questions still remain with regard to this new technology in the management of diseases of the colon and rectum. First, the number of laparoscopic colon and rectal resections necessary to surpass the learning curve has not yet been established. Second, current resident training has not been definitively established. However, a 1-day course does not constitute adequate knowledge and safety to perform all types of resections. Third, the so-called significant cost-savings analyses never include the cost of the expensive instruments, including the cameras, video, insufflator, monitors, recorders, printers, and cables. Nor does cost analysis ever include the expensive extra operating room time needed during the setup and takedown of the myriad of equipment necessary to perform so-called cost-effective, minimally invasive surgery. Fourth, the cost-effectiveness of both reusable and disposable instruments must be assessed.

Finally, it is of paramount importance that science prevail and adequate prospective randomized trials be performed to answer the question of acceptability of the technology for the cure of cancer.

REFERENCES

1. American Society of Colon and Rectal Surgeons. Policy statement, American Society of Colon and Rectal Surgeons. Dis Colon Rectum 35:5A, 1992
2. Falk PM, Beart RW, Wexner SD et al: Laparoscopic colectomy: a critical appraisal. Dis Colon Rectum 36:28, 1992
3. Wexner SD, Johansen OB: Laparoscopic bowel resection: advantages and limitations. Ann Med 24:105, 1992
4. Blenkinsopp WK, Stewart-Brown S, Blesovsky L et al: Histopathology reporting in large bowel cancer. J Clin Pathol 34:509, 1988
5. Jacobs M, Verdeja JC, Goldstein MS: Minimally invasive colon resection (laparoscopic colectomy). Surg Laparosc Endosc 1:144, 1991
6. Dodson RW, Cullado MJ, Tangen LE et al: Laparoscopic-assisted abdominoperineal resection. Contemp Surg 42:42, 1993
7. Cohen SM, Wexner SD: Laparoscopic colorectal resection for cancer: the Cleveland Clinic Florida experience. Surg Onc 2:35, 1993
8. Shida H, Ban K, Matsumoto M et al: Prognostic significance of location of lymph nodal metastases in colorectal cancer. Dis Colon Rectum 35:1046, 1992
9. von Mikulicz J: Small contributions to the surgery of the intestinal tract. Boston Med Surg J 148:608, 1903
10. Fusco MA, Paluzzi MW: Abdominal wall recurrence after laparoscopic-assisted colectomy for adenocarcinoma of the colon and rectum. Dis Colon Rectum 36:858, 1993
11. Alexander RJT, Jaques BC, Mitchell KG: Laparoscopically-assisted colectomy and wound recurrence, letter. Lancet 341:249, 1993
12. O'Rourke, Price PM, Kelly S et al: Tumor inoculation after laparoscopy. Lancet 342:368, 1993
13. Nduka CC, Monson JRT, Menzies-Gow N et al: Abdominal wall metastases following laparoscopy. Br J Surg 86:648, 1994
14. Wexner SD, Cohen SM: Port site metastases after laparoscopic colorectal surgery for cure of malignancy. Br J Surg 82:295, 1995
15. Tate JJ, Kwok S et al: Prospective comparison of laparoscopic and conventional anterior resection. Br J Surg 80:1396, 1993
16. Darzi A, Lewis C, Menzies-Gow N, Guillou PJ, Monson JRT: Laparoscopic abdominoperineal excision of the rectum. Surg Endosc 9:414, 1995
17. Kmiot WA, Reiver D, Cohen SM: A prospective comparison of laparoscopic and open procedures in colorectal surgery, abstracted. Dis Colon Rectum 37:p22, 1994
18. Senagore AJ, Luchtefeld MA, Macheigan JM et al: Open colectomy versus laparoscopic colectomy: are there differences? Am Surg 59:549, 1993
19. Vayer AJ, Larach SE, Williamson PR et al: Cost effectiveness of laparoscopic colectomy. Dis Colon Rectum 36:34, 1993
20. Pfeifer J, Reissman P, Wexner SD et al: Laparoscopic versus open colon surgery: cost and outcome. Surg Endosc (in press)
21. Uddo JF: Intestinal intracorporeal anastomosis. Presented at the Third International Congress on New Technology and Advanced Techniques in Surgery. Luxembourg, June 11–17, 1995
22. Larach SW, Salomon MC, Williamson PR et al: Laparoscopic-assisted colectomy: experience during the learning curve. Coloproctology 1:38, 1993
23. Milsom JW, Lavery IC, Bohm B et al: Laparoscopic assisted ileocolectomy in Crohn's disease. Surg Laparosc Endosc 3:77, 1993
24. Schmitt SL, Cohen SM, Wexner SD et al: Does laparoscopic-assisted ileal pouch anal anastomosis reduce the length of hospitalization? Int J Colorect Dis 9:134, 1994
25. Monson JRT, Darzi A, Carey PD et al: Prospective evaluation of laparoscopic-assisted colectomy in an unselected group of patients. Lancet 340:831, 1992
26. Binderow SR, Cohen SM, Wexner SD et al: Must early postoperative oral intake be limited to laparoscopy? Dis Colon Rectum 37:584, 1994
27. Reissman P, Teoh TA, Cohen SM et al: Is early oral feeding safe after elective colorectal surgery. Ann Surg (in press)
28. Peters WR, Bartels TL: Minimally invasive colectomy: are the potential benefits realized? Dis Colon Rectum 36:751, 1993
29. Phillips EH, Franklin M, Carroll BJ et al: Laparoscopic colectomy. Ann Surg 216:703, 1992
30. Lauroy J, Champault G, Risk N, Boutelier P: Metastatic recurrences at the cannula site: should digestive carcinomas still be managed by laparoscopy?, abstracted. Br J Surg, suppl. 81:31, 1994
31. Jacobi C, Keller HN, Said S: Implantation metastasis of unsuspected gall bladder carcinoma after laparoscopy, abstracted. Br J Surg, suppl. 81:82, 1994
32. Fleshman J, Fry R: Laparoscopic assisted and mini-laparotomy approaches to colorectal diseases are similar in early outcome, abstracted. Dis Colon Rectum 38:p23, 1995

Editorial Comment I

Norman S. Williams

The past few years have seen an explosion in laparoscopic colorectal surgery. Articles appear almost weekly describing how yet another classical colorectal procedure has been conquered by the laparoscope. Authors write about how they have performed a relatively small number of difficult technical maneuvers via the laparoscope, allowed the patients to eat on the night of the procedure, discharged them home the next day, and found them back at work the next week.

Drs. Cohen and Wexner ask the uncomfortable question as to whether laparoscopic surgery is justifiable in the colorectal field. I share their concerns. Having performed a reasonable number of laparoscopic procedures and presented my successes, I believe it is necessary to look critically at what we are trying to achieve.

I am convinced that laparoscopic colorectal surgery is here to stay, and its use will expand. The motive for critical assessment such as Drs. Cohen and Wexner's and this commentary is not to seek the banning of the laparoscope in colorectal surgery but to ensure its responsible use within the specialty. Just because a technique is feasible does not mean it should be used across the board. Selectivity is an issue that has not received the attention it deserves.

Drs. Cohen and Wexner concentrate on laparoscopic surgery for colorectal cancer, yet, as can be seen from the rest of this book, the laparoscope has been used for other diseases, and similar questions need to be asked. The type of procedures in which the laparoscope can be used in the colorectal field may be classified as follows:

1. Nonexcision (e.g., formation of stoma, rectopexy, diagnosis and staging of malignancy)
2. Excision for benign disease (e.g., diverticular disease, polyp, inflammatory bowel disease)
3. Excision for carcinoma

Too often, surgeons have described their experience in all three categories, and it is often difficult to distinguish one from the other. However, if we take each of these categories and pose the question of justifiability, we may obtain different answers. Thus, nonexcisional laparoscopic surgery for colorectal disease is more akin to the more conventional laparoscopic operations, such as fundoplication or herniorrhaphy. There is little need for intraoperative repositioning of instruments, ports, monitors, or personnel. There is no division of mesenteric blood vessels; a specimen does not need retrieval, and an anastomosis is not required. These are ideal criteria for a laparoscopic maneuver. Thus, our unit has performed 25 defunctioning or end stomas for a variety of indications with a relatively low morbidity. Patients have been fully mobilized within 24 hours of the operation, and if it had not been for the teaching of stoma care, they would have been home within several days. Numerous other groups have obtained similar results.[1] Is this procedure justifiable? Certainly. Should it be subjected to a prospective controlled trial? Probably. Is such a trial likely to be performed? Doubtful. The benefits of this procedure are so striking, it is unlikely that any group will have the inclination to perform a study in which they are convinced of the answer beforehand. The same cannot be said of rectopexy. The rectum can be mobilized laparoscopically and can be fixed by Marlex mesh or similar material, which is either stapled or tacked to the sacrum.[2,3] In some skilled hands, Marlex can be dispensed with, and the rectal serosa can be sutured to the sacrum. However, it is not at all clear how secure the fixation is using the laparoscopic technique. Nevertheless, the learning curve is relatively short, and many groups are using the technique. This procedure cries out for a prospective controlled study. The main end point, that is, recurrence, is easily defined, and such a trial should be relatively simple to mount.

The second category, excisional surgery for benign disease, covers a wide range of pathology and procedures. At one end of the spectrum is restorative proctocolectomy for ulcerative colitis. This technique demands extraordinary technical skill and takes an inordinate amount of operating time. It is clearly feasible, but what is to be gained? The specimen has to be removed, and although a Pfannenstiel incision improves the cosmetic result, it is doubtful if this benefit alone would justify the hours required to mobilize the colon and divide its mesentery, particularly if a covering ileostomy is still required at the end. It is very doubtful, therefore, with the level of technological development now available, whether surgeons should continue laparoscopic restorative proctocolectomy.

At the other end of the spectrum is the limited resection that is required for Crohn's disease in the distal ileum.[4] Here, it is relatively simple to mobilize the right colon, exteriorize the diseased segment through a small right iliac fossa incision, resect the segment, form the anastomosis, and then return it to the peritoneal cavity. If necessary, more proximal strictures can be delivered and dealt with either by resection or strictureplasty through the same incision. Such a laparoscopically assisted maneuver is the sensible way to use the technology. Although an intracorporeal anastomosis is quite feasible, it seems totally unnecessary when the specimen in any case must be delivered through the abdominal wall. A prospective controlled trial is probably required to demonstrate the benefits; but this procedure is being performed in ever increasing numbers and is likely to be accepted by the surgical community long before a trial is mounted, let alone completed.

Finally, we come to the question of excisional laparoscopic surgery for colorectal cancer. Many of the pros and cons have been elegantly set out by Drs. Cohen and Wexner. Nevertheless, a few points bear emphasis. A laparoscopic abdominoperineal resection for rectal cancer is far easier to perform than a laparoscopic low anterior resection. It is of some concern, therefore, that some enthusiasts seem to have a high incidence of abdominoperineal resections in their series.[5] Whereas this may be due to referral patterns, concern must be expressed that sphincters may be sacrificed unnecessarily for the sake of ensuring that the procedure can be performed without a laparotomy. Of even greater concern is the degree of clearance that can be achieved around the tumor, particularly for low rectal cancer. Whereas the posterior dissection of the rectum in the "holy plane" of Heald[6] is relatively simple using the laparoscope, anterior and lateral dissection are more problematic. With a large rectal tumor in a narrow pelvis, safe and radical laparoscopic dissection may be impossible.

Even when the tumors are entirely mobile, and even when they are not in the rectum and are more accessible, the problem of port site recurrence must be addressed. This complication has only recently been described following laparoscopic surgery for a variety of cancers, including colorectal.[7] Whether the incidence of port site recurrence is higher compared to abdominal wound metastases following open laparotomy remains to be seen, but the suspicion is that this is the case. Dealing with a tumor that is adherent to surrounding structures, the surgeon may release malignant cells into the peritoneal cavity where they may be implanted into the tracks left when the cannulas are removed. Similarly, if a large tumor after mobilization is exteriorized with difficulty through a small incision, it is likely that cells will be implanted unless appropriate precautions are taken. Now that this complication has been recognized, strategies are evolving to prevent it.

The above points highlight the need for selection of patients for laparoscopic excision of colorectal cancer. There should be no sense of failure, if for good reasons, a laparoscopic resection has to be abandoned. On the contrary, the decision should be applauded. However, such selection underlines the difficulty in mounting prospective controlled trials. The difficulties are compounded by the length of the learning curve, and the latter raises ethical and moral issues. Nevertheless, I believe that it is essential to set up carefully controlled multicenter trials for laparoscopic colorectal surgery, particularly when performed for cancer. This generation of surgeons has a duty not only to ensure that this form of surgery is safe and effective but to determine in which patients it is contraindicated.

REFERENCES

1. Khoo RE, Montrey J, Cohen MM: Laparoscopic loop ileostomy for temporary fecal diversion. Dis Colon Rectum 36:966, 1993
2. Berman IR: Sutureless laparoscopic rectopexy for procidentia: technique and implications. Dis Colon Rectum 35:689, 1992
3. Cuschieri A, Shimi SM, Vander Velpen G et al: Laparoscopic prosthesis fixation rectopexy for complete rectal prolapse. Br J Surg 81:138, 1994
4. Milsom JW, Lavery IC, Bohm et al: Laparoscopically-assisted ileocolectomy in Crohn's disease. Surg Laparosc Endosc 3:77, 1993
5. Phillips EH, Franklin M, Carroll BJ et al: Laparoscopic colectomy. Ann Surg 216:703, 1992
6. Heald RJ: The "holy plane" of rectal surgery. J R Soc Med 81:503, 1988
7. Nuduka CC, Monson JRT, Menzies GOW et al: Abdominal wall metastases following laparoscopy. Br J Surg 81:648, 1994

Editorial Comment II

John Northover

Polemical questions such as "How long is a piece of string?" never can be answered in simple terms. Similarly, "Is laparoscopic colorectal surgery justifiable?" is a complex matter with no answer simpler than "Yes (or no), but. . . ." After all, what does *justifiable* mean? According to the *Oxford English Dictionary*, one rather interesting meaning is "Made inherently righteous by the infusion of grace." Stand that next to Cohen and Wexner's warnings about enthusiasts (the oldest *OED* definition is "One who is, really or seemingly, possessed by a god"), and we have much food for thought. In laparoscopic terms, will those thus "possessed" bypass scientific method, surreptitiously infusing grace to make laparoscopic colorectal surgery (LCRS) "inherently righteous" by default—with a little help from a rampant therapeutic-industrial complex—actively promoting the easily induced addiction of the surgical gizmophile?

An even-handed, even critical, appraisal by authors such as Cohen and Wexner, who are very active in LCRS (I hesitate to imply enthusiasm on their part) is worth much more to the advancement of our understanding of its merits than a dozen "me-too" series of cases. The self-evident attractiveness of (almost) incisionless surgery is a trap for the unwary. It is no surprise that solid evidence for the superiority of LCRS is hard to come by. As Drs. Cohen and Wexner point out, most studies so far are not closing down debate on even the most straightforward questions such as length of stay, postoperative pain, or lymph node counts in cancer surgery.

I am sure few would argue with the need for good randomized trials, but let us not fall into the trap of seeing the randomized trial as the automatic answer to the difficult questions in laparoscopic cancer surgery. Cohen and Wexner bemoan the lack of trial data to demonstrate "either the superiority or even the equivalence of laparoscopic colectomy (in the treatment of cancer)." In the classical randomized trial, the null hypothesis is tested, that is that there is no difference between two treatments. In this example—open cancer surgery compared to LCRS—if equivalence could be shown, the enthusiast would argue that LCRS is preferred because of all its other obvious advantages (e.g., shorter stay, less pain). But to show true equivalence is statistically very demanding, because much larger numbers of patients are needed than those required to show a difference in favor of one treatment. Given the difficulties in recruiting large numbers, the alternative, therefore, is to design a trial aimed at testing for superiority of one treatment. Would anyone but the most "possessed" enthusiast argue today that LCRS is likely to be superior to open surgery in terms of local recurrence, cancer-free survival, or overall survival? It is much more likely to be the other way around, in which case we find ourselves contemplating design of a trial in which we try to define the proportionate *inferiority* of the novel treatment (i.e., LCRS). But I thought new modalities were expected to be better than the old. Nevertheless, let us press on. Given that this would be the pragmatic question, how big a deficit in survival after LCRS would we be prepared to accept as the price of less postoperative pain or shorter stays (always assuming these can be demonstrated ultimately). Five percent, ten maybe? If in the end it was shown that such a deficit truly occurred, we would have lost the putative increment in survival seen by many to accrue from the use of postoperative adjuvant therapy.

I have outlined this circuitous argument not to decry the use of the randomized trial, or even LCRS, but to indicate that the mere deployment of randomized comparison does not automatically defuse the controversy. Unless port site recurrence, or some other as yet unreported bizarre phenomenon, becomes of such detractive importance that the LCRS bandwagon goes into reverse, I expect that laparoscopic cancer surgery will become less cumbersome and more widely applied outside of trials. Ultimately, there is likely to be an inexorable and informally developed broad acceptance of its "inherent righteousness," just as sphincter-saving surgery in all its forms grew out of the early heresies (as they were then seen by many) of Claude Dixon in the 1930s.

So is the widespread use of LCRS justified? No, not yet anyway. But that will not stop it.

27
Credentialing

James W. Fleshman, Jr.

Laparoscopic surgery is not a new process. Laparoscopic approaches to gynecologic and obstetric diseases have been used over the past decades since fiberoptic technology became available. The granting of privileges for laparoscopy was afforded to any surgeon who could document knowledge and adequate technique in each of these fields. In the past decade, however, videolaparoscopy has become available, and the widespread use of laparoscopic approaches to multiple diseases has made the granting of privileges more complicated.[1] It is impossible for a single institution, board, or society to credential physicians to perform laparoscopic surgery. The American Society of Gastrointestinal Endoscopists (ASGE) and the Society of American Gastrointestinal Endoscopic Surgeons (SAGES) have developed guidelines to help individual institutions develop methods of granting privileges for endoscopy and laparoscopic surgery.[2–5] There are numerous implications to credentialing for laparoscopy. These include method of training, overall experience, overall technical skill, knowledge and ability to treat diseases requiring laparoscopic approaches, and an adequate continuing education in the use of laparoscopic approaches.

The unfortunate result of the lack of a Board of Laparoscopy has been that individual hospitals must rely on their own experts within their medical community to give recommendations for laparoscopic privileging. In certain circumstances, these recommendations have been based more on achieving a competitive edge than the real attainment of skill and knowledge. The hospitals and institutional privileging committees must use objective criteria to conclude whether a physician is capable of treating disease with a laparoscopic approach. These objective criteria may include a specified number of cases. It is the hope of SAGES and the American Society of Colon and Rectal Surgeons (ASCRS) that numbers of cases will not become the ultimate criteria. However, the use of a number of proctored cases may be adequate to overcome the numbers game. As residents leave their training programs, the question remains of what is an adequate number of cases to qualify them to perform laparoscopic surgery. This question applies not only to laparoscopy. The number of pancreatic and head and neck cases performed by general surgeons is continuing to decrease, even though general surgeons are reported to be qualified at the completion of a certified residency training program. Another example of the incongruity in the numbers game is the low number of abdominoperineal resections done by general surgeons in the community each year. The American College of Surgeons has published data that are based on a survey and indicate that each general surgeon will perform 0.8 abdominoperineal resections a year. Continued expertise in this technique is therefore questionable at this level of ongoing practice.

The issue of proctoring is a difficult one. The standards task force for the SAGES has suggested that proctoring should be limited to objective observation without participation on the part of the proctor. This procedure eliminates the underlying medicolegal risk to the proctor and also ensures that the surgeon under scrutiny is performing the entire procedure. A preceptorship, by contrast, involves the teaching surgeon in the operative case as the trainee gains skill and knowledge with the preceptor's instruction. A proctor may be an imported surgeon from another area or neighboring hospital as well as a member of the local institutional staff. This method provides the flexibility for small community hospitals to establish a credentialing program even though they do not have a large medical staff from which to draw expertise.

As more complicated procedures become available to the laparoscopic surgeon, it is sometimes difficult to specify privileging. It is helpful to divide the procedures used in laparoscopy into basic, advanced, and experimental. Basic procedures would thus include cholecystectomy and appendectomy. Advanced procedures would include small bowel and colon resection and fundoplication. Experimental procedures would include hernia repair, adrenalectomy, nephrectomy, and the like. The labeling of each procedure in these levels may change as time, experience, and scientific data prove the efficacy of the procedures. The credentialing to perform each procedure must be individualized by the Chairman of the Department of Surgery in each institution because no proctor will be available for some of the experimental procedures. In these cases, adequate experience in the animal laboratory and evidence of preceptorship may suffice.

The use of weekend training courses to obtain adequate skill and knowledge to perform procedures was used initially in training surgeons to perform laparoscopic cholecystectomy. It is difficult to state categorically that this is inadequate training. Training surgeons in practice is always a difficult problem. However, the use of weekend courses and animal laboratory experience seems to have worked fairly well. The use of a proctor in these circumstances becomes essential. Residency training programs that include laparoscopic experience would certainly obviate the need for weekend courses, unless a new procedure is developed after the resident leaves training. Once again, the institution will be required to decide whether proctoring is necessary before that individual can perform new procedures in the hospital.

Credentialing for laparoscopic procedures should not be considered a sanctioning of the laparoscopic approach to particular diseases. For example, laparoscopic hernia may or may not be efficacious for the repair of inguinal hernias. Experimental data are pending. The credentialing committee therefore is advised to establish certain criteria for the performance of experimental procedures. An approved investigational review board protocol should be submitted, and a human studies committee consent form should be signed by each patient undergoing experimental procedures. These precautions benefit both the patient (by informing the patient) and the physician (by providing medicolegal protection). Once the procedure has proven to be safe in the hands of the investigator and/or proven to be the method of choice for this particular disease, the investigational review board human studies consent form can be dropped. The credentialing committee in each institution should be aware of its responsibility in the control of new techniques in the hospital and operating room.

Because the individual institutions remain autonomous in their granting of privileges and none of the national societies or organizations have assumed the credentialing responsibility, the individual institutions should take advantage of the advice and help of the national organizations in developing their credentialing process. For this reason, some of the organizations have developed proctor lists and guidelines for granting of hospital privileges in laparoscopic surgery; they have experts who will assist individual institutions in developing the privileging document and give advice on the need for investigational review protocol consent. The autonomy of the institutions is therefore protected. The national organizations do not assume the overwhelming responsibility of certifying each individual surgeon through a very expensive examination process, and individual surgeons retain their rights to advance their skills, knowledge, and sphere of practice. Laparoscopic colorectal surgery is an evolving field and will obviously change as government policy changes along with the attitude of national organizations and the climate of the medical/legal profession. Individual hospitals and surgeons must protect themselves by ensuring a strict credentialing process in each local institution, thus showing the patients and community their concern for an excellent quality of medical care.

REFERENCES

1. Delineation of Privileges in Laparoscopic and Thoracoscopic Surgery. Approved by the Endoscopic Surgery Credentialing Committee, Jewish Hospital of St. Louis, 1993
2. Guidelines for granting of privileges for laparoscopic (peritoneoscopic) general surgery. Society of American Gastrointestinal Endoscopic Surgeons guidelines. Surg Endosc 7:67, 1993
3. Guidelines for Hospital Credentialing for Laparoscopic Colectomy. American Society of Colon and Rectal Surgeons, 1991
4. Guidelines for General Surgery Resident Education in Gastrointestinal Endoscopy. SAGES Publication No. 0015, Society of American Gastrointestinal Endoscopic Surgeons, 1992
5. Society of American Gastrointestinal Endoscopic Surgeons Position Statement. Approved by the Board of Governors of the Society of American Gastrointestinal Endoscopic Surgeons, 1992

Editorial Comment I

Thomas L. Dent

When scalpels, scissors, and hemostats were the basic surgical tools, and operations learned during residencies remained the same throughout surgeons' careers, the issue of who should be permitted to perform specific operations was fairly simple. With the explosion of modern technology, however, surgeons are now performing new and very different operations from those they learned as residents. Laparoscopic surgery, almost overnight, has created a new paradigm for general surgery. As a department chairman, the director of a residency program in general surgery, the chairman of our hospital's credentials committee, and a member of the Board of Directors of the Society of American Gastrointestinal Endoscopic Surgeons (SAGES), I have given the matter of training, credentialing, and privileging for laparoendoscopic procedures a great deal of thought.

Dr. Fleshman summarizes the general credentialing issues in laparoscopic surgery very nicely. I especially like his categorization of procedures into basic, advanced, and experimental, which mirrors my own thinking.[1] I also agree with him that proctoring by an unbiased observer is a better way of determining and documenting competence in a surgical procedure than that done by preceptors.[2] Preceptors, because they are also acting as teachers (as do program directors of residency programs), have a vested interest in seeing that their trainees are granted privileges. This attitude may bias their judgment in favor of the trainee when they evaluate competence in a particular procedure. Many hospitals, including ours, are beginning to increase the use of proctors. Proctoring, however, is expensive, time-consuming, and cumbersome. Also, it is difficult to find proctors who are completely unbiased (either for or against) in the local community.

Unfortunately, the terms *credentialing* (which means documentation of training, experience, and competence) and *privileging* (which means permission, granted by the individual hospital, to care for patients and to perform specific procedures) frequently are used interchangeably. The distinction between them is more than semantic. Dr. Fleshman implies that the American Board of Surgery reports all general surgeons to be "qualified [i.e., credentialed] at the completion of a certified residency training program" to perform pancreatic surgery, head and neck surgery, and abdominoperineal resection, despite low numbers of these cases done by some of them during training, and that hospitals, therefore, automatically privilege general surgeons to perform such procedures. Although this may happen in some hospitals, the American Board of Surgery[3] specifically refutes this interpretation by stating:

> It is neither the intent nor the purpose of the Board to define the requirements for membership on the staff of hospitals or institutions involved in the practice or teaching of surgery. Its principal objective is to certify the education, experience and knowledge of broadly qualified and responsible surgeons and not to designate who shall or shall not perform surgical operations or any category thereof.

Hospitals still do (or should) review numbers within categories of similar operations and require documentation of competence before granting specific privileges. For the future, the Executive Director of the American College of Surgeons (ACS) has suggested that national "portable" privileges (presumably granted by the ACS) might be an alternative to individual hospital privileging, especially in a managed care setting that requires surgeons to practice at multiple hospitals and to change hospitals frequently.[4,5]

Dr. Fleshman does not discuss the issue of whether laparoscopic colorectal surgery is appropriate for surgeons to perform on a regular basis. Before a hospital decides to grant privileges to perform a particular procedure, not only does it have to determine whether a surgeon's training is adequate, it also has a responsibility to determine whether the procedure in question should be performed. There are those, including myself, who believe that surgeons are moving too quickly to incorporate laparoscopic colorectal procedures into their practice before their safety and advantages have been demonstrated adequately.[6,7]

Another important training issue specific to laparoscopic colon surgery not addressed by Dr. Fleshman is the difficulty for colorectal surgeons currently in practice to find enough basic laparoscopic procedures to be able to progress to the more advanced laparoscopic colorectal procedures. This lack of experience is less a problem for general surgeons who can hone their laparoscopic skills by performing cholecystectomies before progressing to laparoscopic colectomy, but there are no basic colorectal laparoscopic procedures. Currently, there is no easy solution to this problem. Obviously, this problem will present less difficulty to future colorectal fellows who will have obtained some basic laparoscopic training and experience during their general surgery residency.

With the technology explosion and the increasing scrutiny of methods of training and credentialing by the public, the media, the government, and the legal profession, the issues discussed in the chapter are important both to surgeons and hospitals. We must first be sure that new procedures are safe and appropriate and then be sure that only surgeons who are competent to perform them are permitted to offer them to their patients.

REFERENCES

1. Dent TL: Training and credentialing. In MacFadyen BV Jr, Ponsky JL (eds): Operative Laparoscopy and Thoracoscopy. Raven Press, New York (in press)
2. Society of American Gastrointestinal Endoscopic Surgeons: Framework for Post-Residency Surgical Education and Training. Society of American Gastrointestinal Endoscopic Surgeons, Los Angeles, 1994
3. American Board of Surgery: Booklet of Information, July 1993–June 1994. Philadelphia, American Board of Surgery, 1994
4. Ebert PA: As I see it. Am Coll Surg Bull 78(8):2, 1993
5. Ebert PA: As I see it. Am Coll Surg Bull 78(11):2, 1993
6. Colons and keyholes, editorial. Lancet 340:824, 1992
7. Wexner SD, Cohen SM, Johansen OB et al: Laparoscopic colorectal surgery: a prospective assessment and current perspective. Br J Surg 80:1602, 1993

Editorial Comment II

Lester Rosen

The process of primary or secondary credentialing of colorectal surgeons for colorectal laparoscopic surgery is undergoing transformation. Currently, the basic requirements may include training in an accredited colorectal residency with a laparoscopic program (primary) or a training seminar endorsed by a specialty society such as the American Society of Colon and Rectal Surgeons (secondary). Evidence of training in the form of a certificate or letter should be sent directly to the applicant's institutional surgical chairman.

The chairman should be familiar with current colorectal laparoscopic guidelines that are endorsed by national specialty societies and with the specific institutional process for the granting of surgical privileges. For cases in which the applicant is a practicing surgeon (within or from another institution), it would be useful for the chairman to know the institution's colorectal quality assurance and use data for present or future recommendations, such as continuation of colorectal laparoscopic privileges.

Privileges should be gradational and may include a proctorship in which the applicant serves as first assistant and then surgeon, with the proctor assisting or in attendance. Independent colorectal laparoscopic privileges should be granted by the Chairman of Surgery when competency is established. The interval until competency may vary according to the skill or experience of the applicant as well as the proctor. Advanced laparoscopic courses may be required.

The Surgical Chairman should elucidate the recommended privileges of the applicant to the appropriate medical staff committee that assumes the responsibility for processing requested privileges.[1]

Specific issues relating to risk management, including informed consent and medical ethics, should be addressed within the process. Following institutional approval of the applicant's privileges, a monitoring process should be initiated. Renewal or revision of privileges based on the monitoring of surgical outcomes should be performed in a timely manner in accordance with the policies set forth by the Department of Surgery and the institution.

REFERENCES

1. Forde KA: Hospital credentialing. p. 686. In Ballantyne GH, Leahy PF, Modlin IM (eds): Laparoscopic Surgery. WB Saunders, Philadelphia, 1994

Editorial Comment III

Rama M. Jager

Proper credentialing through a standardized peer review process should protect patients from abuse by unskilled or hazardous surgeons, either from their negligence or ignorance. Granting laparoscopic privileges to a surgeon with inadequate training and skills obviously has important patient-care, economic, legal, and moral ramifications. Each surgeon-applicant undergoes evaluation of the training and experience to conduct the procedure competently, safely, and appropriately. This standard is particularly difficult to uphold when privileges involve new invasive procedures such as laparoscopic colectomy. Despite the use of most sophisticated models and strategies, matching patient needs with laparoscopic surgeons' capabilities remains imperfect. Hospitals in the United States currently have systems—the credentialing and privileging committees and their programs—(although less than ideal) to guide surgeons with dissimilar training and skills to work according to their degree of competence.[1–3]

Credentialing is more than an entry permit and an initiation rite. It is a fundamental and indispensable professional self-regulation process that reflects the ability of the profession to self-discipline.[4] It aims to realize the ultimate goal of patient welfare and simultaneously increases the accountability of the surgical profession. Surgeons cannot afford to surrender their obligation to self-impose strict educational standards. If they do so—because of the expediency, their zeal toward an innovation, or simply from lack of time—it is only a question of time before the credibility of the profession is lost. In return for their initial investment of time and effort in systematized credentialing, surgeons will see improved surgical care, a more responsive professional staff, and increased patient trust and satisfaction.

The ideal credentialing process should not only improve total patient care but also require a small investment of surgeons' time. The medical staff should receive it willingly. Formal, nonpunitive, and prompt feedback to surgeons regarding their progress will foster remedial education. It should also include stringent monitoring of the entire credentialing process itself. Matching all these objectives at times is difficult and can lead the credential committees into undesirable entanglements. It is especially so in credentialing a procedure such as laparoscopic colectomy in which most surgeons in practice are untrained during their formal surgical residency.

As Dr. Fleshman points out, development of a structured protocol to grant laparoscopic colectomy privileges is difficult. There is no stringent published and accepted list of required skills for laparoscopy.[2] The epistemic uncertainty makes it difficult to design a perfect credentialing process but should not prevent us from the quest for a reasonable model. For example, the skills in laparoscopic colorectal surgery include the use and understanding of various laparoscopic dissection techniques and their application. The properly trained and educated laparoscopic surgeon is familiar with the pros and cons of various techniques, their limitations, tissue reactions, and safety features. Various guidelines published by specialty societies, including the American Society of Colon and Rectal Surgeons and Society of American Gastrointestinal Endoscopic Surgeons, may also be useful in formulating acceptable criteria.

Currently, very few surgeons acquired the surgical skills needed to do laparoscopic colorectal surgery during residency training. The entry into laparoscopic colorectal surgery should not be so difficult as to prevent any postgraduate abdominal surgeon who is well trained in open colorectal surgery from offering patients the benefits of the minimally invasive techniques after proper training. The didactic and animal laboratory experience will help to reduce complications during initial experience.[5] However, no amount of bench training or laparoscopic surgery on pigs and dogs will make one an expert laparoscopic surgeon. The multiple studies exploring the learning curves in laparoscopic surgery show the superiority of proctoring and learning from experience.[6,7] Assisting a more experienced laparoscopic surgeon and having a proctor watch during the initial operations may hasten acquisition of laparoscopic skills.

Credentialing is not a static process. It requires periodic re-examination of all policies, plans, and formalities—past, present, and future—for their pertinence, practicality, and fulfillment. It does not mean that the entire list of credentials and privileges for every surgeon needs yearly review and revisitation. Such stringent requirements pose an unreasonable burden not only for the reviewing committee but also for the surgeon in practice who has to provide necessary documentation. However, new surgical procedures such as laparoscopic colectomy require careful analysis, review of indications, and delineation of skills necessary to grant privileges regularly. The periodic review process should help identify surgeons whose quality of care is below reasonable thresholds and ensure that these surgeons receive suitable remedial training.

Apart from getting proper training, the surgeons should not ignore the credentialing process. The surgeons should get involved actively with their hospital Credentials Committee. The never-ending changes in health care and other demands on our time constantly challenge those of us in active clinical practice or in academic medicine. Active interest and participation will help surgeons maintain control of this important process. Those not able to be active members of the Credential Committee should be sure some laparoscopic surgeons are on the committee who can represent surgical interests. Credentialing of laparoscopic skills should optimally be done by laparoscopic surgeons and not by nonprocedural physicians. Surgeons have an obligation and a need to participate in the development, administration, and monitoring of all types of regulatory activities affecting surgical education and practice.

The process of credentialing can lead to potential abuse by some. It may become a tool to limit use of even those surgical advances that improve patient care if those advances impose additional, nonreimbursable costs to the health care facility. Economic credentialing is a looming threat,[8] and especially so for laparoscopic surgeons, because laparoscopic surgery involves instrumental expenses that are nonreimbursable by Medicare or the medical insurance industry. A small number of hospitals are currently evaluating physicians' economic practice patterns to control the surgeons' clinical practices through the credentialing process to reduce the cost of care. Some hospital administrators believe that economic credentialing improves physicians' hospital practice, performance, and patient care. Whether the derived improvement is for the hospital's fiscal benefit or patient's welfare is unclear and debatable. As the hospitals continually face competitive and economic factors forcing cuts in costs and overhead, the economic credentialing of the hospital surgical staff will accelerate. What recourse do surgeons on staff have when hospital administration restricts access to instrument-intensive therapies such as laparoscopic surgery? There should be formal, documented, regulations for the due process of appeal. The medical staff by-laws should support the surgeons' right to a hearing so that the administrative committee can hear the surgeons' arguments as well as the arguwments of those who criticize the procedure solely on the basis of cutting costs. Cost control is here to stay in medical practice but not at the cost of compromising patient care and deterring medical progress.

Certain pragmatic aspects are also involved in credentialing and privileging. Compliance with federal and state guidelines and requirements is a definite necessity for health care facilities with regard to proper accreditation, certification, and reimbursement.[9,10] Proper attention to credentialing also protects institutions from legal exposure induced by inadequate credentials checks. Credentialing is also important for surgeons in our litigious environment. No credentials protect a surgeon from the assault by a plaintiff's attorney, but the lack of credentials magnifies a surgeon's responsibility in any technical mishap or expected poor outcome.

REFERENCES

1. Asbun HJ, Reddick EJ: Credentialing in laparoscopic surgery: a survey of surgeons. J Laparoendosc Surg 2:27, 1992
2. Dent TL: Credentialing, evaluation, and training in laparoscopic surgery. Surg Clin North Am 72:1003, 1992
3. Dorsey JH: Education and credentialing of the gynecologic laparoscopic surgeon. Obstet Gynecol Clin North Am 18:661, 1991
4. Wilson FC: Credentialing in medicine. Ann Thorac Surg 55:1345, 1993
5. Stovall TG, Ling FW, Lipscomb GH et al: A model for resident surgical training in laparoscopic sterilization. Obstet Gynecol 83:470, 1994
6. Guazzoni G, Montorsi F, Bergamaschi F et al: Open surgical revision of laparoscopic pelvic lymphadenectomy for staging of prostate cancer: the impact of laparoscopic learning curve. J Urol 151:930, 1994
7. See WA, Cooper CS, Fisher RJ: Predictors of laparoscopic complications after formal training in laparoscopic surgery. JAMA 270:2689, 1993
8. Koska MT: Hospital CEOs divided on use of economic credentialing. Hospitals 65:42, 1991
9. Maher VF: International migration and medical credentialing. Med Law 11:275, 1992
10. Gabel RA: Quality assurance/peer review for recredentialing/relicensure in New York State. Int Anesthesiol Clin 30:93, 1992

28

Economics of Instrumentation

David F. Canal

Laparoscopic surgery has revolutionized the field of surgery and has numerous advantages over conventional surgery; decreased length of hospitalization, decreased pain, and earlier return to regular activity or employment. Can this be improved? What else can we as physicians and surgeons do?

One area that requires more attention, especially in our present medical climate, is the financial responsibility of physicians in dispensing patient care. Put more simply, physicians must make cost-responsible decisions. Total medical costs have been shown to be higher for laparoscopic surgery than for standard surgery.[1–4] The increased charges are incurred despite a shortened length of stay. The patient does return to work sooner after laparoscopic surgery and is therefore less of a burden to co-workers and society, but the hospital bill is still higher.

The medical costs can be separated into hospital charges and physician charges, both of which are higher for laparoscopic surgery than for open surgery. Most would agree that laparoscopic surgery is not necessarily more difficult to perform, but it is quite different from standard surgery. Laparoscopy is a technical skill that needs to be acquired, but once acquired—or if acquired in residency training—is the increased fee still justified? The time required (or the learning curve) to develop expertise in laparoscopy is significant, but that time is usually spent operating on patients, not toiling away in a laboratory. Surgeons must act responsibly when setting fees for laparoscopic surgery.

What factor in the hospital charges is causing this increase in cost? Several studies addressing this question all point toward the same answer. The operating room costs seem to be the culprit. These are not simply the operating room charges based on time, because laparoscopic cases are neither longer nor shorter than the open counterpart.[1–6] Initial costs of purchasing the laparoscopic equipment or standard instruments are not usually reflected directly in the room charges; however, some institutions do charge a higher fee for rooms using laparoscopic technology.

Trying to review the charges for surgical procedures is very difficult and quite variable from institution to institution. Each hospital has its own formulas for calculating what the patient will be charged for each required item. Unfortunately, there seems to be quite a markup on the disposable purchases used in the operating rooms. This markup usually includes countable items such as sutures, sponges, drains, and gloves, as well as disposable instruments.

Numerous studies have tried to examine and compare the cost of the laparoscopic hand-held instruments, disposable and reusable. The comparison of disposable versus reusable instruments is neither simple nor straightforward. Many significant factors must be considered. The initial cost, the cost of labor, the cost of cleaning, the level of disinfection or sterility, and the cost of instrument repair are factors that must be considered when evaluating the costs of maintaining reusable instruments. For the disposable instruments, one needs to look at the dollar expenditure for each instrument, the costs of manufacturing, sterilizing, transporting, storing, and disposing, as well as the cost to the environment.

Some advantages of disposable hand-held laparoscopic instruments include ease in preparation for each case and ease of cleanup after each use, as well as some advantages noted in instrument use. A disposable Veress needle should always be sharp and may provide some margin of safety. Using a disposable trocar with a retracting safety shield for the initial insertion site is desired by many, but is the retracting shield (and expense) really necessary for the additional puncture sites?[7,8] The safety of inserting any foreign body into the peritoneal cavity depends much more on the technique and expertise of the surgeon than on the type of instrument being used. Scissors are another particularly sensitive instrument. They can lose their cutting ability after repetitive use or misuse. Inadvertently cutting against a metallic clip can easily dull scissors (laparoscopic, as well as Metzenbaum scissors). In my own personal practice, I alternate between two reusable hook-type scissors and have had no problems in over 500 laparoscopic cholecystectomies. No particular advantage in function has been noted when comparing disposable and reusable grasping or dissecting instruments. Disposable clip appliers for ligating blood vessels or stapling devices for securing mesh have the advantage of repetitive application. The disposable clip applier obviates the need to remove the instrument for each fire, and exposure is therefore readily maintained. Of course, neither time nor effort are required to clean or sterilize disposable instruments at the conclusion of a case.

Surgeons who use reusable instruments believe that reusable instruments, with the exception of scissors, function as well as their disposable counterparts. Most of the advantages of reusable laparoscopic instruments are related to economic issues.[2–4,6] An example is the clip applier used to clip blood vessels or the cystic duct. A reusable clip applier is easy to use, easy to clean, can be steam sterilized, applies clips that are secure, and uses clips that cost only dollars. This is in stark contrast to the cost for a disposable clip applier. Reusable instruments can be used repeatedly and do maintain their function.[9] Many other reusable instruments have similar advantages.

Another area of concern between disposable and reusable instruments is the sterility and cleanliness of reusable instruments. Sterility is defined as the complete elimination or destruction of all forms of microbial life. Disinfection, on the other hand, means the elimination of many or all pathogenic organisms except bacterial spores. Disinfection can be divided into three levels: high, intermediate, and low. The goal of any instrument that traverses sterile tissue or the vascular space is sterility or high-level disinfection. For years, arthroscopes, cystoscopes, and laparoscopes have been cleaned then soaked to achieve high disinfection. They have been scrutinized to determine if any infectious complications could be attributed to the instrument. The process of cleaning and soaking instruments in appropriate disinfectant for the appropriate length of time has proved acceptable—provided the process is performed correctly.[10,11] That is the key. The personnel cleaning surgical instruments—whether it is orthopedic hammers and screwdrivers, neurosurgical clips and suckers, vascular clamps and needle drivers, or laparoscopic instruments—must be trained and must perform the task well.

When operating room personnel were queried about the difficulties encountered cleaning reusable laparoscopic instruments, they all responded in a similar fashion. Cleaning laparoscopic instruments requires meticulous attention, but there are few instruments to clean, compared with a standard laparotomy pan of instruments. The nurses and technicians thought that the time taken to clean laparoscopic instruments adequately was not different from standard procedure, and the time spent cleaning instruments neither delayed the operating schedule nor contributed to overtime work. They reported that they usually had the laparoscopic instruments clean and prepared for steam sterilization or high-grade disinfection before the patient left the operation suite. Concerns have been raised about foreign debris not being cleaned adequately from laparoscopic instrumentation before disinfection.[5] These concerns are valid and must be addressed by having conscientious, capable people performing the task of cleaning instruments correctly. The incidence of infectious complications after various laparoscopic procedures is very low, and it has been next to impossible to implicate instrumentation as a source for the infection.[5,10,11]

Several reviews have tried to calculate all the variables and then make some sort of definitive statement about which method—disposable instrumentation or reusable instrumentation—is best. No blanket statement can be made over such a complex issue. The surgeon must evaluate each procedure individually because procedures now performed via the laparoscope vary drastically. The surgeon must decide if the institution's operating room personnel are able and willing to provide the care and service necessary to clean and process laparoscopic instruments. Surgeons must make themselves aware of the sensitive issues, but only when they are armed with appropriate and complete information should they make a cost-responsible decision.

REFERENCES

1. Stoker ME, Vose J, Omara P et al: Laparoscopic cholecystectomy: a clinical and financial analysis of 280 operations. Arch Surg 127:589, 1992
2. Rutkow IM: Laparoscopic hernia repair: the socioeconomic tyranny of surgical technology. Arch Surg 127:1271, 1992
3. Basso N, Chang TM, Howard TJ et al: Laparoscopic surgery: a difference. Arch Surg 127:1269, 1992
4. Voyles CR, Petro AB, Meena AL et al: A practical approach to laparoscopic cholecystectomy. Am J Surg 161:365, 1991
5. Reichert N: Laparoscopic instruments, patient care, cost issues. AORN 3:637, 1993
6. Voyles CR: The laparoscopic dividend. JAMA 11:146, 1992
7. Yuzpe AA: Pneumoperitoneum needle and trocar injuries in laparoscopy: a survey on possible contributing factors and prevention. J Reprod Med 5:485, 1990
8. Nezhat FR, Silfen SL, Evans D et al: Comparison of direct insertion of disposable and standard reusable laparoscopic trocars and previous pneumoperitoneum with Veress needle. Obstet Gynecol 1:148, 1991

9. Deardorf MA: Increasing multipuncture laparoscopic instrument longevity. AORN 2:357, 1991
10. Duppler DW: Laparoscopic instrumentation, videoimaging, and equipment disinfection and sterilization. Surg Clin North Am 5:1021, 1992
11. Marshburn PB, Rutala WA, Wannamaker NS et al: Gas and steam sterilization of assembled versus disassembled laparoscopic equipment—microbiologic studies. J Reprod Med 7:483, 1991

Editorial Comment I

Sergio W. Larach

Economic issues in medical practice are quickly becoming the leading concern. In general, however, physicians have little or no specific training in the professional analysis of complex medical economics.

Dr. Canal sharply addresses the subject of the economics of instrumentation and brings up the continuous controversy on the use of reusable versus disposable instruments.

The role of the surgeon in the future of laparoscopy is vital in guiding the development of new instruments, promoting the safety for patients, and achieving cost containment. These objectives involve the difficult task of conciliating a quality of care and low cost that usually do not run a parallel course, in the new cost-conscious health care environment.

In this chapter, Dr. Canal discusses what is the only cost element that is familiar to a surgeon: the cost of surgical instruments. It is true that total costs are much more important parameters, but to properly calculate total cost/benefit parameters of laparoscopic versus open surgery requires a deeper analysis of the entire subject that I believe should not be done by physicians alone.

Instrumentation clearly plays a key role in the future of laparoscopic procedures. At the present we believe that the use of most disposable laparoscopic instruments, if charged responsibly, represents a good cost-responsible decision. There are concerns on the feasibility of proper cleaning of the reusable instruments, and at the present time, many instruments for advanced laparoscopy (i.e., EndoGIA) are only available in disposable forms. I agree with Dr. Canal that physicians, as well as all the other health-related workers, should make a decision that is cost responsible.

Editorial Comment II

Steven D. Wexner

Dr. Canal has certainly provided an excellent overview of the problem of economics of instrumentation. He has thoroughly delved into the argument of reusable versus disposable instrumentation. However, far more fundamental to the subject and far more controversial are the arguments contained in the first few paragraphs. Dr. Canal begins by stating that "Laparoscopic surgery has revolutionized the field of surgery and has numerous advantages over conventional surgery." Because this textbook is about colorectal surgery, that particular statement does require a combination of good measures of faith and emotion. Although laparoscopic cholecystectomy certainly has numerous advantages, including decreased length of hospitalization, decreased pain, and earlier return to regular activity or employment, no prospective randomized trials have proven these advantages for colorectal surgery. Certainly, all of us who routinely perform laparoscopic colorectal surgery believe that these advantages do indeed exist. However, the belief of a surgeon who performs laparoscopic surgery can hardly replace scientific data collected (even if that surgeon is me). The other variable in this first sentence is that the advantages may well be seen when the surgery is performed in appropriately selected patients by appropriately trained surgeons. Unfortunately, at the time of this writing, neither of these categories has been defined in a universally acceptable way. Each and every article and textbook of laparoscopic colorectal surgery, including this one, lists virtually all disease entities and conditions as potential indications. Each textbook and every professional society has its own guidelines for credentialing and its own policy statements on appropriate training. The uniform thread throughout this otherwise Gordian nexus of debate and uncertainty is that results are better in certain situations than in others. Specifically, the skills requisite to perform laparoscopic cholecystectomy and appendicectomy are not directly translatable to the skills requisite to perform a laparoscopic colectomy. These details are discussed in much greater detail in Chapter 27. As a result of these differences, two separate schools of surgery have developed. One school employs the laparoscope to treat a wide variety of disorders that may on occasion include colorectal disorders. The other group treats, exclusively, disorders of the colon, rectum, and anus and may, when appropriate, employ the laparoscope to facilitate a procedure. Is the group of surgeons who tries to use the laparoscope for each and every operation better equipped to diagnose and manage disorders of the distal alimentary tract? Is the group of individuals who treats exclusively disorders of the distal alimentary tract able to satisfactorily employ the laparoscope when needed? The answers to these questions, unfortunately, do not exist. The former group of surgeons would argue that expertise in the instrument is more important than understanding the disease process or the organ system. They would certainly argue that the skills are translatable. Alternatively, the latter group would argue that a thorough understanding of the pathology, pathophysiology, pharmacology, and surgical and medical management skills play a more important role than the selection of the instrument. This group would also argue that the last two decades have allowed the development of videocolonoscopy and that those skills indeed are helpful when performing laparoscopy. Once again, in the absence of answers, no data are available. Most probably, it is irrelevant as to which group one belongs provided that one's judgment is sound, one's skills are well honed, and one's ego is not easily bruised.

Dr. Canal notes that total medical costs have been higher for laparoscopic surgery when compared to standard surgery. He intimates that an increased fee may indeed be generated or at least billed by the surgeon when performing a laparoscopic colectomy. I think that this practice is reprehensible in the absence of proof that we are indeed providing a superior service to the patient. Early in the learning curve, such an increased fee was justified by many surgeons because of the increased time necessary to perform the procedure. However, such an increase is unjustifiable because it is the surgeon's own decision to spend that additional time, and therefore, a bill should not be generated for learning. If anything, one could easily justify the patient charging the surgeon for being used as a teaching model. This role reversal, in fact, highlights what I believe is Dr. Canal's error in stating that the time should not be spent in a laboratory. To safely perform laparoscopic colorectal surgery, it is not only advisable but *mandatory* for the surgeon to develop skills in an animal model. Although in certain countries, such laboratories are not permitted, fortunately, in the United States, they are encouraged and are easy to find. Many corporate-sponsored laboratories exist, and surgeons are more than welcome to hone their skills using instruments of a corporation who would be more than happy to subsequently sell those instruments to the practicing surgeon's hospital. It is, therefore, both immoral and unjustifiable to embark on laparoscopic colorectal surgery without first working in a laboratory.

Can one justify an increased fee after having surpassed the learning curve? Again, after the learning curve has been surpassed, the time required to perform a laparoscopic colectomy should not be statistically significantly different from the time required to perform a similar open colectomy. Therefore, because there is no additional time taken, the fee should be the same.

Finally, one might argue that an increased fee is justifiable because the patient has an earlier return to work and, as Dr. Canal mentions, is "less of a burden to coworkers." Again, although such statements may be true for patients who have undergone a cholecystectomy or an appendectomy, the same cannot be said of the typical patient who undergoes a colectomy. Most patients who undergo colectomies in this country do so for either carcinoma, diverticulitis, rectal prolapse, or inflammatory bowel disease. The vast majority of patients in the former three groups are elderly and very likely retired by the time of surgery. The latter group of patients are generally young but, because of protracted illness, are often receiving disability compensation. Therefore, very few of the patients within the four mentioned groups, which comprise the majority of colorectal surgical patients, can be analyzed in the same manner as patients with calculous cholecystitis or acute appendicitis. The staunch laparoscopic proponent might argue that, although the majority of such patients are either retired or disabled, they return to regular activity earlier than they otherwise would (mentioned by Dr. Canal). In point of fact, because the insurance company and not the patient is paying the bill, it is highly unlikely that the insurance company is interested in the patient's activity after discharge from the hospital.

The last issue I address here concerns operating room charges. Dr. Canal states that "laparoscopic cases are neither longer nor shorter than the open counterpart." He offers six references on the topic. Once again, however, this textbook is about laparoscopic colorectal surgery. To date, authors have noted an increased operative time, at least on the ascendancy of the learning curve, if not permanently.[1–12] Regardless of the authors' views and conclusions in any of these papers relative to benefits or lack thereof, increased time is universally accepted. Regardless of ubiquitous reporting of longer operative times, none of the authors have discussed the additional time required to set up the operating room and to clean it after a laparoscopic procedure. While certain institutes may have dedicated laparoscopic rooms, the majority of hospitals need more flexibility in their operating rooms. Thus, one must account for the time required to bring the monitors, video cables, suction and irrigation tubing, as well as other accoutrements into the operating room before the procedure. My colleagues and I are in the middle of a study looking at this issue and, although our actual laparoscopic operative time is not statistically different from that for a comparable open procedure, the setup and takedown times remain approximately double those seen in the open situation. Once again, the issue is raised to as to whether it is justifiable to bill the patient for this extra time. To date, no data condone such a practice. The obvious problem with increased setup and takedown times is that another patient cannot be in the operating room getting operated on and, therefore, hospital revenues decrease. Clearly, many issues of economics of instrumentation remain unanswered. I hope that this devil's advocate editorial comment offers a balance to Dr. Canal's well-written chapter.

REFERENCES

1. Cohen SM, Nogueras JJ, Wexner SD: Laparoscopic colorectal surgery: ascending the learning curve. World J Surg (in press)
2. Hoffman GC, Baker JW, Fitchett CW, Vansant JH: Laparoscopic-assisted colectomy: initial experience. Ann Surg 219:732, 1994
3. Milsom JW, Lavery IC, Bohm B, Fazio VW: Laparoscopically assisted-ileocolectomy in Crohn's disease. Surg Laparosc Endosc 3:77, 1993
4. Monson JRT, Darzi A, Carey PD, Guillou J: Prospective evaluation of laparoscopic-assisted colectomy in an unselected group of patients. Lancet 340:831, 1992
5. Musser DG, Boorse RC, Madera R, Reed JF III: Laparoscopic colectomy: at what cost? Surg Laparosc Endosc 4:1, 1994
6. Peters SR, Bartels TL: Minimally invasive colectomy: are there potential benefits realized? Dis Colon Rectum 36:751, 1993
7. Scoggin SD, Frazee RC, Snyder SK et al: Laparoscopic-assisted bowel surgery. Dis Colon Rectum 36:747, 1993
8. Senagore AJ, Luchtefeld MA, Macheigan JM et al: Open colectomy versus laparoscopic colectomy: are there differences? Am J Surg 59:549, 1993
9. Tate JJ, Kwok S et al: Prospective comparison of laparoscopic and conventional anterior resection. Br J Surg 80:1396, 1993
10. Vara-Thorbeck C, Garcia-Caballero M, Salvi M et al: Indications and advantages of laparoscopic-assisted colon resection for cancer in elderly patients. Surg Laparosc Endosc 4:110, 1994
11. Vayer AJ, Larach SW, Williamson PR et al: Cost effectiveness of laparoscopic-assisted colectomy. Coloproctology 16:190, 1994
12. Wexner SD, Cohen SM, Johansen OB et al: Laparoscopic colorectal surgery: a prospective assessment and current perspective. Br J Surg 80:1602, 1993

29

Role of Randomized Clinical Trials

Rama M. Jager

New revolutions, religions, and democratic heads of state inspire some to convert immediately and others to condemn incessantly. Technologic breakthroughs and paradigm shifts cause similar reactions. Some surgeons cheered the introduction of pelviscopic therapeutic surgery and laparoscopic cholecystectomy as the dawn of a new era of minimal invasion, while many chided the same as being dangerous and untested. A similar debate is occurring with laparoscopic colorectal surgery.

Some surgical techniques are true therapeutic breakthroughs. They signify a revolutionary advance from existing treatment. Their superiority is unmistakably obvious, and evidence of their superiority requires no randomized trials.[1] Laparoscopic cholecystectomy is one such example. Most new therapies, however, are minor modifications of existing treatments and require randomized comparative clinical trials to prove their equivalency or superiority. Is laparoscopic colectomy similar to laparoscopic cholecystectomy in its superiority over existing techniques? The debate and disagreement as to the value of laparoscopic colorectal surgery and whether it represents a major therapeutic breakthrough or only a modest incremental technical improvement is evident in the previous chapters of this book.

Drs. Cohen and Wexner, in Chapter 26, take a balanced look at current published data and their own extensive experience with laparoscopic colorectal surgery. As they cogently and convincingly point out, no valid statistical data from randomized clinical trials are currently available to support the superiority or equivalency of laparoscopic colorectal surgery in comparison with conventional open techniques. They question whether the laparoscopic cancer resection is adequate or even meets the standards of current oncosurgical dogma. Controversy regarding the putative reduction in operative blood loss, cost, and hospitalization from laparoscopic colorectal surgery is presented. They propose randomized clinical trials to compare laparoscopic colorectal surgery with conventional open techniques before adaption of the former.

NECESSITY

Are randomized clinical trials imperative to evaluate laparoscopic colorectal surgery? Based on the number of randomized clinical trials—whether well designed or ill conceived—that are published in medical journals, the answer seems self-evident. No new drug enters the market without a few randomized trials proving its benefit. By contrast, randomized controlled studies dealing with new surgical techniques are less common.[2] The hazards of embracing a new surgical technique without strict comparison with existing techniques prove the need for randomized clinical trial. Some may argue that laparoscopic colorectal cancer resection should not be done without proving its superiority or equivalency to the open resection by randomized clinical trials. Is that view a necessarily cautious approach to safe surgical care or stiflingly rigid constraint that is nonenforceable? To resolve the quandary, the methodology of clinical trials in surgery and the potential limitations with the different study techniques need a review.

Significance of Proper Sample Size

Not all randomized clinical trials are equally designed. The efficacy of any randomized comparative clinical trial depends on the size of the sample and the degree of difference in treatment effect (effect size) between the compared groups. The larger the difference in treatments, the smaller is the sample size needed to prove the difference. Thus, sample size in any randomized clinical trial is crucial. The power of a randomized trial increases if the sample population is large or if the treatment effect size is high from reduction in the variation inside the group.[3]

Inadequate sample size is the major flaw in many published randomized clinical trials.[4] Clinical researchers usually select sample sizes that can identify only large treatment effects, thus risking type II error, ignoring smaller treatment effects that may be clinically beneficial.[5] When the treatment difference is estimated from 10 to 15 percent, and the significance level fixed under 0.05, the ideal needed sample size exceeds 1,000. These standards assume that intragroup variation from multiple prognostic factors is minimal to absent. What if the treatment difference is less than 10 percent? A trial with a sample size of 1,000 may fail to show the superiority of laparoscopic technique over the conventional open technique if the former achieves only 10 percent improvement (depending on the end point selected) over the latter. Were laparoscopic colectomy to differ significantly from the open technique, small sample sizes would be adequate. By contrast, more subtle differences demand recruitment of larger numbers of patients, preoccupying the investigators and their institutions with temporal, administrative, and financial burdens.[6]

When the sample size is small, general comparison of survival time between the treatment groups may only show a biased estimate even when the study is well designed. Some investigators use multivariate analysis of various known prognostic factors and consider the possible treatment–co-variate interactions to reduce this bias.[7] The problem with small sample size is magnified by unavoidable heterogeneity of patient population in their cancer stage and their natural prognosis. These are known prognostic factors. What about prognostic factors that have yet to be identified and thus possibly unevenly distributed in the groups? The smaller the sample size, the more heterogeneous the groups are regarding both known and unknown prognostic factors and the less generalizable the outcome of the trial. Data from these studies are valid for the tested groups but not for the entire reference population. Stratification of the patient population based on cancer stage also further reduces the sample size for each stratum and makes it difficult to interpret the subtle differences in survival. Treatment allocation in multicenter, stratified randomized clinical trials may produce significant difference in the number of patients per treatment arm, biasing the final data.[8] As for any other methodology, proper designing and analysis of randomized clinical trials are essential to extrapolate the conclusions to the population in reference.

Problems

The randomized, controlled, comparative clinical trial is the current gold standard for evaluation of new treatments and medications. However, many statisticians remind us of the problems with extrapolation and generalization of results from a randomized clinical trial.[9,10] Heterogeneity of both the sample patient population and of the surgical technique plague the validity of data in surgical trials, despite attempts to remove the selection bias by pretreatment randomization.

In spite of randomization, the group treated by laparoscopic surgery may differ from the group treated by conventional surgery in innumerable respects. Both the known and unknown tumor-related prognostic factors, as well as surgical technique factors that may be uneven between the groups, bias the results. Fisher's original proposal for randomization in comparative trials to reduce the differences in the groups[11] dealt with trials where the subjects were in matched pairs. The matched subjects were assigned at random to either one treatment or the other. Most randomized clinical trials fail to randomize matched pairs and thus magnify the uneven distribution of prognostic factors in the compared groups.

The other problem is difficulty with recruitment of patients. Patients may complain about randomized trials and show reluctance to participate. They often complain of being guinea pigs. Despite the noble end, randomized clinical trials do limit and diminish the role of patient's choice in medical decision making. If the patients are given a detailed explanation that the type of treatment of the cancer will be decided by chance, many patients might be unwilling to be recruited into the trial. Most of our patients in the 1990s are well informed. If they perceive that they may receive the surgeon's less preferred technique, whether the surgeon prefers laparoscopic or open technique, they may be unwilling to participate in the trial.[12]

Even if a medical center participates in the clinical trial whole-heartedly, it may not recruit all the eligible patients into the trial. It is not uncommon that only a small portion of eligible patients enters a randomized clinical trial. In many oncologic clinical trials, less than 3 percent of all eligible patients enter a clinical trial.[13] Are the data from the 3 percent of patients who entered the randomized clinical trial to be extrapolated to all potential patients who may need the treatment, or should we consider clinical comparative but retrospective data from the 97 percent of eligible patients who did not undergo pretreatment randomization? When do we consider it invalid to extrapolate the results from a small study sample beyond the specific study patient population? There are no definite answers. Limited enrollment into a randomized trial can compromise the appropriateness of generalization. The data obtained from the trial may be meaningful for the patient population of the trial but cannot be generalized to the entire patient population with colorectal cancers. It is reasonable to assume that the comparison of data from the randomized prospective trials and retrospective, systematic comparative observation of nonrandomized clinical experience may help us decide the validity of extrapolation and generalization.[14]

Surgical fundamentalists may argue that any data from any nonrandomized study are inherently less valid than the collective and comparative but retrospective clinical experience. The consequences of such scientific prejudice hinder testing of new operative techniques and reduce the therapeutic potential of the innovation.[15] The detriment from randomized clinical trials stems from the widespread belief in the infallibility of the methodology of randomized clinical trials. Data from an ill-designed or ill-analyzed randomized clinical trial may relegate a potentially beneficial surgical technique to oblivion—solely based on the strength of methodology used. A review of 58 randomized clinical trials with negative conclusions, published in three prestigious British medical journals, highlights this handicap.[16] The review showed that 43 of the 44 evaluable trials had a greater than 10 percent chance of missing a 25 percent relative treatment difference, and that 31 of the trials had a greater than 10 percent risk of missing a 50 percent relative treatment difference. The negative results reported from the studies were compatible with a 25 percent beneficial relative treatment effect in 36 studies and a 50 percent treatment benefit in 22 studies. Of the total 44 studies, 23 studies had an incorrect interpretation of the findings.

The prestige of the methodology is also its peril. Many treatments with potential benefit may be incorrectly eliminated from clinical practice by a faulty study,[17] solely because the study carried the prestige of being a randomized clinical trial.

ARE RANDOMIZED CLINICAL TRIALS THE FINAL ANSWER

Are the data from nonrandomized clinical data of any value? If an operative technique was not efficacious in a randomized clinical trial, should it be untested by other methods of study? Randomization may partially nullify the selection bias in treatment groups. The need for large sample size to show subtle differences between the treatments may make it inappropriate in many surgical scenarios. Comparative clinical observation by surgeons in practice does suffer from a selection bias influenced by the patient's choice of treatment and the surgeon's zeal. By contrast, it has the advantage of massive sample size, avoiding the problem of inappropriate generalization and extrapolation. If we view all the retrospective clinical data as invalid mainly because of the probable selection bias, the specter of the best—namely, the randomized clinical trials—becoming the enemy of the good—namely, the data from systematic comparative clinical observation[18]—has been raised. The discussion in the cited reference is worth reviewing in entirety by all surgical researchers.

Other problems of relying on randomized clinical trials alone as a sole methodology to test the equivalency or superiority of laparoscopic colectomy need elaboration. Limitations—such as time constraints, the difficulty with patient recruitment, and the intragroup cancer-stage variation—render it difficult to evaluate the laparoscopic colectomy using the randomized controlled clinical trials. If the difference in treatment effect is less than 10 percent, the sample size of more than 1,000 patients is necessary. It is possible that the differences are large and significantly more than 10 percent. If so, the sample size is not an issue. If the differences in treatment results are dramatic, an argument can be made that such differences become manifest rapidly in clinical observation even before completion of randomized clinical trials.[19] Other problems with clinical trials need attention. Some workers point to the mislaid total reliance on all-important *P* value.[20] A trend or a difference with a *P* value greater than 0.05 may be statistically and possibly clinically significant. The concept is that if *P* is not less than 0.05, the treatment is ineffective and deserves abandonment. This is especially so if the clinical comparative data point to the benefit of the tested treatment.

APPROPRIATENESS IN EVALUATING SURGICAL TECHNIQUES

Are randomized clinical trials appropriate in surgical studies? Randomized clinical trials are common in pharmaceutical industry and in medical oncology. The use and ease of use of randomized clinical trials in surgery may differ from that in medical oncology or the pharmaceutical industry. The standard pharmaceutical practice of randomized, placebo-controlled, double-blind efficacy trials is neither pragmatic nor ethical for testing surgical treatments.[21] For the past decade, comparative trials have become more frequent than placebo trials, even in the pharmaceutical industry and, by necessity, in surgical studies. However, the number of randomized controlled trials published in journals such as *The British Journal of Surgery* has declined, suggesting the reluctance of many patients to relinquish their right to choose their surgical treatment and leave it to chance.[22] The value of a randomized clinical trial in surgical treatment is well accepted, but the value of other methods in surgical research should not be ignored. Comprehensive, accurate, and objective comparison of results from a new technique such as laparoscopic colorectal surgery with that of traditional open surgery done by the same surgeon in previous years, or by another group of surgeons, provides useful data to improve our current surgical practices.

In addition, designing a randomized trial needs pertinent clinical data. A randomized clinical trial cannot be done in a vacuum or in isolation from other nonrandomized clinical experience. Past clinical experience is useful not only in designing but also in monitoring and reporting results of the trial.[23,24]

SIGNIFICANCE OF RETROSPECTIVE STUDIES

A rigid approach in any scientific discipline is hazardous. Most clinicians, including surgeons, firmly believe that retrospective clinical data are "inherently fallacious."[25,26] My submission that retrospective clinical trials with comparative historical controls provide adequate data may appear anti-intellectual and politically incorrect. Realizing the ethical and pragmatic aspects of randomized clinical trials, even some statisticians debating the scientific methodology concede that nonrandomized retrospective trials with historical control groups are useful and appropriate.[27–31] Some well-respected statisticians argue that proper collection of data from nonrandomized clinical experience for future studies using historical controls and Baysean concepts provides adequate and useful information comparable to the current gold standard, the randomized clinical trial.[32]

ADVANTAGES OF META-ANALYSIS

A few randomized clinical trials or a few retrospective comparative studies cannot dispel our collective ignorance and medical uncertainty in our day-to-day surgical practice.[16] The systematic overview or meta-analysis of previously published clinical trials is a reliable technique to analyze data from variegated trials. Because meta-analysis combines and synthesizes evidence from multiple randomized trials, excessive variation in the quality of the included trials may limit the value of the overview. Such overviews of limited or ill-designed trial data are more probably biased.[33] On the other hand, cumulative meta-analysis of well-designed clinical trials enables determination of clinical efficacy of a treatment and its side effects. It also helps in planning future trials.[34]

NEED FOR CENTRALIZED REGISTRY OF TRIALS FOR RAPID DATA DISTRIBUTION

The design and execution of clinical trials, whether randomized clinical trials or retrospective trials with historical controls, are not enough. Rapid distribution of results from the clinical trial to the practicing surgeon is needed. New data from randomized clinical trials, even if valid, may not be incorporated immediately into clinical practice. An example often cited is the use of thrombolytic therapy to reduce the mortality of acute myocardial infarction. Even after publication of several large trials, less than 50 percent of patients with acute myocardial infarction were receiving thrombolytics.[35,36] Electronic dissemination of such invaluable information through various popular data bases such as Medlars and Internet is one immediately apparent avenue. Such wide promulgation of the data will help both patients and surgeons make intelligent and informed decisions by giving them access to a reliable and authoritative review of currently available knowledge bases.[37] The knowledge base is also indispensable in planning future clinical studies.

CONCLUSION

Laparoscopic colorectal surgery is in evolution. Techniques are changing, and so are the indications. Surgeons are still learning to master the technical aspects of this new approach. Well-designed randomized clinical trials—the gold standard in clinical study techniques—and the clinical data from practicing surgeons will decide the future role of laparoscopic techniques in management of colorectal diseases.

It is a poignant question. Is laparoscopic colorectal surgery justifiable? My answer is a qualified "yes." As is the case with any surgical technique, no one approach is suitable for all our patients. Proper clinical judgment plays a role in effective management of patients with colorectal cancer and deciding who can benefit from the new minimally traumatic surgical techniques. Given the current published clinical experience, some laparoscopic colorectal surgical procedures are superior to the open technique. Here is my list of such laparoscopic procedures: diagnostic laparoscopy, laparoscopic appendectomy, segmental colectomy for benign disease and for advanced cancer, laparoscopic enterostomy, laparoscopic repair of iatrogenic colon injury, and possibly proctopexy.

The laparoscopic resection of malignant colorectal disease is currently being done in many centers. Multiple North American and European randomized clinical trials are in the design stage. Over the next few years, the systematic observational comparison of results from the laparoscopic experience with those of historical controls, as well as randomized clinical trials, and, more important, meta-analysis of these trials will answer the question as to the adequacy of the laparoscopic resection of colorectal cancer. A centralized electronic disseminated registry of clinical trials dealing with treatment of colorectal diseases helps rapid distribution of information to practicing surgeons and thus improves our patient care.

REFERENCES

1. Kaufman D: Cancer therapy and the randomized clinical trial: good medicine? CA Cancer J Clin 44:109, 1994
2. Buyse M: Randomized clinical trials in surgical oncology. Eur J Surg Oncol 17:421, 1991

3. Kraemer HC: To increase power in randomized clinical trials without increasing sample size. Psychopharmacol Bull 27:217, 1991
4. Vandekerckhove P, O'Donovan PA, Lilford RJ et al: Infertility treatment: from cookery to science. The epidemiology of randomized controlled trials. Br J Obstet Gynaecol 100:1005, 1993
5. Raju TN, Langenberg P, Sen A et al: How much "better" is good enough? The magnitude of treatment effect in clinical trials. Am J Dis Child 146:407, 1992
6. Whitehead J: Interim analyses and stopping rules in cancer clinical trials. Br J Cancer 68:1179, 1993
7. Schmoor C, Ulm K, Schumacher M: Comparison of the Cox model and the regression tree procedure in analyzing a randomized clinical trial. Stat Med 12:2351, 1993
8. Signorini DF, Leung O, Simes RJ et al: Dynamic balanced randomization for clinical trials. Stat Med 12:2343, 1993
9. Bailey KR: Generalizing the results of randomized clinical trials. Controlled Clin Trials 15:15, 1994
10. Urbach P: The value of randomization and control in clinical trials. Stat Med 12:1421, 1993
11. Fisher RA: The Design of Experiments. 4th Ed. Oliver and Boyd. Harvard University Library, Edinburgh, 1947
12. McIntyre IMC: Tribulations for clinical trials. BMJ 302:1099, 1991
13. Benson AB III, Pregler JP, Bean JA et al: Oncologists' reluctance to accrue patients onto clinical trials: an Illinois cancer center study. Clin Oncol 9:2067, 1991
14. Davis CE: Generalizing from clinical trials. Controlled Clin Trials 15:11, 1994
15. Sullivan MD: Placebo controls and epistemic control in orthodox medicine. J Med Philos 18:213, 1993
16. Williams HC, Seed P: Inadequate size of "negative" clinical trials in dermatology. Br J Dermatol 128:317, 1993
17. Rabeneck L, Viscoli CM, Horwitz RI: Problems in the conduct and analysis of randomized clinical trials. Are we getting the right answers to the wrong questions? Arch Intern Med 152:507, 1992
18. McPherson K: The Cochrane lecture. The best and the enemy of the good: randomized controlled trials, uncertainty, and assessing the role of patient choice in medical decision making. J Epidemiol Community Health 48:6, 1994
19. Thompson SG: Controversies in meta-analysis: the case of the trials of serum cholesterol reduction. Stat Methods Med Res 2:173, 1993
20. Chalmers TC, Lau J: Meta-analytic stimulus for changes in clinical trials. Stat Methods Med Res 2:161, 1993
21. Stirrat GM, Farrow SC, Farndon J et al: The challenge of evaluating surgical procedures. Ann R Coll Surg Engl 74:80, 1992
22. Pollock AV: Surgical evaluation at the crossroads. Br J Surg 80:964, 1993
23. Spiegelhalter DJ, Freedman LS, Parmar MK: Applying Bayesian ideas in drug development and clinical trials. Stat Med 12:1501, 1993
24. Urbach P: The value of randomization and control in clinical trials. Stat Med 12:1421, 1993
25. Cranberg L: Do retrospective controls make clinical trials "inherently fallacious?" BMJ 1265, 1979
26. Urbach P: The value of randomization and control in clinical trials. Stat Med 12:1421, 1993
27. McPherson K: The Cochrane lecture. The best and the enemy of the good: randomized controlled trials, uncertainty, and assessing the role of patient choice in medical decision making. J Epidemiol Community Health 48:6, 1994
28. Byar DP et al: Design considerations for AIDS trials. N Engl J Med 323:13443, 1990
29. Ottenbacher K: Impact of random assignment on study outcome: an empirical examination. Controlled Clin Trials 13:50, 1992
30. Platt R: Methodologic aspects of clinical studies of perioperative antibiotic prophylaxis. Rev Infect Dis, suppl. 10:S810, 1991
31. Leber P: Is there an alternative to the randomized controlled trial? Psychopharmacol Bull 27:3, 1991
32. Howson C, Urbach P: Scientific Reasoning: The Bayesian Approach. 2nd Ed. Open Court. Chicago, 1993
33. Sandercock P: Collaborative worldwide overviews of randomized trials. Ann NY Acad Sci 703:149, 1993
34. Lau J, Antman EM, Jimenez-Silva J et al: Cumulative meta-analysis of therapeutic trials for myocardial infarction. N Engl J Med 327:248, 1992
35. Ketley D, Woods KL: Impact of clinical trials on clinical practice: example of thrombolysis for acute myocardial infarction. Lancet 342:891, 1993
36. Chalmers TC: An international registry of published randomized clinical trialws such as "Cochrane Database of Systematic Reviews" will aid meta-analyses. Ann NY Acad Sci 703:156, 1993
37. Silagy C: Developing a register of randomized controlled trials in primary care. BMJ 306:897, 1993

Editorial Comment

Robin S. McLeod

Clinicians are frequently faced with the necessity of making a decision about which therapy (medical or surgical) is most appropriate for their patient. Several strategies may be used to make these decisions, ranging from anecdotal experience, checking with known experts in the field, or seeking scientifically based evidence. The latter is usually drawn from published reports in the literature and, depending on the study design, one may have more or less confidence in the strength of the evidence.

The randomized controlled trial is accepted as the best trial design for comparing two medical therapies.[1] It is analogous to the experiment performed by the scientist in the research laboratory. It has a rigorous design so that both random error and systematic error (bias) are minimized and the likelihood of making incorrect conclusions or generalizations about the effectiveness of a treatment is minimized. Several essential components of the randomized controlled trial lead to its rigorousness. First, subjects are randomly allocated to two groups: usually a treatment group (in which the new treatment is being tested) and a control group (in which the standard therapy or placebo is administered). Thus, the control group is concurrent and subjects are randomly allocated to the two groups. Second, the interventions and follow-up are standardized and performed prospectively. Thus, both groups (it is hoped) are similar in all respects, except for the single factor being studied. Not only does this guard against differences in factors known to be important, it also ensures that differences due to other factors that have not been identified are not present.

The major trial designs, other than the randomized controlled trial, used in clinical medicine are cohort studies, case control studies, and case series and reports.[2] By far, case series are the most common studies found in the surgical literature, accounting for more than 50 percent of published articles in one series.[2] However, all these designs are less rigorous than the randomized controlled trial; this is especially true of case series. Because there is no concurrent control group, data are collected retrospectively, and the intervention is uncontrolled, they are subject to both known and unknown biases that may lead to incorrect conclusions about the efficacy of treatment.

Dr. Jager discusses many problems related to randomized controlled trials. Although much has been written about the difficulties of performing randomized controlled trials, especially surgical trials, it is my belief that many of those issues—particularly methodological issues—are not as great impediments as has been claimed.[3]

Dr. Jager argues that results from randomized controlled trials may be biased because "factors that have yet to be identified [may be] unevenly distributed in the groups" and "treatment allocation...may produce significant differences in the number of patients per treatment arm, biasing the final data." In fact, this is precisely the strength of the randomized controlled trial. By randomizing patients, the treatment groups should be similar in all known and unknown factors. Having said that, there is always a risk that by chance alone, there will be imbalance even with randomization. If this means that one group has significantly more patients with blue eyes than the other, one would be unconcerned. However, if a significantly higher proportion of patients in one group had an anterior resection, one might be concerned. To ensure that such imbalances do not occur, patients can be stratified according to the most important prognostic factors before randomization. For instance, in a trial in which duration of hospital stay is the primary outcome variable, patients might be stratified according to whether they are scheduled to have a colon or a rectal resection (assuming that these are variables that have a major impact on hospital stay).

Dr. Jager also points out that there may be "heterogeneity of both the sample patient population and of the surgical technique." This issue should not impact on the credibility or acceptance of the trial results (internal validity), but it may impact on the generalizability (external validity) of the results. In designing a trial, the investigator must set down inclusion criteria. These may be rather unrestricted so that most patients are eligible for entry or they may be restricted so that a relatively small proportion of patients are eligible for entry. Thus, in a trial comparing survivorship following laparoscopic or open surgery, one might include all patients with a colorectal cancer or only those with cancers of the colon. Provided the trial was methodologically sound, the results of both trials would be equally valid (internal validity). However, the results of the former trial would be more generalizable. The disadvantage of a trial with unrestricted inclusion criteria is that there is a greater risk of missing a treatment effect or of being uncertain which subgroups may benefit from the treatment. Decisions regarding inclusion criteria depend on what question is being asked and, although generalizability of the trial results may vary, the internal validity of the results is not affected.

The issue of surgical procedure standardization is difficult and one that must always be addressed in a surgical trial. Variations in surgical technique may occur because of surgeons' variable experience and ability and individual preferences in performing the procedure, as well as technical modifications that may occur as the procedure evolves. Certain strategies may be employed to ensure a minimum standard of surgery, such as ensuring that all surgeons agree on the performance of critical aspects of the procedure, providing teaching sessions, requiring that the surgeon has performed a certain number of cases, and obtaining documentation that the procedure has been performed satisfactorily (e.g., operative videos or pathology specimens to document the extent of resection). Beyond that, the investigators can decide whether only a limited number of surgeons known to be experts will participate or whether a large number of surgeons, with perhaps a wide range of experience, will be asked to participate. If fewer surgeons are involved, standardization is more likely. By contrast, the advantage of many participating surgeons or centers is that the results may have greater generalizability. Again, whether a few surgeons or a large number participate, the internal validity of the trial is not affected. The issue of standardization is important in the context of a laparoscopic trial, since surgeons vary in their competence of this relatively new technique. However, this is a methodologic issue that can be addressed in the design of the trial.

Although well-designed randomized controlled trials usually provide valid results to important questions, poorly designed randomized controlled trials are of little value and may, as suggested by Dr. Jager, lead to incorrect abandonment of efficacious treatments. Calculation of sample size is only one aspect to consider in designing a trial. Where the clinically significant difference in treatment effect is small, sample size tends to be large. Although this makes the performance of a trial more difficult, it is in these situations that a randomized controlled trial is even more necessary. Large treatment differences are often obvious and results are less likely to be confounded by biases, whereas small differences may be missed or incorrectly attributed to the treatment unless extraneous factors are controlled. Recruitment of patients may be difficult, especially if the sample size is large, and multicenter trials may be necessary. However, that many trials comparing surgical to medical therapies have been completed suggest that patients will participate in these trials and surgeons should not assume that a trial is infeasible.[4–6] Surgeon reluctance rather than patient reluctance may be a greater obstacle to the performance of a randomized controlled trial.

SHOULD TRIALS ASSESSING LAPAROSCOPIC COLORECTAL TECHNIQUES BE PERFORMED

Although Dr. Jager may be somewhat uncertain whether randomized controlled trials are necessary, to me, the answer is an unequivocal "yes." As long as uncertainties exist about the effectiveness of laparoscopic procedures, randomized controlled trials are needed. These uncertainties do exist. For instance, are we certain that an adequate resection for cancer can be achieved laparoscopically? Are recurrence rates and mortality similar following open and laparoscopic colectomy for colorectal cancer? Are hospital stay and costs reduced with laparoscopic colectomy? Answers to these questions may be derived from case series but if so, doubts will always be present about the validity of the results because of concerns of patient selection biases, differences in surgical technique, and other patient care factors. Although randomized controlled trials are more costly to perform and results are not readily available, they also tend to have great impact. As examples, the results of the EC-IC Bypass Study and the North American Symptomatic Carotid Endarterectomy Trial (NASCET) have had a major impact on the surgical treatment of stroke.[5,6]

It is quite likely that trials assessing laparoscopic colorectal procedures would also have a major impact. However, any trial would have to be methodologically sound, with adequate sample size, strict inclusion criteria, well-defined outcome measures, and compliance with surgical techniques. In addition, participating surgeons should be equally skilled in both open and laparoscopic colorectal techniques. Adequate funding is necessary to ensure reliable data collection and analysis. The investigators should have a strong commitment to the trial and should be uncertain about which treatment alternative is superior (equipoise). This is because it is unlikely that surgeons who have definite opinions regarding the superiority of a technique would be able to recruit patients, since that bias would probably be transmitted to the patient. Furthermore, one could argue that from an ethical standpoint, surgeons who do not have a reasonable amount of uncertainty about which treatment is superior, should not enter patients into a trial.

ROLE OF CASE SERIES IN DOCUMENTING THE RESULTS OF LAPAROSCOPIC COLORECTAL PROCEDURES

I believe that there is a role for case series in documenting the results of laparoscopic colorectal procedures, but that does not mean that results from case series alone are adequate and randomized controlled trials are unnecessary. Rather, results from case series should be considered observations to stimulate the thoughtful surgeon to generate hypotheses and ask further questions that can then be tested by more rigorous studies (i.e., a randomized controlled trial). Rigorously collected data from series of patients may also be helpful in improving the generalizability of results from randomized controlled trials. The problem of randomized controlled trial results not being generalizable because of under- or overrepresentation of groups or poor patient recruitment has been recognized in medical pharmacology. The Agency for Health Care Policy and Research was established by the U.S. Congress to address this issue.[7] Their suggestion has been to combine the results of randomized controlled trials, which determine the direction of effectiveness, with data from large groups collected by database analysis. This combines the internal validity of randomized controlled trials with the external validity of database analyses to determine whether a treatment is effective across a range of patients where a large randomized controlled trial is not possible. Finally, one must accept that in certain situations a randomized controlled trial cannot be performed (e.g., because the condition or disease is sufficiently rare to preclude adequate numbers of patients) and evidence from case series may be the only source on which to base treatment decisions.[8]

In summary, there is a role for randomized controlled trials in assessing laparoscopic colorectal techniques. One accepts that there may be difficulties in performing these trials. However, laparoscopic surgery is perhaps one of the biggest innovations in modern surgery and surgeons should accept the challenge of testing this modality in rigorous experiments.

REFERENCES

1. Guyatt GH, Sackett DL, Cook DJ, Evidence-Based Medicine Working Group: Users' guide to the medical literature. How to use an article about therapy or prevention. Are the results of the study valid? JAMA 270:2598, 1993
2. Solomon MJ, McLeod RS: Clinical studies in surgical journals. Have we improved? Dis Colon Rectum 36:43, 1993
3. McLeod RS, Wright J, Solomon MJ et al: Randomized controlled trials in surgery—issues and problems. Surgery 1995 (in press)
4. Spechler SJ, The Department of Veterans Affairs Gastroesophageal Reflux Disease Study Group: Comparison of medical and surgical therapy for complicated gastroesophageal reflux disease in veterans. N Engl J Med 326:786, 1992
5. EC-IC Bypass Study Group: Failure of extracranial–intracranial arterial bypass to reduce the risk of ischemic stroke: results of an international randomized trial. N Engl J Med 313:1191, 1985
6. North American Symptomatic Carotid Endarterectomy Trial Collaborators: Beneficial effect of carotid endarterectomy in symptomatic patients with high-grade carotid stenosis. N Engl J Med 325:445, 1991
7. U.S. Government Accounting Office: Cross design synthesis: a new strategy for medical effectiveness research. GAO/PEMD-92-18, Washington, DC, 1992
8. Solomon MJ, McLeod RS: Should we be performing more randomized controlled trials? Surgery 1995 (in press)

30

Cost Analysis

Sergio W. Larach and Andrea Ferrara

Laparoscopy is becoming an increasingly prevalent approach for a wide variety of surgical procedures. The time to prove its feasibility as a technique has now elapsed, and the cost of its spreading use has become a very important issue.

This surgical technique relies on the evolving fields of video imaging, stapling devices, and the development of instruments for endoscopic use. Laparoscopic surgery therefore has high costs in start-up, maintenance, and replacement.

The cost of health care is a multifaceted problem. Every area has a wide variety of parameters that make standardization of values a very difficult problem. Moreover, local cost analysis can be extrapolated to a national picture only with caution. The responsibility of evaluating fully the costs and benefits of laparoscopic surgery therefore must be shared by hospital administrators, supply companies, and physicians. Only a concerted move by these forces will ensure the progress of this field.

A preliminary and superficial cost analysis shows that obvious charges are often higher for laparoscopic cases than for open surgery and that the excess expense is largely secondary to excess charges applied to the disposable instruments used in laparoscopic surgery. To identify the total cost of one versus another technique, consideration must be given not only to the cost-shifting practice currently used by major medical centers to offset nonproductive operations but also to the frequently mentioned earlier return to work issue. It is not a surprise to find that many patients do not expect or desire an early return to work. By contrast, patients do enjoy other benefits of laparoscopic surgery (i.e., less pain, smaller scars) that are difficult to express in terms of saved dollars. These issues alone make total cost analysis very difficult.

Although numerous authors have evaluated the cost-effectiveness of laparoscopic cholecystectomy,[1–5] only one author[6] has examined the charges involved with laparoscopic-assisted colectomy. To establish the cost-effectiveness of laparoscopic-assisted colectomy, we evaluated the various charges that constitute the total cost of a laparoscopic resection and compared these costs with those of open colectomies.

METHODS

Between October 1991 and February 1993, we performed 38 laparoscopic-assisted colectomies. We compared these patients with a group of 38 patients operated on between February 1990 and February 1993. Patients were matched for age, sex, hospital, concomitant medical illness, resection, and pathology.

Patient characteristics are shown in Table 30-1. All patients were admitted to the hospital the day before operation. Bowel preparation was by polyethylene gylcol (PEG) solution lavage and oral antibiotics. A second-generation cephalosporin was administered intravenously on call to the operating room. After anesthetic induction, a Foley catheter and a Salem pump nasogastric tube were placed, and the abdomen was prepared and draped.

Table 30-2 lists the equipment used for the laparoscopic-assisted resections. A small periumbilical incision was made into the peritoneal cavity. A Hassan port was placed, and the abdomen was inflated with carbon dioxide. The laparoscope was inserted, and a laparoscopic exploration was made with special attention to the liver in case of cancer resection. Other ports were inserted under direct laparoscopic vision. Mobilization of the colon to be resected was then done in a fashion similar to those in open cases, and the mesentery was divided intracorporeally.

RESULTS

The cost analysis comparison of 38 patients who have had laparoscopic-assisted colectomies with the matched group of open resections is shown in Table 30-3.

Table 30-1. Patient Characteristics

	Laparoscopic Resection	Open Resection
Age	65.8	64.7
Sex	14 men, 24 women	15 men, 23 women
Hospital	30 ORMC/SLH, 8 LMC	30 ORMC/SLH, 8 LMC
Medical illness	Hypertension (8)	Hypertension (7)
	CAD (10)	CAD (8)
	Diabetes (5)	Diabetes (1)
	CLL (1)	CLL (0)
	COPD (3)	COPD (3)
	Weight loss (2)	Weight loss (1)
	UC (0)	UC (1)
Resection	Right colectomy (9)	Right colectomy (9)
	Left colectomy/LAR (21)	Left colectomy/LAR (21)
	APR (5)	APR (5)
	Total proctocolectomy (1)	Total proctocolectomy (1)
	Sigmoid colostomy (1)	Sigmoid colostomy (1)
	Sigmoidectomy, pexy (1)	Sigmoidectomy, pexy (1)
Pathology	Adenocarcinoma (25)	Adenocarcinoma (25)
	Squamous carcinoma (0)	Squamous carcinoma (1)
	Melanoma (1)	Melanoma (1)
	Villous adenoma (6)	Villous adenoma (4)
	Diverticulosis (4)	Diverticulosis (5)
	Ulcerative colitis (0)	Ulcerative colitis (1)
	Constipation (1)	Constipation (1)
	Prolapse (1)	Prolapse (1)

Abbreviations: APR, abdominoperitoneal resection; CAD, coronary artery disease; CLL, chronic lymphocytic leukemia; COPD, chronic obstructive pulmonary disease; LAR, low anterior resecton; LMC, Lucerne Medical Center; ORMC/SLH, Orlando Regional Medical Center/Sand Lake Hospital; UC, ulcerative colitis.

Obviously, although the total cost is not significantly different, charges for operating room time, operating room equipment, and anesthesia are significantly higher for laparoscopic-assisted colectomies. A significant difference is seen in the time to return of bowel function. Return of bowel sounds, flatus, and first postoperative bowel movement were much earlier in the patients who had laparoscopic-assisted resections. The day of discharge was also earlier but did not achieve statistical significance. The laparoscopic-assisted resections were longer in duration, although this difference did not reach statistical significance.

CONCLUSION

Based on the data presented, laparoscopic-assisted colectomy is cost-effective, because the total hospital cost for laparoscopic-assisted versus open resection did

Table 30-2. Laparoscopic Equipment Used

Equipment	
Automatic Xenon Flash Generator and Light Source	Karl Storz 610
Supercam Beamsplitter Camera	Karl Storz 9050 B
Hopkins Telescope (0 degree, 10 mm × 35 cm)	Karl Storz 26033 AP
Electronic Laparoflator (10 L/min flow, LE and analog display)	Karl Storz 26012 C
Nezhart Dorsey Hydro Dissection Pump System	American Surgical Instruments
High-resolution video monitor and video cassette recorder	
Laparoscopic instruments	
Endo right angle clamp	Ethicon, Inc.
Endo Babcock clamp	Ethicon, Inc.
Endopath disposable Hassan (10/11-mm trocar)	Ethicon, Inc.
Endopath disposable surgical trocars with attached	Ethicon, Inc.
Endopath adjustable stability threads (10/11- and 12-mm sizes)	
Ligaclip endoscopic multiple clip applier with 360-degree rotation (EMCA)	Ethicon, Inc.
5-mm Endopath disposable scissors with cautery	Ethicon, Inc
Endopath 60-mm endoscopic linear cutter device	Ethicon, Inc.
EndoGIA stapler with vascular or thick tissue cartridges, 30 or 60 mm	United States Surgical Corp.
Pursestring device	United States Surgical Corp.
Endo Babcock clamp	United States Surgical Corp.

Table 30-3. Cost Comparison: Open Resection Versus Laparoscopy

	Open Resection	Laparoscopic Resection	*P* Value
Charges			
Total cost	$22,938	$26,662	0.30
Operating room time	$ 3,371	$ 4,227	0.011
Operating room equipment	$ 2,610	$ 5,478	<0.001
Anesthesia	$ 669	$ 918	0.002
Length of procedure	167 min	196 min	0.10
Return of bowel function			
POD bowel sounds	2.87	1.71	<0.001
POD flatus	5.11	3.13	<0.001
POD bowel movement	6.32	4.45	<0.001
POD discharge	8.45	7.05	0.075

Abbreviation: POD, postoperative day.

Table 30-4. Comparison of Complications

Complications	Open Resection	Laparoscopic Resection
Minor		
Atelectasis		1
Atrial fibrillation		1
Ileus	4	2
Bleeding	2	1
Fever	1	2
Urinary tract infection	1	1
Pneumaturia		1
Major		
Perforation, multiple system organ failure[a]		
Pneumonia	2	1
Congestive heart failure	2	1
Incisional hernia, reoperation		1
Ureteral injury		1

[a]Patient expired.

not differ significantly. In this series, one patient died (total hospital charges of $129,591). Comparing the costs of only the other patients reveals that the total charges are almost identical ($22,938 open vs. $23,881, P = 0.68). The finding that the operating room time charges and anesthesia charges were higher with laparoscopic-assisted colectomies is explained by the increased duration of the laparoscopic procedure. These findings are consistent with those of Falk.[6,7] As stated in other papers,[8–16] the operative time does decrease as the surgeon becomes more proficient with the technique. A comparison of our first 19 with our last 19 cases shows the average operative time decreasing from 231 minutes to 161 minutes (P = 0.009).

Another significant difference, as expected, was the difference in operating room equipment charges. Laparoscopic cases had an average added cost of about $3,000, largely a consequence of two factors: (1) the current lack of dependable reusable trocars and laparoscopic staplers and (2) the hospital markup charges for all reusable items are very high.

Our 13-percent conversion rate (laparoscopic to open resection) is lower than that reported by Falk (41 percent).[2] This difference reflects a patient selection bias. Because this study was concerned with those cases in which a laparoscopic-assisted resection was performed, we did not include those cases that were opened after laparoscopic exploration only (as a result of dense adhesions, tumor invasion of contiguous structures, or other factors).

Although our postoperative day of discharge did not achieve statistical significance, if one compares only those patients from each group who did not have any complications, the average postoperative day of discharge was 7.6 for open resections as compared with 5.6 for laparoscopic-assisted resection (P<0.001).

The complication rate encountered (34 percent) was not much higher than after open resections (24 percent). Our complication of incisional hernia with small bowel strangulation was completely avoidable. We currently close all port sites with figure-of-eight sutures. The complication of ureteric stricture occurred despite adequate visualization of the ureter and was attributed to an area of skeletonization with resultant loss of blood supply. A comparison of the complications that occurred with the two procedures is given in Table 30-4.

In conclusion, laparoscopic-assisted colon resection is technically feasible, safe, and cost-effective. Actual cost savings may be obtainable once operative time decreases as proficiency with the laparoscopic technique is obtained and once lower cost laparoscopic instrumentation is introduced. Laparoscopic-assisted colectomy will be a useful tool in the colon and rectal surgeon's armamentarium.

REFERENCES

1. Stoker ME, Vose J, O'Mara P et al: An early review of 800 laparoscopic cholecystectomies: a clinical and financial analysis of 280 operations. Arch Surg 127:589, 1992
2. Baird DR, Wilson JP, Mason EM et al: An early review of 800 laparoscopic cholecystectomies at a university affiliated community teaching hospital. Am Surg 58:206, 1992
3. Peters JH, Ellison C, Innes JT et al: Safety and efficacy of laparoscopic cholecystectomy: a prospective analysis of 100 initial patients. Am Surg 58:206, 1992
4. Voules CR, Petro AB, Meena AL et al: A practical approach to laparoscopic cholecystectomy. Am J Surg 161:365, 1991
5. Grace PA, Quereshi A, Coleman J et al: Reduced postoperative hospitalization after laparoscopic cholecystectomy. Br J Surg 78:160, 1991
6. Falk PM, Beart RW, Wexner SD et al: Laparoscopic colectomy: a critical appraisal. Dis Colon Rectum 36:28, 1993
7. Jacobs M, Verdeja JC, Goldstein HS: Minimally invasive colon resection (laparoscopic colectomy). Surg Laparosc Endosc 1:144, 1991
8. Phillips EH, Franklin M, Carroll BJ et al: Laparoscopic colectomy. Ann Surg 216:703, 1992
9. Larach SW, Salomon MC, Williamson PR et al: Laparoscopic-assisted colectomy: experience during the learning curve. Coloproctology 15:38, 1993
10. Wexner SD, Johansen OB, Nogueras JJ et al: Laparoscopic total abdominal colectomy: a prospective trial. Dis Colon Rectum 35:651, 1992
11. Wexner SD, Johansen OB: Laparoscopic bowel resection: advantages and limitations. Ann Med 24:105, 1992
12. Dodson RW, Cullado MJ, Tangen LE et al: Laparoscopic-assisted abdominoperineal resection. Contemp Surg 42:42, 1993
13. Sharpe DR, Redwine DB: Laparoscopic segmental resection of the sigmoid and rectosigmoid colon for endometriosis. Surg Laparosc Endosc 2:120, 1992
14. Cooperman AM, Zucker KA: Laparoscopic guided intestinal surgery. p. 295. In Zucker KA (ed): Surgical Laparoscopy. Quality Medical Publishing, St. Louis, 1991
15. Beart RW: Laparoscopic-assisted colon resection. p. 554. In Corman MI (ed): Colon and Rectal Surgery. JB Lippincott, Philadelphia, 1993
16. Schrock TR, Bailey HR, Coller JA et al: Laparoscopic colectomy. Perspect Colon Rectal Surg 5:171, 1992

Editorial Comment

Steven D. Wexner

Drs. Larach and Ferrara are both to be commended on their skill and expertise as laparoscopic surgeons. In this chapter, they share with us a cost analysis in a group of 38 patients who underwent laparoscopic-assisted colorectal surgery and compared costs in these patients to patients matched for age, sex, hospital concomitant medical illness, resection, and pathology.

First, and not surprisingly, they noted that the cost of operating room time, operating room equipment, and anesthesia were all statistically significantly higher in the laparoscopic than in the standard open group. Despite these additional charges, the hospital stay was not statistically significantly shorter in the laparoscopic group. Accordingly, the total cost was not statistically significant between the two groups: $22,938.00 in the standard group and $26,662.00 in the laparoscopic group. One of the reasons for the lack of a cost advantage in this series is that Larach and Ferrara discharge their standard open patients in only 8.45 days; therefore, the gain by laparoscopy was only 1.40 days. This failure to find a statistically significant savings in length of hospitalization was quite different from the series by Ortega and colleagues.[1] One of the multiple advantages reported by Ortega et al was a discharge savings of more than 50 percent. However, close analysis reveals that while Ortega and colleagues discharge their laparoscopic patients at a mean of 5 days, they discharge their standard open patients in a mean of 11 days. Therefore, it is very difficult to compare their data with the data of Larach and Ferrara. In point of fact, as cited in other portions of this textbook, in two separate prospectively randomized studies at Cleveland Clinic Florida, we have shown a reduction in the length of hospital stay merely by the routine use of early oral intake after laparotomy. In the original study, 64 patients were prospectively randomized to either early oral feeding or standard postoperative intake after laparotomy.[2] A 1.3-day reduction in hospitalization was realized from a mean of 8.0 days in the standard intake group to a mean of 6.7 days in the early oral intake group. In a more recent series, 162 patients were prospectively randomized to either early oral feeding or standard postoperative oral intake. The date of discharge was accelerated from 6.8 to 6.2 days merely by the addition of early intake.[3] Immediately noticeable from the brief discussion of these data, however, is that even in a standard setting, our patients are discharged home after only 6 days, not the 11 days cited by Ortega and colleagues. Thus, it would be very difficult to show as appreciable a difference in discharge with a current routine 6-day discharge after laparotomy with colectomy. A 1-day difference is hardly as impressive as is a 6-day difference. Similar to the relatively brief hospitalizations noted in the studies by Binderow et al[2] and Reissman et al,[3] Rajagopal and colleagues[4] from Omaha, Nebraska, studied the postoperative lengths of stay after laparotomy and colectomy between 1984 and 1993. They noted a reduction from a mean stay of 9.4 days to a mean stay of 6.3 days (P<0.0001) without the use of laparoscopy. A recent review assessed 24 published English language reports on laparoscopic colectomy in which the length of stay was analyzed. These 808 patients remained in the hospital a mean of 7.1 days.[5] Subsequent to that review article, a large multicenter French series analyzed the 4-year experience of 275 cases of laparoscopic or laparoscopic-assisted colorectal surgery. In this study, Boulez[6] noted an 8.9-day mean length of hospitalization.

More specifically relevant to cost, the fact is that no data exist relative to the *cost* of laparoscopic or laparoscopic-assisted colorectal surgery. All articles to date have merely recounted *charges* to the patient rather than the actual cost of the procedure. Certainly, with changes in the health care system, cost rather than charges will be the important variable and will begin to be measured. We are in fact in the process of performing an outcomes analysis study to include the actual cost rather than the charges for the procedure. However, as of this writing, very few data are available to address the issue. Other than the article cited by Larach and Ferrara, only six studies report cost.[7] In the study by Senagore and colleagues,[8] 26 patients who underwent laparoscopic or laparoscopic-assisted colorectal surgery were compared to 12 patients who underwent laparoscopic converted procedures and ultimately to 105 patients in whom standard laparotomy was performed. The mean ages in the groups were somewhat different and, not surprisingly, the lengths of surgery progressively increased from a mean of 2.1 to 2.9 hours in the laparoscopic group to 3.4 hours in the converted group. Also not surprisingly, because the standard open patients were kept in the hospital for a mean of 9.9 days, the mean 6.0 days of hospitalization after laparoscopic surgery appeared to be a significant savings. Ultimately, the statistical validity of this study is tremendously flawed. Specifically, the 12 patients in whom laparoscopy was converted to laparotomy were separately analyzed. Therefore, the mean cost of \$17,583.00 ± \$731.00 was separate from the mean cost in the laparoscopic group of \$12,131.00 ± \$612.00. Therefore, the 26 patients in the laparoscopic group appeared to have a cost advantage as compared to the mean \$14,449.00 ± \$696.00 in the 102 patients in whom laparotomy was performed. Hence, editorial license in writing this critique has allowed me to merge the two groups in the Senagore et al study.[8] When the 38 patients in whom laparoscopic surgery was attempted (regardless of whether the procedure was technically completed or not), the mean charge was \$13,884.00, which was not statistically significantly different from the \$14,449.00 in the standard open group. Similarly, Musser and associates[9] found that while laparoscopic procedures cost a mean of \$9,811.00, standard open procedures cost \$11,207.00. In a previous study from our center, 40 patients who underwent laparoscopic-assisted colorectal surgery were compared to 40 age-, sex-, diagnosis-, hospital-, surgeon-, and procedure-matched controls. No statistically significant differences were found in either mean operating room time (3 versus 2 hours, respectively), mean duration of ileus (4 versus 5 days, respectively), mean length of hospital stay (7 versus 7 days, respectively), or total cost (\$23,294.00 versus \$19,384.00, respectively).[10] A much larger, more recent study from our department reached the same conclusion. Unlike the studies by Senagore et al[8] and by Musser et al,[9] Larach and Ferrara's study parallels ours in that the groups were of identical size and the patients in the two groups were matched for all potentially matchable variables. Thus, the two studies in which no cost advantage was noted are more statistically valid than the two studies in which a cost advantage was found. Specifically, Hoffman and co-workers[12] attempted the method of Senagore and colleagues.[8] However, despite this statistical sleight of hand, both the laparoscopic-assisted and laparoscopic-converted procedures cost more than the open procedures. Specifically, the mean operating room charges were \$7,351.00 in the assisted group, \$7,148.00 in the converted group, and only \$3,990.00 in the open group ($P < 0.005$). Similarly, the mean total hospital charges were \$12,464.00 in the assisted group, \$13,956.00 in the converted group, and \$10,213.00 in the open group.

In conclusion, Larach and Ferrara are to be commended for their academic honesty. They have done an admirable job of data analysis and have shown that at least at the present time, laparoscopic colorectal surgery does not offer savings in patient billable charges. I do agree with their conclusion that as we become more proficient in our techniques and perhaps use more cost-effective equipment, ultimately, a savings will be realized. However, unfortunately, such a statement is now unproven.

REFERENCES

1. Ortega A, Beart R, Anthone G, Schlinker R: Laparoscopic bowel resection and consecutive series, abstracted. Dis Colon Rectum 37:22, 1994
2. Binderow SR, Cohen SM, Wexner SD et al: Must early postoperative oral intake be limited to laparoscopy? Dis Colon Rectum 37:584, 1994
3. Reissman P, Teoh TA, Cohen SM et al: Is early oral feeding safe after elective colorectal surgery? Ann Surg (in press)
4. Rajagopol AS, Thorson AG, Sentovich T et al: Decade trends in length of postoperative stay following abdominal colectomy, abstracted. Dis Colon Rectum 37:26, 1994
5. Bernstein M, Wexner SD: Laparoscopic colorectal surgery for colorectal cancer—techniques and results: the USA experience. In Williams N (guest ed): Seminars in Laparoscopy. WB Saunders, London (in press)
6. Boulez J: Multicentric analysis of laparoscopic colorectal surgery in FDCL group: 274 cases, abstracted. Surg Endosc 8:944, 1994
7. Falk PM, Beart RW, Wexner SD et al: Laparoscopic colectomy: a critical appraisal. Dis Colon Rectum 36:38, 1993
8. Senagore AJ, Luchtefeld MA, Macheigan JM, Mazier WP: Open colectomy versus laparoscopic colectomy: are there differences? Am Surg 59:549, 1993
9. Musser DJ, Boorse RC, Madera F, Reed JF III: Laparoscopic colectomy: at what cost? Surg Laparosc Endosc 4:1, 1994
10. Reiver D, Kmiot WA, Cohen SM et al: A prospective comparison of laparoscopic and open procedures in colorectal surgery, abstracted. Dis Colon Rectum 37:22, 1994
11. Pfeifer J, Reissman P, Wexner SD et al: Laparoscopic vs. open colon surgery. Surg Endosc (in press)
12. Hoffman GC, Baker JW, Fitchett CS, Vansant JH: Laparoscopic-assisted colectomy: initial experience. Ann Surg 219:732, 1994

Index

Numbers followed by *f* indicate figures; those followed by *t* indicate tables.

I

K

L

M

N

O

S

T

U

V

W

X

Y